A Q&A Approach to Organic Chemistry

A Q&A Approach to Organic Chemistry

Michael B. Smith

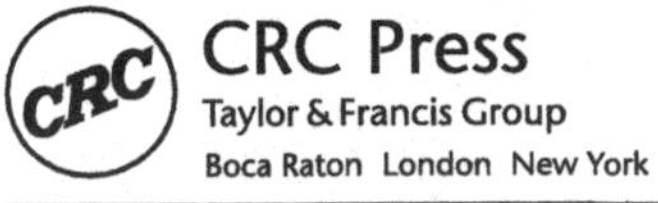

CRC Press is an imprint of the
Taylor & Francis Group, an **informa** business

First edition published 2020
by CRC Press
6000 Broken Sound Parkway NW, Suite 300, Boca Raton, FL 33487-2742

and by CRC Press
2 Park Square, Milton Park, Abingdon, Oxon, OX14 4RN

First issued in paperback 2021

CRC Press is an imprint of Taylor & Francis Group, an Informa business

Publisher's Note
The publisher has gone to great lengths to ensure the quality of this reprint but points out that some imperfections in the original copies may be apparent.

ISBN 13: 978-1-03-224068-8 (pbk)
ISBN 13: 978-0-367-22427-1 (hbk)

Typeset in Times
by Deanta Global Publishing Services, Chennai, India

Contents

Preface ix
Common Abbreviations xi
Author xiii

Part A A Q&A Approach to Organic Chemistry

1 **Orbitals and Bonding** 3
1.1 ORBITALS 3
1.1.1 Atomic Orbitals 3
1.1.2 Electron Configuration 5
1.1.3 Molecular Orbitals 5
1.2 BONDING 6
1.2.1 Ionic Bonding 6
1.2.2 Covalent Bonding 7
1.3 HYBRIDIZATION 12
1.4 RESONANCE 15
END OF CHAPTER PROBLEMS 18

2 **Structure of Molecules** 19
2.1 BASIC STRUCTURE OF ORGANIC MOLECULES 19
2.1.1 Fundamental Structures 19
2.1.2 Structures with Other Atoms Bonded to Carbon 22
2.2 THE VSEPR MODEL AND MOLECULAR GEOMETRY 23
2.3 DIPOLE MOMENT 25
2.4 FUNCTIONAL GROUPS 26
2.5 FORMAL CHARGE 28
2.6 PHYSICAL PROPERTIES 28
END OF CHAPTER PROBLEMS 32

3 **Acids and Bases** 33
3.1 ACIDS AND BASES 33
3.2 ENERGETICS 35
3.3 THE ACIDITY CONSTANT, K_a 38
3.4 STRUCTURAL FEATURES THAT INFLUENCE ACIDITY 40
3.5 FACTORS THAT CONTRIBUTE TO MAKING THE ACID MORE ACIDIC 45
END OF CHAPTER PROBLEMS 48

4 **Alkanes, Isomers, and Nomenclature** 49
4.1 DEFINITION AND BASIC NOMENCLATURE 49
4.2 STRUCTURAL ISOMERS 50
4.3 IUPAC NOMENCLATURE 52
4.4 CYCLIC ALKANES 57
END OF CHAPTER PROBLEMS 58

5 Conformations 61
5.1 ACYCLIC CONFORMATIONS 61
5.2 CONFORMATIONS OF CYCLIC MOLECULES 67
END OF CHAPTER PROBLEMS 75

6 Stereochemistry 77
6.1 CHIRALITY 77
6.2 SPECIFIC ROTATION 81
6.3 SEQUENCE RULES 83
6.4 DIASTEREOMERS 87
6.5 OPTICAL RESOLUTION 89
END OF CHAPTER PROBLEMS 90

7 Alkenes and Alkynes: Structure, Nomenclature, and Reactions 93
7.1 STRUCTURE OF ALKENES 93
7.2 NOMENCLATURE OF ALKENES 95
7.3 REACTIONS OF ALKENES 98
7.4 REACTION OF ALKENES WITH LEWIS ACID-TYPE REAGENTS 107
7.4.1 Hydroxylation 107
7.4.2 Epoxidation 111
7.4.3 Dihydroxylation 113
7.4.4 Halogenation 114
7.4.5 Hydroboration 117
7.5 STRUCTURE AND NOMENCLATURE OF ALKYNES 122
7.6 REACTIONS OF ALKYNES 124
END OF CHAPTER PROBLEMS 129

8 Alkyl Halides and Substitution Reactions 133
8.1 STRUCTURE, PROPERTIES, AND NOMENCLATURE OF ALKYL HALIDES 133
8.2 SECOND-ORDER NUCLEOPHILIC SUBSTITUTION (S_N2) REACTIONS 134
8.3 OTHER NUCLEOPHILES IN S_N2 REACTIONS 143
8.4 FIRST-ORDER SUBSTITUTION (S_N1) REACTIONS 151
8.5 COMPETITION BETWEEN S_N2 vs. S_N1 REACTIONS 156
8.6 RADICAL HALOGENATION OF ALKANES 158
END OF CHAPTER PROBLEMS 162

9 Elimination Reactions 165
9.1 THE E2 REACTION 165
9.2 THE E1 REACTION 172
9.3 PREPARATION OF ALKYNES 176
9.4 SYN ELIMINATION 178
END OF CHAPTER PROBLEMS 180

10 Organometallic Compounds 183
10.1 ORGANOMETALLICS 183
10.2 ORGANOMAGNESIUM COMPOUNDS 183
10.3 ORGANOLITHIUM COMPOUNDS 185
10.4 BASICITY 187
10.5 REACTION WITH EPOXIDES 188
10.6 OTHER METALS 188
END OF CHAPTER PROBLEMS 190

11 Spectroscopy 191
11.1 THE ELECTROMAGNETIC SPECTRUM 191
11.2 MASS SPECTROMETRY 192
11.3 INFRARED SPECTROSCOPY (IR) 196
11.4 NUCLEAR MAGNETIC RESONANCE SPECTROSCOPY (nmr) 201
END OF CHAPTER PROBLEMS 215

12 Aldehydes and Ketones. Acyl Addition Reactions 219
12.1 STRUCTURE AND NOMENCLATURE OF ALDEHYDES AND KETONES 219
12.2 REACTION OF ALDEHYDES AND KETONES WITH WEAK NUCLEOPHILES 221
12.3 REACTIONS OF ALDEHYDES AND KETONES. STRONG NUCLEOPHILES 230
12.4 THE WITTIG REACTION 233
END OF CHAPTER PROBLEMS 235

Part B A Q&A Approach to Organic Chemistry

13 Oxidation Reactions 239
13.1 OXIDATION REACTIONS OF ALKENES 239
13.2 OXIDATION OF ALKENES: EPOXIDATION 244
13.3 OXIDATIVE CLEAVAGE: OZONOLYSIS 247
13.4 OXIDATIVE CLEAVAGE. PERIODIC ACID CLEAVAGE OF 1,2-DIOLS 250
13.5 OXIDATION OF ALCOHOLS TO ALDEHYDES OR KETONES 251
END OF CHAPTER PROBLEMS 255

14 Reduction Reactions 257
14.1 CATALYTIC HYDROGENATION 258
14.2 DISSOLVING METAL REDUCTION: ALKYNES 264
14.3 HYDRIDE REDUCTION OF ALDEHYDES AND KETONES 265
14.4 CATALYTIC HYDROGENATION AND DISSOLVING METAL REDUCTIONS. ALDEHYDES AND KETONES 269
END OF CHAPTER PROBLEMS 273

15 Carboxylic Acids, Carboxylic Acid Derivatives, and Acyl Substitution Reactions 275
15.1 STRUCTURE OF CARBOXYLIC ACIDS 275
15.2 PREPARATION OF CARBOXYLIC ACIDS 280
15.3 CARBOXYLIC ACID DERIVATIVES 283
15.4 PREPARATION OF ACID DERIVATIVES 290
15.5 HYDROLYSIS OF CARBOXYLIC ACID DERIVATIVES 301
15.6 REACTIONS OF CARBOXYLIC ACIDS AND ACID DERIVATIVES 305
15.7 DIBASIC CARBOXYLIC ACIDS 310
END OF CHAPTER PROBLEMS 312

16 Benzene, Aromaticity, and Benzene Derivatives 315
16.1 BENZENE AND NOMENCLATURE OF AROMATIC COMPOUNDS 315
16.2 ELECTROPHILIC AROMATIC SUBSTITUTION 319
16.3 SYNTHESIS VIA AROMATIC SUBSTITUTION 335
16.4 NUCLEOPHILIC AROMATIC SUBSTITUTION 337
16.5 REDUCTION OF BENZENE AND BENZENE DERIVATIVES 344
16.6 POLYCYCLIC AROMATIC COMPOUNDS AND HETEROAROMATIC COMPOUNDS 347
END OF CHAPTER PROBLEMS 353

17 Enolate Anions and Condensation Reactions 357
17.1 ALDEHYDES, KETONES, ENOLS, AND ENOLATE ANIONS 357
17.2 ENOLATE ALKYLATION 361
17.3 CONDENSATION REACTIONS OF ENOLATE ANIONS AND ALDEHYDES OR KETONES 366
17.4 ENOLATE ANIONS FROM CARBOXYLIC ACIDS AND DERIVATIVES 372
END OF CHAPTER PROBLEMS 383

18 Conjugation and Reactions of Conjugated Compounds 385
18.1 CONJUGATED MOLECULES 385
18.2 STRUCTURE AND NOMENCLATURE OF CONJUGATED SYSTEMS 387
18.3 REACTIONS OF CONJUGATED MOLECULES 391
18.4 THE DIELS–ALDER REACTION 393
18.5 [3+2]-CYCLOADDITION REACTIONS 401
18.6 SIGMATROPIC REARRANGEMENTS 403
18.7 ULTRAVIOLET SPECTROSCOPY 406
END OF CHAPTER PROBLEMS 409

19 Amines 413
19.1 STRUCTURE AND PROPERTIES 413
19.2 PREPARATION OF AMINES 416
19.3 REACTIONS OF AMINES 420
19.4 HETEROCYCLIC AMINES 424
END OF CHAPTER PROBLEMS 426

20 Amino Acids, Peptides, and Proteins 429
20.1 AMINO ACIDS 429
20.2 SYNTHESIS OF AMINO ACIDS 435
20.3 REACTIONS OF AMINO ACIDS 437
20.4 PROTEINS 441
END OF CHAPTER PROBLEMS 447

21 Carbohydrates and Nucleic Acids 449
21.1 CARBOHYDRATES 449
21.2 DISACCHARIDES AND POLYSACCHARIDES 457
21.3 SYNTHESIS OF CARBOHYDRATES 459
21.4 REACTIONS OF CARBOHYDRATES 461
21.5 NUCLEIC ACIDS, NUCLEOTIDES, AND NUCLEOSIDES 464
END OF CHAPTER PROBLEMS 471

Appendix: Answers to End of Chapter Problems 473

Index 505

Preface

What is organic chemistry?

Organic chemistry is the science that studies molecules containing the element *carbon*. Carbon can form bonds to other carbon atoms or to a variety of atoms in the periodic table. The most common bonds observed in an organic chemistry course are C—C, C—H, C—O, C—N, C—halogen (Cl, Br, I), C—Mg, C—B, C—Li, C—S and C—P.

This book is presented in the hope that it will provide extra practice to students taking organic chemistry for the first time and also serve as a cogent review to those who need to refresh their knowledge of organic chemistry. This book of questions began life as *Organic Chemistry* in 1993 to assist those students taking undergraduate organic chemistry and was part of a HarperCollins Outline series that was never completed. My book, along with those other books in the series that were completed, was sold as a reference book rather than a textbook. In 2006, a second edition of *Organic Chemistry* was published and marketed more or less the same way. The book laid fallow for several years until this version became possible. With this book, published by CRC Press/Taylor & Francis Group, I continue the idea of teaching organic chemistry by asking leading questions.

A Q&A Approach to Organic Chemistry is intended as a supplement to virtually any organic chemistry textbook rather than a stand-alone text and it will allow a "self-guided tour" of organic chemistry. Teaching organic chemistry with a Q&A format uses leading questions along with the answers and is presented in a manner that allows a student to refresh and renew their working knowledge of organic chemistry. Such an approach will also be of value to those reviewing organic chemistry for MCATs (Medical College Admission Test); graduate record exams (a standardized test), which is an admissions requirement for many graduate schools); the PCAT (Pharmacy College Admission Test), which identifies qualified applicants to pharmacy colleges before commencement of pharmaceutical education; and so on.

This Q&A format was classroom-tested here at the University of Connecticut for many years where one of the earlier versions of this book was used as a supplement. Indeed, the book was not required for purchase and used only on a voluntary basis by students. According to their end-of-semester evaluations, students who wanted or needed additional homework found the book very useful and helpful. Classroom experience and comments from students have been used for the preparation of this new student-friendly book.

This book is organized into 21 chapters and will supplement most of the organic textbooks on the market. In all chapters, there are leading questions to focus attention on a principle or reaction and the answer is immediately provided. The organization of the book provides an initial review of fundamental principles followed by reactions based on manipulation of functional groups. The intent in all cases is to provide a focused question about a specific principle or reaction and the answer immediately follows. There is also a chapter on spectroscopy as well as chapters on amino acid and peptide chemistry and carbohydrate and nucleoside chemistry. Each chapter ends with several homework questions for that chapter, and the answers are provided in an Appendix at the end of the book.

I thank all of the organic chemistry students I taught over the years. They provided the inspiration for the book as well as innumerable suggestions that were invaluable. I thank Ms. Hilary Lafoe and Ms. Jessica Poile, the Taylor & Francis editors for this book, and also Dr. Fiona Macdonald, the publisher. This book would not have been possible without their interest in chemistry and their help as the book was written. I thank Professor John D'Angelo of Alfred University who provided a very useful and helpful review of the manuscript. I thank PerkinElmer who provided a gift of ChemDraw Professional (Version 18.0.0.231[4318]). All the reactions and figures were done with ChemDraw except for those images that use molecular models and the artist-rendered drawings. All molecular models were rendered with Spartan'18 software and I thank Warren Hehre and Sean Ohlinger of Wavefunction,

Inc., who provided a gift of Spartan'18 software, version 1.2.0 (181121). I thank Ms. Christine Elder (https://christineelder.com), graphics design artist, for her graphic arts expertise to render the drawings on pages 14 (C1), 66 (C5), 93 and 122 (C7), 208 and 209 (C11), 280 (C15), 315 and 342 (C16). Finally, I thank my wife, Sarah, for her patience and understanding while I was putting this book together.

Where there are errors, I take complete responsibility. Please contact me at michael.smith@uconn.edu if there are questions, problems, or errors.

Michael B. Smith
Professor Emeritus
December 2019

Common Abbreviations

Other, less common abbreviations are given in the text when the term is used.

Abbreviation	Meaning	Structure
Ac	Acetyl	O, Me
AIBN	azobisisobutyronitrile	
aq	aqueous	
AIBN	Azobisisobutyronitrile	
AMP	Adenosine monophosphate	
ATP	Adenosine triphosphate	
Ax	axial	
9-BBN	9-Borabicyclo[3.3.1]nonane	
Bn	Benzyl	$-CH_2Ph$
Boc	*tert*-Butoxycarbonyl	O, O*t*-Bu
Bu	*n*-Butyl	$-CH_2CH_2CH_2CH_3$
Bz	Benzoyl	
°C	Temperature in Degrees Celsius	
^{13}C NMR	Carbon Nuclear Magnetic Resonance	
cat	Catalytic	
Cbz	Carbobenzyloxy	O, OCH_2Ph
CIP	Cahn–Ingold–Prelog	
mCPBA	3-Chloroperoxybenzoic acid	
DCC	1,3-Dicyclohexylcarbodiimide	$c\text{-}C_6H_{11}\text{-}N{=}C{=}N\text{-}c\text{-}C_6H_{11}$
DEA	Diethylamine	$HN(CH_2CH_3)_2$
DMAP	4-Dimethylaminopyridine	
DMF	*N,N′*-Dimethylformamide	O, H, NMe_2
DMSO	Dimethyl sulfoxide	
EDTA	Ethylenediaminetetraacetic acid	
ee or % ee	% Enantiomeric excess	
Equiv	Equivalent(s)	
Et	Ethyl	$-CH_2CH_3$
Ether	diethyl ether	$CH_3CH_2OCH_2C_3$
Eq	equatorial	
FDNB	Sanger's reagent, 1-fluoro-2,4-dinitrobenzene	
FMO	Frontier molecular orbitals	
FVP	Flash Vacuum Pyrolysis	
GC	Gas chromatography	
h	Hour (hours)	
^{1}H NMR	Proton Nuclear Magnetic Resonance	
HMPA	Hexamethylphosphoramide	
HOMO	Highest occupied molecular orbital	
hv	Irradiation with light	
IP	Ionization potential	

***i*Pr**	Isopropyl	$-CH(Me)_2$
IR	Infrared	
IUPAC	International Union of Pure and Applied Chemistry	
K	Temperature in kelvin	
LCAO	Linear combination of atomic orbitals	
LDA	Lithium diisopropylamide	$LiN(i\text{-}Pr)_2$
LUMO	Lowest unoccupied molecular orbital	
mcpba	*meta*-Chloroperoxybenzoic acid	
Me	Methyl	$-CH_3$ or Me
min	minutes	
MO	Molecular orbital	
mRNA	Messenger ribonucleic acid	
MS	Mass spectrometry	
NMR	nuclear magnetic resonance	
N.R.	No reaction	
NAD^+	Nicotinamide adenine dinucleotide	
NBS	*N*-Bromosuccinimide	
NCS	*N*-Chlorosuccinimide	
Ni(R)	Raney nickel	
NMO	*N*-Methylmorpholine *N*-oxide	
Nu (Nuc)	Nucleophile	
PCC	Pyridinium chlorochromate	
PDC	Pyridinium dichromate	
\PES	Photoelectron spectroscopy	
Ph	Phenyl	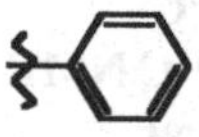
PhMe	Toluene	
PPA	Polyphosphoric acid	
Ppm	Parts per million	
Pr	*n*-Propyl	$-CH_2CH_2CH_3$
Py	Pyridine	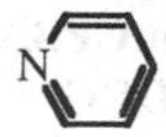 N
RNA	Ribonucleic acid	
rt	Room temperature	
s	seconds	
$(Sia)_2BH$	Disiamylborane (Siamyl is *sec*-Isoamyl)	
sBuLi	*sec*-Butyllithium	$CH_3CH_2CH(Li)CH_3$
S_EAr	Electrophilic aromatic substitution	
SET	Single electron transfer	
S_NAr	Nucleophilic aromatic substitution	
SOMO	singly occupied molecular orbital	
T	Temperature	
***t*-Bu**	*tert*-Butyl	$-CMe_3$
TBHP (*t*-BuOOH)	*t*-Butylhydroperoxide	Me_3COOH
TFA	Trifluoroacetic acid	CF_3COOH
$ThexBH_2$	Thexylborane (*tert*-hexylborane)	
THF	Tetrahydrofuran	
TMEDA	Tetramethylethylenediamine	$Me_2NCH_2CH_2NMe_2$
Tol	Tolyl	$4\text{-}(Me)C_6H_4$
Ts(Tos)	Tosyl = *p*-Toluenesulfonyl	$4\text{-}(Me)C_6H_4SO_2$
UV	Ultraviolet spectroscopy	
VIS	visible	
VDW	van der Waals	

Author

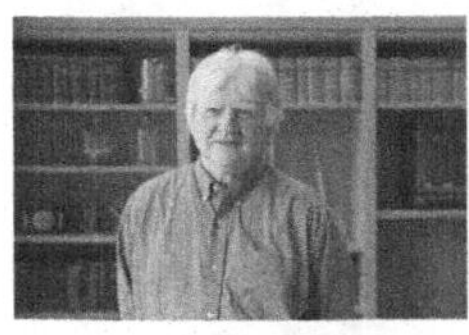

Professor Michael B. Smith was born in Detroit, Michigan, and moved to Madison Heights, Virginia, in 1957. He graduated from Amherst County High School in 1964. He worked at Old Dominion Box Factory for a year and then began studies at Ferrum Junior College in 1965. He graduated in 1967 with an AA and began studies at Virginia Tech later that year, graduating with a BS in Chemistry in 1969. He worked as a chemist at the Newport News Shipbuilding & Dry Dock Co., Newport News, Virginia, from 1969 until 1972. In 1972, he began studies in graduate school at Purdue University in West Lafayette, Indiana, working with Professor Joseph Wolinsky, graduating in 1977 with a PhD in Organic Chemistry. He took a postdoctoral position at Arizona State University in Tempe, Arizona, working on the isolation of anti-cancer agents from marine animals with Prof. Bob Pettit. After one year, he took another postdoctoral position at MIT in Cambridge, Massachusetts, working on the synthesis of the anti-cancer drug bleomycin with Prof. Sidney Hecht.

Professor Smith began his independent career as an assistant professor in the Chemistry department at the University of Connecticut, Storrs, Connecticut, in 1979. He received tenure in 1986, and spent six months on sabbatical in Belgium with Professor Leon Ghosez at the Université Catholique de Louvain in Louvain la Neuve, Belgium. He was promoted to full professor in 1994 and spent his entire career at UConn. Professor Smith's research involved the synthesis of biologically interesting molecules. His most recent work involved the preparation of functionalized indocyanine dyes for the detection of hypoxic cancerous tumors (breast cancer), and also the synthesis of inflammatory lipids derived from the dental pathogen, *Porphyromonas gingivalis*. He has published 26 books including *Organic Chemistry: An Acid-Base Approach*, 2nd edition (Taylor & Francis), the 5th–8th edition of *March's Advanced Organic Chemistry* (Wiley), and *Organic Synthesis*, 4th edition (Elsevier), which is the winner of a 2018 Texty Award. Professor Smith has published 96 peer-reviewed research papers and retired from UCONN in January of 2017.

Part A

A Q&A Approach to Organic Chemistry

What is organic chemistry?

Organic chemistry is the science that studies molecules containing the element *carbon*. Carbon can form bonds to other carbon atoms or to a variety of atoms in the periodic table. The most common bonds observed in an organic chemistry course are C—C, C—H, C—O, C—N, C—halogen (Cl, Br, I), C—Mg, C—B, C—Li, C—S, and C—P.

1

Orbitals and Bonding

This chapter will introduce the carbon atom and the covalent bonds that join carbon atoms together in organic molecules. The most fundamental properties of atoms and of covalent bonds will be introduced, including hybridization, electronic structure, and a brief introduction to using molecular orbital theory for bonding.

1.1 ORBITALS

1.1.1 Atomic Orbitals

What is the electronic structure of an atom?

A given atom has a fixed number of protons, neutrons, and electrons, and the protons and neutrons are found in the nucleus. The electrons are located at discreet energy levels (quanta) away from the nucleus. The nucleus is electrically positive, and electrons are negatively charged.

What is the Schrödinger wave equation?

The Schrödinger equation, $H\psi = E\psi$, is a linear partial differential equation that describes the wavefunction or state function of a quantum-mechanical system. The motion of an electron is expressed by a wave equation, which has a series of solutions and each solution is called a *wavefunction*. Each electron may be described by a wavefunction whose magnitude varies from point to point in space. The equation is a partial differential equation that describes how the *wavefunction* of a physical system changes over time.

What are atomic orbitals?

An atomic orbital is a mathematical function that describes the wave-like behavior of either one electron or a pair of electrons in an atom. If certain simplifying assumptions are made, it is possible to use the Schrödinger equation to generate a different wavefunction for electrons with differing energies relative to the nucleus. A particular solution to the so-called Schrödinger wave equation, for a given type of electron, is determined from the Schrödinger equation, and a solution for various values of ψ that correspond to different energies shows the relationship between orbitals and the energy of an electron. The wavefunction is described by spatial coordinates $\psi(x,y,z)$, and using Cartesian coordinates a point is defined that describes the position of the electron in space.

What is a node?

A node is derived from a solution to the Schrödinger equation where the wavefunction changes phase, and it is taken to be a point of zero electron density.

What is the Heisenberg uncertainty principle?

The *Heisenberg uncertainty principle* states that the position and momentum of an electron cannot be simultaneously specified so it is only possible to determine the probability that an electron will be found at a particular point relative to the nucleus. The probability of finding the electron in a unit volume of three-dimensional space is given by $|\psi(x,y,z)|^2$, or $|\psi|^2 d\tau$, which is the probability of an electron being in a small element of the volume $d\tau$. This small volume can be viewed as a charge cloud if it contains an electron, and the charge cloud represents the region of space where we are most likely to find the electron in terms of the (x,y,z) coordinates. These charge clouds are *orbitals*.

What is a s-orbital?

Different orbitals are described by their distance from the nucleus, which formally corresponds to the energy required to "hold" the electron. One solution to the Schrödinger equation is symmetrical in that the wave does not change phase (zero nodes; a node is the point at which the wave changes its phase). This corresponds to the first quantum level and known as a *s-atomic orbital*. The 1s-orbital represents the first energetically favorable level where electrons can be held by the nucleus. The space in which the electron may be found is spherically symmetrical in three-dimensional space. All spherically symmetrical orbitals are referred to as *s-orbitals*. The nucleus is represented by the "dot" in the middle of the sphere.

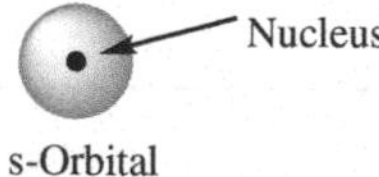

s-Orbital

What is a p-orbital?

When the solution for the Schrödinger equation has one node (the wave changes phase once), electron density is found in two regions relative to the node. When the space occupied by this electron is shown in three-dimensional space, it is *a p-orbital* with a "dumbbell" shape. In the (x,y,z) coordinate system, the single node could be in the x, the y, or the z plane and all three are equally likely. Therefore, three identical p-orbitals must be described: p_x, p_y, and p_z relative to the nucleus, as shown. Identification of three identical p-orbitals means that there are three p-wavefunctions that describe three electrons that are found at the same energy.

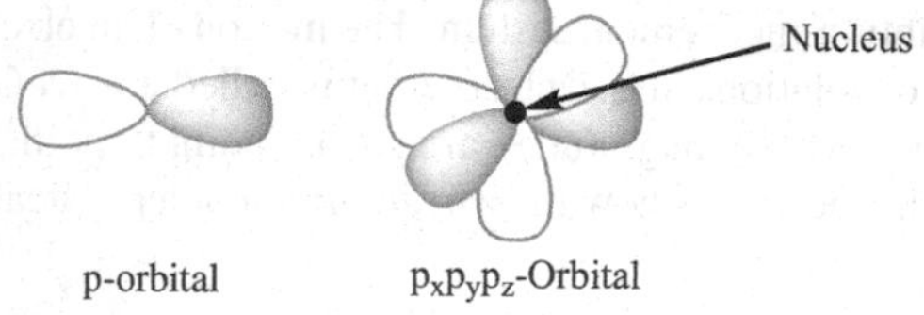

p-orbital $p_xp_yp_z$-Orbital

What is a degenerate orbital?

Orbitals with identical energies are said to be *degenerate*, and the three 2p-orbitals shown in the preceding question are degenerate orbitals. The three electrons in different orbital lobes have the same energy and have the same charge. Due to the presence of like charges, the orbital lobes repel and will assume positions as far apart as possible in a tri-coordinate system. In other words, the three orbitals will be directed to the x-, y-, and z-directions in a three-dimensional coordinate system as shown.

Do the electrons in a p-orbital migrate from one lobe to the other?

No! The picture of the p-orbital represents the uncertainty of where to find the electrons. The diagram shows an equal probability of finding the electrons in each of the three dumbbell-shaped orbitals, above and below a node, which is taken as a point of zero electron density and corresponds to the position of the nucleus in the diagram. Therefore, the electrons are found in the entire p-orbital (*both* lobes), and the diagram simply indicates the uncertainty of their exact location.

How many orbitals are there in each valence shell?

Each orbital can hold two electrons. For the first valence shell containing H and He, there is one s-orbital. For the next valence shell (containing B, C, N, O, F), there is one 2s orbital, but three 2p-orbitals. The 2p-orbitals have different spatial orientations, correlated with the x, y and z axes of a three-dimensional coordinate system. In other words, the three p-orbitals are p_x, p_y, and p_z.

1.1.2 Electron Configuration

What is electron configuration?

The electron configuration is the distribution of electrons of an atom or molecule in atomic or molecular orbitals. Electrons are distributed in shells, each of which has different types of electrons: s, p, d, f. Each orbital (energy level) occurs further from the nucleus; the electrons are held less tightly. Each orbital can hold a maximum of two electrons and each energy level will contain different numbers of electrons (one electron for the $1s^1$ and two electrons for the $1s^2$ orbital, as shown. There are six electrons for p-orbitals; two each is possible for each of the three-degenerate p-orbitals. There are ten electrons for d-orbitals; two each for the five d-orbitals. Orbitals will fill from lowest energy to highest energy orbital, according to the order shown in the mnemonic for the electronic filling order of orbitals.

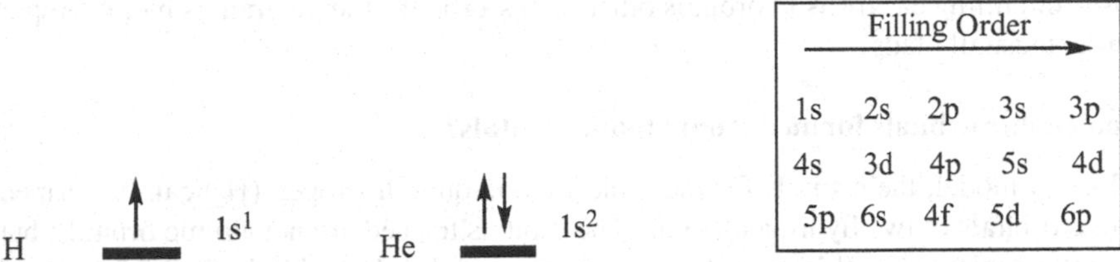

What is the Aufbau principle?

Orbitals "fill" according to the *Aufbau principle*. The principle states that *each orbital* in a sublevel s, p, or d *will contain one electron before any contains two.* Orbitals containing two electrons will have opposite spin quantum numbers (they are said to be *spin paired*, ↑↓). An example is helium in the preceding question.

What is the order in which the three degenerate p-orbitals fill with electrons through the 2p level? Ignore the 1s and 2s levels.

The order for the 2p-orbitals will be $2p_x \rightarrow 2p_y \rightarrow 2p_z \rightarrow 2p_x \rightarrow 2p_y \rightarrow 2p_z$:

↑ _ _ → ↑ ↑ _ → ↑ ↑ ↑ → ↑↓ ↑ ↑ → ↑↓ ↑↓ ↑ → ↑↓ ↑↓ ↑↓

1.1.3 Molecular Orbitals

What is the difference between a molecular orbital and an atomic orbital?

An atomic orbital is a mathematical function that describes the wave-like behavior of either one electron or a pair of electrons in an atom. A molecular orbital (MO) is a mathematical function describing the wave-like behavior of an electron in a molecule.

An atomic orbital is associated with a specific atom. The electrons found on an individual atom of an element are in atomic orbitals whereas the electrons found in an atom that is part of a covalent bond are in molecular orbitals. A molecular orbital is formed once two atoms are joined in a covalent bond. Much of the electron density is shared between the two nuclei of the two atoms rather than being exclusively on the nuclei of the two atoms. This energy level for the electrons found in the molecular orbital is different from electrons that are on an individual atom such as that found in an element.

What is the Linear Combination of Atomic Orbitals (LCAO) model?

The LCAO model is the superposition of atomic orbitals that constitutes a technique for calculating molecular orbitals in quantum chemistry. The LCAO model is a mathematical model that is used to mix the atomic orbitals of two atoms to get new orbitals for the resulting bond between those two orbitals. In the LCAO method, the atomic orbitals of each "free" atom are mixed to form molecular orbitals. The model requires that there can be no more or no less orbitals and no more or no less electrons in the orbitals for the new bond than are found in the atomic orbitals for the two atoms. These new orbitals must be of a different energy than the atomic orbitals in a non-degenerate system. In other words, when mixing two atomic orbitals, one new orbital is formed that must be lower in energy and one is formed that is higher in energy relative to the atomic orbitals.

How does the LCAO model apply to covalent bonds in simple diatomic molecules such as hydrogen?

Two atoms are combined to form a covalent bond, and the atomic orbitals of each atom are combined to form a molecular orbital. Assume that the electrons in each atomic orbital are transferred from energy levels near the atom to different energy levels that correspond to electron density between the nuclei of the bonded atoms. A molecular orbital is an orbital associated with the molecule rather than the individual atoms, as shown below for H_2. For molecules containing more electrons than hydrogen or helium, and for those containing electrons in orbitals other than s-orbitals, the diagram is more complex and the LCAO approach usually fails.

How are molecular orbitals formed from atomic orbitals?

Using the LCAO model, the orbitals for the molecule diatomic hydrogen (H_2) can be formed by mixing the atomic orbitals of two hydrogen atoms. The orbitals formed are not atomic orbitals, but they are associated with a molecule, in this case H_2, and are called *molecular orbitals.* Each of the two hydrogen 1s atomic orbitals (H atomic orbital) contains one electron, and these orbitals have the same energy. When mixed to form the molecular orbital, the molecular orbital electrons have a different energy, and those orbitals are in a different position relative to atomic orbitals, as shown for the molecule H—H. Therefore, if the two atomic orbitals mix, two molecular orbitals are generated, one higher in energy and one lower than the original atomic orbitals. It is noted that *this model does not work well for atoms that have degenerate p-orbitals.*

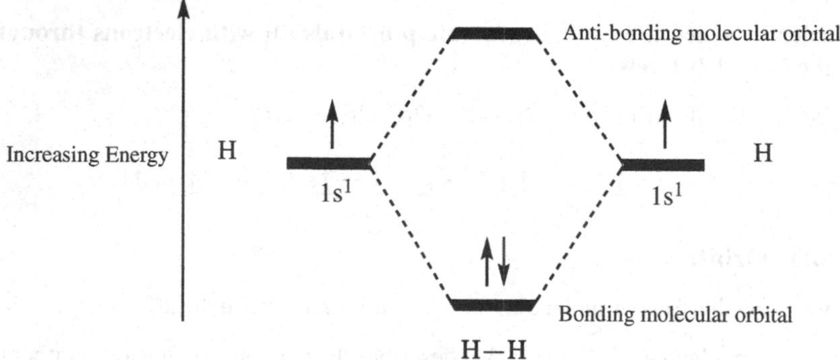

1.2 BONDING

1.2.1 Ionic Bonding

What is a Lewis dot structure?

A Lewis electron dot formula generates a bond between two atoms by simply using dots for electrons for the two electrons that comprise a bond. In other words, each bond is represented by two dots between the appropriate atoms, and unshared electrons are indicated by dots (one or two) on the appropriate atom.

What is the Lewis dot structure of lithium fluoride? Add the charges!

$$\mathrm{Li}^{+}\ :\!\ddot{\underset{\cdot\cdot}{\mathrm{F}}}\!:^{-}$$

What is an ionic bond?

An ionic bond occurs when two atoms are held together by electrostatic forces, where one atom or group assumes a positive charge and the other atom or group assumes a negative charge. Sodium chloride (NaCl), for example, exists in the solid state as $Na^{+}Cl^{-}$.

$$\overset{+}{Na}\ \vdots\ \ddot{\underset{\cdot\cdot}{Cl}}{:}^{-}$$

Why does sodium assume a positive charge in NaCl?

If the valence electrons associated with each atom are represented as dots (one dot for each electron), the structure for NaCl will be that shown above. Sodium chloride has an ionic bond, and in an ionic bond all of the electrons are on chlorine and none are on sodium. Sodium (Na) is in Group 1 and has the electronic configuration $1s^22s^22p^63s^1$. If one assumes that the sodium atom can react, it can either lose one electron (*ionization potential*) or gain seven electrons (the ability to gain one electron is called *electron affinity*) in order to achieve a "filled" shell. The loss of one electron gives the electronic configuration $1s^22s^22p^6$, which is a filled shell and very stable, and requires much less energy than gaining seven to give another filled shell. After transfer of one electron, sodium has no electrons around it. In other words, it is Na^+, which is missing one electron relative to atomic sodium; this means it is electron deficient and so assumes a positive charge (see *formal charge* in Section 2.5).

Why does chlorine assume a negative change in NaCl?

In the ionic bond for NaCl, the chlorine atom has eight electrons around it. The chlorine (Cl) atom has the electronic configuration $1s^22s^22p^63s^23p^5$. If one imagines that the Cl atom reacts, and since chlorine is in Group 17 with seven electrons in the outmost shell, it can either gain one electron or lose seven electrons. Clearly, the loss of seven electrons will require a great deal of energy. Energetically, it is far easier for Cl to gain an electron, leading to formation of a negatively charged atom. Therefore, Cl gains an electron in contrast to Na, which loses an electron. With an excess of electrons, given that electrons carry a negative charge, the Cl will take a negative charge. The strong electrostatic attraction between the positive sodium and the negatively charged chlorine binds the two atoms together into an ionic bond.

1.2.2 Covalent Bonding

What is a covalent bond?

A covalent bond has two electrons that are shared between two atoms. In the case of hydrogen (H_2), the covalent bond can be represented as H:H or H—H, where the (:) or the (—) indicates the presence of two electrons. In a covalent bond, the bulk of the electron density is localized between the hydrogen nuclei. This type of bond usually occurs when the atom cannot easily gain or lose electrons. Another way to view this is that there is a small electronegativity difference between atoms. A model of fluorine (F—F or F_2) shows the electron density around both atoms, but significant electron density is clearly between the two fluorine nuclei that represent the covalent F—F bond.

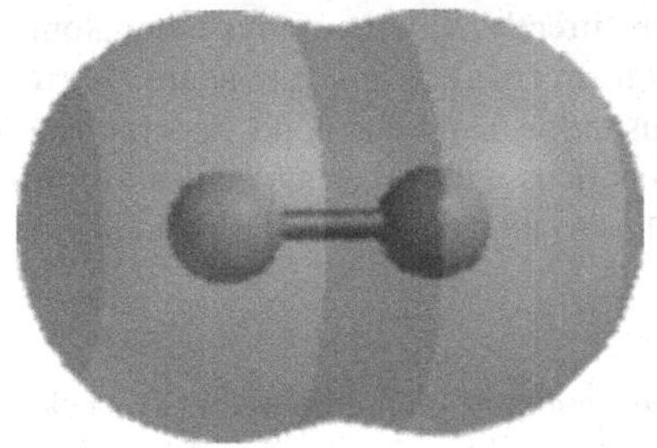

What is the Lewis dot structure of diatomic hydrogen?

H : H

What is the octet rule?

The octet rule states that every atom wants to have eight valence electrons in its outermost electron shell.

What is valence?

Valence is the number of bonds an atom can form to satisfy the octet rule and remain electrically neutral. Valence is not to be confused with valence electrons, which are the number of electrons in the outermost shell. In the second row from C to F, the valence is (*8 – the **last digit** of the group number*): C: 8 – 4, or 4; N: 8 – 5, or 3; O: 8 – 6, or 2; F: 8 – 7, or 1. Boron is an exception. There are only three electrons and, therefore, boron can form no more than three covalent bonds and remain neutral. In other words, an atom can form only as many bonds as there are electrons available to share. Note that the valence of boron is three and it is electron deficient.

What is the Lewis dot structure of a carbon–carbon bond when drawn as a covalent bond but ignoring all other electrons and the other valences of each carbon?

C : C

What is a Lewis acid?

A Lewis acid is any substance that can accept a pair of nonbonding electrons, so it is an electron-pair acceptor. An example is boron, which has only three electrons in the outermost shell, can only form three covalent bonds but is electron deficient because it requires two more electrons to satisfy the octet rule. These two electrons are gained by reaction with an electron-rich molecule and trivalent boron compounds are Lewis acids.

What is a Lewis base?

A Lewis base is any substance that can donate a pair of nonbonding electrons, so it is an electron-pair donor. Electron donation to a hydrogen atom is not included in the Lewis base definition, however. In other words, a base that donates two electrons to a hydrogen atom is a Brønsted–Lowry base not a Lewis base.

Why does carbon have a valence of four?

Carbon is in Group 14 so there are four valence electrons. Therefore, carbon forms a total of four covalent bonds by sharing the electrons with many other atoms, including another carbon atom. With carbon (C: $1s^2 2s^2 2p^2$), there are four electrons in the highest valence shell. The gain of four electrons or the loss of four electrons would require a prohibitively high amount of energy. In a thought experiment, assume that a carbon atom can form bonds directly with up to four other atoms. In such an experiment, carbon, because it is lower in energy, will form covalent bonds to share electrons with another atom rather than "donate" or "accept" four electrons to form an ionic bond. A carbon atom with appropriate functionality attached can undergo chemical reactions with other molecules to form covalent bonds to other carbon atoms, to hydrogen atoms, as well as to many atoms in the periodic table.

What is covalent bond?

In a covalent bond, the electrons are mutually shared between two nuclei in that bond, so each nucleus has a filled shell (eight in the case of carbon and two in the case of hydrogen). The most common way to show mutual sharing of electrons for two carbon atoms is to draw a single line between the two atoms (C—C) rather than using the Lewis dot structure, C:C. The two electrons are equally distributed between the two carbon atoms and the resultant bond has a symmetrical distribution of electron density between the two atoms.

What does a covalent bond between two hydrogen atoms look like in the molecule H_2?

The two hydrogen atoms are identical, the mutual sharing of electrons leads to a symmetrical distribution of the electron density between the two hydrogen nuclei, as shown in the accompanying molecular model (an electronic potential map)

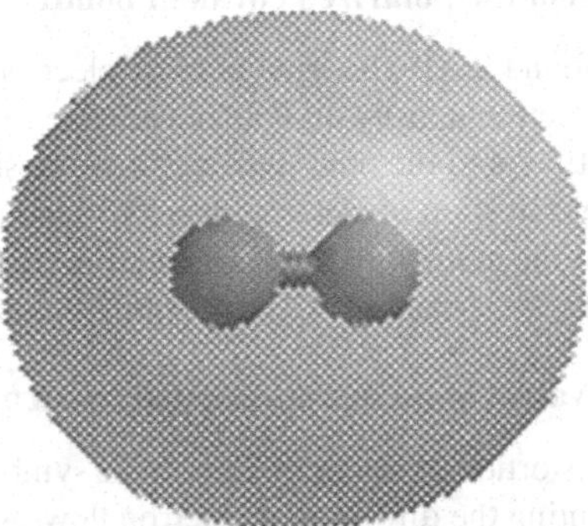

What does a covalent bond between two carbon atoms with identical atoms attached?

If the two carbon atoms are identical, the mutual sharing of electrons leads to a symmetrical distribution of the electron density between the two carbon nuclei.

What is electronegativity?

Electronegativity is a measure of the attraction that an atom has for the bonding pair of electrons in a covalent bond. A more electronegative atom will attract more electron density toward itself than a less electronegative atom.

What is a polar covalent bond?

If two atoms are part of a covalent bond, and one atom is more electronegative than the other, the shared electron density is distorted toward the more electronegative atom, as shown in the molecular model of H—F, rather than the symmetrical distribution found in H—H. The shaded area on the far right indicates higher electron density, which is clearly on the more electronegative fluorine atom.

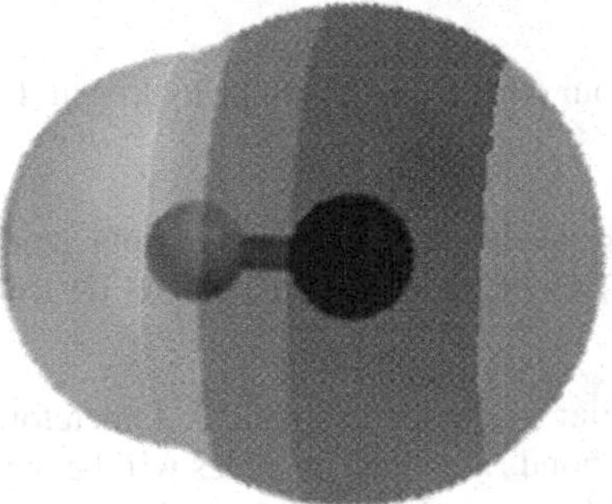

When a bond is formed between two atoms that are not identical, the electrons do not have to be equally shared. If one atom is more electronegative (electronegativity is the ability of an atom to attract electrons to itself; the electronegativity is higher), it will pull a greater share of electrons from the covalent bond toward itself. The larger the difference in electronegativity, the greater the distortion of electron density in the covalent bond toward the more electronegative atom.

What is an example of a molecule with a polar covalent bond?

An example is H—F (see the molecular model in the preceding question), where the fluorine is significantly more electronegative than the hydrogen atom. This difference in electronegativity will lead to electron distortion in the covalent bond toward the fluorine, away from hydrogen, and an unsymmetrical covalent bond will form that has less electron density between the nuclei. In other words, it is a weaker bond. The model shown indicates this electron distortion, with the shaded area on the far right (higher electron density) toward the fluorine and the shaded area on the far left (lower electron density) toward the hydrogen atom.

How can HF be drawn to represent the polarized covalent bond?

In a polarized bond such as that found in HF, fluorine is more electronegative, and the bond density is distorted such that there is more electron density on fluorine relative to the hydrogen. The more electronegative atom will be "more negative" and the other will be "more positive." The molecule is neutral so there are no ionic charges, but the distortion of electron density in the polarized covalent bond is represented by a "partial charge" (δ^+) at the atom with the least electron density and (δ^-) at the atom with the most electron density. Therefore, the polarization of HF is represented as $^{\delta+}$H—F$^{\delta-}$.

Can the dipole of a polarized covalent bond be represented by an appropriate symbol?

A common way to represent this distortion of electrons is with the symbol $+\!\!\longrightarrow$, with the + representing the positive atom and $\longrightarrow$ representing the direction of electron flow. As noted in the previous question, it is perhaps more common to use a δ^+ at the atom with the least electron density and δ^- at the atom with the most electron density, as shown for H—F. Such a covalent bond is polarized, and this disparity in electron density leads to a dipole moment. Any covalent bond between two atoms where one is less electronegative, and the other is more electronegative, will be a polar covalent bond.

What is dipole moment?

Bond dipole moment is a measure of the polarity of a chemical bond, generally induced by differences in electronegativity of the two atoms in that bond. The bond dipole symbol is μ and the unit of measurement is the Debye (D).

Is the C—H bond considered to be polarized?

No! Although C and H have different electronegativities (H = 2.1 and C = 2.5 on the Pauling electronegativity scale), the C—H bond is not considered to be polarized. This assumption is based on the polarity of molecules containing only C—H bonds, but the chemical reactivity of molecules that contain only C—H bond will support this view.

What is a heteroatom?

A heteroatom is defined as any atom other than carbon or hydrogen. Examples are O, N, S, P, Cl, Br, F, Mg, Na, etc.

Which of the following are polar covalent bonds? For the polarized bonds, identify the negative and positive poles: (a) C—O (b) C—C (c) O—H (d) H—H (e) Br—Br (f) C—N (g) N—N (h) O—O (i) H—Br (j) NaCl

Only those bonds between dissimilar atoms will be polarized, therefore (a), (c), (f), (i), and (j) are polarized covalent. NaCl (j) is an ionic bond. The negative poles will be oxygen in (a) and (c), nitrogen in (f), and bromine in (i). The positive poles are carbon in (a) and (f), hydrogen in (c) and (i).

What is van der Waals attraction?

When there are no polarizing atoms in the molecules, the only attraction between molecules results from the electrons of one molecule being attracted to the positive nuclei of atoms in another molecule. This interaction is known as *van der Waals attraction* (sometimes called *London forces*).

What are dipole–dipole interactions?

The intermolecular electrostatic interaction between polarized atoms in one molecule with polarized atoms in a nearby molecule is referred to as a dipole–dipole interaction. The net result of this $\delta+ \longleftarrow \delta-$interaction is that these molecules will be associated together, and some energy will be required to disrupt this association.

How does the physical size of the group that is attached to the heteroatom influence dipole–dipole interactions?

The electrostatic interaction of the two dipolar molecules is diminished by the physical size imposed by the carbon groups since the molecules cannot come as close together. As the molecules approach each other, larger groups compete for the same space (this is called *steric hindrance*) and repel each other, counteracting the electrostatic attraction to some extent.

What causes two molecules with C—O or C=O bonds to associate together in the liquid phase?

When two molecules, each with a polarized covalent bond, come into close proximity, the charges for one bond will be influenced by the charge on the adjacent molecule. In the example shown with two molecules of propane-2-one (acetone), the negative oxygen of one molecule is attracted to the positive carbon of the second molecule. Likewise, the positive carbon of that molecule is attracted to the negative oxygen of the other. In general, the greater the dipole moment, the stronger the interaction and the greater the energy will be required to disrupt that interaction between the molecules.

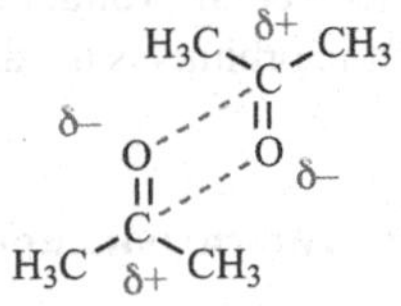

H_3C δ+ CH_3
δ– O C=O δ–
H_3C C δ+ CH_3

What are hydrogen bonds?

When hydrogen forms a polar covalent bond with heteroatoms (atoms other than carbon or hydrogen, the most common are O—H, N—H, S—H), the hydrogen takes the δ^+ charge of the dipole. There is a strong interaction with a negative heteroatom that is brought into close proximity to a positive polarized hydrogen of another molecule. The interaction shown in the figure for the O—H units of methanol is referred to as a *hydrogen bond.*

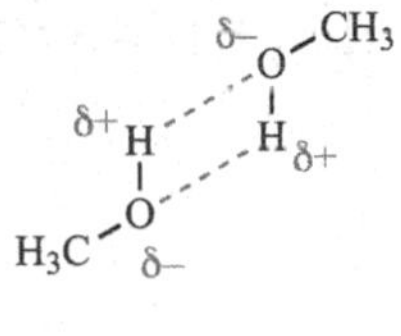

δ– O CH_3
δ+ H H δ+
H_3C O δ–

Which is stronger, a dipole–dipole interaction or a hydrogen bond?

The attraction between a polarized hydrogen atom and a heteroatom in a hydrogen bond is generally significantly stronger than the dipole–dipole attraction between the two atoms in a polarized covalent bond (not involving H). The bond polarization of an X—H bond is generally greater, so there is more attraction with a negative dipole, and the hydrogen atom is small. Due to the small size of hydrogen, there is minimal steric hindrance due to intramolecular interactions with another nearby atoms.

Why is the attraction between two molecules of methanol, each with an O—H unit, stronger than the attraction between two molecules of acetone (see above), each of which bears a C=O group?

The electronegative oxygen atom makes the O—H bond in methanol more polarized than the C=O bond in acetone. The hydrogen atom is also smaller, so it is easier for the oxygen atom on a methanol molecule to approach the hydrogen atom in another molecule of methanol. As the carbon atom of one acetone molecule approaches the oxygen atom of another acetone molecule, there is a significant intermolecular steric interaction of the methyl groups between the different molecules. Therefore, it is anticipated that the intermolecular hydrogen bond interaction of one methanol molecule for another is stronger than the intermolecular dipole–dipole interactions of one acetone molecule for another.

1.3 HYBRIDIZATION

What are "core" electrons?

Electrons that are close to the nucleus that they are too tightly bound to be shared with another atom to form a covalent bond. Such electrons are referred to as *core electrons*; *they are not the valence electrons.* Core electrons are not involved in chemical reactions and so they are not involved in covalent bonding.

What are valence electrons?

Valence electrons are electrons in the outermost electronic shells of an atom, and they are available for chemical reactions and thus for sharing with another atom to form a covalent bond.

What is a molecular orbital and what is a molecular orbital diagram?

A molecular orbital is a mathematical function that describes the wave-like behavior of an electron in a molecule. Another way to look at a molecular orbital is as a function that describes the electronic behavior of electrons in a covalent bond. A molecular orbital diagram describes the chemical bonding in molecules and the linear combination of atomic orbitals is used to generate the molecular orbital diagram for a particular bond.

How is the LCAO method used to combine two carbon atoms to give the molecular orbital diagram for C—C?

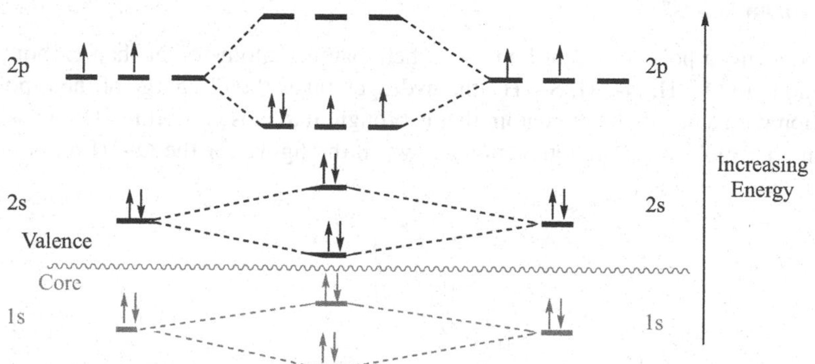

Atomic carbon has an electronic configuration of $1s^22s^22p^2$. The molecular orbital diagram is shown. Using the LCAO method to form a carbon–carbon single bond, the two 2s orbitals and the three, degenerate p-orbitals of two carbon atoms are combined to give six molecular orbitals in a C—C molecule. The total number of orbitals remains constant, but the molecular orbitals must be of a different energy relative to the atomic orbitals and they are split into high energy and low energy components. The orbitals are symmetrically split, as shown. The total number of electrons cannot change, and they are added and spin-paired, beginning with the lowest energy orbitals. The three, degenerate p-orbitals on the carbon atoms lead to three lower energy degenerate molecular orbitals as well as three degenerate higher energy orbitals, as shown in the diagram. Note that when the four "p" electrons are added to the molecular orbitals, the LCAO method suggests two unshared electrons, which is not the case in real molecules.

Why does the molecular orbital diagram for diatomic carbon give an incorrect result?

The attempt to mix s- and p-atomic orbitals leads to the discrepancy. The LCAO-generated molecular orbital diagram shown for a C—C bond suggests more than one type of bond. The 2s molecular orbitals combine to form one type of bond; the p-orbitals combine to form another type of bond, and there appear to be unshared electrons in the orbitals. The prediction of two different kinds of bonds is a result of trying to mix s- and p-orbitals, and *this prediction is not correct.* In fact, it is known from many years of experiments that one type of bond is formed by each carbon atom. Indeed, CH_4 (methane) forms four identical bonds to four hydrogen atoms, for example.

A new model that generates a better description of a C—C bond is required that recognizes all four bonds as the same type in the final molecule.

How is the LCAO model used to give the molecular orbital diagram for C—C by mixing two sp³-hybrid orbitals?

When these identical orbitals (they are the same energy, therefore, degenerate) from two "hybridized" carbon atoms are mixed to form a molecular orbital, the core electrons remain the same, but the covalent orbitals now show four identical bonds (two electrons per bond). Since the correct answer was known in advance, the modified model must give the correct answer.

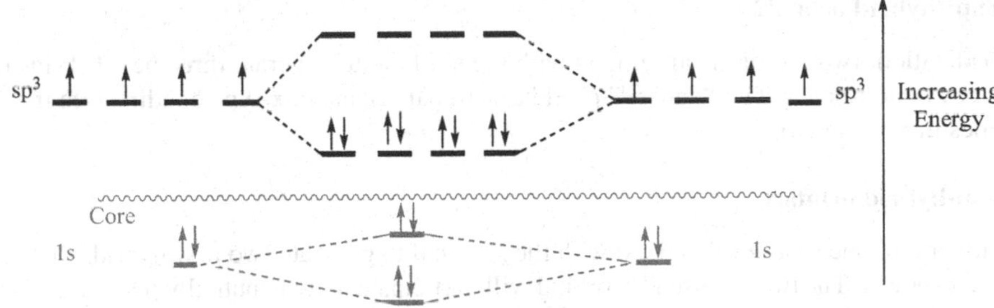

Can one gain or lose orbitals during hybridization?

No! The number of hybrid orbitals that are formed cannot be more or less than the total number of atomic orbitals.

Can one gain or lose the total number of electrons during hybridization?

No! The number of electrons in the molecular orbitals cannot be more or less than the total number of electrons in the atomic orbitals.

What is a sp³-hybrid orbital?

In sp³-hybridization, all three p-orbitals are mathematically mixed with the s-orbital to generate four new hybrids that can form four covalent bonds of the same type.

What is a sigma bond?

A sigma (σ) bond is the usual covalent bond between two atoms such as C—C, C—H, C—O, or C—N, where the electron density is concentrated between the two nuclei (essentially on a "line" between the two nuclei). The σ-bond is associated with what is known as a "single covalent bond."

How is a σ-bond normally drawn between two sp³-hybridized carbon atoms?

A carbon–carbon σ-bond is drawn as C—C. When drawn with a single line to represent the covalent bond between two carbon atoms, that bond is assumed to be a covalent σ-bond.

What is the classification for the bond in a C—C unit?

When drawn with a single line to represent the covalent bond between two carbon atoms, that bond is assumed to be a covalent σ-bond: e.g., C—C.

How is hybridization applied to a covalently bound atom?

When the s- and p-atomic orbitals of an atom are mathematically "mixed," four identical hybrid orbitals are formed. Since one 2s and three 2p are mixed, the resulting hybrid orbitals are called sp^3-hybrid orbitals. When these sp^3-hybrid orbitals for two carbon atoms are used in the Linear Combination of Molecular Orbitals model, four identical bonding molecular orbitals are formed. When the atomic orbitals are rearranged, mixtures of them (hybrids) are formed and used for bonding. For carbon and other elements of the second row, the hybridization is limited to mixing one 2s and one or more of the three 2p-orbitals.

How are hybrid orbitals different when using different numbers of 2p-orbitals?

There are three basic types of hybridization: sp^3, sp^2, and sp^1 (or just sp). In each case, the sp refers to the hybridization of the atom where the superscript indicates the number of p-orbitals used to form hybrids in combination with the 2s-orbital.

What is a sp^2-hybrid orbital?

In sp^2-hybridization, two p-orbitals are mixed with the s-orbital to generate three new hybrids that can form three covalent σ-bonds. The "unused" p-orbital will participate in π-type bonding (see the chemistry of alkenes in Section 7.1).

What is a sp-hybrid orbital?

In sp-hybridization, one p-orbital is mixed with the s-orbital to generate two new hybrids that can form two covalent σ-bonds. The two "unused" p-orbital will participate in two, mutually perpendicular π-type bonds (see the discussion of alkynes in Section 7.5).

What is a π-bond?

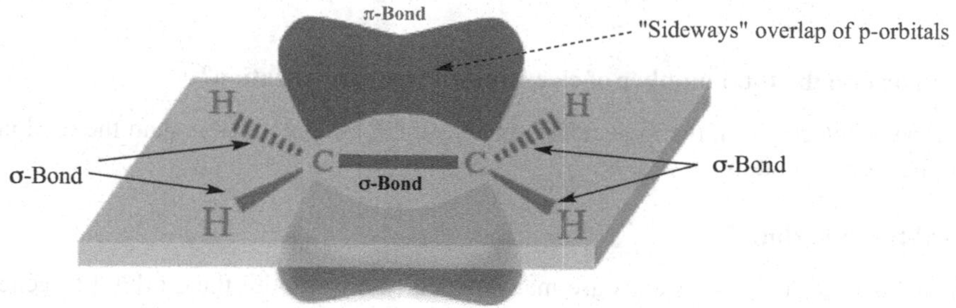

A pi- (π) bond occurs when two sp^2-hybridized are connected by a covalent bond, and each atom has an "unused" p-orbital, as described above. Sigma bonds using sp^2-hybrid orbitals connect the two carbon atoms and all four C—H bonds. Each sp^2-hybridized carbon has a "unused" p-orbital. When these p-orbitals are parallel and on adjacent atoms, they can share electron density via "sideways" overlap to form a new bond (called a π-bond) that is much weaker than the σ-bond. Effectively, there are two bonds between the carbon atoms, a strong σ-bond, and a weak π-bond, as shown for ethene.

How is the double bond between two carbon atoms represented, ignoring the other bonds to carbon?

A carbon–carbon double bond is represented as C=C. Note that in the C=C representation it is not possible to indicate which is the σ-bond and which is the π-bond, and it is not necessary to do so. One line represents the σ-bond and the other line represents the π-bond.

1.4 RESONANCE

What is a carbon–carbon single bond?

A C—C single bond is a normal covalent σ-bond between two carbon atoms, involving mutual sharing of two electrons between the two carbon nuclei.

What is a carbon–carbon double bond?

A C=C unit contains one σ-bond and one π-bond between the two carbon atoms (see the figure of ethene in Section 1.3 and see Section 7.1)

Is it possible to form a double bond between other atoms?

Yes! A double bond can form between carbon and other atoms, or between atoms other than carbon. Examples are C=O, C=S, C=N, as well as N=N, O=O, N=O, S=O.

What is the structure of a molecule with an oxygen–oxygen double bond, one with an N=O bond, and one that contains a S=O bond?

An example of a molecule with an oxygen–oxygen double bond is diatomic oxygen, O_2. An example of a molecule that contains a nitrogen–oxygen double bond (N=O) is nitric acid. An example of a molecule that contains a sulfur–oxygen double bond (S=O) is sulfuric acid.

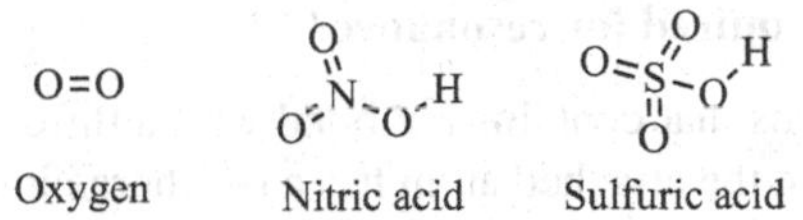

O=O

Oxygen

Nitric acid

Sulfuric acid

What is a point charge?

A point charge is a charge that is completely localized on a single atom. In the chloride ion (Cl^-), for example, the two electrons that comprise the negative charge are in an orbital localized on the chlorine atom.

Can bonds be formed that are "in-between" single and double bonds?

In some cases, it is possible for electron density to be delocalized in such a way that the actual bond is in between a single and a double bond. In such a bond, electron density is delocalized over several atoms rather than localized on a single atom. This phenomenon occurs most commonly when a charge is present in an atom and is also commonly associated with the presence of π-bonds.

What is resonance?

Resonance occurs when the electron density of bonds is not localized between two atoms but rather delocalized over three or more atoms. In other words, bonds between two atoms can be intermediate between single and double bonds, due to the sharing of electrons by several atoms, which is described as delocalizing the electron density over several atoms. In effect, the electron density is "smeared" over several atoms.

Which is more stable, a point charge or a delocalized charge?

If a charge is delocalized over several atoms rather than localized on a single atom, the charge density on each atom is diminished. Lower charge density is usually associated with lower energy, so a delocalized charge should be more stable (less reactive) than a localized charge.

How is resonance in a molecule represented?

Resonance delocalization for a molecule is represented by drawing two or more resonance contributors, with different localized bonds and charges as required. The double-headed arrow shows that the resonance contributors are linked to represent a single, delocalized structure. An example is the oxocarbenium ion where the positive charge is delocalized over the O and the C, and this delocalization is represented by the two structures shown with the double-headed arrow. The different structures represent the extent of electron delocalization in the actual structure.

What are the resonance contributors for the allylic carbocation?

There are two resonance contributors as shown. The positive charge is not localized on the two structures but delocalized over three atoms. The double-headed arrow represented links the two structures with the positive charge on the first and third carbon atoms to represent the delocalization. Likewise, the π-bond is not localized on the two structures, but the resonance contributors linked by the double-headed arrow are used to show that the π-electrons are delocalized.

What structural features are required for resonance?

A molecule of three or more atoms that contains a π-bond with a third atom that has a (+) charge, a (–) charge, or a single electron. When the attached atom has a (+) charge it is a cation. When the third atom has a (–) charge it is an anion, and when it has a single electron it is a radical. When there are two atoms with a (+) charge on one atom and an attached heteroatom such as O, S, or N has at least one unshared electron, resonance can occur.

$X{=}Y{-}Z^{+}$	$X{=}Y{-}Z^{-}$	$X{=}Y{-}Z^{\bullet}$	$:Y{-}Z^{+}$
Cation-1	Anion	Radical	Cation-2

What is the energetic consequence of resonance?

The delocalization of the point charge to dispersal of charge over several atoms (a greater surface area) leads to greater stability of the molecule. In general, the greater the point charge, the less stable (more reactive), and the lesser the point charge, the more stable (less reactive) the molecule. Resonance enhances the stability of a molecule and the term "resonance stability" is common. A resonance-stabilized structure is more stable and therefore less reactive.

What is a resonance contributor?

The two cation structures (cation-1 and cation-2) are used as an example. Cation-1 type structures are characterized by a X=Y unit (C=C, C=O, etc.) attached to an atom with a p-orbital (a cation, an anion, or a radical). A cation is essentially an empty p-orbital, an anion is essentially a filled p-orbital, and a radical is a p-orbital with a single electron.

Note the use of a *double-headed arrow* to indicate the involvement of two electrons to delocalize electron density (resonance) over the three atoms in X—Y—Z. Indeed, the curved arrow in cation-1 is used to show electron dispersal over the X—Y—Z unit. The arrow in cation-1 indicates dispersal of the electron density from X=Y to the Z^{+} orbital, leaving behind a positive charge on X. The actual structure of cation-1 is not X=Y—Z^{+} or is it $^{+}$X—Y=Z. In the actual structure, the electron density is delocalized over all three atoms, so *both* structures are used to represent the actual structure. This phenomenon is called *resonance* and the two structures are *resonance contributors* to the actual structure. Similar structures can be drawn as resonance contributors for the anion and the radical shown in a preceding question.

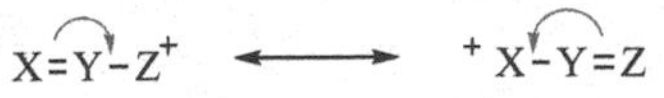

$$X{=}Y{-}Z^+ \longleftrightarrow {}^+X{-}Y{=}Z \qquad :Y{-}Z^+ \longleftrightarrow {}^+Y{=}Z$$

Cation-1 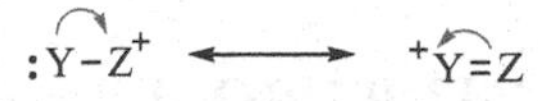 Cation-2

Cation-2 type structures have a positive charged carbon attached to an atom that has lone electron pairs, such as O, S, Cl, Br, etc. In cation-2, the lone electron pair on Y is shared with the orbital of Z^+ (see the use of the curved arrow to indicate the dispersal of two electrons). The resulting resonance contributor has a double bond between Y=Z with a positive charge on Y. If the two electrons in the double bond are donated back to the positively charged Y^+, the original resonance contributor with Z^+ is regenerated. Therefore, molecules with this structural motif have the two resonance contributors shown.

Are the two structures shown as resonance contributors in equilibrium with each other?

No! They are *not* equilibrating structures, but rather two structures in resonance with one another that, taken together, represent the bonding between the atoms. Such a molecule has bonds in-between single and double bonds due to delocalization of the charge. The two structures are *not* in equilibrium.

What are the resonance contributors for the nitrate anion, NO_3^-? For the perchlorate anion (ClO_4^-)?

The nitrate anion has three resonance contributors and the perchlorate anion has four resonance contributors, as shown in the figure.

Nitrate anion

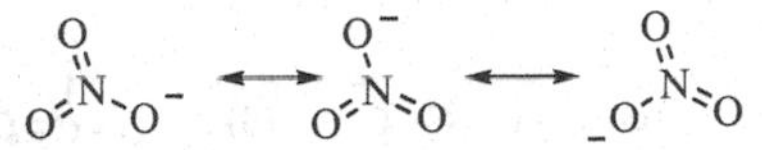

Perchlorate anion

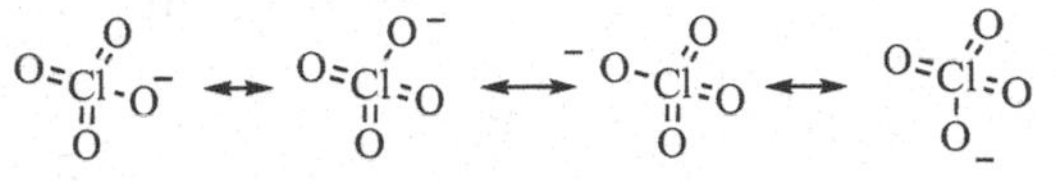

What are the resonance contributors for (a) and for (b)?

$$\text{(a)}\ H_2C{=}CH{-}\overset{+}{C}H_2 \qquad \text{(b)}\ H{-}\overset{\overset{O}{\|}}{C}{-}O^-$$

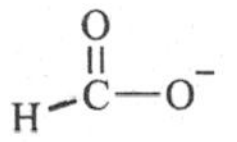

The so-called allylic cation (a) has the two resonance contributors shown, which the positive charge delocalized over the three carbon atoms. The formate anion (the anion of formic acid) has the two resonance contributors shown with the negative charge delocalized over the two oxygen atoms and the carbon.

$$\text{(a)}\ H_2C{=}CH{-}\overset{+}{C}H_2 \longleftrightarrow H_2\overset{+}{C}{-}CH{=}CH_2 \qquad \text{(b)}\ H{-}\overset{\overset{O}{\|}}{C}{-}O^- \longleftrightarrow H{-}\overset{\overset{O^-}{|}}{C}{=}O$$

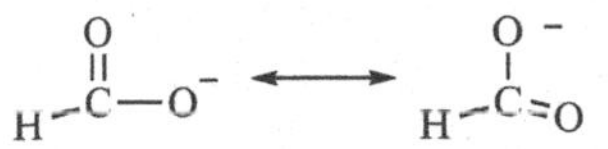

In example (b) in the immediately preceding question, is the negative charge equally distributed over all three atoms, or is the charge density higher on some atoms?

In the formate anion, the oxygen atoms are more electronegative and attract electron density more than carbon, so the negative charge (the two electrons) are more concentrated on the oxygen atoms than on the carbon atom.

What are two types of systems with a charge or a radical that exhibit resonance?

The resonance structures shown for cation-1 in the preceding question represent one type of resonance involving a three-atom array with one π-bond between two atoms and the third atom attached with a (+), a (–) charge, or a single electron (a radical). The second type of structure is cation-2, with one atom that has a positive charge and the attached atom (usually O, S, or N) has a lone electron pair.

END OF CHAPTER PROBLEMS

1. Describe a 3s-orbital and a 3p-orbital.
2. What is the difference between a $2p_x$ and a $2p_y$ orbital?
3. Give the electronic configuration for each of the following: O, F, Cl, S, Si.
4. Identify each of the following molecules as having an ionic bond, a covalent bond or both: (a) K–Cl (b) Na–C≡N (c) H_3C—Br (d) H_2N—H (e) N–Na (f) HO–Na (g) HO—H.
5. Give the number of covalent bonds each atom can form and remain electrically neutral: (a) C (b) N (c) F (d) B (e) O.
6. Why is BF_3 considered to be a Lewis acid?
7. Which of the following bonds is most polarized: C—C, C—N, C—O, C—F?
8. Identify the valence electrons in each of the following (also identify the atom involved): (a) $1s^22s^22p^3$ (b) $1s^22s^22p^63s^1$ (c) $1s^2$ (d) $1s^22s^22p^63s^23p^3$
9. Indicate which bonds are consistent with hydrogen bonding, which are consistent with dipole–dipole interactions, and which would be consistent with only van der Waals interactions: (a) C—O—H (b) C—F (c) C—C (d) N—H
10. Indicate which structures are likely to have resonance contributors. In those cases where there is resonance, draw the resonance contributors.

(a) $C=C-C^+$ (b) $\overset{+}{Cl}=C$ (c) $C-C=C-\overset{-}{C}$ (d) H–O–C(=O)–C

2

Structure of Molecules

This chapter will describe the fundamental structures of organic molecules, the properties associated with those structures, and the structural features that lead to important functional groups.

2.1 BASIC STRUCTURE OF ORGANIC MOLECULES

2.1.1 Fundamental Structures

What is valence?

Valence is a whole number that represents the ability of an atom or a group of atoms to combine with other atoms or groups of atoms. The valence is determined by the number of electrons that an atom can lose, add, or share. Therefore, valence is the number of electrons available for chemical bond formation for each atom. Valence also relates to the number of bonds an atom can form and remain neutral. Valence is 8-#, where # is the *last digit* of the group number for an atom: # is 4 for Group 14, 5 for Group 15, 6 for Group 16, and 7 for Group 17.

What is the valence of each of the following: C, H, N, O, F?

The valence of each atom is determined by subtracting the last digit of group number from 8 for C, N, O, F since these atoms are in the second row. Therefore, C = 4, N = 3, O = 2, and F = 1. The valence is the number of bonds that can be formed to each of these atoms and the resulting atom will be neutral (no charge). In other words, carbon can form four bonds, nitrogen can form two, oxygen can form two, and fluorine can form one. In all cases, the resulting molecule is neutral.

What is a simple molecule that satisfies the valence of oxygen and a simple molecule that satisfies the valence of nitrogen?

Oxygen has a valence of two, and H—O—H (water) satisfies the valence of oxygen. Nitrogen has a valence of three, and NH_3 (ammonia) satisfies the valence of nitrogen.

H–O–H Water

H–N(–H)–H Ammonia

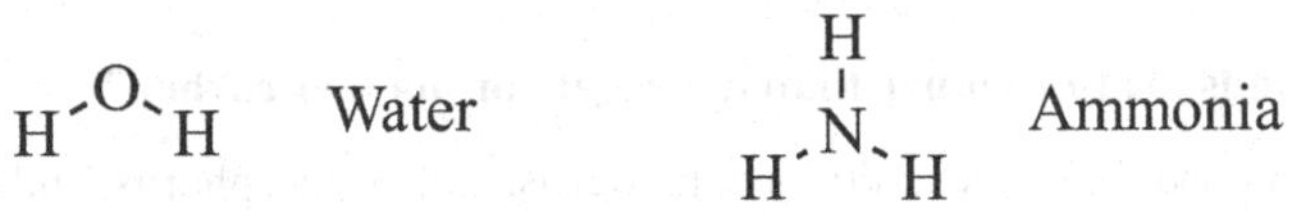

What are valence electrons?

Valence electrons are outer shell electrons that are associated with an atom and participate in the formation of a chemical bond. Valence electrons can participate in the formation of a chemical bond if the outer shell is not full. As practical matter, valence electrons are the number of electrons in the outermost shell of an atom that are available to form a covalent bond with another atom. Boron has three valence electrons, carbon has four valence electrons, nitrogen three, oxygen two, and fluorine has one.

How many valence electrons does N have? O?

Since the valence electrons for N and for O are those in the second electronic shell, nitrogen has five valence electrons while oxygen has six.

What is the structure of the molecule with one carbon connected to four hydrogen atoms by σ-covalent bonds?

```
    H
    |
H - C - H     Methane
    |
    H
```

What is the experimentally determined geometry of methane (CH_4)?

Experiments have determined that CH_4 has the structure with the four hydrogen atoms in a tetrahedral array about a central carbon atom, and the H—C—H bond angles are 104°28′ (104.47°). All four of the bond angles are identical, consistent with the tetrahedral shape.

The use of a solid wedge and a dashed line represents the three-dimensional shape of methane. The solid wedge indicates the bond and the attached atom is projected out of the page, and the dashed line indicates that the bond and the attached atom are projected behind the page. The normal lines are used to indicate that the bonds and the attached atoms are in the plane of the paper. This convention is used to indicate the three-dimensional shape of molecules about a specific atom.

Based on the geometry of methane, what can be inferred about the geometry of organic molecules based on carbon?

With a valence of four, and four other atoms attached, each carbon atom in an organic molecule should be tetrahedral, as they are in methane. The bond angles will vary with the attached atom, but each carbon should have a tetrahedral-type geometry.

Can carbon form bonds to itself?

Yes! Carbon can form linear chains of carbon atoms or chains of carbon with carbon atoms or carbon chains branched from a carbon chain. This property of carbon, to form covalent bonds to other carbon atoms, leads to a huge number of different molecules. Carbon can also form covalent bonds to many other atoms in the periodic table, leading to a huge variety of molecules that contain carbon.

Can carbon form bonds to atoms other than hydrogen, or another carbon?

Yes! Carbon can form bonds to oxygen, nitrogen, halogens, sulfur, phosphorus, and other atoms, and to various metals.

How can five carbon atoms be connected together in as many different ways as possible? Complete all of the remaining valences on each carbon with a hydrogen atom.

There are three different possibilities. There is one possibility with five carbon atoms in a linear chain, one four-carbon liner chain with a one-carbon branch, and one three-carbon linear chain with two branched carbon atoms.

$CH_3{\cdot}CH_2{\cdot}CH_2{-}CH_2{-}CH_3$ $\quad$ $CH_3{-}CH(CH_3){-}CH_2{-}CH_3$ $\quad$ $CH_3{-}C(CH_3)_2{-}CH_3$

Note that the linear chain of carbon atoms is drawn in such a way that each carbon has four attached atoms. However, the attachments are not drawn in a way that shows all the bonds. The CH_3–C unit means that the first carbon is connected to three hydrogen atoms and one carbon. The three hydrogen atoms are shown to the right of the carbon, indicating that the three hydrogen atoms are attached to that carbon, and the carbon that is also attached is shown to the right. The C—CH_2—C unit means that the central carbon has four bonds, two to the carbon atoms, and two to the hydrogen atoms shown to the right of the carbon. The same protocol is used for every carbon atom.

What is the empirical formula for all of the molecules drawn in the previous question?

In all three cases, the empirical formula is C_5H_{12}.

Two structures have a total of six carbon atoms. One appears to have a linear chain of five carbon atoms and a one-carbon branch at the first carbon and the second structure has a linear chain of six carbon atoms. Are these two structures the same or different?

$CH_3 \cdot CH_2 \cdot CH_2 - CH_2 - CH_2 - CH_3$

CH_3 (attached above the last CH_2)
$CH_3 \cdot CH_2 \cdot CH_2 - CH_2 - CH_2$

Do not be fooled by appearances, the connectivity of these molecules is identical, with six carbons directly connected in a chain. Since both structures have the same connectivity, the two structures shown are the same molecule. In other words, the structure on the left is identical to the one on the right; they are the same. It is not important if the atoms are twisted up or down as long as the connectivity is identical.

What is *line notation*, which is used for drawing organic molecules?

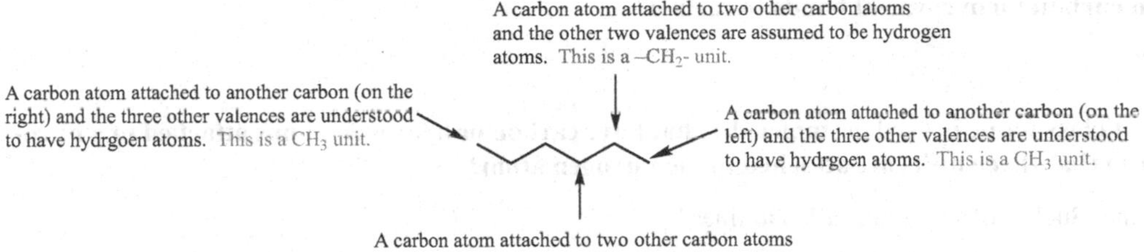

The molecule shown is a linear chain of six carbon atoms, and all other valences for each carbon are understood to be attached hydrogen atoms. Line notation is a shorthand method of drawing organic molecules. Each carbon atom is represented by a "dot," and a line is used to connect each carbon. Only carbon and hydrogen are present, and the hydrogen atoms do not have to be shown; they are understood to be there. In other words, each line represents a bond, and the remaining valences are understood to be hydrogen atoms.

If the connectivity of molecules is different, what can be said about the molecules?

If the connectivity is different, they are different molecules.

What is a five-carbon linear chain with a one-carbon branch on carbon 2 and a four-carbon linear chain with two one-carbon branches on C2 using line notation, both with the empirical formula C_6H_{14}?

Both molecules shown in the preceding question have the same empirical formula, C_6H_{14}, but different connectivity of the atoms, so they are different molecules. What is their relationship?

These two molecules with the same empirical formula but different connectivity are said to be *isomers*.

What is the term for molecules that have the same empirical formula but different connectivity for the carbon atoms?

Isomers. Specifically, *constitutional isomers*.

Which are of the following are isomers?

(a) 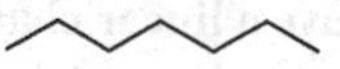 (b) 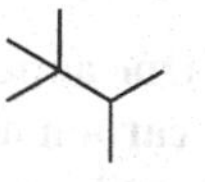 (c) 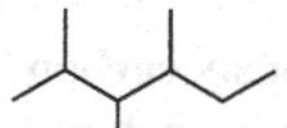 (d)

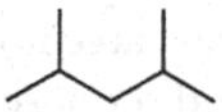

The empirical formula of (a), (b), and (d) are the same, C_7H_{16}, but they have different connectivity and are different molecules. Therefore, (a), (b), and (d) are constitutional isomers, or just isomers. Note that (c) has a different empirical formula, C_9H_{20}, so it is a different molecule, but it is not an isomer of (a), (b), or (d).

(a) 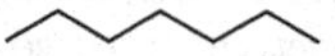 C_7H_{16} (b) C_7H_{16} (c) C_9H_{20} (d) C_7H_{16}

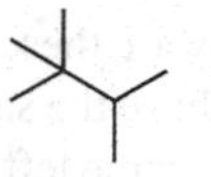

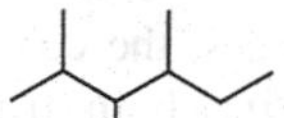

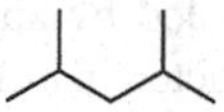

2.1.2 Structures with Other Atoms Bonded to Carbon

Can carbon form covalent bonds to carbon?

Yes!

What class name is used for molecules that have carbon or hydrogen atoms attached to a nitrogen so that three units are attached to the nitrogen atom?

Amine. Such molecules are called amines.

What is the molecule that has three carbon atoms attached to a nitrogen atom, and each carbon has three hydrogen atoms?

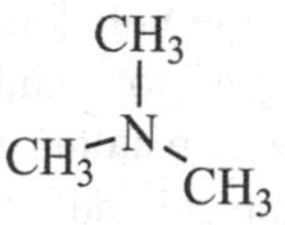

CH_3–N(CH_3)–CH_3

This molecule is known as an amine, specifically trimethylamine (see Sections 2.4 and 19.1). Note that there is an electron pair on nitrogen that is not used to form covalent bonds in this structure. The lone electron pair is not included in the structure shown, but it is understood to be there.

What is the molecule that has two carbon atoms attached to a nitrogen atom, a hydrogen on the nitrogen, and three hydrogen atoms of each of the carbon atoms?

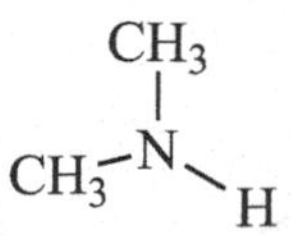

CH_3–N(CH_3)–H

Nitrogen can form covalent bonds to C or H. The molecule shown is an amine, specifically dimethylamine (see Sections 2.4 and 19.1). As with the preceding question, the lone electron pair is not shown in the structure but is understood to be there.

Can carbon form covalent bonds to oxygen?

Yes!

What is the molecule that has one carbon attached to an oxygen atom, one hydrogen atom attached to oxygen, and three hydrogen atoms attached to the carbon?

$$CH_3{-}O{-}H$$

There are two lone electron pairs on the oxygen, which has a valence of two and forms two covalent bonds, but the lone electron pairs are not shown. This molecule has an O—H unit and it is classified as an alcohol. Specifically, this molecule is methanol (see Sections 2.4, 7.4, and 8.3). In alcohols, oxygen forms bonds to both H and to C.

Another way to draw the structure given as an answer to the previous question is CH_3OH. How is this possible?

The three hydrogen atoms on each carbon are "condensed" to CH_3. Drawing CH_3O means that the carbon atom is bonded to the three H atoms to its right, as well as to the oxygen to complete the fourth valence. Likewise, the oxygen is understood to be bonded to C, not to H.

What is the molecule that has two carbon atoms connected to an oxygen atom, and each of the carbon atoms has three hydrogen atoms attached?

This molecule with a C—O—C structure is called an ether, specifically dimethyl ether (Sections 2.4 and 8.3). There are also two lone electron pairs on the oxygen, which has a valence of two, and forms two covalent bonds, but the lone electron pairs are not shown.

Another way to draw the molecule shown in the previous question is CH_3OCH_3. How is this possible?

In CH_3OCH_3, the oxygen is bonded to the carbon on its left, and the one on its right. Remember, the valence of O is two. The carbon to the right of O is bonded to the O, as well as to the three hydrogen atoms to its right. The valence of carbon is four.

What is the class of molecule with a carbon attached to oxygen and also a hydrogen atom?

Alcohol. Compounds such as this are known as alcohols, ROH, where R is any carbon group. Alcohols will be discussed in Sections 2.4 and 13.5.

What is the class of molecule with two carbon groups attached to oxygen?

Ether. Compounds such as this are known as ethers, ROR, where R is any carbon group.

2.2 THE VSEPR MODEL AND MOLECULAR GEOMETRY

What model is used determine the shape of a molecule when the atoms are found in the first row of the periodic table?

All molecules have a three-dimensional structure, of course. A simple model that will predict the approximate shape of a given molecule *formed from atoms in the second row of the periodic table* is the

***V**alence **S**hell **E**lectron **P**air **R**epulsion* (*VSEPR*) model. In this model there are two key components: (1) carbon, oxygen, and nitrogen are assumed to be at the center of a tetrahedron, (2) atoms bonded to carbon, oxygen, and nitrogen form a tetrahedral array of atoms around each central atom, and (3) electron pairs occupy space and are counted as "groups" attached to the central atom. The shape of the molecule is determined by the relative position of the atoms, assuming that the lone electron pairs are not seen.

What is meant by the shape of a molecule?

The shape is the three-dimensional shape of a molecule, which is determined by the bond angles and bond distances of the atoms directly connected to a given atom. Shapes can be determined in some cases using various experimental techniques or inferred in other cases by indirect methods. Using carbon as an example, the tetrahedral array of atoms attached to a given carbon leads to the tetrahedral shape or tetrahedral geometry that is associated with organic molecules.

How can the shape of a molecule be probed?

Organic chemists use a simple model, the VSEPR model, for a preliminary prediction of the three-dimensional structure of molecules that contain atoms in the second row of the periodic table. This model is used to estimate the structure and properties of that molecule. The model is overly simplistic, and the bond angles and bond distances are not taken into account, as the nature of the atoms or groups attached to carbon changes. Nonetheless, it is a useful tool to estimate the three-dimensional shapes of organic molecules.

How is the VSEPR model used?

The electrons in each bond around the central atom (C, N, O) will repel (like charges repel), but the bonds are connected to a central locus and the attached atoms or groups attached cannot dissociate from the central atom. Lone electron pairs are similarly "connected" to the central atom. The most efficient spatial arrangement that minimizes electronic repulsion is to put each atom or electron pair at the corner of a regular tetrahedron (bond angles are 109°28′). Using this observation, the model assumes a tetrahedral array of atoms and electrons around the atoms in the second row, specifically carbon, oxygen, and nitrogen.

Can the VSEPR model be used for boron compounds?

Boron has only three groups around it since there are only three valence electrons. When the electrons in the bonds repel, they distribute to the corners of a planar triangle. Therefore, molecules of boron tend to be planar. In other words, the tetrahedral VSEPR model is not used for boron compounds.

How can the VSEPR model be used to predict the three-dimensional shape of CH_4, CH_2Cl_2, H_2O, and NH_3?

For methane (Section 4.1) the four hydrogen atoms are distributed to the corners of a regular tetrahedron with carbon as the central locus. There are no unshared electron pairs on the carbon and the "shape" of the entire molecule is dictated by the covalent bonds and is *tetrahedral*. When two of the hydrogens are replaced with chlorine (dichloromethane), there are no unshared electron pairs on carbon and the overall shape remains *tetrahedral*. When water is analyzed, there are two hydrogens and two lone electron pairs, distributed to the corners of a tetrahedron. When viewing the molecule, however, only the *atoms* are observed (H—O—H), and these atoms assume an *angular* or *bent* shape for the water molecule. When ammonia is analyzed, the three hydrogens and one lone pair distribute to the corners of the tetrahedron. On viewing the *atoms*, however, the atoms assume a *pyramidal* shape, with nitrogen at the apex of the pyramid.

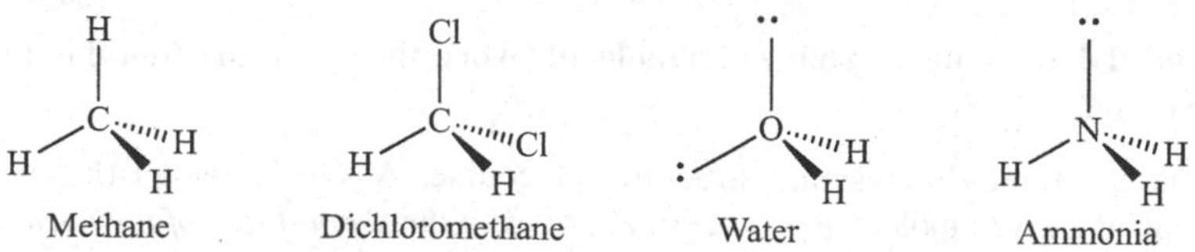

Methane Dichloromethane Water Ammonia

What are the main shortcomings of the VSEPR model?

This VSEPR model is flawed since it does not predict differences in shape due to the size of the various atoms and ignores attractive and repulsive forces that are present in some molecules. It does a reasonable job for simple molecules, however, and it usually used for a "first guess" of the shape of a molecule.

2.3 DIPOLE MOMENT

What is a dipole?

A dipole is the separation of charges within a molecule between two covalently bonded atoms or atoms that share an ionic bond. A dipole is the unsymmetrical dispersion of electron density in a covalent bond toward a concentration of higher electron density in one atom of that bond, in a molecule that has at least one polarized covalent bond. A polarized covalent bond has a partial negative charge on one atom and a partial positive charge on the other. The term dipole can also be used in connection with an entire molecule, where the electron density is not symmetrically dispersed.

What is dipole moment?

Dipole moment is the quantity that describes two opposite charges separated by a distance. Dipole moment for a bond is determined by discovering the size of the partial charges on the molecule and the bond length. The dipole moment for a bond (the bond dipole moment) is defined as the product of the total separation of positive or negative charge and the distance between the atoms. If there is a difference in electronegativity of the elements involved in the bond ($3.0 - 2.1 = 0.9$, for example), there is a shift in electron density toward the more electronegative atom, leading to polarization of the bonding electrons, and of the whole molecule. The dipole moment can therefore be associated with an individual bond, and also with the entire molecule.

Dipole moment, μ, is calculated by the equation $\mu = \delta\ d$, and measured in units of Debye, where 1 Debye = 3.34×10^{-30} coulomb/meter. The charge difference is measured in coulombs and the bond distance is measured in meters. In this equation, μ is the dipole moment in Debye, d is the bond distance, and δ is the charge difference between the atoms.

The dipole moment of C—F is 1.847 Debye and that of C—Cl is 1.860 Debye. Why does the C—Cl bond have a larger dipole moment relative to C—F?

The bond distance between the C and Cl atoms is 174 pm whereas the bond distance between the C and F atoms is 134 pm, due to the larger size of the chlorine atom relative to the fluorine atom. The atomic radius of Cl is 175 pm and the atomic radius of F is 147 pm.

What is the dipole moment for the C—F bond using both the arrow notation and the partial charge notation?

$$\overset{\delta+}{\mathrm{C}}\overset{\longmapsto}{\text{———}}\overset{\delta-}{\mathrm{F}}$$

The dipole moment is indicated by the +-arrow and also by δ^+ and δ^- are used to indicate the dipole. The point of the arrow is pointed toward the more electronegative fluorine atom, which is labeled with the δ^-. The less electronegative carbon atom is positioned by the + end of the arrow and it is labeled with the δ^+.

How can the VSEPR model be used to predict the dipole moment for a molecule rather than a single bond?

A molecule will have several bonds and each carbon atom, for example, may have up to four single covalent bonds. Each bond will have a dipole moment called a bond moment. Dipole moments are additive, and the dipole moment for a molecule is the additive value of all individual bond moments and the sum of the individual bond moment direction. The VSEPR model can be used to approximate the three-dimensional shape of molecules. The individual dipole moment of each bond in that molecule is superimposed on the VSEPR model, the direction and the magnitude of each bond moment is determined, and the dipole moment for the molecule can be estimated. Using the dipole moment for the molecule, the relative polarity (polar vs. non-polar) of the molecule can be estimated.

How can the VSEPR model be used to predict the direction of the dipole moment of methane (CH_4) and of dibromomethane (CH_2Br_2), if any?

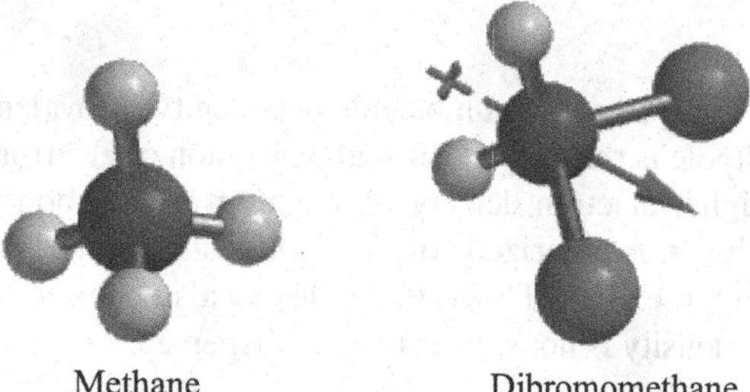

Methane Dibromomethane

In a molecule such as methane, the C—H bond is not considered to be polarized (the electronegativity of C and H are assumed to be the same, although they are not the same). Since there is no dipole moment for any bond and the dipole moment for the molecule is the sum of all bond dipole moments, the bond moment is zero. In other words, there is no dipole moment for methane.

For dibromomethane, there are two bond moments, along the C—Br bonds. The dipole moment for the molecule is the sum of all bond dipole moments. The negative pole of each of those bonds is the bromine. Since dipole moments are directional, *the dipole moment for the molecule is the vector sum of all the individual bond moments.* The vector sum of the two C—Br bond moments is in the direction that bisects the Br—C—Br bond as shown in the model. The dipole moment for dibromomethane will be equal in magnitude to the vector sum of the two individual bond moments. The experimental dipole moment is calculated to be 1.32 Debye. Note that the unit for dipole moment is the Debye, and has both magnitude and direction

What is the direction of the dipole moment for the molecule $CHCl_3$ (known as chloroform)?

The dipole moment for each C—Cl bond is shown. There are three dipole moments for the bonds (bond moments are adjacent to each bond) and with the tetrahedral shape of the molecule, the vector sum (bond distance and direction; see the simple model) of the three C—Cl bond moments bisects the base of the "tetrahedron" in the direction shown in the model. Note that the unit for dipole moment is the Debye and has both magnitude and direction.

Chloroform

2.4 FUNCTIONAL GROUPS

What is a functional group?

When atoms other than carbon or hydrogen are incorporated into an organic molecule, certain collections of heteroatoms taken as a unit have unique chemical and physical properties and are called *functional groups.* Functional groups include the hydroxyl unit (OH), an amine unit (a nitrogen atom with three attached atoms or groups), and the thiol unit (SH). Other functional groups include collections of atoms that contain π-bonds, including C=C, C≡C, and C=O, C=N, and C≡N.

Why are functional groups important?

Certain collections of atoms have chemical and physical properties that are unique. Further, when such collections of atoms appear in different organic molecules, those molecules often have similar chemical and physical properties. For this reason, it is convenient to categorize organic molecules by such collections of atoms, which are called *functional groups.* The functional group is the basis used to name most organic molecules. These functional groups are also part of various classes of compounds, such as alcohols, ethers, amines, etc.

What functional groups involve only carbon and hydrogen?

The C=C and C≡C units in a molecule are functional groups that define the alkene and alkyne classes of compounds, respectively.

What functional groups involve oxygen and carbon and/or hydrogen?

These functional groups include OH (hydroxyl), C–O–C (ether), C=O (carbonyl), CO_2H (carboxyl). The class of compounds with a hydroxyl group are the alcohols; with an ether unit are called ethers; the carbonyl is found in aldehydes and ketones; a carboxyl group defines the class of compounds known as carboxylic acids.

What functional groups involve nitrogen, carbon, and/or hydrogen?

Amines are the class of compounds that have one, two, or three carbons attached to a nitrogen atom, with hydrogen attached to nitrogen when there are only one or two carbon groups. In addition, C≡N (cyano) is another nitrogen-containing functional group that is attached to carbon molecules. Molecules with a cyano functional group are called nitriles.

What functional groups involve sulfur, carbon, and/or hydrogen?

These include SH (thioxy) is found in the class of compounds known as thiols (the older name is mercaptan) and the C—S—C unit is found in sulfides.

What functional group correlates with the following names: hydroxyl, thiol, carbonyl, carboxyl, amino, cyano, alkene, alkyne, and ether?

When these functional groups are incorporated into a molecule, they usually form a *class* of molecules that tend to have unique chemical and physical properties. Examples of each type of functional group are obtained by attaching one or more *R* group to each functional group, where *R* is a generic carbon group. The key functional groups are:

O—H	hydroxyl	S—H	thiol	C=O	carbonyl
H—O—C=O	carboxyl	C—N	amino	C≡N	cyano
C=C	alkene	C≡C	alkyne	C—O—C	ether

What functional group is found in each of the following classes of molecule: alcohol, thiol, aldehyde, ketone, carboxylic acid, amine, nitrile, alkene, alkyne, and ether?

When the functional group OH (hydroxyl) is in a molecule, the class is called *alcohols.* When the carbonyl (C=O) is incorporated, there are two structural variations. The carbonyl can be connected to both a hydrogen atom and a carbon group (use R as a generic abbreviation) to give an *aldehyde* or the carbonyl can be connected to two carbon groups (R) to give a *ketone.* If the carbonyl also contains a hydroxyl (H—O—C=O, or it is abbreviated –COOH), the molecule is called a *carboxylic acid.* If a trisubstituted nitrogen is in the molecule, the class is called an *amine.* If there is one R group and two hydrogens, it is a primary amine (1° = primary). If there are two R groups and one H, it is a secondary (2°) amine, and three

R groups give a tertiary (3°) amine. The class of compounds that contains a cyano group (C≡N) is called a *nitrile*. If the molecule contains a carbon–carbon double bond (C=C), it is an *alkene* and if it contains a carbon–carbon triple bond (C≡C), it is an *alkyne*. A compound characterized by a C—O—C unit is an *ether*. These are the major functional groups that will be discussed, and a few others will be added later.

2.5 FORMAL CHARGE

What is formal charge?

In a given structure, an atom that has one less bond than its valence it will have a (–) charge, whereas if it has one more bond it usually will have a (+) charge. Formal charge can reside on individual atoms, and the sum of all the formal charges on the individual atoms leads to the formal charge for the overall molecule.

What is the formula used to determine formal charge?

The formula is:

$$\text{Formal Charge} = \Omega = (\text{Valence Number}) - (\text{Number Unshared Electrons}) - \frac{1}{2}(\text{Number Shared Electrons})$$

Determine the formal charge of each atom and also for the entire molecule of dimethylamine, $(CH_3)_2NH$.

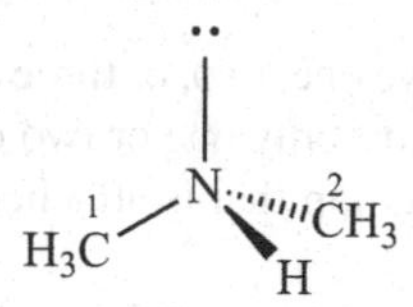

Dimethylamine

Before determining the formal charge for the entire molecule, first determine the formal charge for each atom. The sum of all atomic formal charges will give the formal charge for the molecule. For both carbon atoms, the valence number is the group number (four for C). There are no unshared electrons and eight covalently shared electrons. For C^1, $\Omega = 4 - 0 - ½(8) = 0$. For C^2, Ω also = 0. For the nitrogen, the valence (group) number is 5 (since N is in Group 15) and Ω is 5 – (1) – ½(8)) = 0. The formal charge for each hydrogen is 0 [1 – 0 – ½ (2)]. To determine the formal charge for the molecule Ω_{mol}, the sum of the formal charge for all atoms is used: $\Omega_{mol} = \Sigma\ (\Omega_{atom})$. For this example, $\Omega_{mol} = 0 + 0 + [8 \times 0] + 0 = 0$. Therefore, dimethylamine exists as a neutral species.

What is the criterion for a "real" molecule based on formal charge?

For the molecules encountered in the first organic course, it is very unusual for a molecule to exist as anything but a neutral compound (formal charge = 0), a mono-cation (formal charge of +1), or a mono-anion (formal charge of –1). For the purposes of structures encountered in a first-year organic chemistry course, if a structure is drawn and has a charge of greater than +2 or less than –2, that structure is likely to be very high in energy and should be questioned.

2.6 PHYSICAL PROPERTIES

How are functional groups related to the physical properties of a molecule?

The presence or absence of a functional group in an organic molecule has a profound effect on the boiling point, melting point, adsorption characteristics, etc. These parameters are physical properties, commonly measured to help identify a unique molecule.

What is a physical property?

A physical property is a parameter associated with a pure molecule that is unique and assists in the identification of that molecule. Examples are dipole moment, polarity, boiling point, melting point, adsorptivity, refractive index, and solubility. While some of these physical properties may overlap with other similar or related molecules, it is highly unusual for *all* of the physical properties to overlap. This set of physical properties allows each molecule to be identified as unique.

What is the definition of boiling point?

Boiling point is formally defined as the temperature at which the molecules in the gas phase (over a liquid phase) and the molecules in the liquid phase are at equilibrium.

What are the factors that influence boiling point?

To get molecules into the gas phase, the intermolecular forces holding them together in the liquid phase must be disrupted, which requires heat. In general, the greater the mass of the molecule, the higher the boiling point, and larger molecules (more atoms) should have a higher boiling point than smaller molecules (less atoms). Intermolecular interactions of the molecule are very important. Three examples will illustrate this statement: (a) $CH_3CH_2CH_3$ (*propane*; molecular weight = 44), (b) $H_3C–O–CH_3$ (*dimethyl ether*; molecular weight = 46), and (c) CH_3OH (*methanol*; molecular weight = 32). The molecular weights are not significantly different, although methanol has the lowest molecular weight. However, methanol has the highest boiling point.

In case (a) there are no dipole interactions and the only intermolecular forces are *van der Waals forces* (sometimes called *London forces*). These are quite weak, and the boiling point of propane is –42°C for a molecular weight of 44.10. For case (b), the polarized C–O bonds lead to a stronger intermolecular interaction relative to London forces, and the dipole-dipole interactions help keep the molecules associated. It takes more energy to disrupt these interactions and the boiling point is –24°C for a molecular weight of 46.07. The modest increase in mass cannot account for the 17.3°C increase in temperature required to boil dimethyl ether. When methanol in case (c) is examined, the boiling point of 64.7°C for a molecular weight of 32.04 is far higher than either propane or dimethyl ether. This large increase is due to the hydrogen bonding interactions between the oxygen and the hydrogen atom attached to oxygen, which are much stronger than the dipole interactions found in dimethyl ether.

What are van der Waals interactions?

The *van der Waals force* is a distance-dependent interaction between atoms or molecules. This force arises when adjacent atoms come close enough that their outer electron clouds just barely touch, inducing charge fluctuations that result in a nonspecific, nondirectional attraction. Part of this interaction is the *London dispersion force,* which is a temporary attractive force that occurs when the electrons in two adjacent atoms occupy positions that make the atoms form temporary dipoles. An example is the associative interaction of one nonpolar molecule, such as butane, with a second nonpolar butane molecule.

What are dipole–dipole interactions?

Dipole–dipole interactions result from the through-space interaction of two molecules and can have polarized covalent bonds. In this interaction, the partially negative portion of one of the polar molecules is attracted to the partially positive portion of the second polar molecule. An example is the through-space interaction of the carbonyl on one ketone with the carbonyl of a second ketone molecule.

What is hydrogen bonding?

A hydrogen bond results from the attraction of a hydrogen atom that is part of a polarized bond such as O—H, S—H, N—H, etc. In all cases, the hydrogen will have a δ^+ dipole. The through-space interaction of such a hydrogen atom with any electronegative atom (O, N, S, Cl, Br, etc.) is not a covalent bond, and is weak and easily broken. A hydrogen bond is one of the strongest associative interactions and hydrogen bonding is strong enough to hold molecules together by a strong associative between atoms within a molecule or between two separate molecules. The strength of a hydrogen bond is dependent on the strength of the dipole of the X—H bond.

Why are intermolecular associative forces important for the boiling point of a molecule?

Boiling point is the temperature at which enough energy is added for an equilibrium to be established between molecules in the liquids phase and molecules in the gas phase. For this to occur, the intermolecular associative forces such as van der Waals, dipole–dipole, or hydrogen bonding must be disrupted. In other words, sufficient energy must be added to overcome to attractive energy of these associative forces.

Which of the following is likely to have the highest boiling point: CH_3CH_3, $CH_3CH_2CH_3$, or $CH_3CH_2CH_2CH_2CH_3$?

Since all three compounds have only carbon and hydrogen atoms, and no functional groups that are capable of dipole–dipole interactions or hydrogen bonding, all will have only van der Waals interactions; the mass of the compounds must be considered as more important to boiling point. The molecule with five carbon atoms (molecular weight = 72) has a higher mass than the compound with three carbon atoms (molecular weight = 44), which is higher than the molecule with only two carbon atoms (molecular weight = 30). The five-carbon compound has the highest boiling point: 2C = –89°C, 3C = –42°C, 5C = +36.1°C.

Which of the following is likely to have the highest boiling point: $CH_3(C{=}O)CH_3$, CH_3OH, or CH_3CH_3?

There is not a large difference in molecular weight for each of the molecules, so differences in intermolecular interactions are expected to dominate. Since CH_3OH (molecular weight = 32; boiling point = 64.7°C) is the only molecule with an OH unit, which is capable of hydrogen bonding, it is likely to have the highest boiling point. Acetone (molecular weight = 58; boiling point = 56°C), with the carbonyl group, has dipole–dipole interactions, which are weaker intermolecular interactions relative to hydrogen bonding, and has the next highest boiling point. Ethane (molecular weight = 30; boiling point = –89°C), with no functional groups, has only van der Waals interactions and has the lowest boiling point.

What is the definition of melting point?

Melting point is defined as the temperature at which the molecules in the solid phase are in equilibrium with those in the liquid phase.

What factors influence melting point?

An increase in molecular weight often leads to an increase in melting point. The most important feature of a molecule that influences melting point is, however, more difficult to describe. The more symmetrical a molecule, the higher the melting point. Conversely, the more amorphous a molecule, the lower the melting point.

Which has the higher melting point, A or B?

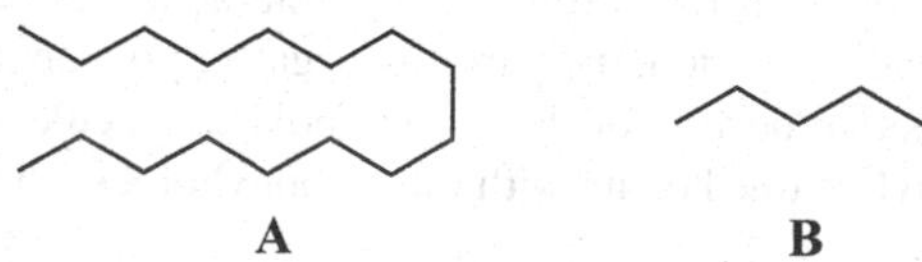

Both ***A*** (hexadecane) and ***B*** (pentane) have only C and H and no functional groups. Neither ***A*** nor ***B*** are "compact," and mass is probably the dominant factor. The molecular weight of ***A*** is 226 and the molecular weight of ***B*** is 72, and ***A*** is expected to have the higher melting point (+18°C for ***A*** vs. –129.8°C for ***B***).

Which has the higher melting point, A or B?

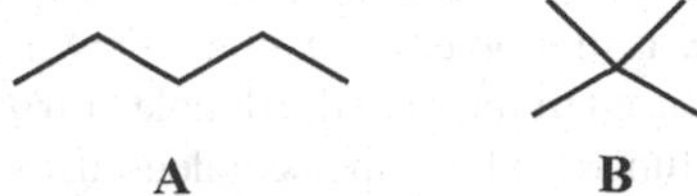

Comparing ***A*** (pentane) with ***B*** (2,2-dimethylpropane), the melting points are –129.8°C for pentane and –16.6°C for dimethylpropane. Both molecules have the same empirical formula (same number and kind of atoms), so they clearly have the same mass. Note that 2,2-dimethylpropane is more compact, however, and will "fit" into a crystal structure better than the "floppy" linear molecule, pentane. Such enhanced "packing" leads to a lower melting point for pentane, ***A***.

What is solubility?

Solubility is the property of one molecule (a solid, a liquid, or a gas called the *solute*) to dissolve into another molecule that is in the liquid state, called the *solvent.* Solubility is measured by the maximum amount of solute dissolved in a solvent at equilibrium, and the result is a saturated solution.

Is a ten-carbon molecule with only C and H likely to be soluble in water?

No! Water is highly polar, and a ten-carbon hydrocarbon is very nonpolar. Therefore, they are not expected to be mutually soluble.

Is a two-carbon alcohol, CH_3CH_2OH, likely to be soluble in water?

Yes! The OH unit can hydrogen bond so there will be strong associative interactions between water and the alcohol. The result of these interactions is an increased solubility for alcohols that have only a few carbon atoms. In general, alcohols of less than five carbons are soluble in water. Molecules of five to eight carbon atoms may be partially soluble in water and molecules of more than eight carbon atoms are generally insoluble.

How does solubility give information about the structure of a molecule?

The old axiom "like dissolves like" can be used with remarkable accuracy. In general, non-polar molecules will dissolve well in non-polar liquids such as hydrocarbons but not in polar liquids such as water. Conversely, a polar molecule will not dissolve in a non-polar liquid but will dissolve in a polar liquid. If a molecule contains one or more C-heteroatom bonds (a heteroatom is an atom other than C or H) it is considered to be polar. If it contains no polarized bonds, it is considered to be non-polar. There are exceptions to this latter statement that use the qualifying statement for the heteroatom case. A molecule such as CCl_4 has a net dipole moment of zero for the molecule and is non-polar. The actual test of polarity (and usually solubility) is, therefore, the dipole moment for the molecule. There are degrees of polarity and degrees of solubility. Molecules that undergo extensive hydrogen bonding are very polar and very soluble in polar liquids such as water. A molecule with a small dipole (CH_3Cl) will be less polar than one with more dipole interactions ($CHCl_3$) and this will be reflected in partial solubilities in polar solvents but some solubility in non-polar solvents. Solubility in water is suggested when a molecule can hydrogen bond to water. If there are more than five to eight carbon atoms, however, the one hydrogen bond is counteracted by the carbon atoms (with the attached hydrogen atoms).

END OF CHAPTER PROBLEMS

Line notation will be used for these and subsequent problems. When atoms other than C and H are present, the atom or group will be shown, as in problem 1. A line is drawn to the Br, OH, etc. Where there is a multiple bond, two or three lines are used to indicate the double or triple bond, respectively. An example is in problem 1b. In some cases, the functional group is condensed, as in the COOH unit shown in problem 1b and in 6c, drawn in two different ways.

1. For each series of compounds, identify the one of the following that has the highest boiling point? Explain.

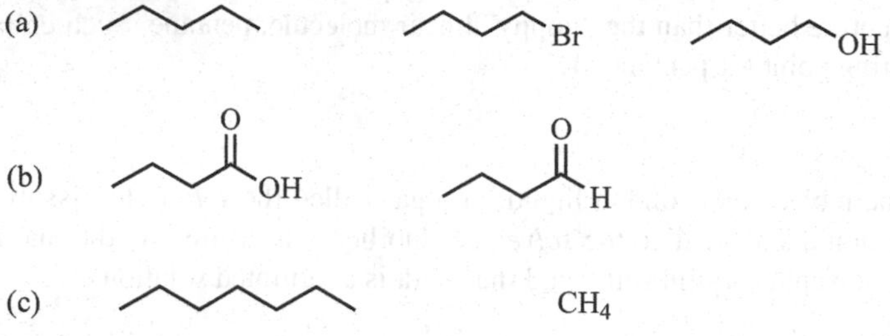

2. Predict the shape of each of the following: (a) the C–O–C unit of CH_3OCH_3 (b) the four atoms about carbon in Cl_3CH (c) the C–O–H unit of CH_3OH (d) the N and three carbon atoms in $NH(CH_3)_2$.
3. Indicate the direction of the dipole moment on the VSEPR model for each of the following: (a) CH_3OCH_3 (b) Cl_3CH (c) CH_3OH (d) NH_3 (e) CHBrCl.
4. What is the functional group identified with each of the following: (a) alcohol (b) ketone (c) alkyne (d) aldehyde (e) thiol (f) nitrile?
5. Determine the formal charge for all atoms in each molecule. Calculate the final charge for each molecule.

O_2, H_{11}, C^1, C^2, O_1, H_2, $N-H_3$, H_5 H_4

(a)

$:\ddot{O}:$ H_3 H_4

$H_{11}-C_1-C_2-C_3-N{\equiv}C_4$

H_2 H_5 H_6

(b)

6. Indicate which molecule has the higher boiling point in each of the following pairs. In each case explain your answer.

(a) OH (b) OH OH OH (c) CO_2H HO

7. Which molecule has the higher melting point? Explain.

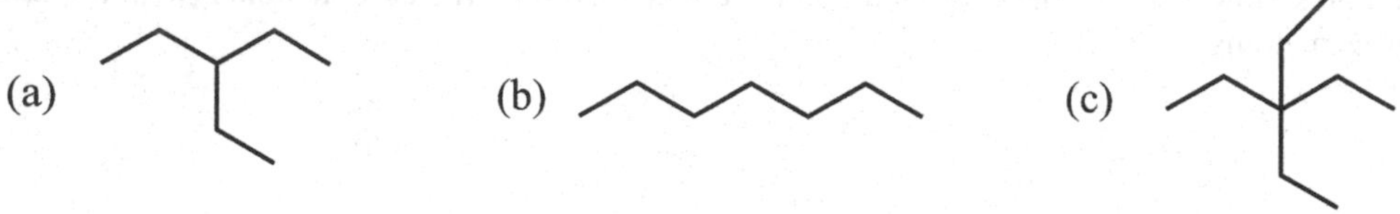

3

Acids and Bases

Acid–base reactions are perhaps the most important category of chemical reactions in all of organic chemistry. It will be seen that many, if not most, organic reactions have an acid–base component. Seeing this relationship usually requires modifying the traditional concept of what is an acid and what is a base.

3.1 ACIDS AND BASES

There are two fundamental definitions of acids and bases, the Lewis definition and the Brønsted–Lowry definition. Both definitions will be viewed through the lens of electron donation and electron acceptor ability.

What is the generic symbol for an acid?

The proton, which is usually represented by H^+.

What is a Brønsted–Lowry acid?

A Brønsted–Lowry acid is defined as a hydrogen ion donor. As a practical matter, a Brønsted–Lowry acid must have a hydrogen atom with a δ^+ dipole.

What structural feature makes a molecule able to donate a hydrogen ion?

The hydrogen atom must be polarized at H^+ or $H^{\delta+}$. In the neutral HCl molecule, not in water, the H has a positive dipole and can be donated to a base by the Brønsted–Lowry acid definition. Another way to say this, and arguably more correct, is that the base donates two electrons to the hydrogen atom and "pulls it off." An alcohol, which has a C—OH unit, is a Brønsted–Lowry acid since the H has a positive dipole.

What are four examples of mineral acids that qualify as Brønsted–Lowry acids?

Four examples are hydrochloric acid (HCl), sulfuric acid (H_2SO_4), nitric acid (HNO_3), and perchloric acid ($HClO_4$).

Do different molecules differ in Brønsted–Lowry acid strength?

Yes! Assuming that a structure such as C—X—H, where X is O, S, N, or another atom other than C or H, the atoms or groups attached to C will "push" or "pull" electron density from the X—H bond, which makes it more difficult or less difficult for the H to be removed. In other words, C—X—H is a weaker acid or a stronger acid, respectively. This analysis is overly simplistic, and it ignores the products formed after the hydrogen is donated and, of course, does not mention the base to be used. A stronger base will remove the hydrogen more easily than a weaker base. This analysis is a simple illustration that different molecules can be stronger or weaker Brønsted–Lowry acids.

What is a Lewis acid?

The classical definition of a Lewis acid is an electron pair acceptor.

What is the structural difference between a Lewis acid and a Brønsted–Lowry acid?

A Brønsted–Lowry acid has a polarized hydrogen atom, such as X—H, whereas a Lewis acid does not have a polarized hydrogen atom but rather has an electron deficient atom such as boron that can accept electrons from another molecule.

What are two common examples of a Lewis acid?

Both BCl_3 (boron trichloride) and $AlCl_3$ (aluminum trichloride) are Lewis acids. Both boron and aluminum are in Group 13 of the periodic table. They can form three covalent bonds, using the three valence electrons, to generate a neutral molecule. These atoms can attain the octet only by accepting an electron pair from another molecule (a Lewis base). Therefore, both B and Al are electron deficient in these compounds.

What is a Brønsted–Lowry base?

The classical definition of a Brønsted–Lowry base is a hydrogen atom acceptor.

What is a Lewis base?

A Lewis base is an electron pair donor. A Lewis base is a molecule that can donate two electrons to an atom other than hydrogen or carbon.

What is an "ate" complex?

An "ate" complex is the product of a Lewis acid–Lewis base reaction, which is the Lewis acid–Lewis base adduct.

What is the product when the Lewis acid $AlCl_3$ reacts with ammonia (NH_3)?

The product of a Lewis acid–Lewis base reaction is a Lewis acid–Lewis base adduct. More commonly, this product is called an *"ate" complex*. The reaction of ammonia and $AlCl_3$ is the ate complex shown. The arrow between N and Al in the figure represents the dative bond of the ate complex. This bond can also be shown as a line with the nitrogen assuming a positive charge and the aluminum assuming a negative charge.

$$Cl_3Al \leftarrow :NH_3 \quad \equiv \quad Cl_3\overset{-}{Al}—:\overset{+}{N}H_3$$

What is a dative bond?

A dative bond is a two-center, two-electron covalent bond in which both electrons come from the same atom. A dative bond is also called a coordinate covalent bond or simply a coordinate bond.

Is it possible to view a Brønsted–Lowry acid in terms of the Lewis acid definition?

Although the definition of a Brønsted–Lowry acid is a hydrogen atom donor, to "donate" a hydrogen atom to another molecule, the elecropositive hydrogen atom of an acid must react with an atom that has an electron pair. In other words, a Brønsted–Lowry acid has a hydrogen atom that is "pulled off" by an atom that donates an electron pair (a base). A Brønsted–Lowry acid reacts with a molecule that can donate an electron pair to H whereas a Lewis acid reacts with a molecule that can donate an electron pair to an atom other than C or H.

How is a Brønsted–Lowry base like a Lewis base?

To accept a hydrogen atom, a Brønsted–Lowry base must donate an electron pair to the hydrogen atom. Therefore, a Brønsted–Lowry base is as a molecule that donates an electron pair to a hydrogen atom. A Brønsted–Lowry base donates an electron pair to a hydrogen whereas a Lewis base donates an electron pair to atoms other than C or H.

What structural features are required for a molecule to be considered an acid?

For a Brønsted–Lowry acid, the molecule must have a hydrogen atom, generally attached to a heteroatom, that has a positive dipole. For a Lewis acid, the atom must be electron deficient, not C or H, and able to accept a pair of electrons from another molecule.

What structural features are required for a molecule to be considered a base?

For a Brønsted–Lowry base, the molecule must be able to form a bond to a hydrogen atom that has a positive dipole by donating a pair of electrons. For a Lewis base, the atom must be electron rich, and able to donate a pair of electrons to another atom other than C or H.

3.2 ENERGETICS

What is the "driving force" for a chemical reaction?

Changes in energy accompany the transformation of starting materials to products in what is known as a chemical reaction.

What is the bond dissociation enthalpy?

The term is the inherent energy (bond dissociation enthalpy), and that energy is released when a bond is broken or is required to form that bond.

What is $H°$?

The term $H°$ is the enthalpy of a given bond or an entire molecule. Formally, enthalpy is a thermodynamic quantity equivalent to the total heat content of a system.

What is the parameter to describe the energy of a chemical transformation?

The parameter is $\Delta G°$, the change in free energy during the reaction.

What is the Gibbs free energy equation?

The *Gibbs free energy equation* is $\Delta G° = \Delta H° - T\Delta S°$.

What is T in the equation in the preceding question?

The term T is the temperature in degrees centigrade.

What is ΔH?

The term $\Delta H°$ is the change in enthalpy.

What is $\Delta S°$?

The term $\Delta S°$ is the change in entropy. The entropy term measures the "disorder" of a given system. Formally, entropy is the lack of order or predictability: gradual decline into disorder. For most of the chemical reactions in this book, the change in disorder is small as a starting material is transformed into a product and the $\Delta S°$ term is very small compared to the $\Delta H°$ term.

What is $\Delta G°$?

This term is the change in free energy for a reaction. If the $\Delta G°$ is positive, the reaction is endergonic (endothermic) and proceeds to the products spontaneously. If the $\Delta G°$ is negative, the reaction is exergonic (exothermic) and proceeds to the products spontaneously.

Why is the term $\Delta S°$ ignored in determining the energy of a reaction?

The entropy term is usually quite small, measured in calories or joules whereas the enthalpy term is much larger, measured in kilocalories or kilojoules. Therefore, ignoring the $T\Delta S°$ term in the Gibbs free energy equation introduces an insignificant error in the energy calculation.

What does the energy curve for an exothermic reaction look like?

The energy curve shows the energy of the starting materials on the left and the energy of the products on the right. Energy is required to initiate the reaction, and for an exothermic reaction the energy of the products is lower than the energy of the starting materials. Enough energy is returned during the reaction to overcome the activation energy, so the reaction is spontaneous and in principle proceeds to completion without the need to continually add heat.

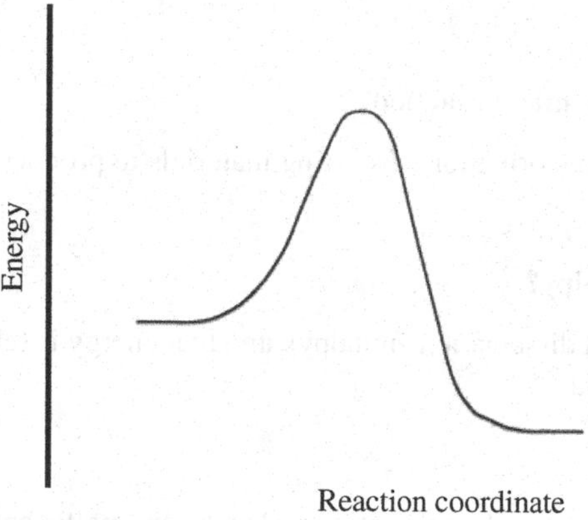

What is the transition state?

The transition state for the reaction is shown. It is the midpoint of the reaction that represents the transition point where the bonds of the starting material are beginning to break, and the bonds of the product are beginning to form. The transition state cannot be isolated or even observed but is taken as the midpoint of the reaction once it is initiated.

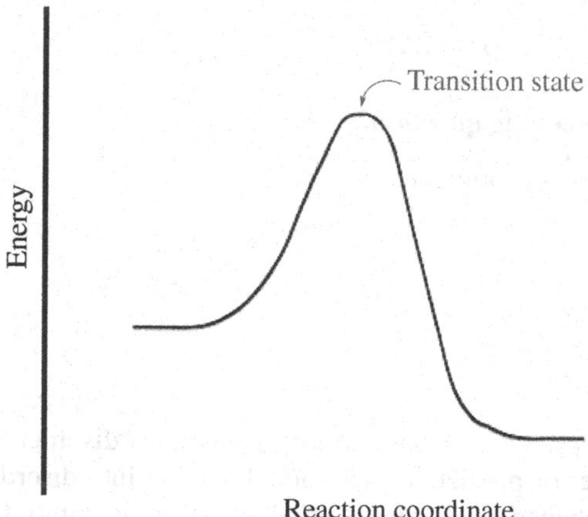

What is the energy of activation?

The activation energy, E_{act}, is shown on the curve and it is the energy required to initiate the reaction. The activation energy is formally the difference in the energy of the starting materials and the energy maximum for the reaction, which is the energy required to begin the bond making–bond breaking process.

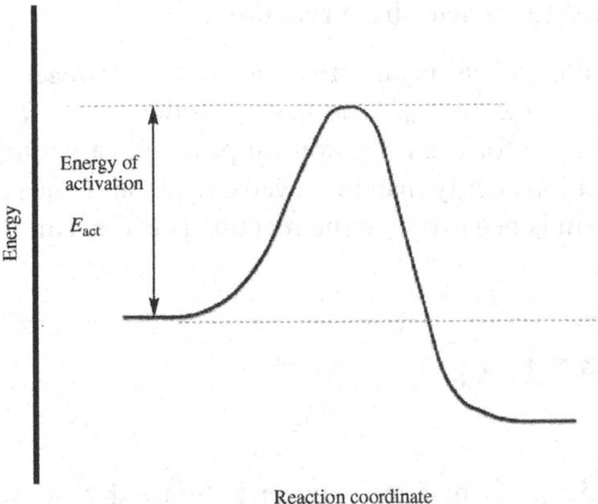

How is the $\Delta G°$ determined from the energy curve.?

The $\Delta G°$ term is calculated by determining the difference in the energy of the starting materials and the energy of the products, as shown in the figure.

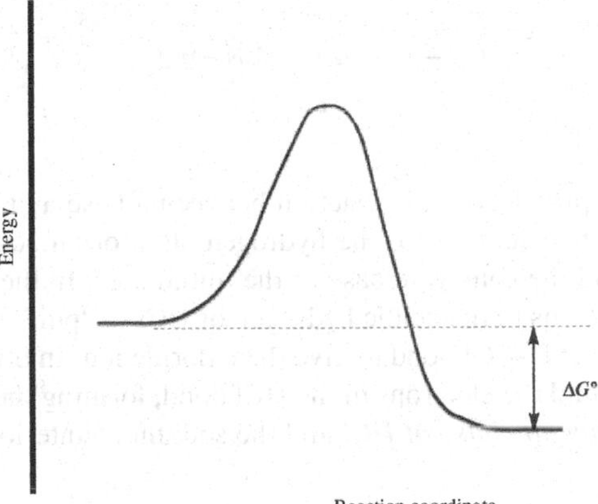

What is the energy curve for an endothermic reaction?

The energy curve shows the energy of the starting materials on the left and the energy of the products on the right. Energy is required to initiate the reaction, and for an endothermic reaction the energy of the products is higher in energy than the energy of the starting materials. Therefore, energy must be continually supplied to keep the reaction going since insufficient energy is returned during the reaction. The energy of activation, the transition state for the reaction, and $\Delta G°$ are also shown.

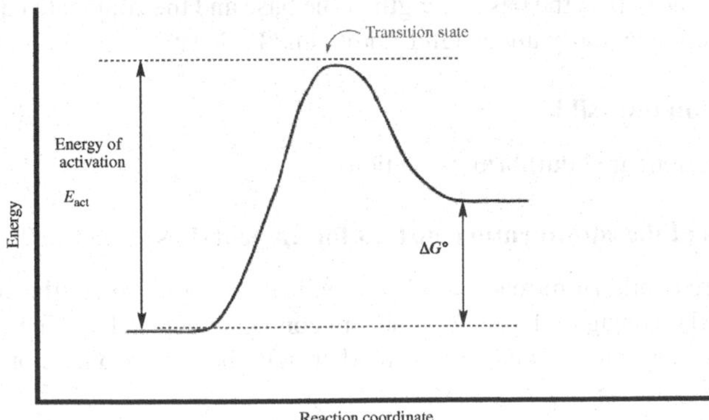

How are these energy curves applied to an acid–base reaction?

An acid–base reaction is an equilibrium. There is an activation energy for reaction of the acid and the base, and another activation energy for the reverse acid–base reaction of the conjugate acid and the conjugate base. There is a transition state for each reaction. In principle, a strong acid reacting with a strong base should have a larger activation energy than the reverse reaction of the conjugate acid with the conjugate base, but only if the ΔG term is negative and the reaction is exothermic.

3.3 THE ACIDITY CONSTANT, K_a

What is a conjugate acid?

A conjugate acid is one of the two products of a reaction between a Brønsted–Lowry base and a Brønsted–Lowry acid. Specifically, when a Brønsted–Lowry base accepts a hydrogen atom, the product will have that hydrogen incorporated in the molecule, and that product is called *the conjugate acid of the initial base*. An example is the reaction of ammonia with the acid HCl, where NH_3 is the base and the product NH_4^+ (the ammonium ion) is the conjugate acid of ammonia. The negative counterion is the chloride ion, which is the conjugate base.

$$H_3N: \quad H{-}Cl \longrightarrow H_3\overset{+}{N}{-}H \quad Cl^-$$

What is a conjugate base?

A conjugate base is one of the two products of the reaction between a base and an acid. Specifically, when a Brønsted–Lowry base donates electrons to the hydrogen atom of an acid, the acid loses that hydrogen to the base, leaving behind the conjugate base of the initial acid. In the reaction, the oxygen atom of hydroxide donates two electrons to the acidic hydrogen of HCl to "pull" the proton away from HCl, with concomitant cleavage of the H—Cl bond to give the chloride ion. In other words, loss of the hydrogen atom from HCl leaves behind the electrons in the HCl bond, forming the *chloride ion*. In this reaction, the *chloride ion is the conjugate base of HCl* and the sodium counterion is transferred from NaOH to NaCl.

$$HO:^- \, Na^+ \quad H:Cl \longrightarrow HO:H \; + \; Na^+Cl^-$$

Which is more important, the acid or the conjugate acid?

This question is nonsense! Both are important. In the reaction of hydroxide with HCl (an acid–base reaction), the products are water and the chloride ion. One can also view chloride as a base, and water as an acid. Only understanding that HCl is a stronger acid than water and that hydroxide is a stronger base than the chloride ion allows for a full understanding of the reaction. As will be seen, the acid strength of the acid and conjugate acid, as well as the base strength of the base and the conjugate base must be examined in every acid–base reaction to really understand acidity and basicity.

Is an acid–base reaction reversible?

Yes! All acid–base reactions are equilibrium reactions.

What is the definition of the equilibrium constant for an acid–base reaction?

Acid–base reactions are equilibrium reactions. For a typical reaction shown, the acid (HA) reacts with the base (B^-) to form the conjugate base (A^-) and the conjugate acid (HB). The reactants HA and B^- constitute an acid/base pair, but A^- and HB is another acid–base pair. Therefore, this reaction is an equilibrium reaction, and the equilibrium constant is K. Since it is an acid–base reaction, the equilibrium constant is given the symbol K_a (the acidity constant).

$$\text{H—A} + \text{B}^- \underset{}{\overset{K_a}{\rightleftharpoons}} \text{A}^- + \text{H—B}$$

In an acid–base reaction, which is the starting material, and which is the product?

In the usual definition of an equilibrium constant, the *products are written on the right* of the equation (in this case the products are the conjugate acid and conjugate base) and the *starting materials are written on the left* of the equation (in this case the starting materials are the acid and the base). This arrangement is taken as the standard definition of an acid.

How do the assumptions about starting material and product influence the K_a term?

For calculating K in general, the concentrations of the products are on top and the concentrations of the starting materials are on the bottom. Therefore, in the equation for K_a, the concentrations of the product are on the top, divided by the concentrations of the reactant.

The equilibrium constant, K_a, is defined as: $K_a = \dfrac{[\text{A}^-][\text{H—B}]}{[\text{H—A}][\text{B}^-]}$

What is the definition of a strong acid?

With the definition of K_a just given, and with the acid/base pair written on the left of the equation, if K_a is large (>1, i.e., HA and B^- reacted to form A^- and HB), then HA is considered to be a strong acid if the HA reacts almost completely with the base and the equilibrium lies strongly toward the conjugate acid and conjugate base. In other words, there is a large concentration of the conjugate acid and the conjugate base, and a low concentration of HA and the base. If K_a is small (<1), then HA and B^- *did not react* to form A^- and HB, but rather A^- and HB reacted to push the equilibrium back toward HA and B^-. In other words, a large value of K_a means there is less starting material than product, and the acid/base pair reacted very well.

What is pK_a?

The pK_a = $-\log_{10} K_a$. Conversely, $K_a = 10^{-pK_a}$.

What is the relationship of pK_a and acidity?

A strong acid will have a small pK_a and a weak acid will have a large pK_a.

What is the relationship between K_a and pK_a?

The pK_a is inversely proportional to K_a and it is the negative base 10 log of K_a. Therefore, a large K_a has a small pK_a and a small K_a has a large pK_a.

If the K_a for an acid is 1.5×10^{-5}, what is the pK_a?

pK_a = $-\log_{10} (1.5 \times 10^{-5}) = 4.8$.

If the pK_a for an acid is 4.35, what is the K_a?

$K_a = 10^{-4.35} = 4.47 \times 10^{-5}$.

How is K_a different from K in a non-acid–base equilibrium?

Except for the fact that K_a is used for an acid–base reaction to distinguish it from other equilibrium reactions, there is no fundamental difference. Remember that K_a indicates that the equilibrium involves a forward acid–base reaction and a reverse acid–base reaction.

3.4 STRUCTURAL FEATURES THAT INFLUENCE ACIDITY

The presence of what types of functional groups lead to that molecule being classified as an acid?

Many classes of organic compounds can be viewed as acids, but they have vastly different acid strengths. Perhaps the most distinguishing feature of carboxylic acids (RCOOH) is that they are Brønsted–Lowry acids and react with a variety of suitable bases. Sulfonic acids (RSO_3H) are also strong organic acids. Alcohols (ROH) are much weaker acids than the carboxylic acids, and with few exceptions they are slightly less acidic than water. For the time-being, carboxylic acids are the focus as the main organic acids.

What is a carboxylic acid?

A carboxylic acid is a class of organic molecule with the structure RCOOH, where R is any carbon group that contains the carboxyl functional group O=C—O—H, and is characterized by an acidic hydrogen atom on the OH unit. In other words, it is a Brønsted–Lowry acid.

What is the structure of a generic carboxylic acid, a generic sulfonic acid, and a generic alcohol, using "R" as the group attached to the carbonyl carbon of the carboxylic acid, the sulfur atom of the sulfonic acid, and the carbon atom of the alcohol?

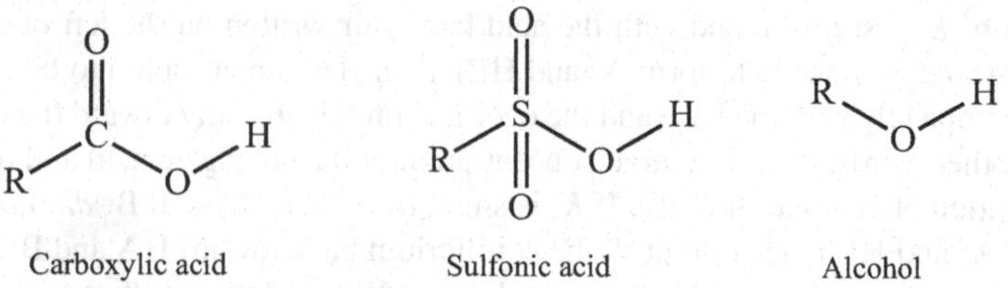

Carboxylic acid Sulfonic acid Alcohol

What is a carboxylate anion?

A carboxylate anion is the conjugate base of a carboxylic acid, formed by the acid–base reaction of a carboxylic acid with a suitable base. The structure of a carboxylate anion is RC(=O)—O⁻.

What is the Brønsted–Lowry acid-base reaction of RCOOH with a generic base, "BASE?"

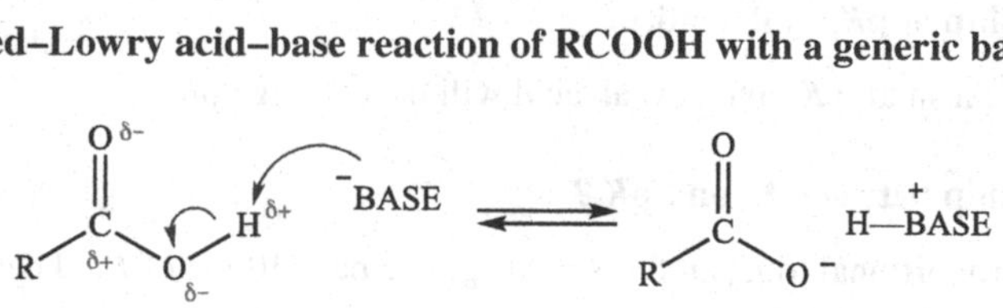

$$RC(=O^{\delta-})–O^{\delta-}–H^{\delta+} + {}^{-}BASE \rightleftharpoons RC(=O)–O^{-} + H–\overset{+}{B}ASE$$

Carboxylic acids have the generic formula shown, where R is any carbon group. Carboxylic acids have the carboxyl group, characterized by the C=O unit (a carbonyl), with an OH unit directly attached to the carbonyl carbon. After reaction with a base, the carboxylate anion is generated as the conjugate base. Carboxylate anions are resonance stabilized, as shown for the formate anion in the answer above.

Why is the carboxylate anion considered to be very stable?

As shown for the carboxylate anion in the preceding question, a carboxylate anion is resonance stabilized. All carboxylate anions are resonance stabilized. The negative charge is delocalized over three atoms (O—C—O). A carboxylate anion is a relatively weak base because it is more difficult to donate electrons as a base if the electrons are delocalized by resonance. Resonance delocalization makes the carboxylate anion *more stable* and therefore *less reactive*.

What is the structure of the anion formed by removal of the acidic hydrogen from formic acid (HCOOH)?

Treatment of formic acid with an undefined base (BASE) generates the resonance stabilized formate anion. With resonance stabilization, the charge is dispersed over three atoms, and is dispersed equally on the two oxygen atoms.

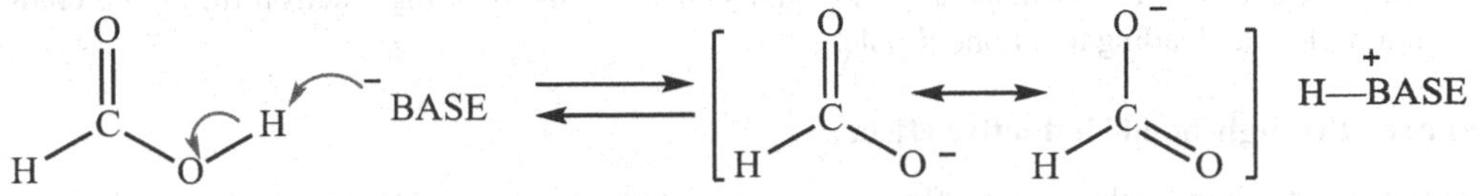

BASE H—BASE

Formate anion

How does the special stability of the carboxylate anion influence acidity?

The carboxylate anion is resonance stabilized and an equilibrium reaction will be influenced by the relative stability of all species that make up that equilibrium. A more stable product indicates that the acid and base reacted efficiently to give that product, which shifts the equilibrium toward that product. If the equilibrium is shifted toward the conjugate base, the carboxylate, K_a, is larger. A large K_a is indicative of a stronger acid.

What is the product when potassium acetate (draw it) is dissolved in aqueous solution at pH 4?

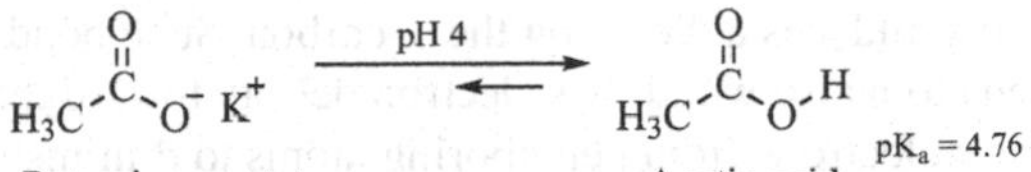

pH 4

Potassium acetate Acetic acid

$pK_a = 4.76$

The relatively weak base (potassium acetate) is protonated in the acidic solution (pH 4) to give acetic acid (ethanoic acid). The equilibrium in the acidic medium is shifted toward the acid.

What is the pK_a of acetic acid (ethanoic acid = CH_3COOH) in water? The pK_a of HCl in water?

The pK_a of acetic acid (ethanoic acid) is 4.76. The pK_a of HCl is –7.

What are the pK_a values of the following carboxylic acids: (a) propanoic acid (CH_3CH_2COOH); (b) butanoic acid ($CH_3CH_2CH_2COOH$); (c) formic acid (HCOOH; also called methanoic acid).

(a) propanoic acid = 4.89; (b) butanoic acid = 4.82; (c) methanoic acid = 3.75.

Why is methanoic acid more acidic than propanoic acid?

The fundamental difference in structure is the "H" attached to the carbonyl in methanoic acid and the carbon group "CH_3CH_2" in propanoic acid. The carbon group is electron releasing relative to hydrogen, so the carbonyl carbon is less "positive" relative to the carbonyl carbon in methanoic acid. This difference in polarization leads to a less polarized O—H bond in propanoic acid relative to the polarization of the O—H bond in methanoic acid. In other words, the acidic proton in methanoic acid is more polarized, has a greater δ^+ dipole, and methanoic acid is more acidic.

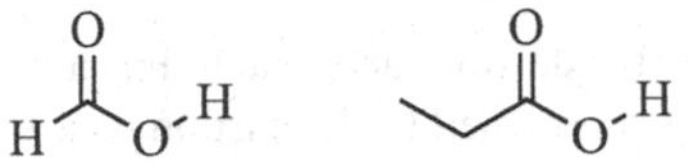

Methanoic acid (formic acid) Propanoic acid

In addition, examination of the conjugate bases $HCOO^-$ versus $CH_3CH_2COO^-$ shows that the electron releasing carbon group in the propanoate anion makes that anion more reactive (less stable), which pushes the equilibrium back toward propionic acid, making that acid less acidic.

What is an inductive effect?

The inductive effect is the transmission of unequal sharing of the bonding electron through a chain of atoms in a molecule, leading to a bond dipole.

What are "through-bond" inductive effects?

Certain electronic bond-polarization effects are transmitted from nucleus to nucleus thorough the adjacent covalent bonds and these are collectively called *"through-bond" effects, a type of inductive effect.* The shifting of electron density described in the discussions for chloroacetic and dichloroacetic acid are examples of "through-bond" inductive effects.

In an O=C—O—H unit, which oxygen has the stronger electron withdrawing effect?

The carbonyl oxygen, O=C, has the stronger bond polarization and the stronger electron withdrawing effect.

When an electron withdrawing group is attached to the carbonyl carbon of a carboxyl, what is the effect on the O—H bond?

The electron withdrawing group induces a δ^+ dipole on the α-carbon, which is adjacent to the δ^+ charge on the carbonyl carbon, which also induces a dipole on the α-carbon. Such bond polarization is destabilizing since the carbonyl oxygen atom also withdraws electron density toward that oxygen. To compensate, the carbonyl carbon withdraws electrons from neighboring atoms to diminish the electron withdrawing effects of the α-carbon, which makes the O—H bond more polarized, the H more positive, and the net effect is greater acidity.

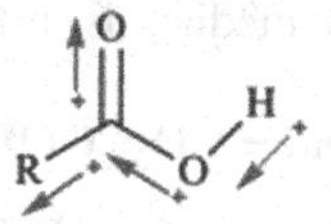

Will an electron withdrawing group attached to a carboxyl increase or decrease acidity?

In general, electron withdrawing groups increase acidity (larger K_a, smaller pK_a).

When an electron releasing group is attached to the carbonyl of a carboxyl, what is the effect on the O—H bond?

The electron releasing group reduces the dipole on the α-carbon, which is adjacent to the δ^+ charge on the carbonyl carbon. Since the carbonyl oxygen atom withdraws electron density toward that oxygen but because of the increased electron density on the α-carbon, the carbonyl carbon withdraws less electron density from neighboring atoms, and the O—H bond is less polarized, the H less positive, and the net effect is diminished acidity.

Why is acetic acid (pK_a 4.76) a weaker acid than formic acid (pK_a 3.75)?

As with propanoic acid in the previous question, acetic acid has a methyl group attached to the electropositive carbonyl. Relative to hydrogen attached to the carbonyl carbon in formic acid (methanoic acid), methyl is an electron releasing group. In other words, that carbon atom attached to the carbonyl is more electron rich relative to the hydrogen attached to the carbonyl. Because of this electron releasing effect, the carbonyl oxygen pulls less electron density from the O—H unit. In other words, the O—H bond is stronger because of the presence of the CH_3 group relative to the H, and that hydrogen is more difficult to break and less acidic (less positive = less like H^+).

Will an electron releasing group attached to a carboxyl increase or decrease acidity?

In general, electron releasing groups decrease acidity (smaller K_a, larger pK_a).

What is a "through-space" field (inductive) effect?

When an electronegative heteroatom group is sufficiently close in space to the acidic hydrogen of the carboxyl, but they are not connected by a covalent bond, the δ^- dipole of the heteroatom and the δ^+ dipole of the hydrogen atom can interact. Due to their proximity in space, an electronegative atom, such as chlorine, attracts the electrophilic hydrogen atom in what for all practical purposes is an intramolecular hydrogen bond, as shown in the figure. The net effect of this through-space inductive effect (sometimes called a field effect) is to weaken the O—H bond and increase the acidity of the molecule. Such through-space effects are usually a stronger influence on the acidity than the through-bond effects. The closer the heteroatom is to the δ^+ hydrogen atom, the stronger the through-space effect, and the further away, the weaker the effect.

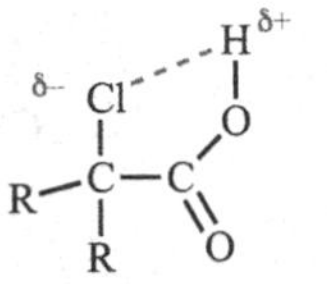

δ– Cl --- H δ+
R—C—C(=O)—O
R

What is an inductive effect?

An inductive effect is the influence on electron density in one portion of a molecule due to electron-withdrawing or electron-donating groups elsewhere in the molecule.

What is the relative acidity of ethanoic acid (acetic acid) and 2-chloroethanoic acid in terms of a through-space effect?

Examination of 2-chloroethanoic acid shows that the chlorine and the H of the OH unit can hydrogen bond (through-space) in what is effectively a five-membered ring: a through-space inductive effect. This interaction polarizes the hydrogen with a greater δ^+ dipole, the O—H bond is therefore weaker, and it is easier to remove the hydrogen by reaction with a base. In other words, chloroacetic acid is a stronger acid because of this through-space interaction; a *through-space inductive effect.* There is no heteroatom substituent in CH_3COOH (ethanoic acid), so such internal hydrogen bonding cannot occur. Therefore, the OH bond is stronger in ethanoic acid and weaker in 2-chloroethanoic acid, which is the stronger acid.

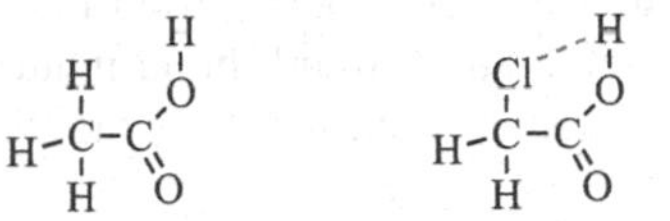

Ethanoic acid　　2-Chloroethanoic acid

The pK_a of chloroacetic acid ($ClCH_2COOH$) is 2.87 and the pK_a of acetic acid (CH_3COOH) is 4.76. Why is chloroacetic acid a stronger acid?

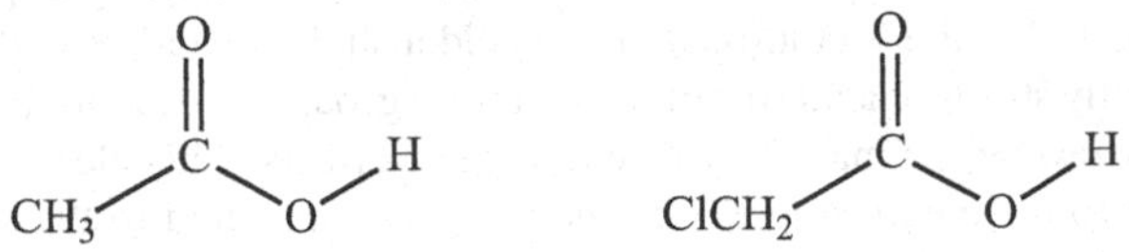

$CH_3C(=O)OH$ acetic acid　　$ClCH_2C(=O)OH$ chloroacetic acid

This question is exactly the same one asked in the previous question but asked in a different way. Clearly, the electronegative carbonyl oxygen pulls electron density away from the carbonyl carbon.

The chlorine is polarized δ^- relative to the α-carbon, however, and the α-carbon is polarized δ^+. This polarization exerts an electron withdrawing effect on the attached carbonyl carbon in addition to the carbonyl oxygen electron withdrawing effect. The presence of the chlorine leads to polarization that puts the δ^+ α-carbon adjacent to the δ+ carbon of the carbonyl group (C=O). The proximity of the two electrophilic carbons leads to an inductive effect in which electron density is pulled away from the oxygen that is attached to H toward the carbonyl carbon. This shift of electron density away from the O—H bond weakens that bond. As the O—H bond is weakened, the hydrogen atom becomes increasingly positive (more like H^+) and more reactive with a base. Therefore, chloroacetic acid is a stronger acid.

The pK_a of chloroacetic acid ($ClCH_2COOH$) is 2.87 and the pK_a of dichloroacetic acid ($Cl_2CHCOOH$) is 1.35. Why is dichloroacetic acid a stronger acid?

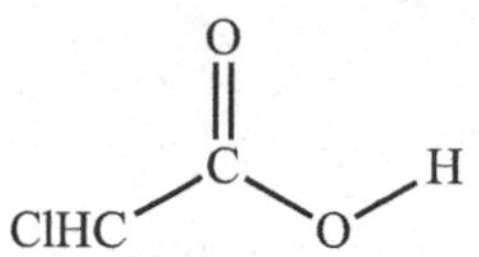

choroacetic acid

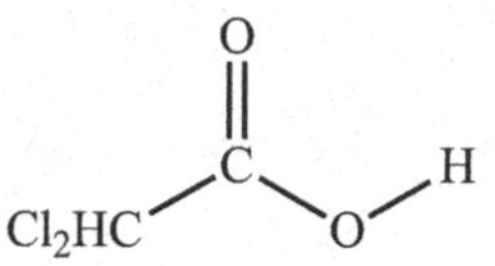

dichloroacetic acid

Each chlorine is polarized δ^- and exerts an electron withdrawing effect on the attached carbon. In other words, the Cl polarizes the α-hydrogen δ^+. If one chlorine atom polarizes the carbon atom attached to the carbonyl and polarizes the O—H bond by shifting electron density away from the hydrogen atom, two chlorine atoms should have a greater effect. Indeed, the two chlorine atoms make the O—H bond more polarized and dichloroacetic acid is a stronger acid than chloroacetic acid.

Is 3-chlorobutanoic acid a weaker acid or a stronger acid than 2-chlorobutanoic acid?

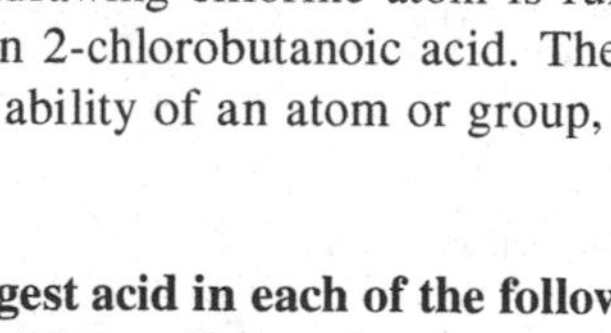

3-Chlorobutanoic acid

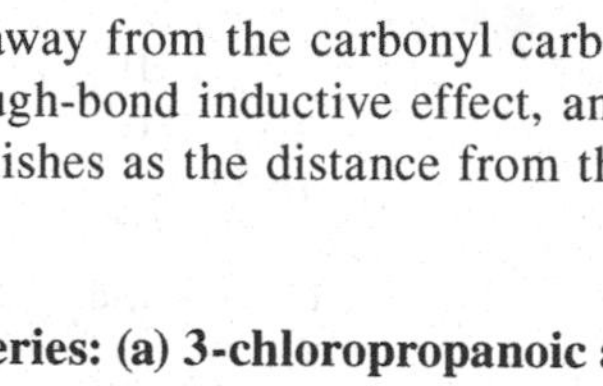

2-Chlorobutanoic acid

The electron withdrawing chlorine atom is further away from the carbonyl carbon in 3-chlorobutanoic acid than in 2-chlorobutanoic acid. The through-bond inductive effect, and hence the electron withdrawing ability of an atom or group, diminishes as the distance from the carboxyl group increases.

What is the strongest acid in each of the following series: (a) 3-chloropropanoic acid or 3-chloropentanoic acid; (b) 2-methoxyethanoic acid or propanoic acid?

In (a) both acids have an electron withdrawing chlorine at C3 but 3-chloropentanoic acid also has an ethyl group attached to C3. The presence of the electron releasing alkyl group, which is missing in 3-chloropropanoic acid, will make 3-chloropentanoic acid a slightly weaker acid. Therefore, 3-chloropropanoic acid is a slightly stronger acid. In (b) the methoxy group attached to the α-carbon renders the α-carbon electron withdrawing, primarily by through-space effects. This electron withdrawing inductive effect is compared to the electron-releasing methyl group attached to the α-carbon in propanoic acid. Since methoxymethyl is electron withdrawing, the O—H bond of that acid is more polarized and 2-methoxyethanoic acid is expected to be the stronger acid (pK_a of methoxyacetic acid = 3.6; pK_a of propionic acid = 4.9).

Why is 2-aminopropanoic acid (alanine) a stronger acid than 3-aminopropanoic acid (β-alanine)?

Alanine β-Alanine

In 2-aminopropanoic acid, the electron withdrawing nitrogen group is closer to the carboxyl group. As shown, the H of the O—H bond is physically close to the electronegative nitrogen of the amino group. A through-space hydrogen bonding effect, effectively through a five-membered ring unit, will further polarize the hydrogen atom and weaken the O—H bond, which makes the molecule more acidic. In 3-aminopropapanoic acid, the nitrogen is positioned farther from the COOH unit, requiring a larger six-membered ring unit for the internal hydrogen bonding. It is more difficult to attain this hydrogen-bonded unit, so the O—H is not weakened as much, and the through-space effect is less. For this reason, 3-aminopropanoic acid is a weaker acid: 2-aminopropanic acid, pK_a 2.34 and 3-aminopropanoic acid, pK_a 3.55. Note that the amino acids are drawn with the free amine and free carboxyl groups rather than the normal zwitterion form due to an internal acid–base reaction (see Section 20.1).

3.5 FACTORS THAT CONTRIBUTE TO MAKING THE ACID MORE ACIDIC

What are four factors that influence acidity?

1. Focusing on Brønsted–Lowry acids, the *bond polarization of the X—H bond in the acid is important.* In this case, X = C, O, N, S, halogen, etc. The more polarized the X—H bond, the more positive the dipole on the hydrogen atom, making it more susceptible to reaction with a base. In one sense, this means that the X—H bond is weaker as it is more polarized, making it easier to break. Therefore C—H is less acidic than N—H, which is less acidic than O–H.
2. The *stability of the conjugate base and conjugate acid is important.* If those products are more stable, the equilibrium is pushed to the right, and the starting acid reacts to a greater extent with the base, and is considered to be more acidic. Conversely, if the conjugate acid and/or base are rather unstable (more reactive), the equilibrium is pushed to the left, the starting acid does not react as much, and it is considered to be less acidic.
3. The relative acidity of the acid and conjugate acid (as well as the base and conjugate base) is important. If the conjugate acid is weaker than the starting acid, the equilibrium is pushed to the right. If the conjugate acid is stronger than the starting acid, the equilibrium is pushed to the left. Similar comments apply to the base and conjugate base.
4. The solvent plays an important role, both in assisting loss of the acidic hydrogen and also in stabilizing the conjugate acid and conjugate base. If the solvent stabilizes the products, the equilibrium is shifted to the right.

Which is expected to be more acidic, HOH or H_2NH, using only bond polarization of the acid as the determining criterion?

Since the O—H unit is more polarized than the N—H unit, based on the electronegative of O versus N, one expects that HOH is more acidic than NH_3 using this single criterion.

Is it reasonable to judge the acidity and basicity of an acid and base completely on the properties of these two molecules, without considering the conjugate acid and base that is formed by the reaction?

No! The acid and base react to form the conjugate acid and conjugate base, but the conjugate acid reacts with the conjugated base to give the original acid and base. It is an equilibrium and both reactions and the concentrations of all four molecules must be known to establish the acidity and basicity of the original pair.

What factors contribute to making the conjugate acid more stable?

If the conjugate acid is more stable, it will be less reactive. Therefore, the X—H bond in the conjugate acid should be stronger and less polarized than the X—H bond in the starting acid.

How does stability of the conjugate acid and the conjugate base contribute to the equilibrium?

If the conjugate acid is more stable (less reactive), the reaction with the conjugate base is less facile relative to the reaction of the original acid and base, and the equilibrium is likely to lie to the right (toward the original acid and base) rather than the left (toward the conjugate acid/base pair). If the equilibrium is shifted toward the conjugate acid and base, the acid is considered to be more acidic, whereas if the equilibrium is shifted back to the original aid and base, they did not react, and the acid is considered to be less acidic. If the conjugate acid is less table (more reactive), it will react with the conjugate base and the equilibrium is shifted toward the starting acid and base (less acidic).

Similar arguments can be made for the conjugate base. If the conjugate base is more stable, it is less reactive, and the equilibrium is shifted toward the conjugate acid/base pair. If the conjugate base is less stable (more reactive), the equilibrium is pushed toward the starting acid and base.

What factors contribute to making the conjugate base more stable?

The conjugate base is often ionized, and large ions tend to be more stable than small ions because they are more easily solvated, and the charge is dispersed over a larger area. An iodide ion is more stable than a chloride ion, for example. If the size of different ionic conjugate bases is compared and the size is relatively close, then the base with the more electronegative atom tends to "hold" electrons. Therefore, it is more difficult to donate those electrons and it is the weaker base. Resonance makes the conjugate base more stable and less reactive by dispersing the charge over several atoms, so resonance stabilized products tend to be more stable than molecules that are not stabilized by resonance. More polarized conjugate bases tend to be solvated to a greater extent in polar media, making them somewhat more stable and less reactive. In general, anything that makes it more difficult for the conjugate base to donate electrons makes it less reactive and therefore a weaker base.

How does the stability of the conjugate base contribute to the equilibrium?

If the conjugate base is more stable (less reactive), the reaction with the conjugate acid is less likely, and the equilibrium is likely to lie to the right rather than the left. In other words, the reaction of the original acid and base is more facile than the reaction of the conjugate acid with the conjugate base.

If the original acid is stronger than the conjugate acid, how is the equilibrium and pK_a influenced?

The equilibrium is pushed to the right, and K_a is larger, making pK_a smaller.

If the conjugate acid is stronger than the acid, how does this influence the equilibrium and pK_a?

The equilibrium is pushed to the left, and K_a is smaller, making pK_a larger. In such a case, the original acid is considered to be a relatively weak acid.

If two reactions are compared, and acid *X* has the structure R—OH and acid *Y* has the structure R_2NH, which is the stronger Brønsted–Lowry acid and why?

Oxygen is more electronegative than nitrogen, so the O—H bond in ROH is more polarized as δ^+ relative to the N—H bond in R_2NH. Therefore, ROH is expected to be more acidic since the H more easily reacts with the base. Since oxygen is more electronegative than nitrogen, the RO^- (alkoxide) unit is less likely to donate electrons, making it a weaker base. In other words, oxygen retains electrons better than nitrogen, so the oxygen cannot donate electrons, and so alkoxide is a weaker base and the amide anion and less reactive. The presence of the weaker base makes the reaction with the conjugate acid poorer, which shifts the equilibrium further to the right for the reaction of ROH, making it more acidic. Oxygen is also larger than nitrogen, so the charge dispersal on oxygen is greater, again making it less able to donate electrons.

If two reactions are compared, and both acid *X* and acid *Y* have the structure R—OH, but acid *X* gives a more stable conjugate base, how does this influence the equilibrium and K_a?

If the conjugate base from acid *X* is more stable, that equilibrium will be pushed further to the right, making K_a larger. In other words, acid *X* is more acidic.

What is the conjugate base formed when formic acid (HCOOH; see structure) reacts with NaOH?

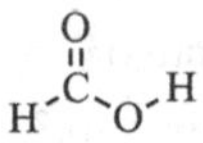

Formic acid

When the hydroxide ion reacts with formic acid by donating two electrons to the δ^+ hydrogen atom, the hydrogen atom is transferred to the oxygen of hydroxide, and the two electrons, since the O—H bond of formic acid are transferred to the formic acid oxygen atom. In other words, the formate anion is formed as the conjugate base of formic acid. Note that the sodium counterion is omitted from this reaction to make it easier to track the electron transfer, but it is transferred from the counterion of hydroxide to the counterion of the formate anion.

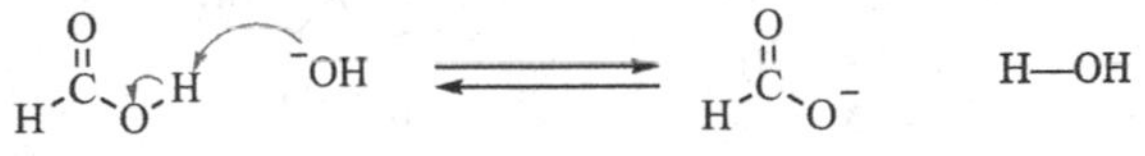

$^-$OH H—OH

Formic acid Formate anion

What are the resonance contributors for the formate anion?

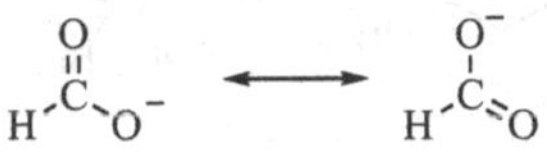

There are two resonance forms of the formate anion, as shown.

Which is the stronger acid, formic acid or methanol (CH_3OH)? Explain your answer!

Formic acid is the stronger acid. When methanol reacts with hydroxide, the product is the methoxide anion, where the charge is localized on the oxygen. Therefore, the electrons are readily available for donation (i.e., it is a good base). The formate anion, however, is resonance stabilized, meaning the electron pair is delocalized over three atoms. Therefore, the oxygen atom is less basic because it is less able to donate electrons. The formate anion is more stable than the methoxide anion, so the equilibrium for formic acid is shifted to the right relative to methanol, making it more acidic.

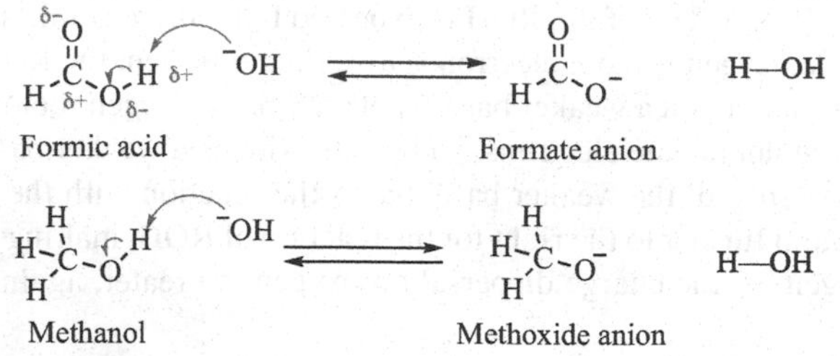

Formic acid ⇌ Formate anion + H—OH

Methanol ⇌ Methoxide anion + H—OH

In addition, the C=O unit in formic acid is polarized as shown, making the O—H unit in formic acid more polarized, and more reactive (i.e., more acidic) relative to the O—H unit in methanol. Note that this simple analysis has ignored any solvent effects, which can play a significant role.

END OF CHAPTER PROBLEMS

1. Which is more acidic, HCOOH or CH_3COOH?
2. Which is more basic, CH_3OCH_3 or CH_3NHCH_3?
3. Convert each of the following K_a values into pK_a.

   (a) 3.4×10^4 (b) 2.33×10^{-9} (c) 5.66×10^{-2} (d) 8.9×10^7

4. Convert each of the following pK_a values into K_a.

   (a) 2.33 (b) 23.55 (c) 17.05 (d) 4.78 (e) 10.15

5. Draw all resonance forms for the carbonate anion in Na_2CO_3.
6. Why is ***A*** a stronger acid than ***B***.

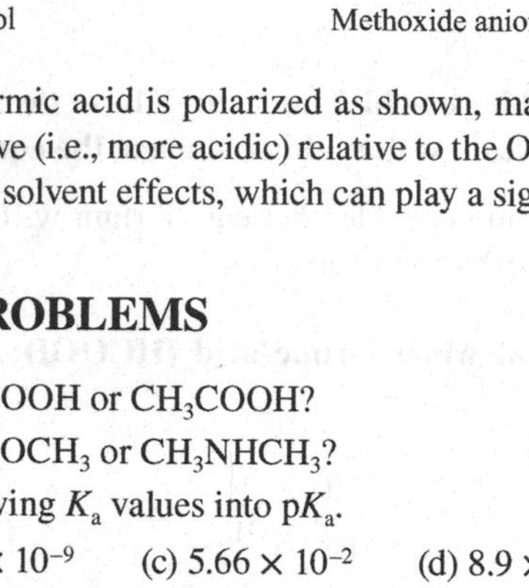

   A **B**

7. Which is the stronger acid, ***A*** or ***B***? Explain!

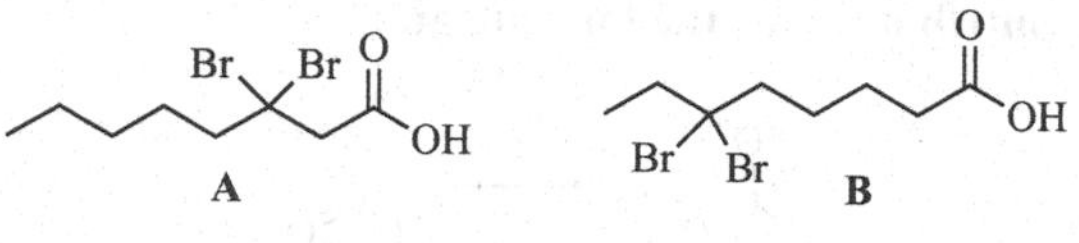

   A **B**

8. Draw a diagram to illustrate a potential through-space inductive effect in 4-chlorobutanoic acid.
9. Why is acetic acid a stronger acid in water than in ethanol?
10. Why is $\Delta S°$ a small number in the Gibbs free energy equation?
11. What is $\Delta G°$ for the following reaction, assuming that $\Delta S°$ is negligible and can be ignored, that $H°$ for the C—I bond is 50.9 kcal, and $H°$ for the C—N bond is 72.9 kcal? Focus only on covalent bonds and ignore any ionic bonds. Is the reaction endothermic or exothermic?

$$CH_3I + NH_3 \longrightarrow H_3\overset{+}{N}{-}CH_3 \; I^-$$

4

Alkanes, Isomers, and Nomenclature

In this chapter the most fundamental of organic molecules, the alkanes, will be discussed. Alkanes are molecules that contain only carbon and hydrogen connected by single covalent bonds. The method for naming alkanes will be introduced as well as their chemical and physical properties.

4.1 DEFINITION AND BASIC NOMENCLATURE

What are two important parameters used to organize and name organic molecules?

Organic molecules are organized according to the number of carbon atoms in the molecule and the presence or absence of functional groups.

What is a hydrocarbon?

A hydrocarbon is a molecule whose structure contains only carbon and hydrogen atoms.

What is the definition of an alkane?

An alkane is a hydrocarbon (composed of only carbon and hydrogen) that possesses the simplest empirical formula for organic molecules and does not contain a functional group.

What is the generic formula for an alkane?

All alkanes have the general formula C_nH_{2n+2}. This formula is also important because it represents the maximum number of hydrogens that can be attached to a given number of carbon atoms. There can be fewer hydrogen atoms than $2n+2$ when functional groups are introduced, but never more.

What is the general approach to naming alkanes?

Alkanes are named according to a set of rules established by the International Union of Pure and Applied Chemistry (IUPAC). The rules define a *prefix* that shows the *number of carbon atoms* and a *suffix* that defines the *functional group*. For alkanes, there is no functional group and the suffix is -ane. Alkanes are taken as the fundamental structure with respect to the number of carbon atoms.

What are the prefixes used to identify the number of carbon atoms in an alkane with a linear carbon chain?

The prefixes used for linear alkanes that contain 1–20 are highlighted in the table and the formal name of each compound is shown, e.g., methane. In each case, the hydrogen atoms are added to each carbon in order to satisfy the valence of four and the C_nH_{2n+2} formula.

C_1	CH_4	**methane**	C_{11}	$CH_3(CH_2)_9CH_3$	**undecane**
C_2	CH_3CH_3	**ethane**	C_{12}	$CH_3(CH_2)_{10}CH_3$	**dodecane**
C_3	$CH_3CH_2CH_3$	**propane**	C_{13}	$CH_3(CH_2)_{11}CH_3$	**tridecane**
C_4	$CH_3(CH_2)_2CH_3$	**butane**	C_{14}	$CH_3(CH_2)_{12}CH_3$	**tetradecane**
C_5	$CH_3(CH_2)_3CH_3$	**pentane**	C_{15}	$CH_3(CH_2)_{13}CH_3$	**pentadecane**
C_6	$CH_3(CH_2)_4CH_3$	**hexane**	C_{16}	$CH_3(CH_2)_{14}CH_3$	**hexadecane**
C_7	$CH_3(CH_2)_5CH_3$	**heptane**	C_{17}	$CH_3(CH_2)_{15}CH_3$	**heptadecane**
C_8	$CH_3(CH_2)_6CH_3$	**octane**	C_{18}	$CH_3(CH_2)_{16}CH_3$	**octadecane**
C_9	$CH_3(CH_2)_7CH_3$	**nonane**	C_{19}	$CH_3(CH_2)_{17}CH_3$	**nonadecane**
C_{10}	$CH_3(CH_2)_8CH_3$	**decane**	C_{20}	$CH_3(CH_2)_{18}CH_3$	**icosane**

What is a linear alkane?

All carbon atoms of the alkane are connected in a linear manner with no branches. As a practical matter, this definition means that for all alkanes of three or more carbon atoms, there is a methyl group (CH_3) connected to some number of methylene units (CH_2), ending in another methyl group (CH_3), so the generic formula for a linear alkane is $CH_3(CH_2)_nCH_3$ (where n is simply an integer, 0, 1, 2, 3…). Ethane ($n = 0$) has two methyl groups connected together, with no intervening methylene unit.

What are typical physical properties of alkanes?

Alkanes are non-polar molecules and generally insoluble in water or other highly polarized liquids. They have no functional group and, therefore, associate in the liquid phase only by van der Waals forces, leading to low boiling points relative to other organic molecules. Once the mass of the alkane is sufficiently large, however, the boiling point also becomes rather high. Indeed, very large alkanes are solids. Linear alkenes do not pack into a crystal structure very well due to conformational mobility (see Section 5.1), and the melting points tend to be rather low relative to other organic molecules, or relative to alkanes that are highly branched. The first number for the following alkanes is the boiling point and that in brackets [ ] is the melting point: propane = −42.1°C [−187.7°C]; pentane = +36.1°C [−129.7°C]; decane = +174.1°C [−29.7°C]; icosane = +343.8°C [+36.4°C].

What is the IUPAC name for the eleven-carbon linear alkane?

Undecane.

Draw dodecane using both condensed notation and line notation.

$CH_3CH_2CH_2CH_2CH_2CH_2CH_2CH_2CH_2CH_2CH_2CH_3$

Dodecane (condensed notation)

Dodecane (line notation)

4.2 STRUCTURAL ISOMERS

What is the valence of carbon?

The valence is four (4) for each carbon, so each carbon in a molecule will form four covalent bonds.

Can carbon form bonds to other carbon atoms as well as non-carbon atoms?

Yes! A carbon atom can form covalent bonds to another carbon, as well as to other atoms.

What is the significance of the fact that carbon can form bonds to other carbon atoms?

This property leads to a very large number of molecules that contain carbon, all with different structures. It also leads to an interesting phenomenon called *isomerism*.

What is an isomer?

An isomer is two or more molecules that have the same empirical formula, but the individual atoms are connected in different ways, leading to *different molecules*.

Are there isomers for the formula C_3H_8?

No! The formula $CH_3CH_2CH_3$ for propane is the only way to attach these atoms and satisfy all valences to keep the molecule neutral. Therefore, propane has no isomers.

Are there isomers for the formula C_4H_{10}? If yes, draw them using line notation.

Yes! There are two isomers. One is the linear connection of carbon atoms, butane. The second isomer is a linear chain of three carbons, with a carbon branch from the middle carbon.

Note the emergence of a pattern. First, make the longest continuous chain. Next, make a structure with one fewer carbon atoms in the longest continuous chain, and attach the extra carbon at different branch points along the longest chain. In this case, there is only one place to attach the extra carbon.

Is the structure shown an isomer of butane, shown in the previous question?

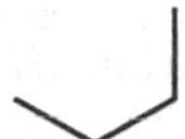

No! The longest continuous chain is four, so butane can be drawn with the carbon atoms "up" or "down," but the linear chain is always four.

How can hexane be drawn in the so-called condensed structure?

In hexane, the six carbons are connected in a linear manner and adding the hydrogens leads to a molecule that satisfies the empirical formula. An expedient way to represent this formula is the *condensed* structure: $CH_3CH_2CH_2CH_2CH_2CH_3$. In this notation, the underlined carbon is connected to two other carbons (one to the right and one to the left). The two hydrogen atoms to the right of the underlined carbon are connected directly to it, whereas the two hydrogen atoms to the left are attached to the previous carbon in the chain. All hydrogen atoms connected to a given carbon are shown to the right.

What are the isomers for the formula C_6H_{14}? Draw them using condensed structures.

Structural isomerism can be illustrated by a molecule with the empirical formula C_6H_{14}. Each carbon will have four bonds and each hydrogen will have one bond. There are, however, five (5) different ways to assemble molecules such that these criteria are satisfied.

$CH_3CH_2CH_2CH_2\,CH_2{\cdot}CH_3$ (1 2 3 4 5 6)

$CH_3{\cdot}CH(CH_3)\,CH_2CH_2\,CH_3$ (1 2 3 4 5) $\equiv$ $CH_3CH_2CH_2\,CH(CH_3){\cdot}CH_3$ (1 2 3 4 5)

$CH_3CH_2\,CH(CH_3){\cdot}CH_2\,CH_3$ (1 2 3 4 5)

$CH_3{\cdot}CH(CH_3){\cdot}CH(CH_3){\cdot}CH_3$ (1 2 3 4)

$CH_3{-}C(CH_3)_2{-}CH_2\,CH_3$ (1 2 3 4)

In hexane, the six carbons are connected in a linear manner and adding the hydrogen atoms leads to a molecule that satisfies the empirical formula. Next, a chain of five linear carbon atoms can be drawn, and there are two different ways to attach the sixth carbon. In one isomer, the one-carbon fragment is attached at the next-to-last carbon. That single carbon can be connected to the "right" or to the "left" but the two structures are identical since they can be completely superimposed, one on the other. A third structure is a different isomer when the single carbon fragment is placed on the "middle" carbon of the five-carbon chain. A structure can be drawn with four carbons placed in a linear chain and a two-carbon fragment is attached to the second carbon, but the longest continuous chain is five, making the structure identical to the five-carbon chain with the one-carbon fragment at the third carbon. A fourth isomer can be drawn where four carbons are placed in a continuous chain and two one-carbon fragments are added at the second and third carbons. The fifth isomer also has the longest continuous chain of four, but the two extra carbon atoms are on the same carbon (C2). These five different molecules are called isomers (molecules with the same empirical formula but different points of attachment for the individual atoms).

Why is the concept of isomerism important for alkanes?

Due to the ability to form isomers, there are literally millions of possible alkanes. The five different isomers of C_6H_{14} were shown in the previous problem. As the number of carbons increase, the number of constitutional isomers increases dramatically: there are 9 for C_7H_{16}, 4347 for $C_{15}H_{32}$ and greater than 62×10^9 for $C_{40}H_{82}$.

Since isomers will all be different molecules (4347 for $C_{15}H_{32}$) with different physical properties (boiling points, melting points, solubility, etc.), a system is required to identify each individual molecule and distinguish it from all other isomers. The first two rules based on the number of carbons and the suffix defining the alkane group are insufficient. Additional rules must be added.

What is a geminal (gem) dimethyl unit?

Two methyl groups on the same carbon are known as a geminal dimethyl, or gem-dimethyl.

What is a vicinal (vic) dimethyl unit?

Two methyl groups on adjacent carbon atoms are known as vicinal dimethyl, or vic-dimethyl.

4.3 IUPAC NOMENCLATURE

What is IUPAC and the relationship to organic chemical nomenclature?

The organization IUPAC is the International Union of Pure and Applied Chemistry. It is an international federation of national organizations that represent chemists in individual countries. IUPAC is the universally recognized authority of chemical nomenclature and terminology, and it establishes an unambiguous and consistent nomenclature and terminology for specific scientific fields. Taken from https://iupac.org/what-we-do/nomenclature/.

What are the IUPAC rules of nomenclature?

The fundamental rules are that a prefix is used to identify the number of carbon atoms in the longest continuous chain, and a suffix that is used to identify the functional group. The first rule must identify the length of the carbon chain, but a rule must be added to locate the number and type of carbon groups attached to that initial carbon chain. To do this, the carbon chain must be numbered. The rules required to distinguish different isomers and indeed different molecules are:

(1) Determine the longest continuous chain of carbon atoms and assign the alkane base name (methane → icosane).

(2) Number the longest chain such that the substituent (atom or groups attached to the longest chain) receives the lowest possible number.

(3) Determine the number of carbon atoms in the substituent and assign a name based on the alkane names but *drop the -ane ending and add -yl.* A one-carbon substituent is meth<u>yl</u>, a two-carbon substituent is eth<u>yl</u>, etc.

What is the IUPAC name of the following molecules?

(a) (b) (c)

(a) 4-Methylheptane (b) 4-Methyloctane (c) 5-Propylhexadecane

What is a substituent?

A substituent is an atom or group attached to the longest continuous carbon chain.

How are substituents named?

Use the prefix to indicate the number of carbon atoms and use the suffix -yl. A one-carbon substituent becomes methyl, a two-carbon substituent, ethyl, etc.

What is an alkyl group?

Any carbon substituent is generically called an alkyl group.

What is the nomenclature rule for naming alkyl groups?

The prefix from the table in Section 4.1 is used to identify the number of carbon atoms in the alkyl group. The suffix is -yl. Therefore, a one-carbon substituent is methyl, a two-carbon substituent is ethyl, three-carbon is propyl, four-carbon is butyl, five-carbon is pentyl, and six-carbon is hexyl.

What is the substituent in *A*?

A

In *A*, the longest continuous chain is six, so this compound is named as a hexane. There is a one-carbon fragment (substituent) attached to the six-carbon chain, which is a *methyl group*.

What is the IUPAC name of *A* in the preceding question?

The IUPAC name of *A* is 3-methylhexane

Why is an isomer of heptane (molecule *A*) in the question above named as a hexane?

Although 3-methylhexane has a total of seven carbons, the longest continuous carbon chain is six carbons and it is, therefore, named as a hexane.

What is the rule for using substituents in a name?

Always place the substituent in front of the base name (alkane ***A*** above is methylpentane, for example) and indicate the position of the substituent with a number. In this case, the longest chain is six, which is a hexane. The substituent is a one-carbon fragment, which is methyl. Number the hexane chain from the closest locant to give the methyl group the lowest number (two rather than four) so ***A*** is named 3-methylhexane.

Why is *A* not named 4-methylhexane?

The nomenclature rule clearly states that the longest continuous chain be numbered to give the substituent the lowest possible number and that the substituent is given the lowest possible number from the closest locant. Therefore, ***A*** is 3-methylhexane and *not* 4-methylhexane.

What is the IUPAC name of the following alkanes?

(a) 4-Ethyloctane (b) Octane (c) 5-Propyltridecane

What is the nomenclature rule when there are more than one of the same groups in the same molecule?

A fourth rule must be added to the original three in order to deal with this situation.

(4) When there are two or more identical substituents, assign each one a number according to its position on the carbon chain and use the prefix di- (two), tri- (three), tetra- (four), penta- (five), etc.

What is the structure and IUPAC name of two isomers of 3-methylhexane that are pentane derivatives?

The empirical formula of 3-methylhexane is C_7H_{16}. Pentane isomers have the longest continuous chain of five atoms and either one two-carbon substituent or two one-carbon substituents. The two examples shown are 2,3-dimethylpentane and 3-ethylpentane.

2,3-Dimethylpentane 3-Ethylpentane

What is the nomenclature protocol if there are more than one of the same substituents?

For multiple substituents use the prefix di, tri, tetra, or penta for 2, 3, 4, or 5, respectively. If there are two methyl groups the name will be dimethyl. Four ethyl groups will be tetraethyl.

If there are more than one of the same substituents, is one number required for all of them, or does each substituent require a number?

A number is required each time a substituent appears in a molecule, even if the same substituent appears multiple times.

What is the IUPAC name of (a), (b), and (c)?

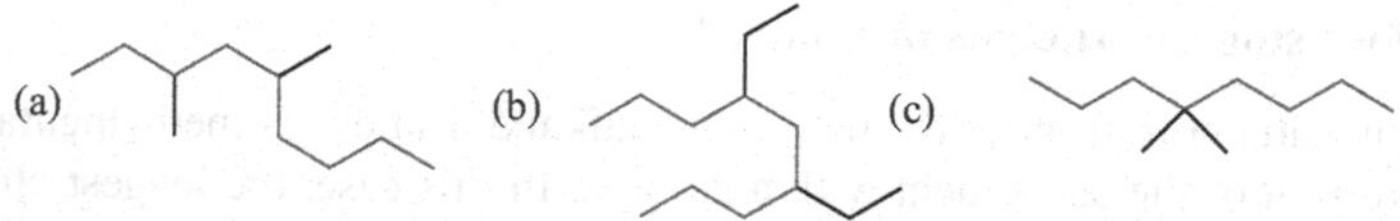

The names are (a) 3,5-dimethylnonane, (b) 4,6-diethylnonane, and (c) 4,4-dimethyloctane. The longest continuous chain in (a) and (b) is nine, and these compounds are nonanes. The longest chain in (c) is eight, so it is an octane. Giving the substituents the lowest combination of numbers leads to 3,5 for (a); 4,6 for (b); and 4,4 for (c). Note that both methyl groups in (a) and in (c) have a number and both ethyl groups in (b) have a number. Further, note that both methyl groups in (c) have a number although they are on the same carbon of the eight-carbon chain and they have the same number. *All substituents are numbered, even if they are on the same carbon.*

How are substituents named when they are not the same, as in *A*?

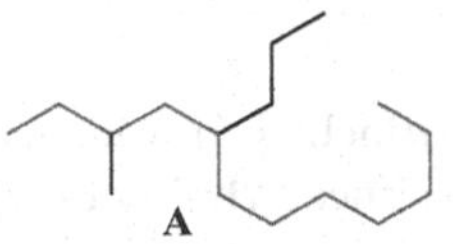

A

The name is 3-methyl-5-propyldodecane. A corollary is necessary for this rule when the substituents are not the same.

(Corollary to Rule 4) When the substituents are different, assign each a number according to its position on the carbon chain and arrange the substituents alphabetically in the final name.

In the case of ***A***, a methyl and a propyl group are substituents, so the methyl (m) comes first, followed by propyl (p). Therefore, the name will be methypropyl: 3-methyl-5-propyldodecane. Once again, the *lowest combination of numbers* is used.

What is the IUPAC name for (a), (b), and (c)?

(a) 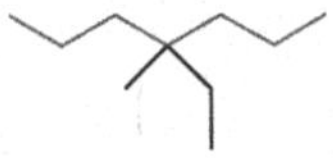 (b) 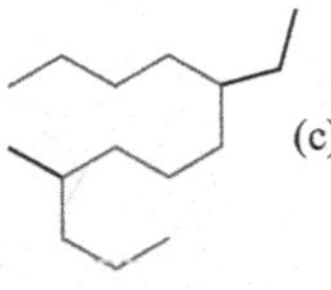 (c)

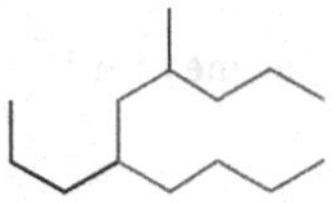

The names are (a) 4-ethyl-4-methylheptane, (b) 8-ethyl-4-methyldodecane, and (c) 4-methyl-6-propyldecane. The substituents are arranged alphabetically based on the first letter of the substituent. Note that in (b), the ethyl group has a higher number than the methyl group, but ethyl comes before methyl in the name.

How are halogen substituents treated in the nomenclature system?

Another modification of the rules is required for fluorine, chlorine, bromine, or iodine.

(5) If a halogen is present in the molecule, treat it as a substituent, dropping its -ine ending and adding -o. Fluorine becomes fluoro, chlorine becomes chloro, bromine becomes bromo, and iodine becomes iodo.

What is the name of (a) and of (b)?

(a) 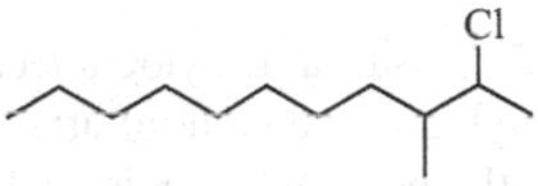 Cl (b) 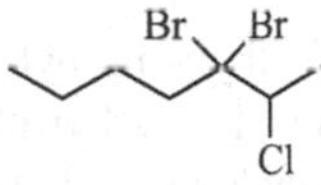 Br Br Cl

The names are (a) 2-chloro-3-methylundecane and (b) 3,3-dibromo-2-chloroheptane. The chlorine atoms in (a) and (b) are treated as a substituent and named chloro. Likewise, the bromine atoms in (b) are named bromo.

How are alkanes named when the substituent is more complex than the simple linear alkyl groups?

In many isomeric alkanes, the substituent is more complex than a simple linear fragment such as methyl, ethyl, etc. As a practical matter, a substituent that has branched substituents is called a complex substituent. The substituent can also be a group or atom other than a carbon group. For carbon substituents containing complex structures, another rule is required that is more complex than others previously cited.

Rule (6) If the carbon substituent is complex (not linear), identify the longest continuous chain of the substituent and use Rules 1 and 3 to determine if it is an ethyl, butyl, hexyl group, etc. Determine the substituents on the substituent chain, number the substituent chain such that the point of attachment to the main chain is always one (1), and assign a number to the secondary substituent. Set apart the complex substituent in brackets.

What is the name fragment *A* that is attached to a longer carbon chain in a molecule? The "squiggle" line represents an undefined linear chain of carbon atoms that constitutes the longest continuous chain!

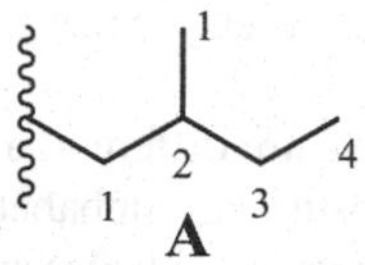

The point of attachment to the longest chain is the first carbon of a four-carbon fragment, or a butyl group. Number the longest carbon chain of the butyl group from *the point of attachment to the longest chain.* At C2 of the butyl substituent, a methyl group is attached. Therefore, this fragment is named 2-methylbutyl.

What is the IUPAC name of *A*?

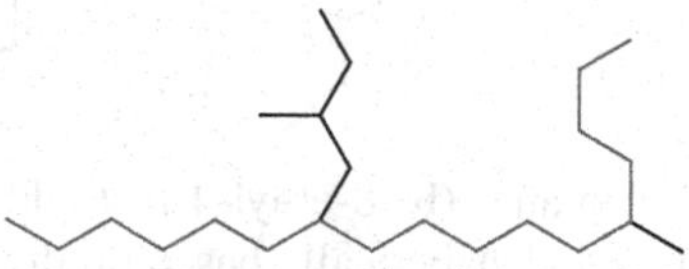

The name is 5-methyl-11-(2-methylbutyl)heptadecane. Note that the ethyl group comes before the methylbutyl group. This arrangement means that the methylbutyl group is categorized as "m" and the ethyl group is of course "e." Note that the complex substituent 2-methylbutyl is set apart from the rest of the name by brackets. The brackets are required in the IUPAC nomenclature.

What is the name of *A*?

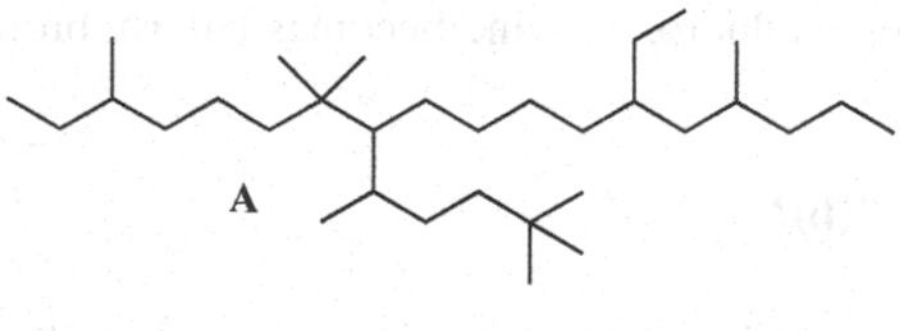

The name is 8-(1,4,4-trimethylpentanyl)-13-ethyl-3,7,7,15-tetramethyloctadecane. Note that the complex substituent, in the brackets, is 1,4,4-trimethylpentanyl, and the point of attachment to the longest chain (octadecane) is at C8 of the longest chain, but C1 of the pentanyl complex substituent.

What are common names?

The IUPAC rules are relatively recent. A system of naming organic molecules developed over many years and persists today for some molecular fragments and small molecules. This system of common names is based on the number of methyl groups on a fragment and their relative position.

Discuss the structural basis for common names.

Many of the common names have a focus on methyl groups. The term *iso-* is used when one carbon at the end of the chain bears a CH and two methyl groups. The total number of carbon atoms dictates the name (isopropyl for three carbons, isobutyl for four carbons, etc.). The *secondary* (or *sec-*) group has a CH, one methyl and an alkyl group (not methyl). This term leads to *sec*-butyl for four carbons and *sec*-pentyl for five carbons. The *tertiary* (*tert-* or just *t-*) group is a carbon with two methyls and one alkyl (which may be methyl). This term leads to *t*-butyl for four carbons, *t*-pentyl for five carbons, etc. When the -$C(CH_3)_3$ group is at the end of the chain, the term *neo*- can be used, as in neopentyl for the five-carbon fragment. Common names are used primarily with simple molecules, although they are used extensively to denote small fragments (an isopropyl group, a *t*-butyl group, etc.).

Give the structure for isopropyl, isobutyl, isopentyl, secondary butyl, secondary pentyl, tertiary butyl, tertiary pentyl, and neopentyl.

-$CH(CH_3)_2$	isopropyl	-$CH_2CH(CH_3)_2$	isobutyl
-$CH_2CH_2CH(CH_3)_2$	isopentyl	-$CH(CH_3)CH_2CH_3$	*secondary* (*sec*)-butyl
-$CH(CH_3)CH_2CH_2CH_3$	*sec*-pentyl	-$C(CH_3)_3$	*tertiary* (*tert*-, *t*-) butyl
-$C(CH_3)_2CH_2CH_3$	*tert*-pentyl	-$CH_2C(CH_3)_3$	neopentyl

4.4 CYCLIC ALKANES

Alkanes can exist as cyclic molecules, where the carbons form a ring. In other words, the continuous chain of carbon atoms forms a ring, which is a cyclic structure. These compounds are known as cyclic alkanes, or cycloalkanes.

What is the general formula for a cyclic alkane?

Cyclic alkanes are a class of alkanes that exist with the two terminal carbons tied together into a ring. Forming the bond to make a ring changes the general formula from C_nH_{2n+2} for an acyclic (no rings) alkane to C_nH_{2n} for a cyclic alkane.

What is the shape of the flat structures of cyclopropane, cyclobutane, cyclopentane, cyclohexane, and cycloheptane using line notation?

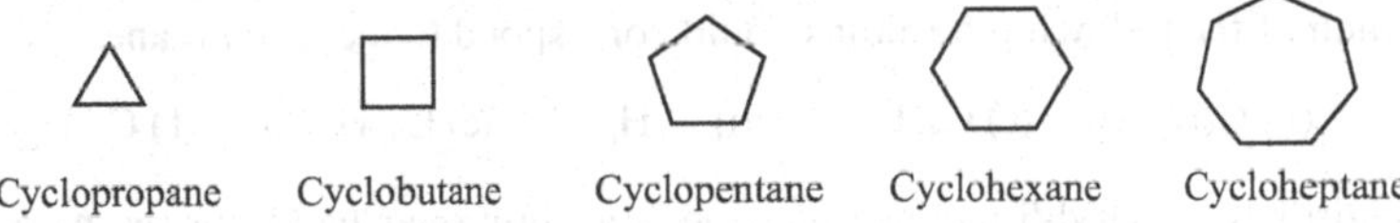

What is the general rule for naming cyclic alkanes?

The nomenclature for cyclic alkanes is similar to that for acyclic alkanes. The total number of carbons dictates the alkane name (propane, butane, pentane, etc.), but the word cyclo- is added to show that it is a ring. This leads to cyclopropane, cyclobutane, cyclopentane, cyclohexane, and cycloheptane, etc.

What is the rule for cyclic alkanes that have substituents?

The rules are the same as with other alkanes. Place the substituent name, with a position number in front of the cycloalkane name. However, with only one substituent, the substituent is always on C1 of the cyclic alkane.

If there is only one substituent, as in methylcyclopentane (draw it), is the number required?

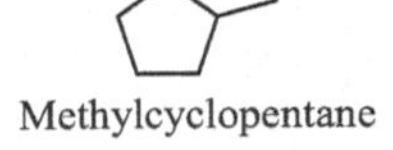

No! Giving the methyl group the smallest number (1) is obvious, and it is not necessary to use it in the name. The molecule shown is simply methylcyclopentane.

How are cyclic alkanes named when there are two or more substituents on the ring?

When there are two substituents, both substituents require a number to specify the position of the groups on the ring and the relationship of the groups, one to the other, because more than one isomer is possible. The ring is numbered from the "top" attached group to give the substituents the lowest possible combination of numbers.

If two different substituents are attached to the ring, list them in alphabetical order, and the first cited substituent is C1. Number the other substituents to give the second substituent the lowest possible number. If there are three or more substituents, the rules are slightly different. List the substituents in alphabetical order, but C1 is chosen so the lowest combination of numbers is obtained.

What is the IUPAC name for (a), (b), (c), and (d)?

(a) 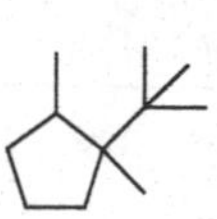 (b) 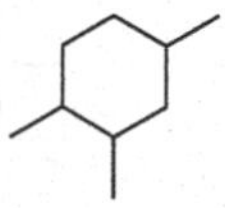 (c) 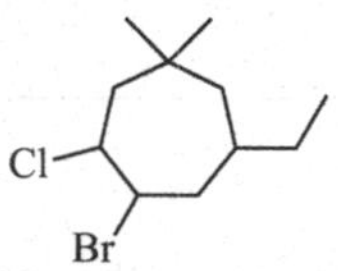 Cl Br (d)

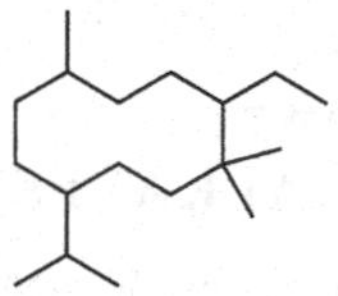

The names are: (a) 1-(*tert*-butyl)-1,2-dimethylcyclopentane; (b) 1,2,4-trimethylcyclohexane; (c) 4-bromo-3-chloro-6-ethyl-1,1-dimethylcycloheptane; (d) 2-ethyl-8-isopropyl-1,1,5-trimethylcyclodecane. In each case, the substituents are numbered to give the lowest combination of numbers. Note that in (a), (c), and (d), C1 is the carbon that bears two substituents.

END OF CHAPTER PROBLEMS

1. Indicate which of the following formulas correspond to an acyclic alkane.

   (a) C_6H_{12} (b) C_8H_{18} (c) C_5H_8 (d) C_6H_6 (e) $C_{40}H_{80}$ (f) $C_{40}H_{82}$

2. Indicate which of the following formulas could correspond to a cyclic alkane.

   (a) C_6H_{12} (b) C_8H_{18} (c) C_5H_8 (d) C_6H_6 (e) $C_{40}H_{80}$ (f) $C_{40}H_{82}$

3. Briefly explain why 3-butyl-5-methylundecane is an improper name for the molecule shown. What is the proper IUPAC name?

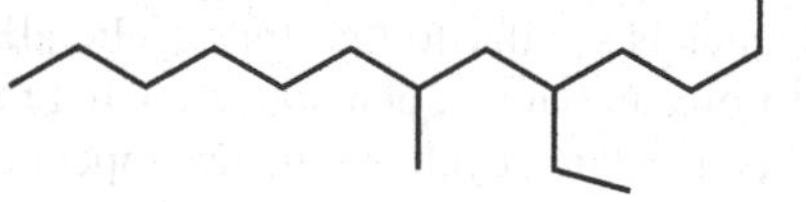

4. Give the IUPAC name for each of the following.

   (a) 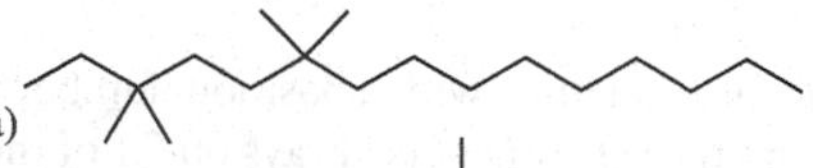 (b) 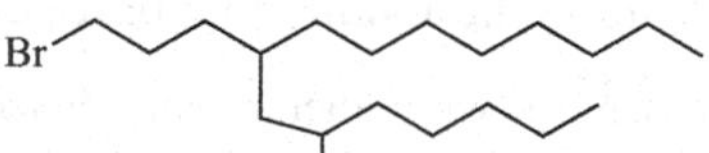 Br (c) 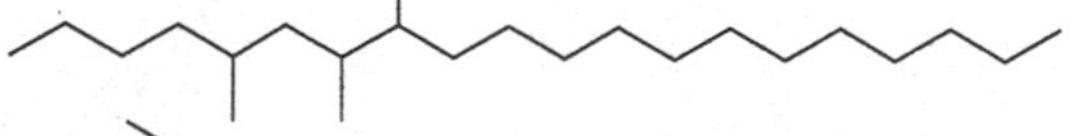 (d) 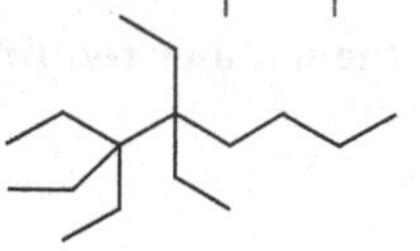 (e)

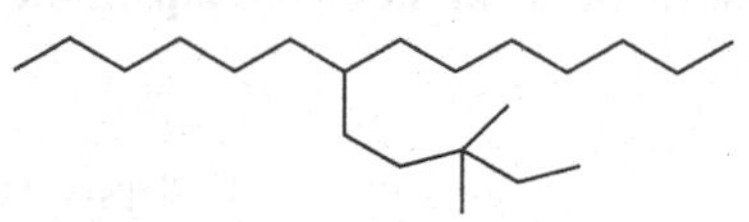

5. Give the structure for each of the following using line notation.

   (a) 3,3,4,4-tetramethylcycloheptane (b) 1-bromo-4-(2,2-dimethylbutyl)cyclodecane
   (c) 5,7,8-tribromocyclononane (d) 3,3,4,4-tetraethylcyclohexane
   (e) 1-(2,2-dimethylpropyl)cyclopentane.

6. Draw the structures of (a) neopentyl bromide (b) isobutane (c) *tert*-pentyl chloride (d) isopentane (e) *t*-butyl iodide.

7. Draw eight different isomers for each of the following: (a) C_8H_{18} (b) C_7H_{16}.

8. Give the IUPAC name for each of the following.

(a) 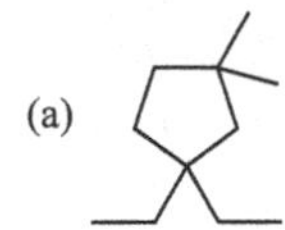 (b) 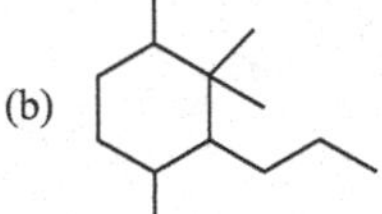 (c) 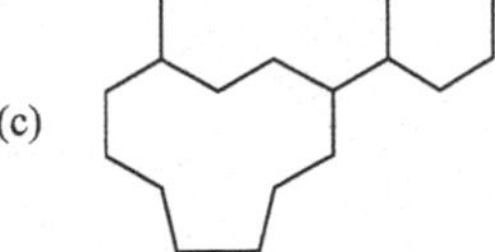

5

Conformations

Rotation about single bonds in acyclic molecules leads to different forms of the molecule, as does pseudorotation of bonds in cyclic compounds that cannot rotate by 360°. Such forms are transient and called rotamers with acyclic compounds. The various form(s) of the molecule leads to conformations of the molecule that are important for reactivity in chemical reactions and in biological systems.

5.1 ACYCLIC CONFORMATIONS

What does the term acyclic mean?

The term is applied to molecules that do not have a ring.

What is the result of a molecule dissipating excess energy by rotation about a single covalent bond?

Molecules absorb energy from the environment, and they dissipate that energy by molecular vibration, translational motion though a medium, collision with other molecules, and so on. One way that a molecule can dissipate energy (heat) is by rotation about atoms in a covalent bond. When the atoms or groups on a carbon–carbon single bond rotate, the spatial arrangement of the atoms or groups changes with the rotations. Such spatial arrangements are called *rotamers.*

What is a rotamer?

Rotation of 360° can occur about covalent carbon–carbon, carbon–heteroatom or heteroatom–heteroatom single bonds. Such rotation leads to different spatial arrangements of the atoms, although it does not change the connectivity. The specific arrangement of the atoms, based on a hypothetical "snapshot" of an arrangement of atoms that is "frozen in space," is called a *rotamer.*

Is there more than one rotamer?

Rotation about a carbon–carbon bond is a dynamic process that leads to a change in arrangement of the atoms that leads to different rotamers, and there are literally an infinite number of possibilities. Although there an infinite number of possible rotamers, due to steric and electronic interactions some rotamers and conformations are lower in energy than others.

What is a conformation for a molecule?

A conformation of a molecule is a spatial arrangement of the atoms in a molecule. There are many conformations that are interconverted by rotation about covalent single bonds. A molecule has a higher percentage of the lowest energy arrangement of the atoms, the lowest energy conformation that corresponds to the low energy rotamer(s).

What is the shape of a given molecule?

The collection of lowest energy rotamers for all the bonds in a molecule is the lowest energy conformation of the molecule, which is taken as the effective shape of the molecule.

What is the structure of ethane?

The three-dimensional structure of the two-carbon alkane, ethane, is shown, along with the condensed notation. Note the tetrahedral arrangement of atoms about each carbon atom.

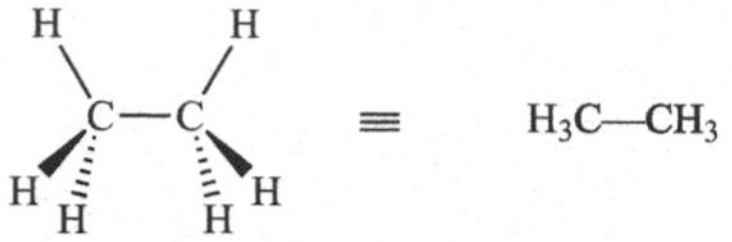

$\equiv$ $H_3C—CH_3$

What occurs if there is rotation about the carbon–carbon bond of ethane?

If the carbon–carbon bond in ethane is examined for rotamers, it is clear there are virtually an infinite number of possibilities. However, attention can focus on just two rotamers, the highest energy where all of the attached hydrogen atoms are close together (they eclipse) and the lowest energy where those hydrogen atoms are as far apart from one another as possible. These two rotamers will determine the barriers to overall rotational motion of the molecule since the highest barrier to rotation is the energy required to rotate past the highest energy rotamer.

What are eclipsed and staggered rotamers?

The high and low energy rotamers of ethane are shown in the figure. The high energy rotamer is the *eclipsed rotamer* and the low energy rotamer is the *staggered rotamer.* In the rotamer in the figure labeled "*eclipsed,*" one hydrogen on the "back" carbon (shown as light gray) is parallel to a hydrogen atom on the "front" carbon (also light gray): they *eclipse.* Starting with the eclipsed rotamer, the rear carbon that has the light gray hydrogen is rotated while the front carbon is held constant. During rotation about the C—C bond, the marked hydrogen atoms pass close to one another in space to generate another eclipsed rotamer and energy is required for the atoms to pass one another. The other rotamer shown is labeled "*staggered*" and the two hydrogen atoms are as far apart as possible; they are "anti" (180° opposite) to one another. As noted, in the rotamer with the hydrogen atoms eclipsed they are as close to each other as possible and this arrangement of atoms is higher in energy than the staggered rotamer where those hydrogen atoms are as far apart from one another as possible.

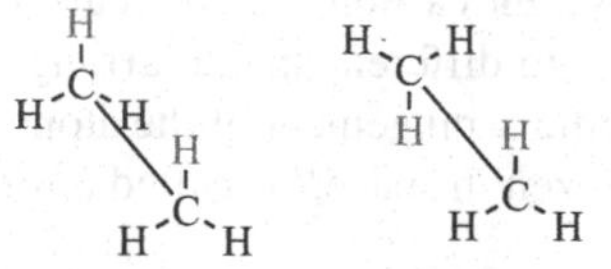

Eclipsed Staggered

Why focus on rotation about the C—C bond rather than one of the C—H bonds?

A hydrogen atom is small and symmetrical, so there is little change in the interaction between atoms during the rotation. Since each carbon has three hydrogen atoms attached, in a tetrahedral array, rotation about the C—C bond will lead to different interactions of the hydrogen atoms, different energy requirements for rotation, and the generation of different rotamers.

What is a sawhorse diagram?

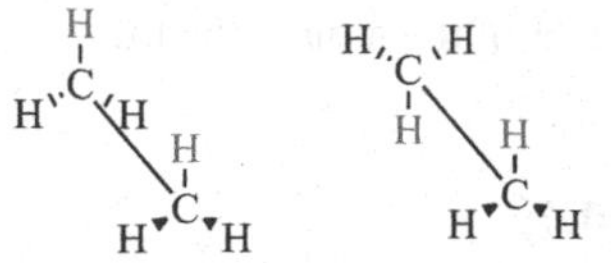

Eclipsed Staggered

A sawhorse diagram is a way to represent a molecule, focusing on a specific bond. In effect, the molecule is turned so that one carbon atom is offset from the other, and the tetrahedral geometry of the remaining bonds is represented by a line, a solid wedge (projected to the front) or a dashed line (projected to the back). Two rotamers for ethane are shown as sawhorse diagrams (eclipsed and staggered) to illustrate.

What is a Newman projection?

A Newman projection is a way to represent a molecule, focusing on a specific bond. The molecule is turned so the sightline is down the C—C bond, with one carbon atom in front and the other carbon atom immediately behind it. For convenience, *the front carbon atom is shown as a dot and the rear carbon as a circle.* The tetrahedral geometry of the remaining bonds is shown by having three bonds projected from the dot and three lines projected from the circle. The eclipsed rotamer of ethane is shown in Newman projection along with the staggered rotamer to illustrate.

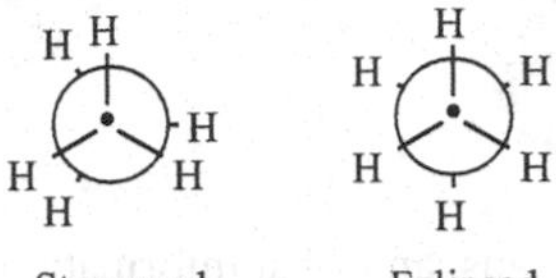

Staggered Eclipsed

What is steric hindrance?

As ethane rotates about the carbon–carbon bond, the hydrogen atoms are in close proximity in the eclipsed or syn rotamer, and as those hydrogen atoms come into close proximity they compete for the same space. The electrons in the bonds repel, and the atoms themselves occupy space and will repel if they get too close. This repulsion is called a *steric interaction,* or *steric hindrance.* If the hydrogen atoms are replaced with carbon groups or heteroatom groups, which are larger, the steric hindrance is greater.

Why is the staggered (anti) rotamer the lowest energy rotamer of ethane?

In principle, rotation about the C—C of ethane can lead to an infinite number of rotamers. Attention can focus on two rotamers of this infinite number, the lowest energy and the highest energy rotamers. The lower energy structure is called the *eclipsed* or *syn* rotamer and the higher energy structure is called the *staggered* or *anti* rotamer. The anti rotamer is the lowest energy since the hydrogens are further apart than in any other rotamer and do not come close together in space upon rotation about the C—C bond. As the molecule rotates about the carbon–carbon bond, the hydrogen atoms come into close proximity in the eclipsed or syn rotamer, and as those hydrogen atoms come into close proximity they compete for the same space. The electrons in the bonds repel, and the atoms themselves repel if they get too close. As noted in the preceding question, this repulsion is called a *steric interaction,* or *steric hindrance.* The staggered or anti rotamer is the lowest energy of all possible rotamers because steric interactions are minimized, whereas the eclipsed or syn rotamer is the highest in energy because steric interactions are maximized.

What are the structures of the anti and eclipsed conformations of ethane in Newman projection? What do the three-dimensional models for these two structures look like?

If these two rotamers are turned so that one "sights" down the carbon–carbon bond, one carbon atom is in front and the other is behind it using a *Newman Projection* to represent each rotamer, as noted above. This view allows the potential steric interactions and especially the high/low energy rotamers to be seen more clearly. The anti rotamer is staggered and the syn rotamer is eclipsed. If the rear carbon of the anti rotamer is imagined to be immobilized and the front carbon is rotated 60° clockwise, the syn rotamer results. In these Newman projections, the anti rotamer clearly shows the hydrogens to be as far apart as possible. Conversely, the hydrogen atoms are very close together in the syn rotamer, illustrating the higher energy of this rotamer.

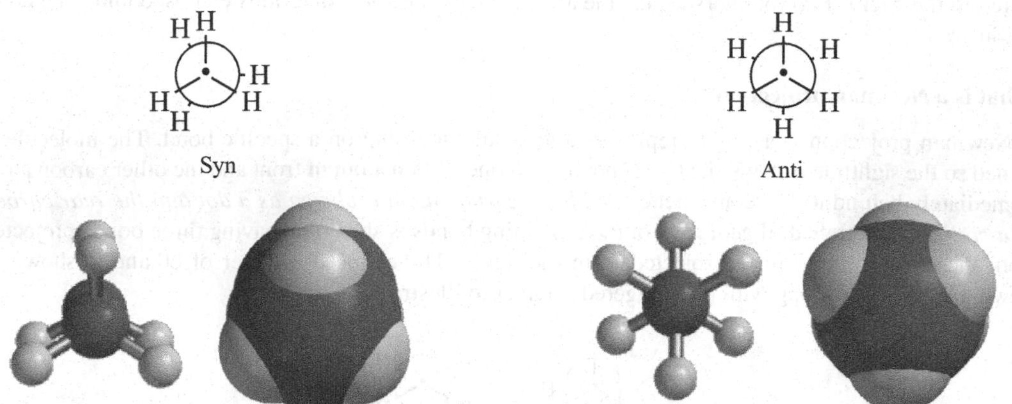

To get a better sense of the size of the atoms, and what information the Newman projection is conveying, the eclipsed rotamer is shown as a ball-and-stick molecular model and also as a space-filling molecular model. Similarly, the staggered or anti rotamer is shown as a ball-and-stick model and as a space-filling model. In the space-filling models, the size of the atoms is conveyed more accurately, and it is clear that the hydrogen atoms are closer together in the syn rotamer than in the anti rotamer. The proximity of the hydrogen atoms in the syn rotamer (the hydrogen atoms eclipse) accounts for the higher energy of that rotamer when compared to the anti rotamer.

Can the rotamers described be isolated?

No! Rotamers such as this are dynamic entities.

What is an energy diagram for rotamers in a molecule?

Rotation about a C—C bond occurs through 360°, the energy of the resulting rotamer increases with increasing steric interactions and decrease as the steric interactions diminish. There will be energy minima and maxima. By plotting the energy of key rotamers at certain angles, a picture emerges of the energy demands for rotation.

Draw the energy diagram for rotation of the carbon–carbon bond of ethane through 360°.

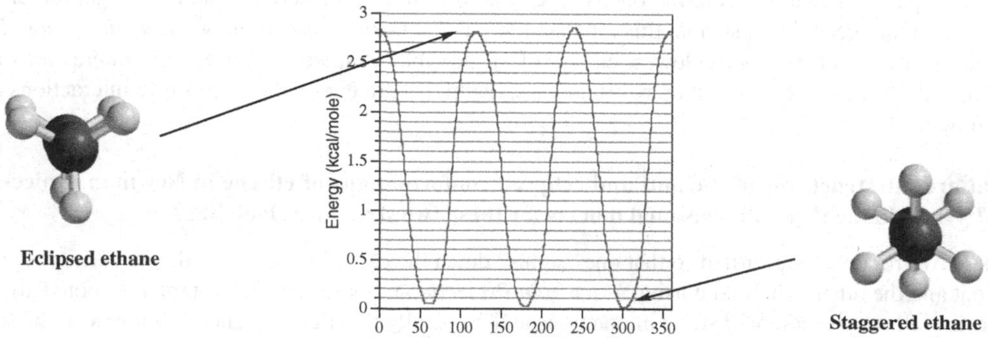

The energy diagram for ethane is shown, and it is clear that the energy rises to a maximum (the eclipsed rotamer) and then falls to a minimum (the staggered rotamer) with each rotation of 60°. There are three hydrogen atoms attached to each carbon, so there are three maxima and three minima.

What does the energy diagram for ethane mean?

When ethane is rotated by 60° about the carbon–carbon bond, a series of three high-energy (syn) and three low-energy (anti) conformations appear as the bond rotates through 360°. This diagram describes the "free" rotation of ethane. Each time the rotation brings the hydrogens together, an *energy barrier* hinders the rotation (slows it down). In other words, *there is an energy barrier for the bonds to pass by each other during rotation*, and rotation is not "free." This barrier is measured to be 2.9 kcal mol^{-1} (12.1 kJ mol^{-1}). Since at least 23 kcal mol^{-1} (96.2 kJ mol^{-1}) of energy are usually available at ambient temperatures, so ethane rotates as shown in the graph and one *cannot* isolate or "freeze" the different rotational isomers.

In the energy diagram for ethane, the energy maximum was measured to be 2.9 kcal mol^{-1} (12.1 kJ mol^{-1}). What does this number mean?

During the rotation, the hydrogen atoms come close together in space. At least 2.9 kcal mol^{-1} (12.1 kJ mol^{-1}) of energy are required for the hydrogen atoms to "pass" each other and continue the rotation about the C—C bond. In effect, the rotation slows down a little as it "climbs" each energy hill and accelerates a little downhill. In other words, rotation about the C—C bond of ethane is not a smooth, continuous rotation, but a "jerky" rotation because of the energy barriers.

What would happen if the molecule was cooled down so that only 2.0 kcal mol^{-1} (8.4 kJ mol^{-1}) were available to the molecule?

There would not be enough energy to pass the 2.9 kcal mol^{-1} (12.1 kJ mol^{-1}) barrier, and the molecule would be essentially frozen since a rotation of 360° would not be possible. In such a situation, the molecule would exist primarily in the anti and near-anti rotamers.

Is the energy diagram for butane the same as ethane with one high-energy and one low-energy conformation?

No! There are four carbons and three C—C bonds, so the energy diagram is predicted to be more complex.

When analyzing the rotamers derived from butane rather than ethane, there are three C—C bonds. Which bond is most important from the standpoint of the highest and lowest energy rotamer?

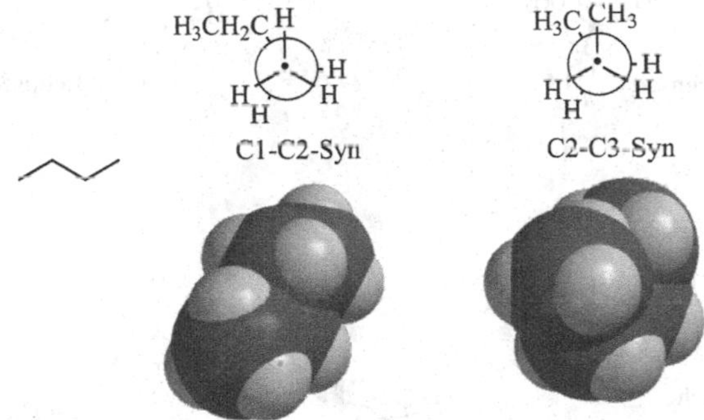

There are three C—C bonds in butane: bonds C1–C2, C2–C3, and C3–C4. The bonds C1–C2 and C3–C4 are identical: a carbon with three hydrogen atoms is connected to a carbon bearing two hydrogen atoms and an ethyl group. The C2–C3 bond is different because each carbon has two hydrogen atoms and a methyl group. *Rotation about the C2–C3 bond leads to an interaction of the two methyl groups* (*C1* and *C4*) that has the maximum energy demand when compared to other rotamers derived from rotation about that bond. This steric interaction is the highest energy interaction for the C2–C3 bond and indeed for the entire molecule.

The Newman projections for the syn rotamers of the C1–C2 bond and of the C2–C3 bond show that there is more steric interaction in the syn rotamer for the C2–C3 bond when compared to any other rotamer. The space-filling model for the C1–C2 syn rotamer shows a steric interaction of a hydrogen atom and the ethyl group, whereas the space-filling model for the C2–C3 syn rotamer shows that the steric interaction of two adjacent methyl groups is significantly higher than the steric interaction of a hydrogen atom and an ethyl group. Remember that rotation about the C2–C3 bond positions the terminal methyl group away from the hydrogen atom at C1 to minimize any steric interaction.

What is the effect on butane when all three C—C bonds are considered rather than just one?

It is clear that molecules, especially those with multiple π-bonds, have different shapes. While all three bonds can exist as their anti-rotamer, syn-syn-syn, syn-syn-anti, syn-anti-anti, and anti-anti-anti rotamers exist for each bond among a nearly infinite array of other rotamers. When the rotamers for all bonds in the molecule are considered, the lowest energy array of atoms gives the molecule as a whole a certain shape, which is known as the low energy *conformation*. Another way to state this observation is that molecules will exist as many conformations since there are many possible rotamers for each bond, but a few conformations and sometimes only one will predominate and this arrangement is taken as the shape of the molecule.

What is a gauche conformation?

A gauche conformation is a staggered rotamer where the two methyl groups are close to each other in space, which makes a gauche conformation higher in energy than the anti rotamer, where the two methyl groups are 180° apart.

Focusing on rotation about the C2–C3 bond of butane, there are three important staggered rotamers. The low energy rotamer is the anti rotamer, but there are two additional staggered rotamers that do not have the methyl groups 180° from one another, but rather the methyl groups are at 60° angles. This increase in steric interaction makes these two staggered rotamers higher in energy than the anti rotamer, but lower than any of the eclipsed rotamers. The staggered rotamers where the methyl groups of butane are proximal but not eclipsing are known as *gauche conformations.*

What are the important conformations for rotation about the C2–C3 bond of butane?

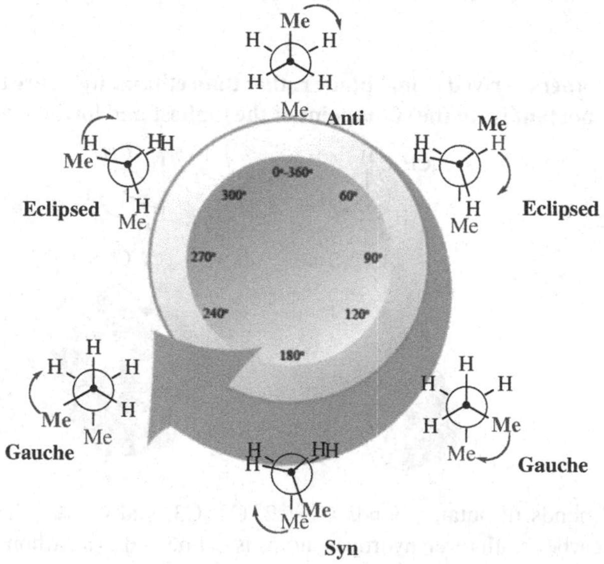

As described in a previous question, the C3–C4 of butane leads to the highest energy steric interaction of the C1 and C4 methyl groups. Both *anti* and *syn* conformations are generated as rotation occurs about the C2–C3 bond, but the relative positions of the two methyl groups are different in different rotamers, leading to rotamers of different energies. Six rotamers are considered to be the most important. There are three anti (staggered) rotamers and three syn (eclipsed) conformations. The anti rotamer is the lowest in energy since the methyl groups are as far apart as possible, and the methyl–methyl interaction is responsible for the greatest steric interaction. Indeed, the syn rotamer is the highest in energy since the methyl–methyl interaction is maximized. This energy barrier has been measured to be 6.0 kcal mol^{-1} (25.1 kJ mol^{-1}). Note, however, that there are two additional *syn* rotamers that are equal in energy (3.4 kcal mol^{-1}; 14.2 kJ mol^{-1}), marked as "eclipsed rotamers" in the diagram. These two rotamers are lower in energy than the syn rotamer but higher in energy than any of the anti rotamers. There are two anti rotamers where the methyl groups are closer together than in the anti rotamer and they are called gauche rotamers. Each gauche rotamer is higher in energy, measured to be (0.8 kcal mol^{-1}, 3.34 kJ mol^{-1}) than the anti rotamer but lower in energy than any syn rotamer. Clearly, rotation about the C2–C3 bond of butane is complex as it rotates 360°, but the maximum barrier to rotation is 6 kcal mol^{-1} (25.1 kJ mol^{-1}) due to the syn rotamer, which is significantly higher than the 2.9 kcal mol^{-1} (12.1 kJ mol^{-1}) barrier encountered in ethane. This difference reflects the greater steric interaction of methyl–methyl vs. hydrogen–hydrogen.

What is a "zig-zag" conformation?

In virtually all alkanes, *the anti- rotamer is assumed to be the lowest energy rotamer for every carbon–carbon bond in the alkane.* Taking decane as an example, assume that every C—C bond exists as the anti rotamer. This assumption leads to a so-called "zigzag" structure shown, which is one *conformation* of decane, as shown in the figure.

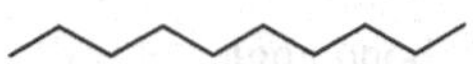

5.2 CONFORMATIONS OF CYCLIC MOLECULES

Is it possible for 360° rotation about a C—C bond when that bond is part of a ring?

No! When a C–C bond is confined to a ring, rotation about 360° is impossible without breaking a bond and disrupting the ring. A twisting motion about the bond occurs, called *pseudorotation,* in order to dissipate excess energy. Pseudorotation of the bonds in rings leads to changes in the shape of the molecule – different conformations.

Is "free rotation" possible around carbon–carbon bonds in cyclic molecules? Why or why not?

No! This question is the same as the preceding question but asked in a different way. Cyclic molecules *cannot* undergo the "free" rotation observed with acyclic alkanes since the bonds are connected in a ring. In order to dissipate excess energy, however, the molecules distort by partial rotation (pseudorotation) of the carbon–carbon bonds, leading to unique conformations for cyclic alkanes. Note that rotation can and does occur about single bonds in groups that are attached to the ring by single covalent bonds but the atoms in those attached groups are not part of the ring.

What is pseudorotation?

Rotation of a C—C bond in a ring cannot proceed by 360° but twisting or pseudorotation of the bond dissipates the energy and minimizes steric interactions of the atoms or groups attached to those carbon atoms. This pseudorotation or twisting motion changes the position of the atoms or groups one to the other when they are attached to the atoms of the ring. Note the relative positions of R^1, R^2, and R^3 in the figure as those positions change with pseudorotation of the six-membered ring.

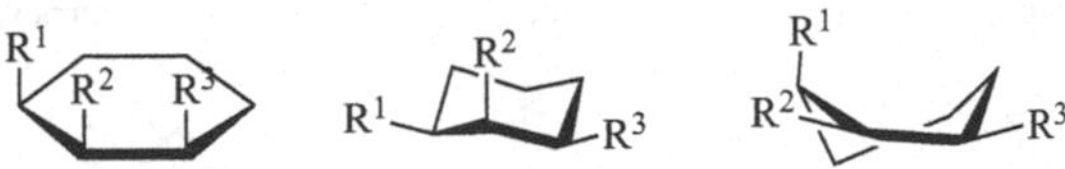

What is angle strain?

When the bond angles in a ring are distorted from the "ideal" tetrahedron of 109°28′ (bond angles for methane), bonds and atoms are in closer proximity, which raises the energy and introduces strain in the molecule. Such strain is called *angle strain* or *Baeyer strain.*

What is Baeyer strain?

Baeyer strain is another name for angle strain.

What is Pitzer strain?

The Newman projections for planar cyclopentane and planar cyclohexane show that all the hydrogen atoms on the "top" eclipse as well as all of the hydrogen atoms on the "bottom," as the structures are drawn. Therefore, there is a significant interaction of these eclipsing hydrogen atoms that destabilizes both planar structures. The steric interactions of these eclipsing atoms (or groups) are referred to as *torsion strain* or *Pitzer strain.*

Cyclopentane Cyclohexane

How do cyclic molecules relieve torsion strain and angle strain in C_4, C_5, and C_6 cyclic alkanes?

In cyclopropane the angle strain is severe (bond angles of 60°), and angle strain is also high in cyclobutane (bond angles of 90°), although less than in cyclopropane. In planar cyclopentane, the bond angles of 108° show little angle strain but significant torsion strain. A planar structure for cyclohexane is also shown and the bond angles are 120° so there is Baeyer strain. The six light gray hydrogen atoms in the figure are on the same side of the planar molecule so all of the C—H bonds eclipse, the hydrogen atoms are relatively close to each other, and there is increased torsion strain.

The steric and electronic interactions in these molecules are relieved by pseudorotation, and the lowest average conformation is known as the so-called "butterfly" conformation for cyclobutane, the "envelope" conformation for cyclopentane, and the "chair" conformation for cyclohexane. Clearly, due to the pseudorotation, *cyclic alkanes do not exist in a planar* conformation because that conformation will be very high in torsion strain and in Baeyer stain. An exception is cyclopropane because pseudorotation is difficult. In the conformations shown, the torsion strain and any Baeyer strain has been relieved. Indeed, the H—C—C bond of cyclohexane resembles the gauche conformation of butane.

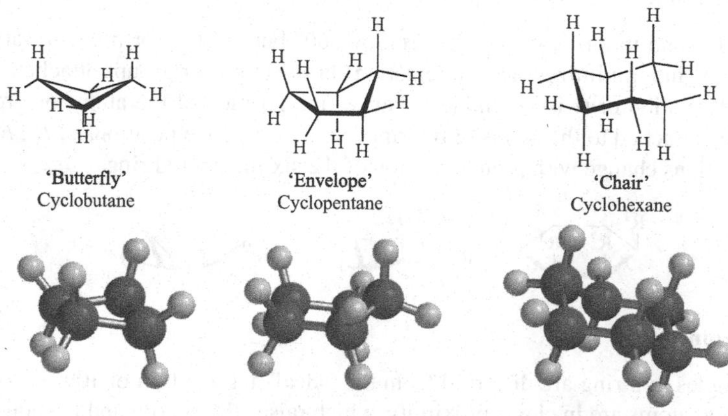

'Butterfly' Cyclobutane 'Envelope' Cyclopentane 'Chair' Cyclohexane

Three-dimensional models are shown to make the actual conformation of each molecule more apparent. The butterfly conformation of cyclobutane, the envelope conformation of cyclopentane, and the chair conformation of cyclohexane are shown. In each case, the distortion from planarity is clear, as is the diminished steric interactions of the hydrogen atoms that leads to less torsion strain.

In the envelope form of cyclopentane, the angle strain is increased relative to the planar form. Why then is the envelope form of cyclopentane the lowest energy form?

In cyclopentane, the angle strain is increased (bond angles of 105°) but the significant reduction in torsion strain makes the envelope conformation much lower in energy than planar cyclopentane.

Why is cyclopropane so high energy when compared to other cyclic alkanes?

The bond angles are about 60° and the molecule is not very flexible. The small bond angle leads to a great deal of Baeyer strain, and the lack of flexibility in the small ring means that pseudorotation is nearly impossible. There is a great deal of torsion strain since the bonds attached to the hydrogen atoms are forced to eclipse.

Why is cyclobutane lower in energy than cyclopropane?

The bond angles in cyclobutane at about 90°, so there is less Baeyer strain, and the extra carbon when compared to cyclopropane gives the molecule more flexibility, so there is more pseudorotation to alleviate torsion strain.

Is cyclohexane more or less flexible when compared to cyclopentane?

The extra carbon atom in cyclohexane gives the molecule increased flexibility for pseudorotation.

What are the bond angles in chair cyclohexane?

In chair cyclohexane, the bond angles are 109°28′ (there is no angle strain) and there is minimal or no Baeyer strain.

Why are there two chair conformations for cyclohexane?

One chair is essentially the mirror image of the other and they are in equilibrium. The two chair conformations are equal in energy for cyclohexane and one is converted to the other by pseudorotation (twisting of bonds), generating the conformation shown in the preceding question.

There are two identical chair conformations of cyclohexane. How is one converted into the other by partial rotation about carbon–carbon bonds?

Cyclohexane is particularly flexible, leading to several different conformations. The lowest energy conformation is the chair, but there are two energetically identical chair conformations for cyclohexane (chair-1 and chair-2). They appear to be the same thing, but if a substituent is placed on the ring, the two chairs become different. This observation will be discussed in a later question.

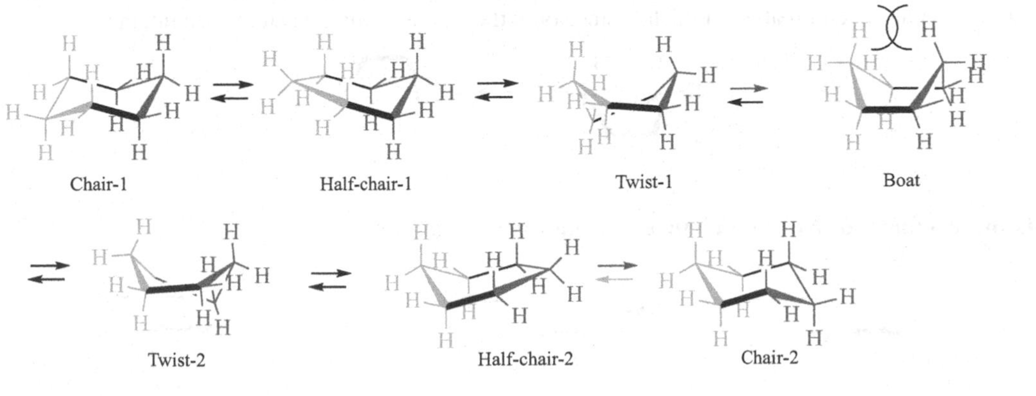

Chair-1 ⇄ Half-chair-1 ⇄ Twist-1 ⇄ Boat

⇄ Twist-2 ⇄ Half-chair-2 ⇄ Chair-2

With a focus on the left side of the six-membered ring, pseudorotation of chair-1 in an "upward" motion leads to half-chair-1, which is particularly unstable, and further pseudorotation leads to a *twist-boat* conformation (twist-1). The pseudorotation of the left side of the molecule leads to a *boat* conformation. Twisting the right side of the boat in a downward motion leads to twist-boat-2, and further pseudorotation leads to the unstable half-chair-2 and finally to the other chair conformation (chair-2). As mentioned, the two half-chair conformations are significantly higher in energy. The twist boat conformations are about 5.5 kcal mol^{-1} (23.0 kJ mol^{-1}) higher in energy than the chairs. The activation energy for the transition of chair-1 to chair-2 is about 10.8 kcal mol^{-1} (45.1 kJ mol^{-1}). The boat conformation is about 5.7 kcal mol^{-1} (23.8 kJ mol^{-1}) higher in energy than the chairs.

What is the energy barrier for chair-to-chair interconversion?

The chair-to-chair interconversion has an energy barrier of 11 kcal mol^{-1} (45 kJ mol^{-1}), but remember that this interconversion is achieved by twisting about the bonds (pseudorotation).

What is a transannular steric interaction?

When atoms or groups that are not connected by a bond come together in space, often due to the conformation of the molecule, there is a steric interaction. In cyclic molecules, such interactions are literally "across the ring," or *transannular.*

What is a flagpole interaction in the boat conformation?

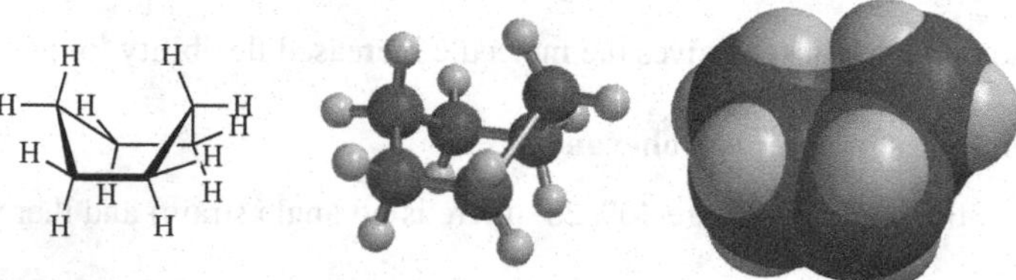

One of the higher energy conformations of cyclohexane is the boat conformation. In the boat conformation, two of the hydrogen atoms, at C1 and C4 (across the ring), are in relatively close proximity. These hydrogens, termed flagpole hydrogens, are close together because of the peculiar conformation of the ring, and there is a transannular steric interaction called a *flagpole interaction.* The flagpole steric interaction contributes to the higher energy of this conformation. The interaction is a little clearer in the molecular model and is particularly easy to see in the space-filling model.

In *cis*-1,4-dichlorocyclohexane, both chlorine atoms are on the same side of the molecule. There are two boat conformations for this molecule, but one is much higher in energy than the other. Why?

The two boat conformations are ***A*** and ***B***. In ***A*** there is clearly a severe transannular (flagpole) steric interaction that makes conformation ***A*** much higher in energy than conformation ***B***, where the flagpole interaction has been greatly diminished since only the smaller hydrogen atoms can interact.

A B

Is there a method to draw a picture of a chair conformation?

-

Yes! First draw two lines that are parallel but offset as shown, make the line in front bold and then place one dot above those lines and ne below as shown. Next, connect those dots to the parallel lines. A chair conformation is drawn again to make it "pretty."

Can a picture of a twist conformation be drawn?

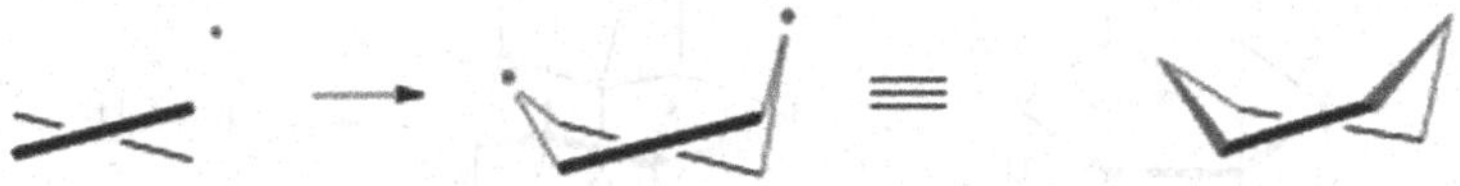

Yes! First draw two lines that are not parallel, make the line in front bold and then place two dots above those lines as shown. Next, connect those dots to the non-parallel lines. A twist conformation is drawn again to make it "pretty."

How many axial hydrogen atoms are there in chair cyclohexane?

Six.

How many axial hydrogen atoms are on each side of a chair conformation?

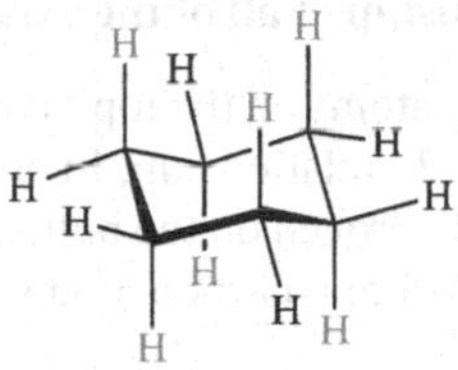

There are *three* axial hydrogen atoms pointed toward the *top* of the chair and *three* hydrogen atoms on the *bottom* of the molecule as it is drawn. In this structure, the axial hydrogen atoms are marked in light gray.

How many equatorial hydrogen atoms are there in chair cyclohexane?

Six.

How many equatorial hydrogen atoms are on each side of a chair conformation?

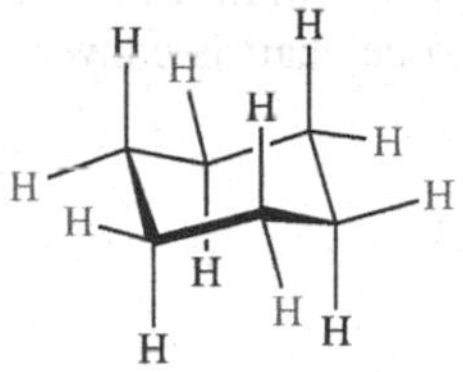

There are six equatorial hydrogen atoms around the "middle" of the molecule, or around the equator of the molecule as it is drawn. In this structure, the equatorial hydrogen atoms are marked in light gray.

Can all of the hydrogen atoms be labeled in planar cyclohexane and also in chair cyclohexane? Label all hydrogen atoms on the "top" of each structure in light gray.

Both planar cyclohexane and chair cyclohexane are shown. Note that these structures have a "top" and a "bottom". Those hydrogen atoms on the "top" side of the structures are marked in light gray. Note that when planar cyclohexane is converted to a chair, the light gray hydrogen atoms are in different relative positions: three in axial positions and three in equatorial positions. Furthermore, the "top" hydrogen atoms alternate axial-equatorial-axial-equatorial-axial-equatorial.

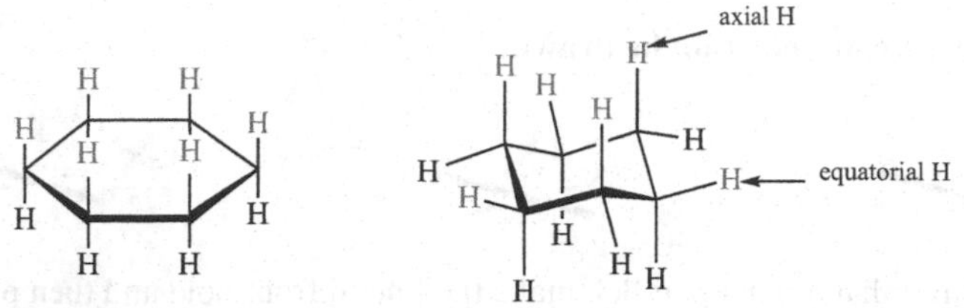

In both structures, all six light gray hydrogen atoms are on "top" of the molecule. In the chair conformation, the top of the chair has three axial hydrogen atoms and three equatorial hydrogen atoms. There are, therefore, three axial bonds and three equatorial bonds on the top side of a chair conformation. Likewise, the "bottom" of the molecule has three axial and three equatorial bonds. *Note that if the top has an axial bond, that carbon will have an equatorial bond on the bottom.* Note that the terms "top" and "bottom" are arbitrary, and simply a device to keep track of the sidedness of the cyclohexane ring.

In chair cyclohexane, what is the relationship of all of the axial hydrogen atoms, one to the other?

Inspection of the light gray axial hydrogen atoms on the top in the previous question shows that the three axial light gray hydrogen atoms have a "1,3" relationship. In other words, there is an axial hydrogen on every third carbon. Similarly, every third hydrogen on the bottom of the chair is axial. Note that the axial hydrogens on top and bottom appear on different carbon atoms.

One chair cyclohexane with the three axial hydrogen atoms on the top is marked in light gray (*A*) and the three axial hydrogen atoms on the bottom are marked in dark gray. What is the other chair (*B*) that results from a "ring "flip?" What is the relationship of the light gray and dark gray hydrogen atoms in *A* relative to *B*?

On the top of ***A***, the light gray axial hydrogen atoms are on C1, C3, C5, whereas the bottom of ***A*** has dark gray axial hydrogen atoms on C2, C4, and C6, where C1 is the carbon on the far left of each chair as it is drawn. In the other chair, ***B***, all six of the axial hydrogen atoms that were axial in ***A*** are equatorial in ***B***. It is clear that the axial-equatorial atoms in one chair are equatorial-axial in the second chair. In this example, the light gray–dark gray hydrogen atoms that are axial in ***A*** become equatorial in ***B***. Similarly, all of the black hydrogen atoms that are equatorial in ***A*** become axial in ***B***. This observation is general. An atom or group in the axial position in one chair is converted to the equatorial position in the other chair that results from pseudorotation.

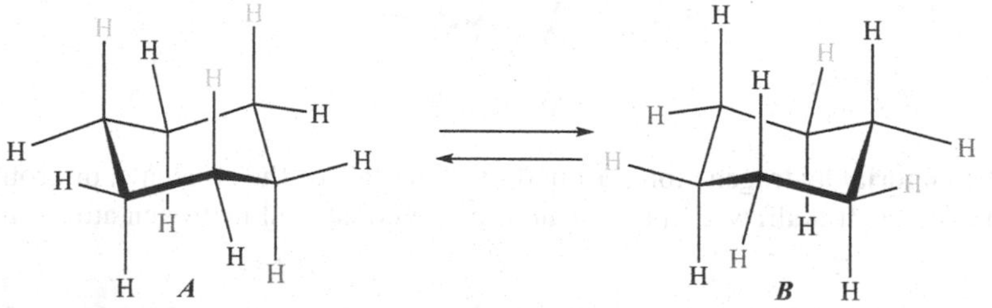

When a hydrogen of cyclohexane is replaced with a methyl group, the molecule is methylcyclohexane and the two chair conformations become non-equivalent. Why?

Remember that there are two chair methylcyclohexanes that are in equilibrium. Further, when the hydrogen atoms of cyclohexane are replaced with alkyl groups (or another group), that group is in an axial position in one chair but because of pseudorotation that group is in an equatorial position in the other chair. Therefore, methylcyclohexane exists in two possible chair conformations, with the methyl in an axial position in one chair conformation as shown and in the other methyl group is in the equatorial position in the other. Therefore, the two chair conformations are different in that one has an axial substituent and the other has an equatorial substituent.

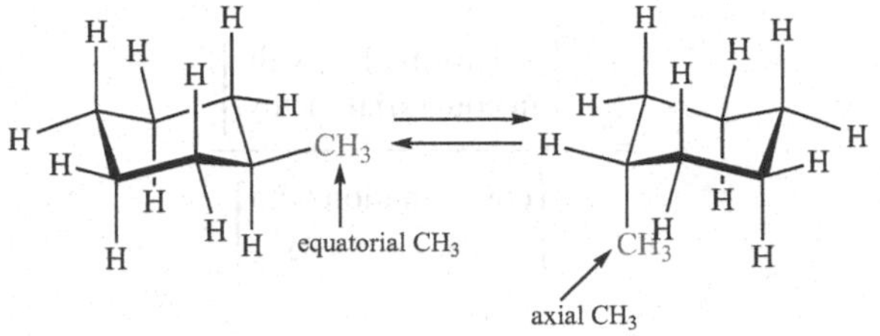

What is A-strain?

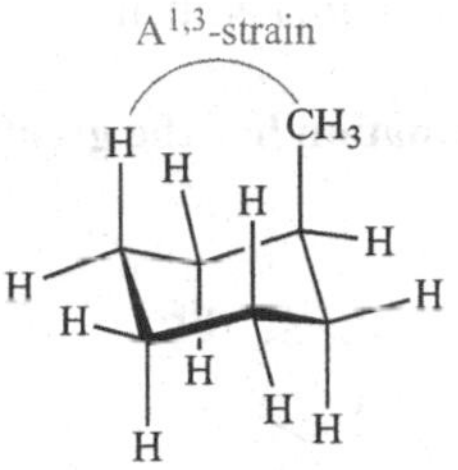

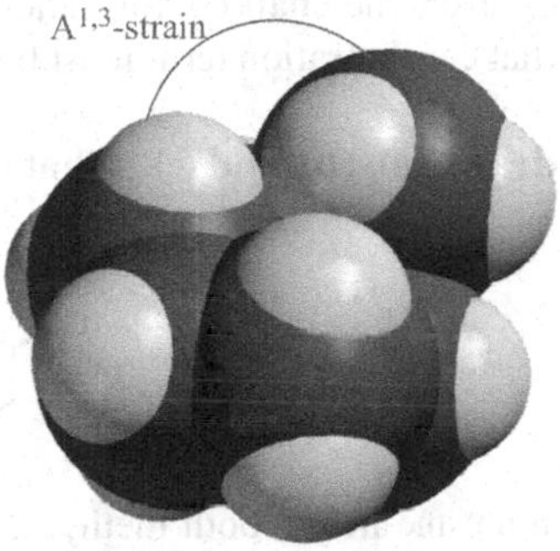

As shown in the figure, the methyl group in methylcyclohexane is in the axial position, which leads to a transannular steric interaction with the other axial hydrogens on that side of the ring. Since every third carbon has an axial bond and therefore an axial hydrogen atom, this transannular interaction is known as a 1,3-diaxial interaction and called *A*^{1,3}*-strain* or just *A-strain*. This interaction known as A-strain only occurs when a hydrogen atom in cyclohexane has been replaced by a different atom or a group. Indeed, the interaction of three axial hydrogens in a chair, as on the "bottom" of the structure is taken as the normal interaction and the is no *A-strain* on that side of the ring. The space-filling model shows the A^{1,3} steric interaction more clearly. The larger the group in the axial position (and the larger number of groups in the axial position), the greater the A-strain and that conformation will have a higher energy. The A^{1,3}-strain due to the methyl group in the axial position makes that conformation higher in energy than the other chair conformation where the methyl group is in the equatorial position. This energy difference (ΔE) for the two chair conformations results in a greater concentration of the conformation where the methyl group is in the lower energy equatorial position.

Which is present in greatest amount at equilibrium, methylcyclohexane with the methyl group in the axial position or in the equatorial position?

Since the chair conformation with the methyl group in the axial position is higher in energy due to A-strain, the equilibrium will shift to favor the lower energy conformation, the chair conformation with the methyl group in the equatorial position.

What parameter is used to determine the position of the equilibrium of the chair conformations in chair cyclohexane?

The equilibrium constant, *K*.

What is the expression for the equilibrium constant for methylcyclohexane as the equilibrium is drawn?

The equilibrium constant expression is:

$$K = \frac{\begin{bmatrix}\text{conformation with} \\ \text{an equatorial methyl}\end{bmatrix}}{\begin{bmatrix}\text{conformation with} \\ \text{an axial methyl}\end{bmatrix}}$$

As presented in the equation for *K* in the preceding question for methylcyclohexane, is *K* larger than 1 or smaller than 1?

Since the equilibrium favors the chair conformation of methylcyclohexane with the methyl group in the equatorial position, that concentration term must be larger, and *K* is greater than 1.

For each molecule drawn (a), (b), and (c). What chair conformation has the greatest amount of A-strain?

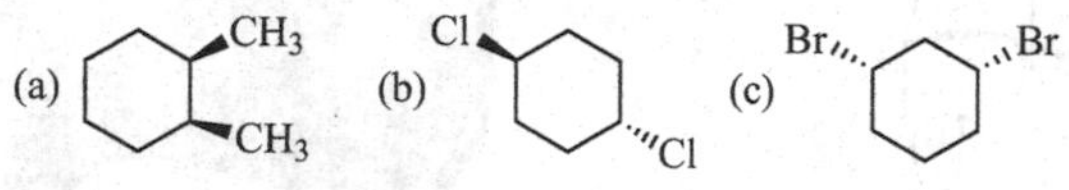

(a) CH_3 CH_3 (b) Cl Cl (c) Br Br

For 1,2-dimethylcyclohexane in (a), both methyl groups are on the same side of the ring, and the two chair conformations are shown. Both structures have one axial methyl and one equatorial methyl group, and they are expected to be equal in energy. In other words, $K = 1$ for this equilibrium.

For 1,4-dichlorocyclohexane in (b), the chlorine units are on opposite sides of the ring, and the two chair conformations are shown. One chair has two axial chlorine atoms whereas the other chair has two equatorial chlorine atoms. Clearly, the A-strain in the chair with two axial chlorine atoms is much greater than the chair with two equatorial chlorine atoms. The equilibrium will favor the di-equatorial chair conformation and $K > 1$ for this equilibrium.

(a) CH_3 CH_3 CH_3 CH_3 ⇌ CH_3 CH_3

(b) Cl Cl Cl Cl ⇌ Cl Cl

(c) Br Br Br Br ⇌ Br Br

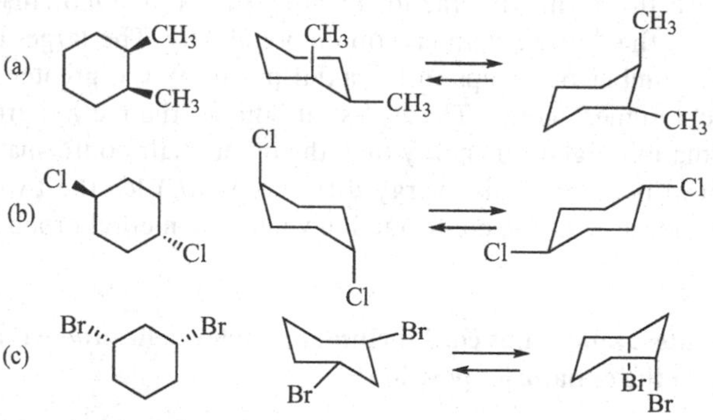

For 1,3-dibromocyclohexane in (c), the bromine units are on opposite sides of the ring, and the two chair conformations are shown. One chair conformation has two axial bromine atoms whereas the other chair has two equatorial bromine atoms. Clearly, the A-strain with the diaxial bromines is much greater than in the conformation with two equatorial bromine atoms. The equilibrium will favor the chair conformation with two equatorial bromine atoms. In other words, $K > 1$ for this equilibrium.

Note that the axial–equatorial relationship of the groups changes when the groups are on the same or opposite sides of the ring, as well as when there is a 1,2-, 1,3-, or 1,4-relationship between the groups.

Attempts to memorize this pattern is possible but can be confusing. It is advised that both chairs be drawn in all questions such as this in order to determine the relationship.

Why do substituted cyclohexane derivatives exist largely in the chair conformation rather than the other conformations available to cyclohexane derivatives?

Chair cyclohexanes predominate as the major conformation of cyclohexane because the boat, half-chair, and twist boat conformations are much higher in energy. Similarly, the envelope form of cyclopentane predominates over the planar form because it is lower in energy. Likewise, methylcyclohexane exists largely in the chair form with the methyl group equatorial.

Why does the equilibrium shift in such a way that for all practical purposes there is only one low energy conformation for *tert*-butylcyclohexane?

The bulky *tert*-butyl group leads to a large amount of A-strain when that group is in the axial position. The 1,3-interaction of the axial *tert*-butyl group with the axial hydrogen atoms is apparent in the molecular model. When the *tert*-butyl group is in the equatorial position, however, three hydrogen atoms are in the axial position, the bulky *tert*-butyl group is in the equatorial position, and there is no A-strain. Therefore, the equilibrium constant for the equilibrium is large and in favor of the chair conformation with the *tert*-butyl groups in the equatorial position. In general, the lowest energy conformation will predominate for any given cyclic alkane. In this case, the energy difference is so large, that *there is much less than 1% of the axial conformation is present at equilibrium.*

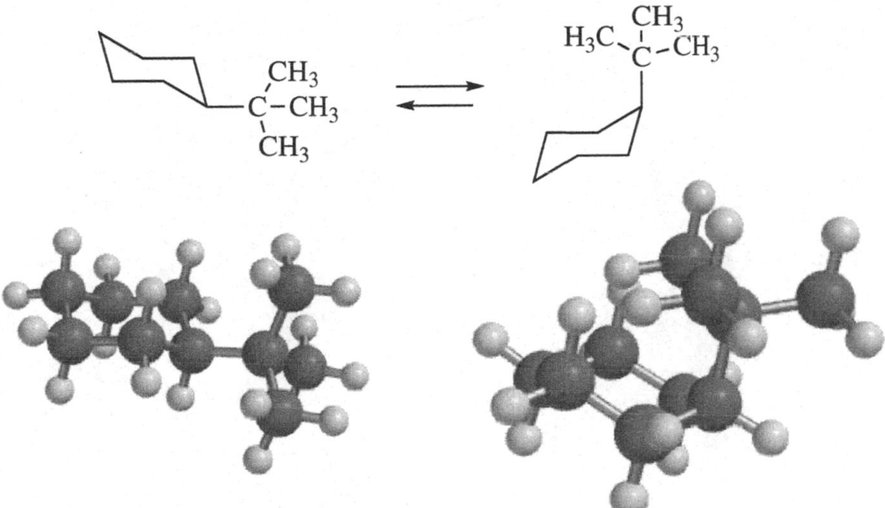

END OF CHAPTER PROBLEMS

1. Draw the highest and lowest energy rotamers for 1,2-dibromoethane, both in sawhorse diagrams and in Newman projection.
2. Draw the two boat conformations that are possible for 1,4-dichlorocyclohexane, where both chlorine atoms are on the same side of the molecules.
3. Of the two boat conformations drawn for Question 2, which is present in higher percentage in the equilibrium mixture? Why?

4. (a) Draw the highest and lowest energy rotamer in Newman projection for the C3–C4 bond of hexane. (b) Draw the highest, lowest, and two different gauche rotamers in Newman projection for 1,2-dibromoethane.
5. Draw the chair form of 1,2,3,4,5,6-hexamethylcyclohexane such that all the methyl groups are equatorial. Now draw the other chair where all methyl groups are axial.
6. Which of the following molecules has the smallest angle strain? Which has the greatest torsion strain? Which has the angle strain greater than the torsion strain?

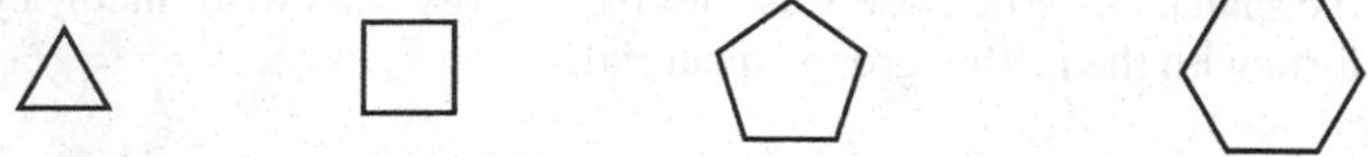

7. Why is the low energy conformation for cyclopentane the envelope rather than the planar conformation when the envelope conformation has more angle strain?
8. Draw both chair conformations for each of the following. Label the highest and lowest energy chair conformation in each case.

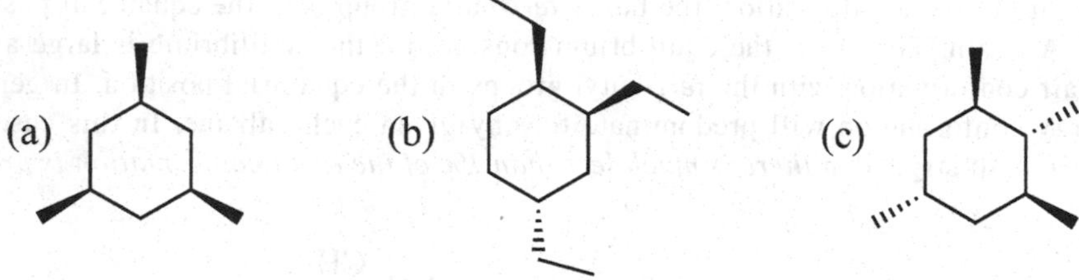

6

Stereochemistry

Organic molecules are three-dimensional, and this property leads to isomers that differ only in their spatial arrangement. Such molecules are called *stereoisomers*, and special properties are associated with stereoisomers that possess stereogenic atoms (an atom that possesses four different groups or atoms). This chapter will introduce the concepts of chirality, including *enantiomers, diastereomers, meso compounds*, and *absolute configuration*. The Cahn–Ingold–Prelog selection rules will be introduced in order to determine the absolute configuration of a stereogenic center. The optical properties of stereogenic molecules will also be discussed, including the highly important physical property, specific rotation.

6.1 CHIRALITY

What is chirality?

When a molecule is asymmetric about a given atom, there is no symmetry in the molecule, and it exhibits a property known as *chirality*. As a result of this asymmetry, the mirror image of such a molecule is a different molecule; that is, the mirror image cannot be superimposed on the original molecule. The property of chirality is important in chemical reactions, and in biological systems.

Is the mirror image of the letter "W" superimposable on another letter of "W?"

Yes! W ⋮ W. The two images are completely superimposable and are, therefore, identical.

Is the mirror image of methane, drawn as a tetrahedron, superimposable on another molecule of methane, also drawn as a tetrahedron?

H H C H H ⋮ H H C H H

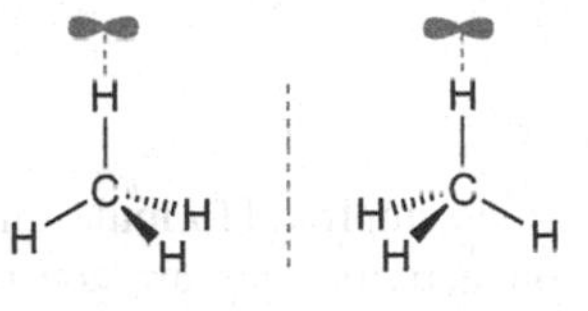

Yes! Simply rotate the mirror image along the axis indicated by 180° and the two structures will superimpose atom for atom. This observation means that the two structures are identical: they are the same molecule.

If 2-bromo-2-chlorobutane is drawn as a tetrahedron with C2 at the center of the tetrahedron, what is the structure of the mirror image of this structure also drawn as a tetrahedron?

Br, H_3CH_2C, C, Cl, CH_3 — Br, Cl, H_3C, C, CH_2CH_3

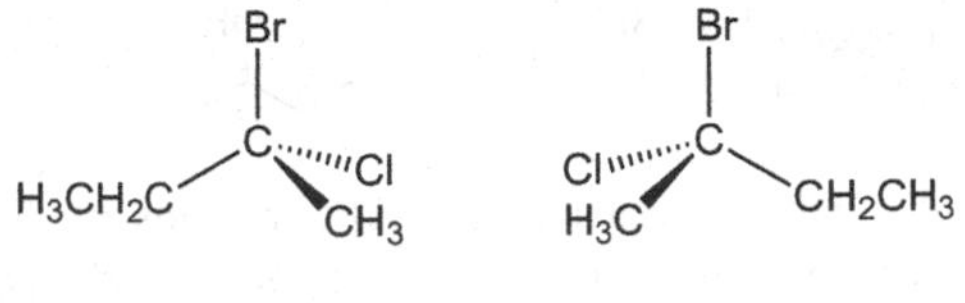

Are the two structures drawn for 2-bromo-2-chlorobutane in the previous question superimposable? Are they the same structure or different structures?

No, the two structures are not superimposable. Models can be made and all attempts to make the superimposition atom for atom will fail. They are different structures. *They are different molecules.*

What is a stereogenic center?

In this book, a *stereogenic center* for carbon (also called an *asymmetric center* or a *chiral center*) is a carbon atom that has four *different* atoms or groups attached to it and possesses no symmetry (it is asymmetric). Any stereogenic atom is asymmetric, including those stereogenic atoms other than carbon. Although a stereogenic atom in this book will be carbon, other atoms may be stereogenic, but they may have a different valence and therefore a different number of atoms or groups attached. An example of a carbon molecule with a stereogenic carbon is 2-bromo-2-chlorobutane in the preceding question. Another example is butan-2-ol: $CH_3CH_2\underline{C}H(OH)CH_3$ where $\underline{C}$ is the stereogenic center. This stereogenic center has a H, an OH, a CH_3, and a CH_2CH_3 attached, so there are four different atoms or groups on the carbon identified as a stereogenic center.

What is the criterion to identify a carbon as a stereogenic carbon?

The carbon atom must have four different atoms or groups, which will give it a mirror image that is not superimposable.

What is an example of a molecule with an atom other than carbon that is stereogenic?

Although this book will focus only on molecules that have a stereogenic carbon atom, stereogenic centers other than carbon are well known. The sulfur molecule shown is known as a sulfoxide. Note that there are three different atoms or groups attached to sulfur and since the valence of sulfur is two, the sulfur takes a positive charge. In this molecule the lone electron pair is counted as a different "group" and the *sulfur is stereogenic.* If an atom has a lone electron pair, it must be considered as a different group, as shown in the example.

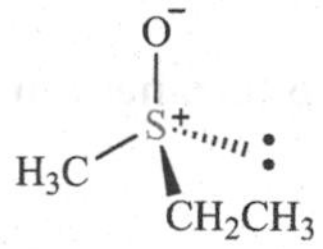

O^- — S^+ (with H_3C, CH_2CH_3, and lone pair :)

What is a stereoisomer?

When two different molecules have the same empirical formula, and they are isomers. If those molecules have the same formula but different connectivity, they are constitutional isomers. If those molecules have the same empirical formula and the same connectivity (all atoms are attached to the same atoms), but they differ in their spatial arrangement about a given atom or point in the molecule, they are called *stereoisomers.* In other words, stereoisomers are isomers with the same empirical formula, the same constitution (the same connectivity), but a different arrangement of atoms in space. The two different molecules 2-bromo-2-chlorobutane and the mirror image discussed in a previous question are stereoisomers.

Which of the following molecules have a stereogenic center?

(a) 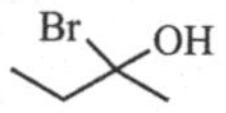 Br, OH (b) 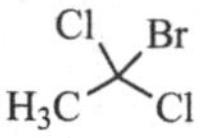 Cl, Br, H_3C, Cl (c) 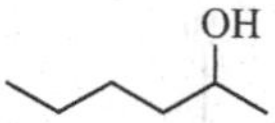 OH (d) 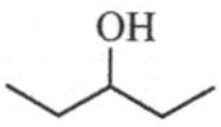 OH

Of these four molecules, (a) and (c) have four different groups or atoms attached to a central carbon atom. Therefore, (a) and (c) have stereogenic centers. Compound (b) has two chlorine atoms and compound (d) has two ethyl groups, and neither (b) nor (d) have a stereogenic center.

What is chirality?

Chirality is a property of molecules where the connectivity and spatial arrangement of atoms lead to asymmetry. The mirror image of that molecule will be a nonsuperimposable and therefore a different molecule. This difference in three-dimensional structure leads to a new type of isomer called a *stereoisomer.* Stereoisomers differ only in the spatial position of their groups. A molecule with this property is said to be *stereogenic* or *chiral.*

What term is used to describe a molecule that has one or more stereogenic centers?

Such molecules are called chiral molecules.

Are there consequences of chirality in a molecule?

Many natural substances are stereogenic, and this property is a key factor in their reactivity, particularly with amino acids and enzymes, saccharides, DNA, and RNA (see Chapters 20 and 21). Stereogenic molecules are also produced by plants and bacteria, and these substances have a variety of properties, including defensive or attractive substances. Differences in stereochemistry in stereogenic molecules are also responsible for the chemicals that trigger odor responses in humans when released into the air from plants or animals. There is an endless list of important chiral molecules.

What is an enantiomer?

Enantiomers are defined as stereoisomers that have non-superimposable mirror images. When a mirror is held up to a molecule possessing a stereogenic center, its *mirror image* is observed. If one tries to superimpose (match every atom in both molecules by laying one on the other), a chiral molecule and its mirror image are *not superimposable.* They are, therefore, *different molecules.* A more precise definition is that two stereoisomers that are non-superimposable mirror images are enantiomers. It is important to understand that recognizing enantiomers as stereoisomers is an important part of the definition.

How can enantiomers of 2-chlorobutane be compared?

In 2-chlorobutane, C2 is stereogenic (a chlorine, a methyl, an ethyl, and a hydrogen are attached to C2). One stereoisomer is ***A*** and its mirror image is ***A′***. They are different molecules because ***A*** and ***A′*** cannot be superimposed. To test superimposability, the molecular models in the figure show the attempt to superimpose ***A*** and ***A′***. The chlorine and hydrogen of C2 of ***A*** and ***A′*** in these models do not match and they are clearly different molecules. Two non-superimposable mirror images of molecules that contain a stereogenic center are called *enantiomers.* Therefore, ***A*** is the enantiomer of ***A′*** and ***A′*** is the enantiomer of ***A***; i.e., ***A*** and ***A′*** are enantiomers!

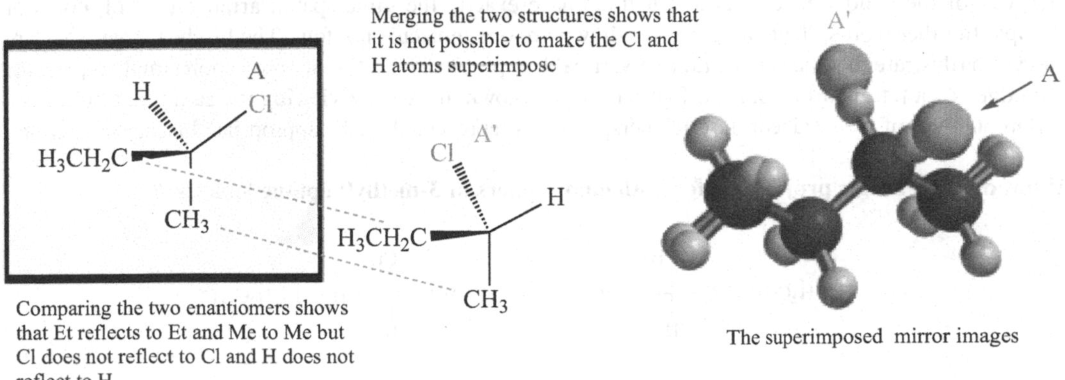

Comparing the two enantiomers shows that Et reflects to Et and Me to Me but Cl does not reflect to Cl and H does not reflect to H

The superimposed mirror images

Are 3-bromopentane and its mirror image enantiomers?

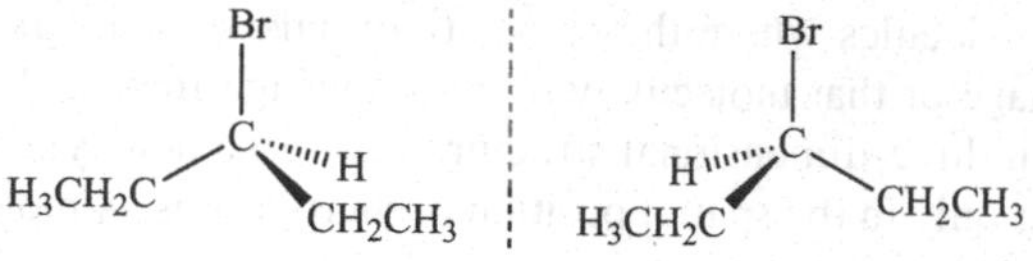

Br, H_3CH_2C, C, H, CH_2CH_3 | Br, H, C, H_3CH_2C, CH_2CH_3

No! Two ethyl groups are connected to the carbon of interest, so that *carbon does not have four different atoms or groups*, and there is no stereogenic center. The two structures shown are the same molecule, not enantiomers. In other words, two molecules that are superimposable are the same.

What is a Fischer projection?

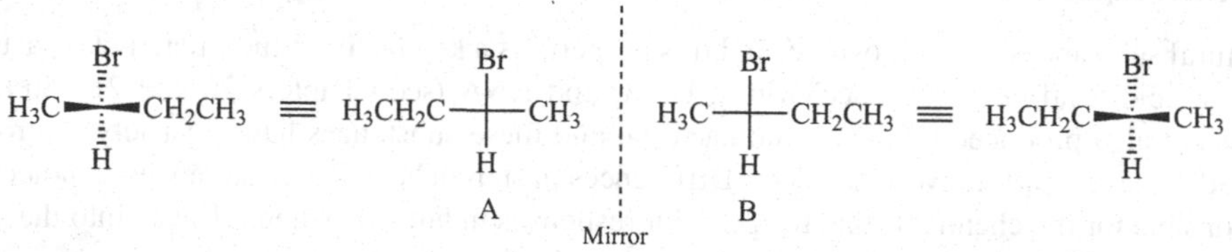

H_3C—C(Br)(H)—CH_2CH_3 ≡ H_3CH_2C—C(Br)(H)—CH_3 (A) | Mirror | H_3C—C(Br)(H)—CH_2CH_3 (B) ≡ H_3CH_2C—C(Br)(H)—CH_3

A convenient notation for molecules containing a stereogenic center involves crossed lines. The horizontal line represents the bonds (and the attached atoms) projected out of the plane of the paper *toward the front.* The vertical line represents bonds projected behind the plane of the paper, *to the rear.* This representation is called a *Fischer projection.* Both enantiomers, ***A*** and ***B***, are drawn with the solid wedges to indicate those atoms/groups are projected in front and with the dashed wedges to indicate those atoms/groups are projected behind. Using this same spatial arrangement, the Fischer projection of both ***A*** and ***B*** is drawn. The solid wedge/dashed wedge structures are shown to indicate the actual stereochemistry represented by the Fischer projection.

What are four different tetrahedron representations of the same stereoisomer of 2-bromobutane? Draw the Fischer projection of each.

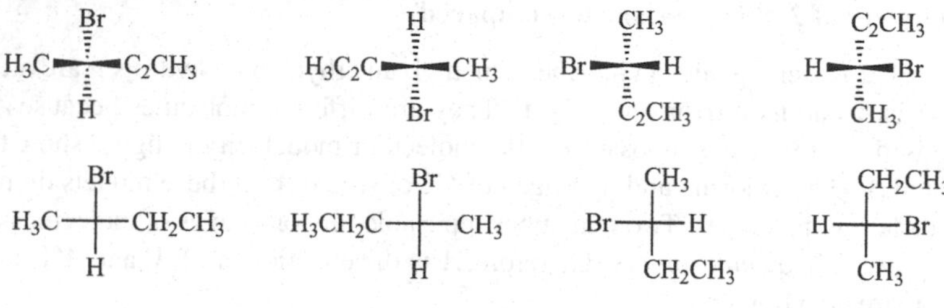

Br / H_3C—C—C_2CH_3 / H; H / H_3C_2C—C—CH_3 / Br; CH_3 / Br—C—H / C_2CH_3; C_2CH_3 / H—C—Br / CH_3

Br / H_3C—C—CH_2CH_3 / H; Br / H_3CH_2C—C—CH_3 / H; CH_3 / Br—C—H / CH_2CH_3; CH_2CH_3 / H—C—Br / CH_3

All four of the solid wedge/dashed structures have exactly the same spatial arrangement of atoms or groups. In other words, the four structures drawn are one molecule not four. The Fischer projections are shown to illustrate that the horizontal line/vertical line protocol for a Fischer projection simply represents the edges of a tetrahedron, and the four structures shown are simply viewing the same molecule from different edges of the tetrahedron. Each perspective is represented by the appropriate Fischer projection.

What do the Fischer projections for both enantiomers of 3-methylheptane look like?

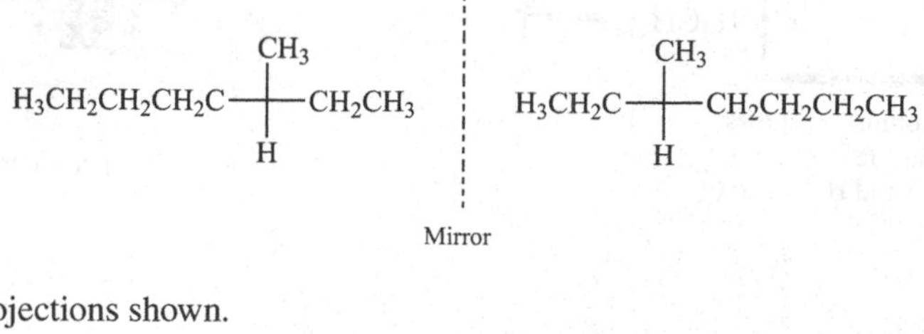

CH_3 / $H_3CH_2CH_2CH_2C$—C—CH_2CH_3 / H | Mirror | CH_3 / H_3CH_2C—C—$CH_2CH_2CH_2CH_3$ / H

The two Fischer projections shown.

6.2 SPECIFIC ROTATION

What is a chiral molecule?

A molecule that does not possess symmetry and rotates plane-polarized light is called a *chiral molecule*. Most of the time, but not always, a chiral molecule will possess one or more stereogenic centers.

What are the physical properties of enantiomers?

Enantiomers have physical properties such as boiling point, melting point, refractive index, etc. that are identical, but they differ in only one physical property. Each enantiomer rotates plane-polarized light in a different direction in what is known as observed rotation. The observed rotation is correlated with the wavelength of light, the concentration, and the physical attributes of the measurement to give a physical property known as specific rotation, which can be used to differentiate enantiomers.

Is it possible to distinguish enantiomers by their physical properties?

This question is essentially the same as that asked in the preceding question. If a molecule contains one stereogenic center, it exists as two enantiomers that are different molecules. They have absolutely identical physical properties (melting point, boiling point, density, solubility, etc.) *except for their ability to interact with plane-polarized light.* One enantiomer will rotate plane-polarized light to the left (counterclockwise), and the other enantiomer will rotate it to the right (clockwise).

What is plane-polarized light?

Plane-polarized light is a light wave in which all photons have the same polarization i.e., the waves oscillate in only one direction. In other words, *polarized light* waves are *light* waves in which the vibrations occur in a single *plane.*

How is the rotation of plane-polarized light measured for a given enantiomer?

The instrument used to measure this property is called a *polarimeter.* The traditional polarimeter that was used prior to the development of electronic polarimeters consisted of a light source with a polarizing filter. The resulting polarized light (i.e., in a single plane) was directed *through* a chamber containing a *solution* of the stereogenic molecule in an appropriate solvent (one that dissolved the stereogenic molecule and did not itself have a stereogenic center). One sighted through the tube containing the sample (in modern instruments this is done electronically), and when compared to a blank (a tube containing only solvent) the angle of the plane-polarized light changed as it passed through the sample. Modern instruments are self-contained, and the sample is placed in the instrument, exposed to plane-polarized light and the angle of rotation is displayed digitally.

In all cases, the angle is measured in degrees (°) and is defined as the *observed rotation, α.*

Can the solvent used in a polarimeter to measure observed rotation for a chiral molecule have a stereogenic center?

No! A solvent with a stereogenic center is a chiral molecule and it would have an observed rotation that was so large, any rotation due to the chiral solute could not be detected. Any solvent used in a polarimeter must not have a stereogenic center. The solvent must be achiral.

If the observed rotation for one pure enantiomer is +60°, can the observed rotation for the enantiomer be deduced?

Yes! The rotation for the mirror image of enantiomer will be equal in magnitude but opposite in sign. If α for a molecule is measured to be +60° for one enantiomer, α for the other enantiomer will be −60°. Note that a (+) denotes clockwise rotation of the plane-polarized light whereas a (−) denotes counterclockwise rotation of the light. The temperature of the experiment (25°C in this case) and the type of light used (sodium D line) are usually included for observed rotation data: i.e., α_D^{25}.

Is observed rotation a physical property of a pure enantiomer?

No! Observed rotation will vary with concentration and solvent and therefore is not a "constant." The physical property is determined using a polarimeter to measure the observed rotation at a specified concentration and path length, at a specified wavelength of the polarized light, and a specified temperature. If these conditions are observed, the observed rotation is converted to *specific rotation*, which is the physical property.

What is specific rotation?

Since the length of the polarimeter tube and the concentration and solvent used may vary, some standardization is required. If the tube is longer, there are more molecules present to interact with plane-polarized light for a given concentration and the observed rotation will be larger. As the concentration increases, there are also more molecules interacting with the light and α increases.

A parameter called *specific rotation* is defined and given the symbol $[\alpha]_D^{25}$ =, measured in degrees (°). The parameters that are important for determination of this physical property are path length (*l*) recorded in decimeters (dm), concentration (c) in g mL^{-1}, and the observed rotation, α. Specific rotation is then given by the expression: $[\alpha]_D^{25} = \frac{\alpha}{(l)(c)}$. Specific rotation is reported with the wavelength of light that is used and also the temperature at which the measurement was made.

If α = +60°, *l* = 5 dm, and c = 1.25 g mL⁻¹, what is the specific rotation at 25°C using the sodium D line?

Using the formula given above, $[\alpha]_D^{25}$ = +9.6°.

If the specific rotation of one enantiomer of butan-2-ol is +13.5°, what is the specific rotation of the other enantiomer?

The magnitude of the specific rotation is the same for both enantiomers. This parameter differs only in sign. If one enantiomer of butan-2-ol has a specific rotation of +13.5°, the other enantiomer must have a specific rotation of –13.5°.

What is a racemic mixture?

The specific rotation of the enantiomers is additive. In other words, the specific rotation of a mixture of the (+) and the (–) enantiomer can be determined by simply adding the (+) term and the (–) terms. A special case arises when there is an equal mixture of the two enantiomers (50:50 mixture of the + and – enantiomer). The (+) term and the (–) term cancel so the specific rotation of the mixture is zero (0). This 50:50 mixture is called a *racemic mixture* (sometimes called a *racemic modification* or simply a *racemate*).

What is the specific rotation of racemic mixture?

The specific rotation = 0 (zero) since the specific rotation of the two enantiomers are additive, equal in magnitude but opposite in sign. The two values must add to zero.

If there are different amounts of two enantiomers (it is not a racemic mixture), are specific rotation values of the two enantiomers additive?

Yes. The specific rotation of the mixture = (value of the + enantiomer) + (value of the – enantiomer).

If one enantiomer has a specific rotation of +60° and its enantiomer is –60°, what is the specific rotation of a 70:30 mixture (+ : –)

Given that the specific rotations are additive, the specific rotation of this mixture can be calculated: $[\alpha]_D^{25} = (+60°)(0.7) + (-60°)(0.3) = +42° + (-18°) = +24°$.

6.3 SEQUENCE RULES

What nomenclature is used to identify different enantiomers?

If enantiomers are different compounds, they must have different names. A set of rules has been devised to allow different names to be assigned to enantiomers. These rules are called the *Cahn–Ingold–Prelog sequence rules.*

Give the IUPAC name for both structures shown.

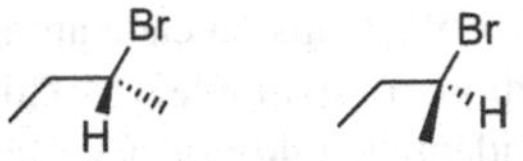

The IUPAC name for *both compounds* is 2-bromobutane. However, they are enantiomers and are different compounds, requiring a different name. Another term must be added to the name in order to distinguish them.

One enantiomer of 2-bromobutane has a specific rotation of –23.1°. Give the structure of the two enantiomers in the previous question; which structure corresponds to this specific rotation?

Examining the specific rotation data for 2-bromobutane raises an interesting question, is the specific rotation of the enantiomer shown + or –? There is *no way* to tell from the structure. Further, *the sign of specific rotation tells nothing about the relative positions of the groups on the stereogenic carbon.* There is an experiment in which the specific rotation is determined over a range of concentrations and temperatures that does give information about the relative positions of groups on a stereogenic center. This phenomenon is called *circular dichroism* but will not be discussed in this book. A protocol will be introduced that can be used to provide a different name to the enantiomers.

What is absolute configuration?

Absolute configuration is the natural spatial arrangement of atoms around a stereogenic center and is an interpretive property, not a physical property. In terms of the importance, this parameter is the parameter used to identify enantiomers as different compounds.

What is a simple method for distinguishing the spatial arrangement of atoms connected to a stereogenic carbon?

Different atoms can be prioritized by their atomic number, where atoms with a higher mass will have a higher priority than atoms with a lower mass.

Is there any correlation between specific rotation and absolute configuration?

No! Specific rotation is a physical property of a molecule that is determined from the interaction of the enantiomers with plane-polarized light. Absolute configuration is the spatial arrangement of atoms around a stereogenic center and prioritizing those atoms is an interpretive property, not a physical property. An enantiomer with a specified absolute configuration could have either a (+) or a (–) specific rotation.

What are the sequence rules used to determine absolute configuration?

A set of rules are used to determine absolute configuration called the *Cahn–Ingold–Prelog selection rules.* The rules are used to assign a designator (*R*) or (*S*) to each enantiomer. The rules assign a priority (a = highest and d = lowest priority) to each *atom* attached to the stereogenic center. It is important to understand that the priority for a group is based on the *atom* attached to the stereogenic center. The first three sequencing rules are as follows:

(1) Working from the point of attachment to the stereogenic center, the first atom encountered is prioritized according to its *atomic number.* Therefore, F > O > N > C > H. (Corollary: If the atoms are the same, higher mass isotopes have a higher atomic number and therefore take the higher priority: therefore, $^{3}H > ^{2}H > ^{1}H$ and $^{18}O > ^{16}O$).

(2) If the atoms are identical (two carbons, for example), proceed outward from the stereogenic center *to the first point of difference*, based on the atoms, not the entire group. Then use Rule 1 to determine the priority.

(3) If the atoms at the first point of difference are identical but the number of substituents on those atoms are different, use the *number* of groups on each atom to determine the priority: (a) three carbons > two carbons > one carbon, for example. (b) This rule is used *only* if the two atoms at the first point of difference are identical and priority cannot be otherwise determined.

What is the "steering wheel" model?

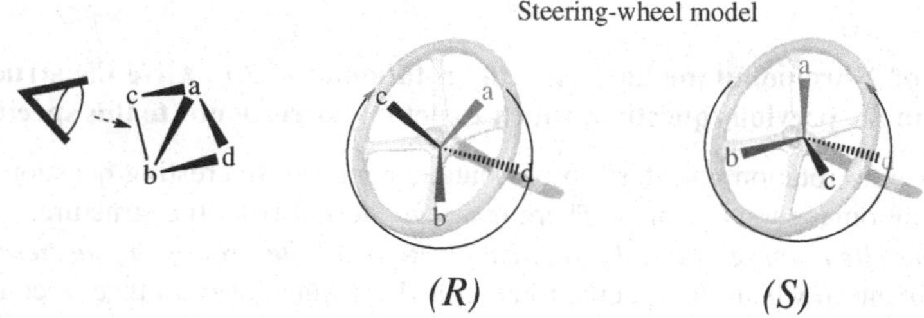

The "*steering wheel*" *model* essentially sights down the base of a tetrahedral array of atoms that "surrounds" the stereogenic carbon. Each point of the tetrahedron (each atom connected to the stereogenic carbon atom) is assigned a priority where (a) is the highest priority and (d) is the lowest priority. The molecule must be turned so that the lowest priority group (d) is *always* to the rear in the model, *before* determining absolute configuration. With the (d) group to the rear, a line is drawn from a → b → c as shown in the "steering wheel" models and if the direction of this line is cl → c → wise, the molecule is assigned the (*R*) configuration. If that line is counterclockwise, the molecule is assigned the (*S*) configuration. The (*R*) or (*S*) absolute configuration, or *handedness*, is part of the name of the enantiomer.

Can the lowest priority atom assume any position in the steering wheel model?

No! The "tetrahedron" must be rotated such that the lowest priority atom is to the rear, which leaves the base of the tetrahedron with the other three atoms or groups projected to the front.

How is the priority from the sequence rules used to name each enantiomer?

With the three rules just cited, many molecules can be assigned as having (*R*) or (*S*) configuration using the so-called "steering wheel" model. In this model, the molecule is rotated to place the lowest priority group away from the viewer. If a line drawn from the highest group (a) → (b) and then to (c) rotates clockwise, the molecules is assigned the (*R*) *configuration.* Therefore, an (*R*)- is placed before the name of that enantiomer. If that line rotates from (a) → (b) → (c) but is counterclockwise, molecules are assigned the (*S*)-configuration. Therefore, an (*S*)- is placed before the name of that enantiomer.

What is the (*R*) and (*S*) absolute configuration of the two enantiomers shown for 2-bromobutane?

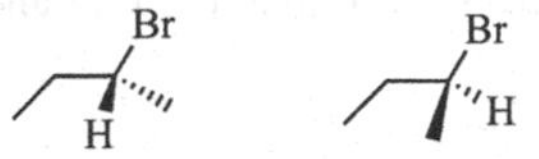

The priority assignments are Br (a), CH_2CH_3 (b), CH_3 (c), and H (d). Using the steering wheel model with (d), which is H, pointed to the rear, the structure on the left is (*R*) and that on the right is (*S*). Therefore, the structure of the left is (*R*)-2-bromobutane and that on the left is (S)-2-bromobutane. Note that the assignment of the ethyl group as higher priority than methyl is based on Rule 2, above.

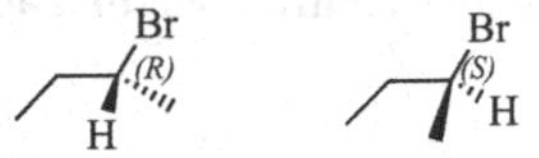

How can the methyl carbon and the ethyl carbon attached to the stereogenic carbon in the preceding question be distinguished?

First, remember that the carbon atoms attached to the stereogenic carbon must be distinguished. A useful method is the identify the atoms attached to each carbon. Therefore, the methyl group can be represented as C^{HHH} and the ethyl group as C^{HHC}, focusing attention on the atoms rather than the group. Since C > H in terms of priority, then C^{HHC} has a higher priority than C^{HHH}.

What is the absolute configuration (*R*) or (*S*) of 1-chloro-1-fluoroethane, giving the proper IUPAC name?

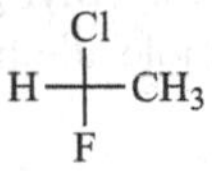

In this example, the atom with the highest atomic number (Rule 1) is chlorine (a), followed by fluorine (b), the carbon of the methyl (c), and, finally, hydrogen (d). These assignments follow Rule 1. This assignment gives a model with the low priority group (d) pointed toward the viewer as shown in the tetrahedron representation. Rotate the molecule to the left to make the (d) group point to the rear in the steering wheel model, and the (c) group is simultaneously rotated to the left by about 120°. This motion *does not break any bonds* and moving (c) moves (a) to the right and (b) rotates to the right. The (a) → (b) → (c) priority is then clockwise, and molecules are assigned the (*R*) configuration. *The IUPAC name is (R)-1-chloro-1-fluoroethane.*

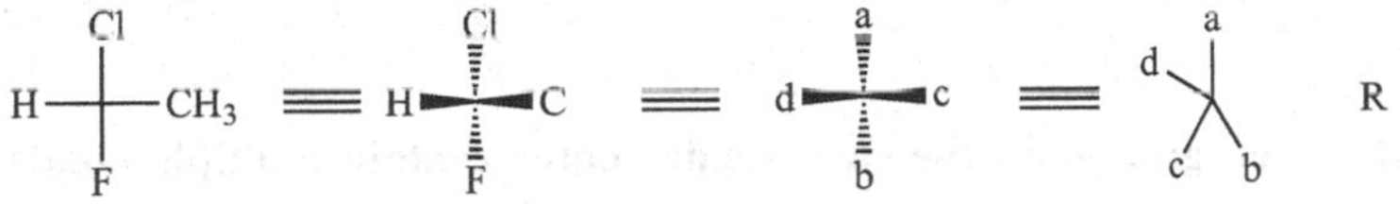

What is the absolute configuration of the enantiomer of hexane-1,3-diol that is shown and what is the proper IUPAC name?

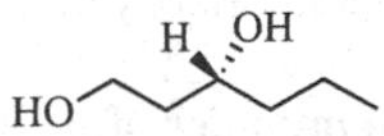

In this example, the highest priority atom is the oxygen of the hydroxyl group (a) attached to the stereogenic carbon, and the lowest priority group (d) is the hydrogen. The next atoms are both carbon, and Rule 1 does not allow for the priority to be assigned. By Rule 2, the first point of difference is the second carbon from the stereogenic center. The first carbons of the two alkyl groups both have one carbon and two hydrogens attached (C^{CHH}) but the next carbons are different (the first point of difference) with one having a C^{CHH} (the propyl) and the other having C^{OCH} (the hydroxyethyl) – see the figure. Since O takes priority over C, the hydroxyethyl group takes priority (b), and the propyl group takes priority (c) (C^{OCH} >

C^{CHH}). This assignment gives a model with the (d) group projected forward. The model must be rotated by 180° to the left to give a model with the (d) group to the rear and this diol has the *R* configuration. *The IUPAC name is (R)-hexane-1,3-diol.*

First point of difference

H OH HO ≡ C^{OHH}-C-C (d, a) C-C-C^{CHH} ≡ (d, a, b, c) ≡ (a, d, c, b) *R*

What is the absolute configuration of the enantiomer of 2-amino-3-ethyl-3-methylbutan-1-ol that is shown, and what is the name?

H_3CH_2C, CH_2OH, $(H_3C)_2HC$, NH_2

In this example, 2-amino-3-ethyl-3-methylbutan-1-ol has the nitrogen attached to the stereogenic carbon as the highest priority (a), but the next three atoms are all carbon. At the first point of difference, the "hydroxymethyl" carbon has two hydrogens and an oxygen (C^{OHH}), and the isopropyl group, C^{CCH}, and the ethyl group, C^{CHH}, are of lesser priority (O > C). The C^{OHH} is clearly higher in priority and takes (b). Using Rules 1 and 2, however, the only atoms available for the (c) and (d) groups are carbon and hydrogen, which are indistinguishable. This situation requires Rule 3, where the number of similar atoms on the carbon at the next point of difference are counted. The C^{CCH} has two carbons to one for the C^{CHH}, so the isopropyl group is (c) and the ethyl group is (d). With this assignment, the model has the (d) group directed to the rear and this molecule has the (*S*)-configuration. *The IUPAC name is (S)-2-amino-3-ethyl-3-methylbutan-1-ol.*

Point of difference

H_3CH_2C, CH_2OH, $(H_3C)_2HC$, NH_2 ≡ HHC_C, C^{OHH}, CCH_C, a ≡ HHC_C, b, CCH_C, a ≡ d, b, c, a *S*

Point of difference

What is the rule when groups on the stereogenic center contain multiple bonds (double or triple)?

Rule (4): If a group on the stereogenic center contains a double or a triple bond, the number of bonds to that atom is taken as the total number of atoms. In other words, a C-C=O is taken to be $\underline{C}^{COO}$, where the underlined carbon is attached to one carbon and *two* oxygens (one O for each bond of the double bond).

What is the absolute configuration the enantiomer of pent-1-en-3-ol that is shown? Assign the name!

H_3CH_2C, CH=CH_2, H, OH

The multiple bond rule is illustrated by the enantiomer shown for pent-1-en-3-ol where the O attached to the stereogenic carbon is the highest priority (a) and the hydrogen is the lowest priority (d). At the first point of difference, the first carbon of the C=C group is assigned to be C^{HCC} due to the double bond (the indicated carbon has one bond to H and two bonds to C where one is the π-bond), so the rule assumes the carbon is attached to two carbon atoms and a hydrogen atom. The ethyl group is C^{CHH}. Rule 3 must be invoked since only carbon and hydrogen are present. In this case, C^{CCH} takes priority (b) over the C^{CHH} which takes priority (c) Rotating the model to the left puts the (d) group to the rear and the molecule has the (*R*)-configuration. *The IUPAC name is (S)-pent-1-en-3-ol.*

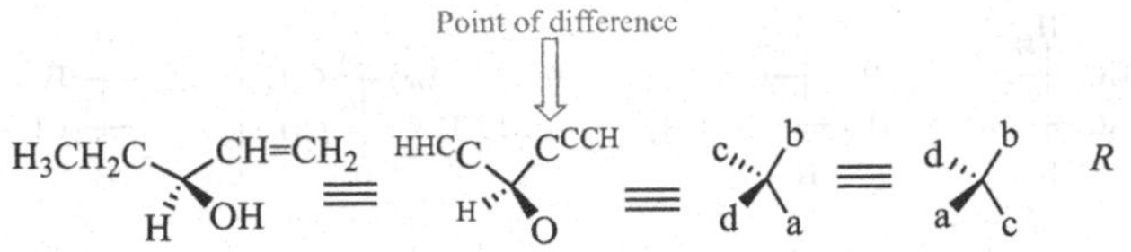

Point of difference

H_3CH_2C $CH{=}CH_2$ H OH ≡ HHC C CCH H O ≡ c b d a ≡ d b a c *R*

6.4 DIASTEREOMERS

What is the consequence for stereoisomers when a molecule has more than one stereogenic center?

When a molecule contains two or more stereogenic centers, it is possible to generate stereoisomers that are different molecules (nonsuperimposable) and are not mirror images. Such stereoisomers are given the term *diastereomer.*

What is a diastereomer?

A diastereomer is defined as a stereoisomer that is a nonsuperimposable, non-mirror image.

Any two different things are nonsuperimposable, non-mirror images, so why is this distinction an important part of the diastereomer definition?

A diastereomer is an isomer of another compound and a stereoisomer of another compound. With the stipulation that compounds must be isomers and stereoisomers, a nonsuperimposable, non-mirror image of another stereoisomer makes sense.

What is the maximum number of stereoisomers for a molecule containing *n* stereogenic centers?

When a molecule has two or more stereogenic centers, there are many more possibilities for stereoisomers. In general, for a stereogenic molecule with n stereogenic centers, there will be a *maximum* of 2^n stereoisomers.

If a molecule has four stereogenic centers, what is the maximum number of stereoisomers that are possible?

For a molecule with four stereogenic centers, the maximum number of stereoisomers is $2^4 = 16$.

For a molecule with 5 stereocenters, can there be more than 32 stereoisomers?

No! There cannot be more than 2^n stereoisomers, which is 32 for 5 stereocenters.

For a molecule with 5 stereocenters, can there be less than 32 stereoisomers?

Yes! There cannot be more than 2^n stereoisomers, which is 32 for 5 stereocenters, but there can be fewer depending on the symmetry of a given structure.

What are all stereoisomers for 2-bromopentan-3-ol?

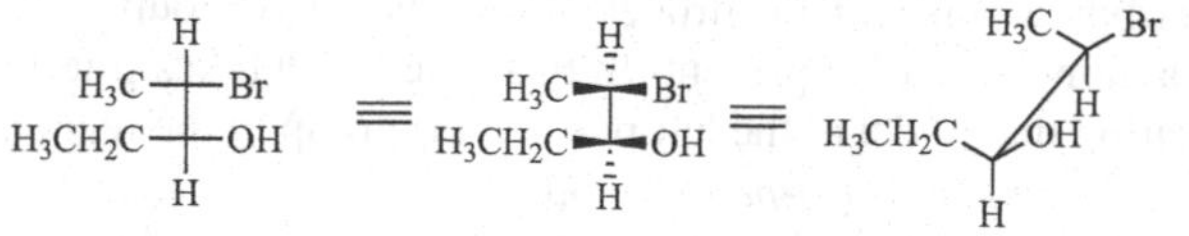

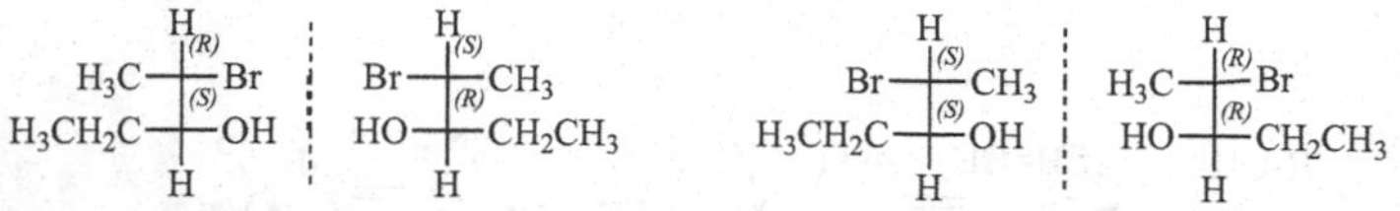

When a molecule has two stereogenic centers, the 2^n rule predicts 2^2, or four stereoisomers. One enantiomer of 2-bromopentan-3-ol is drawn in Fischer projection, but two other representations of this stereoisomer are also given to show the spatial relationship of the atoms or groups. This molecule has an enantiomer, which is shown in Fischer projection. However, these two compounds only constitute two stereoisomers. The initial stereoisomer has the (2*R*,3*S*) configuration and its enantiomer has the (2*S*,3*R*) configuration. If one of the stereogenic centers is *inverted* from 2(*R*) to 2(*S*), giving a diastereomer of the initially drawn stereoisomer, the absolute configuration is now (2*S*,3*S*). This stereoisomer has an enantiomer with the (2*R*,3*R*) configuration. Therefore, there are the four stereoisomers that were predicted. There are two sets of enantiomers, and each enantiomer has two diastereomers.

What is the relationship of (2*R*,3*S*)-, (2*S*,3*R*), (2*S*,3*S*)-, and (2*R*,3*R*)-2-bromopentan-3-ol?

The indicated molecules are clearly stereoisomers, since they have the same empirical formula and the same connectivity. They are, however, non-superimposable, non-mirror image stereoisomers. In other words, they are *different compounds.* The term for stereoisomers that are not superimposable and not mirror images is *diastereomer.* The (2*R*,3*S*) stereoisomer is a diastereomer of the (2*S*,3*S*)- and (2*R*,3*R*)-stereoisomers. The (2*S*,3*R*) stereoisomer is also a diastereomer of these compounds. The (2*S*,3*S*) stereoisomer is a diastereomer of the (2*R*,3*S*)- and (2*S*,3*R*)-stereoisomers. The (2*R*,3*R*) stereoisomer is also a diastereomer of these compounds. Remember both (2*R*,3*S*) and (2*S*,3*R*) are enantiomers, and that (2*S*,3*S*) and (2*R*,3*R*) are enantiomers.

What is a meso compound?

A meso compound is stereoisomer with a *superimposable* mirror image (e.g., the two structures are the same molecule).

Is it possible to have fewer than the number of stereoisomers predicted by the 2ⁿ rule?

Yes! In some cases, a molecule with two or more stereogenic centers will give two stereoisomers that are enantiomers, but the diastereomer (another stereoisomer) will have a *superimposable* mirror image (that is, the two structures are the same molecule). Such a molecule is termed a *meso compound.* Therefore, there are a total of *three* different stereoisomers, *not the predicted four* for two stereogenic centers.

Why does 2,3-dibromobutane have only three stereoisomers?

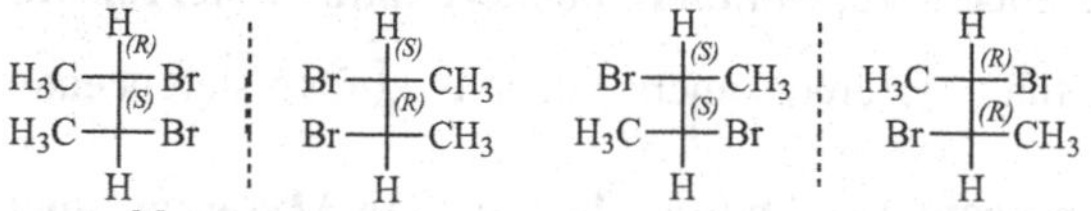

Meso compound

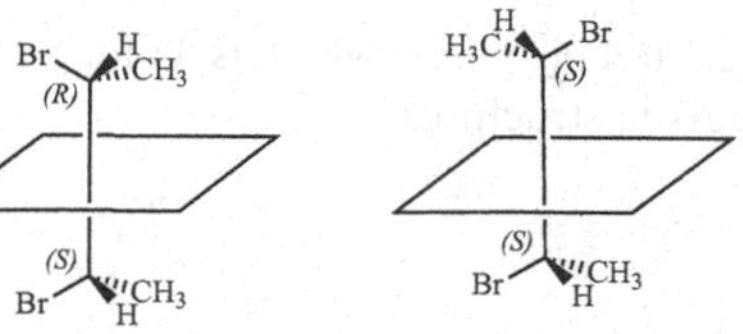

A

Meso compound

B

A simple example of compound with a *meso compound* is 2,3-dibromobutane. The (2*R*,3*S*) stereoisomer has a nonsuperimposable mirror image, (2*S*,3*R*), and they are enantiomers. The diastereomer is the (2*S*,3*S*) stereoisomer, which also has a mirror image, (2*R*,3*R*). However, the (2*S*,3*S*) and (2*R*,3*R*) structures are superimposable mirror images, and therefore identical and a meso compound. They represent only one compound. Therefore, there are only *three stereoisomers*, not four, so the presence of a meso compounds leads to a diminished number of stereoisomers. Close inspection of ***A***, the meso compound, reveals that there is a plane of symmetry that bisects the molecule. In other words, the "top" half of the molecule reflects atom for atom into the "bottom" half *when drawn as the eclipsed rotamer.* Such *symmetry* is characteristic of meso compounds. In other words, if an eclipsed rotamer can be found where every atom superimposes, this will be a meso compound. In examination of ***B***, the model for the (2*R*,3*S*) diastereomer, the enantiomer of (2*S*,3*R*) the Br and H do not superimpose. This lack of symmetry leads to the presence of enantiomers.

Does 1,2-cyclopentanediol have a meso compound?

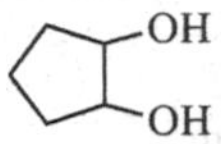

OH
OH

Yes! The (*S*,*S*) and (*R*,*R*) stereoisomers are non-superimposable mirror images and therefore enantiomers. There is a plane of symmetry for the stereoisomer marked (*S*,*R*), where the mirror image of the stereoisomer with both OH groups on one side of the ring is superimposable. There is a plane of symmetry, as marked, and this diastereomer is a meso compound.

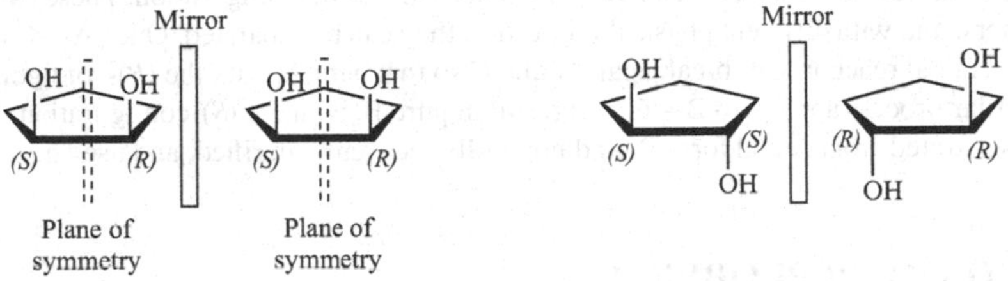

Mirror — Mirror

OH OH — OH OH — OH OH — OH OH
(*S*) (*R*) — (*S*) (*R*) — (*S*) (*S*) — (*R*) (*R*)

Plane of symmetry — Plane of symmetry

6.5 OPTICAL RESOLUTION

Can diastereomers be separated?

Yes! Enantiomers differ only in one physical property, specific rotation. Differences in physical properties are typically used to separate different compounds. Clearly, separation of enantiomers is a problem. A technique has been developed that allows many but not all enantiomers to be separated, but it involves an initial chemical reaction to convert the enantiomers to diastereomers. Since diastereomers are different compounds, they should be separable based on different physical properties, but after separation a second chemical reaction is required to convert the purified diastereomer back to the pure enantiomer.

Is it possible to separate enantiomers one from the other?

No – most of the time! Since enantiomers have the same physical properties of boiling point, melting point, solubility, adsorptivity, etc., it is virtually impossible to physically separate them. Occasionally, the crystal structure of one solid enantiomer is noticeably different enough that it can be selectivity removed (as in Pasteur's separation of tartaric acid by physically picking out the different crystals under a microscope). Most of the time, the only way to separate enantiomers is by a method called optical resolution. Chiral chromatography columns have been developed for the separation of enantiomers. This technique is known as chiral chromatography.

What is optical resolution?

In this technique, the enantiomeric mixture is reacted with another chiral molecule to produce diastereomers as a product of the reaction. Diastereomers are different compounds, with different physical properties. They can, therefore, be physically separated. Once separated, another chemical reaction cleaves the bond between the enantiomer of interest and the second chiral molecule, *resolving* the individual pure enantiomers.

Although chemical reactions have not yet been discussed, is it possible to draw a diagram using A, B, C, etc. to represent molecules in chemical reactions that will illustrate optical resolution?

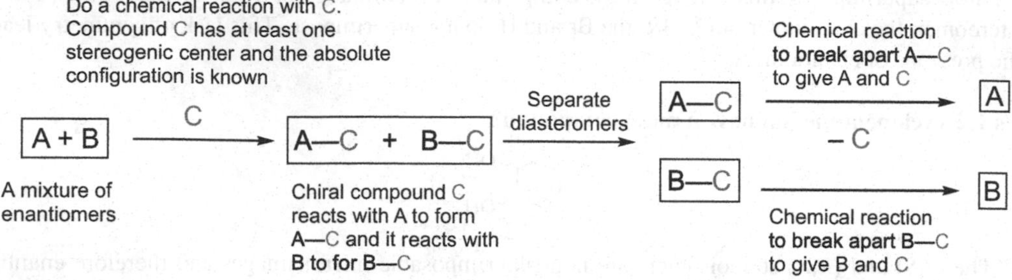

Assume that enantiomer A has the (*R*)-configuration and B has the (*S*)-configuration. For the purpose of illustration, assume that C has the (*R*)-configuration. When C reacts with A, the product A—C will have the (*R*,*R*) configuration, whereas when B reacts, B—C will have the (*S*,*R*) configuration. These two compounds are diastereomers, and with different physical properties, they can be separated. Once A—C is obtained in pure form, a chemical reaction will break apart A and C so that pure A, with the (*R*)-configuration, can be isolated. A similar process applied to B—C will result in pure B, with the (*S*)-configuration. It is assumed that C can be separated from A and form B, and hopefully recovered, purified, and used again.

END OF CHAPTER PROBLEMS

1. Determine the *R* or *S* configuration for each stereogenic center in the following molecules:

(a) CH_2CH_3; Br, CH_3; H, CH_3; CH_3 (b) H, Br; CH_3; Br, H (c) H, OH (d) HO, H; CH_3

(e) CH_3; H; HO, CH_2CH_3 (f) CH_3; H—C≡C—CH_3; OH (g) Cl, Br; CH_3, H (h) H, CH_3; $(CH_3)_3C$, $CH(CH_3)_2$

2. Which of the following are not suitable for use as a solvent in determining the specific rotation of a stereogenic unknown? Explain.

CH_3OH H_2O (CH_3; HO, H) (OH; CH_3) CH_2Cl_2

3. For a polarimeter with a path length of 10 dm, determine the specific rotation for each of the following (concentration is given in brackets with each observed rotation value):

(a) –24.6° (c = 0.47 g/mL) (b) +143.4° (c = 1.31 g/mL) (c) +0.8° (c = 0.65 g/mL)
(d) –83.5° (c = 5.0 g/mL)

4. Calculate the % of *R* and *S* enantiomers present in the following *mixtures* of *R* + *S* enantiomers. In each case, the specific rotation value for the *R* enantiomer is +120°.

   (a) [α] = –14.8° (b) [α] = +109.2° (c) [α] = +4.6° (d) [α] = –18.3°

5. Draw all diastereomers for (a) 2-bromoheptan-3-ol and (b) 4-methyloctan-3-ol using Sawhorse diagrams. Which of the stereoisomers are diastereomers?
6. Draw all different stereoisomers of 2-bromo-3-chloropentane in Fischer projection, and assign the absolute configuration to each stereogenic center. Name each different compound.
7. Discuss the number of stereoisomers possible for butane-2,3-diol and for cyclopentene-2,3-diol.

7

Alkenes and Alkynes: Structure, Nomenclature, and Reactions

Alkenes are a class of compounds characterized by a carbon–carbon double bond (a π-bond), which is highly reactive with a variety of reagents. This π-bond can function as a base in the presence of a suitable acid or as a nucleophile with a suitable electrophile. Reaction of the π-bond with acid generates cations, which can then react with nucleophiles. Alkenes are among the most important of all functional groups due to the versatility of their chemistry. Alkynes react similarly except that only one π-bond will react in most reactions and the product either has a π-bond as part of the structure or reacts to give another product due to the presence of the π-bond.

7.1 STRUCTURE OF ALKENES

What is an alkene?

Alkenes are compounds characterized by one or more C=C units, each comprised of one C—C covalent sigma bond and one π-bond. Alkynes (Section 7.5) are compounds characterized by one or more C≡C units, each comprised on one C—C covalent sigma bond and two π-bonds.

What is a π-bond?

A π bond is a covalent chemical bond formed by the overlap of two lobes of an orbital on one atom with two lobes of an orbital on an adjacent atom.

What is the structure of ethene (the common name is ethylene)?

Ethene (C_2H_4 or $CH_2{=}CH_2$) is the simplest member of the alkene family.

Describe the bonding in ethene.

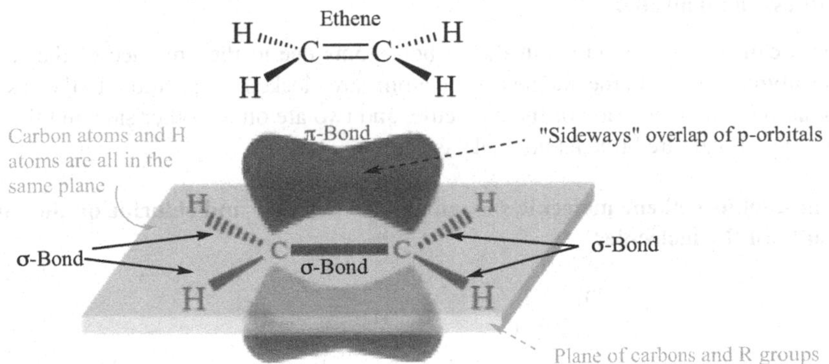

Ethene (C_2H_4 or $CH_2{=}CH_2$) is a planar molecule and has two different kinds of bonds between the carbon atoms: a stronger C—C single bond (called a sigma (or σ-) bond) and a weaker bond called a π-bond. Each type of bond is not apparent when ethene is written as $CH_2{=}CH_2$. To make the bonding between the atoms clearer, the π-bond can be drawn as the "sideways overlap" of p-orbitals, which is represented with electron density above and below the plane of the carbon atoms, as in the figure. The σ-bond (C—C) is a strong bond directed along the line between the two carbon nuclei. The π-bond, however, is formed by overlap of the two parallel p-orbitals on the sp^2 carbons and is therefore much weaker. To be clear, the π-bond is weaker because there is less electron density between the carbon nuclei. It is important to emphasize that only one π-bond is shown in the figure, with lobes above and below the plane of the carbon atoms

Which is the stronger bond in ethene, the σ-bond or the π-bond?

Since the σ-bond has electron density concentrated in a line between the two carbon nuclei, it is very strong. The π-bond has much less electron density concentrated between the carbon nuclei due to the "sideways overlap" of the p-orbitals. Since it has less electron density between the carbon atoms, the π-bond is a weaker bond (more easily broken).

What is the hybridization of the carbon atoms in ethene?

Each carbon of ethene is sp^2-hybridized. Each is trigonal planar, attached to three other atoms and possesses a p-orbital (as part of the π-bond). This sp^2-hybridization is characteristic of the carbon–carbon double bonds of all alkenes.

What is the shape of an sp^2-hybrid orbital?

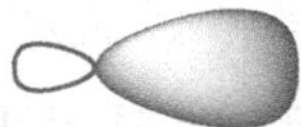

The shape is the same general shape as any other hybrid orbital, with bonding directionality toward the other atom.

Is the sp^2-hybrid orbital used in σ-bonds or in π-bonds?

The sp^2-hybrid orbitals are used to make the σ-bonds of an alkene unit. The π-bonds are the result of sideways overlap of p-orbitals on the sp^2-hybridized carbon atoms.

Is rotation about the C=C unit possible in ethene, or in any alkene?

No! The π-bond effectively prevents rotation about the C=C unit and effectively locks the attached atoms into one position.

Is there sidedness in an alkene?

In ethene, there can be no rotation about the carbon atoms due to the presence of the second bond. Therefore, the atoms attached to the alkene carbon atoms are "locked" in position. In the case of ethene, two hydrogen atoms are on one side of the molecule, and two are on the other side and they cannot be interchanged unless bonds are broken and made again.

In the 1-bromo-2-chloroethene molecule shown, are the bromine and chlorine on the same side or opposite sides of the molecule?

H, Br, C=C, Cl, H — **A**

H, Br, C=C, Cl, H — **B**

In the two representations shown, ***A*** and ***B***, *the bromine and chlorine atoms are on opposite sides.* Both ***A*** and ***B*** show the same molecule. The "sides" are "top" and "bottom" in ***A*** and "front" and "back" in

B. The Br and H are on the bottom side in ***A*** and on the front side in ***B*** (solid wedges). In ***B***, the solid wedges show the Br and H projected to the front, out of the plane of the paper. Similarly, the H and Cl are on the same side, "up" in ***A*** and on the back side in ***B*** (dashed lines). The dashed lines in ***B*** are used to show that the Cl and H are projected behind the plane of the paper. Therefore, Br and Cl are on opposite sides.

It is important to reiterate that there is no rotation about the C=C unit, so the Br and Cl are locked on opposite respective sides in ***A*** or ***B***.

Is a trisubstituted C=C unit more or less stable than a mono-substituted C=C unit?

In general, alkyl groups release electron density to the π-bond of the alkene. This extra electron density strengthens the π-bond, making it more stable. The more highly substituted C=C unit is thermodynamically more stable. Therefore, a tetrasubstituted C=C is more stable than a trisubstituted, which is more stable than a disubstituted, which is more stable than a monosubstituted C=C unit. In principle, the least stable C=C is that in ethene, which has no substituents.

Which alkene is the most thermodynamically stable, 2-methylbut-2-ene or 3-methylbut-1-ene?

The alkene with the most substituents attached to the C=C unit is more stable. A tetrasubstituted alkene is more stable than a trisubstituted alkene, which is more stable than a disubstituted alkene. In this example, 2-methylbut-2-ene is a trisubstituted alkene and is more stable than 3-methylbut-1-ene, a monosubstituted alkene.

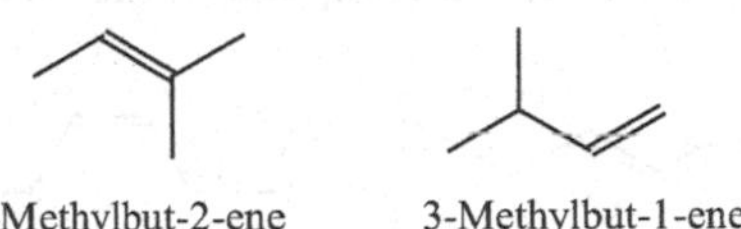

2-Methylbut-2-ene 3-Methylbut-1-ene

7.2 NOMENCLATURE OF ALKENES

What are the IUPAC rules for naming alkenes?

The -ane ending is dropped from the alkane name and replaced with *-ene*. The only rule change that is important involves the C=C unit. The C=C double bond *must* be part of the longest continuous chain and the first carbon of C=C that is encountered must receive the lowest possible number, regardless of the substitution pattern (assuming that C=C is the highest priority functional group).

What is the correct IUPAC name for (a)–(d)?

(a) (b) (c) Br (d)

Alkene (a) has an 8-carbon chain containing the double bond with an ethyl substituent. The name is, therefore, 3-ethyloct-3-ene. Alkene (b) is a cyclic 6-carbon alkene and is called cyclohexene. Numbering for the geminal dimethyl groups (both methyl groups on the same carbon) gives the lowest number 4,4-dimethylcyclohexene (remembering that C1 and C2 of cyclohexene must contain C=C). Alkene (c) is a 7-carbon chain containing one Br, two methyls, and one ethyl. The name is 2-bromo-3-ethyl-4,6-dimethylhept-1-ene. Alkene (d) is a cyclooctene with a methyl and an ethyl group. Since the groups are named and numbered alphabetically, this is 1-ethyl-2-methylcyclooctene.

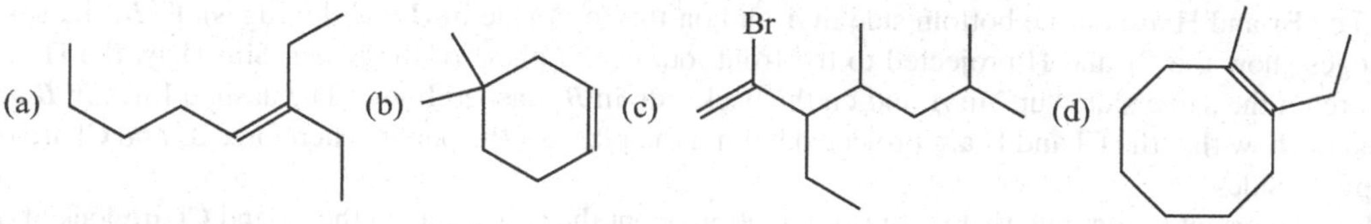

(a) 3-ethyloct-3-ene (b) 4,4-dimethylcyclohex-1-ene (c) 2-bromo-3-ethyl-4,6-dimethylhept-1-ene (d) 1-ethyl-2-methylcyclooct-1-ene

Are alkene isomers based on substituents on the same side or opposite sides stereoisomers?

Yes! The sidedness of alkene substituents leads to a new type of isomer for alkenes. Such positional isomers, where substituents are on the same side or on opposite sides are stereoisomers.

The alkene $CH_3CH_2CH{=}CHCH_2CH_3$ is hex-3-ene, but it exists as two different hex-3-enes. Why are there two different hex-3-enes?

The two different isomers of hex-3-ene are ***A*** and ***B***. The π-bond prevents rotation about the C=C double bond. The two ethyl substituents are, therefore, *locked* in place and cannot be interchanged without breaking and making bonds. In ***A***, the ethyl groups are locked on opposite sides of the molecules, whereas in ***B*** the two ethyl groups are locked on the same side of the molecule. Alkenes ***A*** and ***B*** are different compounds, but they differ only in the relative spatial position of the groups and so they are *stereoisomers*. Since they are different compounds, they require different names to properly identify them.

A B

What is a cis- isomer?

A cis- stereoisomer has two *identical* groups attached to the C=C unit, on the same side of the molecule. Examination of *A* in the previous question shows that there are two *identical substituents* (ethyl) *on the same side of the molecule.* When two identical groups are on the same side of an alkene, the term "cis" is incorporated into the name. Alkene *A* is, therefore, *cis*-hex-3-ene.

What is a trans- isomer?

A trans- stereoisomer has two identical groups attached to the C=C unit, on opposite sides of the molecule. Alkene ***B*** in the previous question has two *identical substituents* (ethyl) *on opposite sides of the molecule.* When two like groups are on opposite sides of an alkene, the term "trans" is incorporated into the name. Alkene ***B*** is, therefore, *trans*-hex-3-ene.

What is the relationship of cis-hex-3-ene and trans-hex-3-ene?

They are stereoisomers. Specifically, they are diastereomers.

Why is there no cis- or trans- designator in the name of 2-methyloct-2-ene?

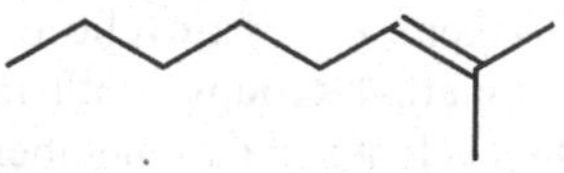

The two identical groups are methyl, but they are both on C1. The cis- and trans- nomenclature is used only when the like groups are on different carbon atoms of the C=C unit. Since the like groups are on the same carbon, there are no cis-/trans- isomers and the name is simply 2-methyloct-2-ene.

Are *A* and *B* stereoisomers?

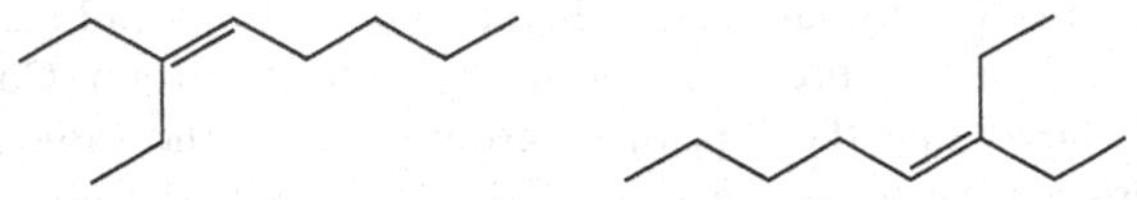

A B

No! Note that both ***A*** and ***B*** are named oct-3-enes with one carbon of the C=C unit that has two attached ethyl groups. Therefore, there will be an ethyl group on each side of the molecule, making the two "sides" identical. In other words, ***A*** and ***B*** are the same molecule (one compound), and not stereoisomers.

What are acceptable names for *A* and *B*?

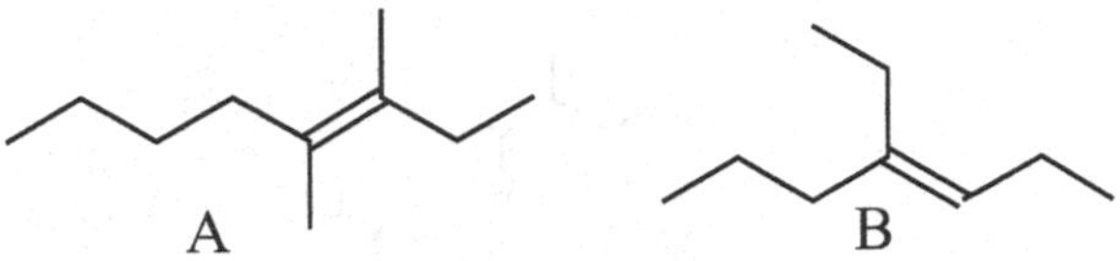

A B

In ***A***, the two identical groups are methyl. Since the methyl on C1 and that on C2 are on opposite sides of the double bond, this is a trans alkene (trans-3,4-dimethyloct-3-ene). In ***B***, the two identical groups are the ethyl groups, and they are on the same side of the double bond. This is a cis- alkene (cis-4-ethylhept-3-ene).

Why do the cis- and trans- names not apply to 2-chloro-3-ethyl-5-methylhex-2-ene?

Cl

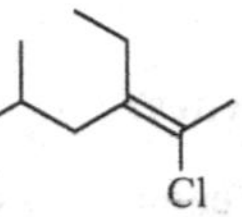

There are no like groups, so the cis- or trans- nomenclature does not apply. Is the Cl cis- to the ethyl or the 2-methylpropyl group, for example? A different nomenclature system is required to properly name compounds such as this.

In 2-chloro-3-ethyl-5-methylhex-2-ene, a methyl and a chlorine atom are on C2. Using the Cahn–Ingold–Prelog selection rules, which is higher in priority?

The chlorine atom is higher in priority relative to the methyl group.

In 2-chloro-3-ethyl-5-methylhex-2-ene, an ethyl and a 2-methylpropyl are on C3. Using the Cahn–Ingold–Prelog selection rules, which is higher in priority?

The 2-methylpropyl group (C^{CCH}) is higher in priority relative to the ethyl group (C^{CHH}).

Are the high priority groups on C2 and C3 in 2-chloro-3-ethyl-5-methylhex-2-ene on the same side or the opposite side?

In 2-chloro-3-ethyl-5-methylhex-2-ene, the chlorine and the 2-methylpropyl are on the same side.

What is the *E-*/*Z-* nomenclature system?

This system is based on a comparison of the substituents of each carbon of the double bond. The substituents are assigned a priority based on the Cahn–Ingold–Prelog selection rules introduced in Section 6.3. Using 2-chloro-3-ethyl-5-methylhex-2-ene as an example, one carbon of the double bond has a chlorine and a methyl substituent. Since Cl > C, the chorine is the highest priority group. The other carbon of the double bond has an ethyl group and a 2-methylpropyl group. Using the sequence rules, 2-methyl-propyl is the higher priority group. Comparing the chlorine and the 2-methylpropyl shows that these priority groups are on the same side of the molecule. When the priority groups are on the same side of the C=C unit, the notation is *Z*- (for *zusammen* = together). If the priority groups are on the opposite side of the C=C unit, the notation is *E*- (for *entgegen* = apart or opposite). The full name for 2-chloro-3-ethyl-5-methylhex-2-ene is 2-chloro-3-ethyl-5-methylhex-2*Z*-ene.

This protocol involves determining the priority of the two groups on one carbon of the double bond, determining the priority of the two groups on the other carbon of the double bond, and then determining if the priority groups are on the same side (*Z*-) or the opposite side (*E*-).

What is the IUPAC name of the molecule shown?

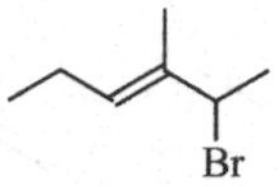

Br

This alkene is an example of an *E*- alkene. The first carbon has a methyl group and a 1-bromoethyl group, with the latter having the higher priority. The other carbon has an ethyl group and a hydrogen, with the ethyl being the higher priority. The ethyl group and the 1-bromoethyl group are on opposite sides of the double bond, making this example an *E*- alkene. The name is 2-bromo-3-methylhex-3*E*-ene.

7.3 REACTIONS OF ALKENES

What types of reactions are common to alkenes?

Acid–base reactions. The π-bond of an alkene can react as a Brønsted–Lowry base in the presence of an acidic compound, or as an electron donor in the presence of an atom that can react as a Lewis acid. When the reaction is with a Brønsted–Lowry acid, an intermediate called a carbocation is formed, which can react with a variety of electron donating species to give new functional groups.

Is the π-bond of an alkene electron rich or electron poor?

The π-bond of an alkene is electron rich. Since the π-bond is much weaker than a covalent σ-bond, the electrons of a π-bond can be donated to an electron deficient atom in many cases.

What is a carbocation?

A carbocation is a trisubstituted positively charged carbon species. A carbocation is a transient product, an intermediate that is an electron-deficient carbon atom bearing a positive charge.

What is the formal charge on a carbocation?

Positive! The formal charge is +1.

What is the structure of a carbocation?

The structure is R_3C^+, R_2CH^+, or RCH_2^+, where R is any alkyl group. The carbon is sp^2-hybridized, and the carbocation has a trigonal planar array of atoms or groups about the positively charged carbon. Note that the planar carbocation has only three substituents on the positive carbon so there is no stereochemistry associated with the carbocation.

Is a carbocation a high energy or a low energy compound?

A carbocation is a high energy intermediate, so it is a highly reactive transient product.

What is an intermediate?

An intermediate is an unstable, highly reactive transient product.

Once formed, is a carbocation usually an isolated product?

No! A carbocation is an unstable, highly reactive species and once formed it is rarely stable enough to be isolated.

If an alkene were mixed with an acid, H^+, what reaction is possible?

The π-bond of the alkene can donate two electrons to H^+. It is therefore a Brønsted–Lowry base. This reaction breaks the π-bond, and a new C—H bond is formed to one carbon of the C=C unit, leaving an electron-deficient carbon with a positive charge on the remaining carbon. The positively charged species is a carbocation, a highly reactive intermediate. Using 2-methylprop-1-ene as an example, reaction with H^+ generates a carbocation.

$$(H_3C)_2C{=}CH_2 \quad H^+ \longrightarrow (H_3C)_2\overset{+}{C}{-}CH_2H$$

A Carbocation

What is H^+?

The symbol H^+ is used for a Brønsted–Lowry acid such as HCl, H_2SO_4, HNO_3, etc. when the acid is dissolved in a solvent that supports ionization, such as water.

The reaction of 2-methylpropene and H^+ is what type of reaction?

The reaction of the π-bond of an alkene with an acid (H^+) is an acid–base reaction, where the alkene reacts as a base.

What is a primary carbocation? A secondary carbocation? A tertiary carbocation?

A primary carbocation has one carbon group and two hydrogen atoms attached to C^+ of RH_2C^+. A secondary carbocation has two carbon groups and one hydrogen atom attached to C^+ of R_2HC^+. A tertiary carbocation has three carbon groups and no hydrogen atoms attached to C^+ of R_3C^+.

Why is a tertiary carbocation more stable than a primary carbocation?

Carbon groups are electron-releasing relative to C^+. Therefore, the more carbon groups attached to the positive carbon of a carbocation "feed" electron density toward C^+. In general, an atom with a high charge is more unstable and more reactive than an atom with a low charge. The more electron density transferred toward C^+ diminishes the net charge and makes the species more stable. In other words, a carbocation with more carbon substituents is more stable than a carbocation with less carbon substituents. Therefore, a tertiary carbocation is more stable than a secondary, which is more stable than a primary. To complete the list, a primary carbocation (RH_2C^+) is more stable than the methyl carbocation (H_3C^+).

When prop-1-ene reacts with H^+, the proton can attach to one of two carbon atoms of the C=C unit. Is one carbocation product preferred?

Yes! The two possible products are ***A*** and ***B***. However, ***A*** is a primary carbocation whereas ***B*** is a secondary carbocation. The secondary carbocation (***B***) is much more stable and is formed preferentially.

Another way to make this statement is that the transition state leading to ***B*** is lower than that leading to ***A***, so the product of this reaction is ***B***.

$$\underset{\mathbf{A}}{H_2\overset{+}{C}-CH(CH_3)H} \longleftarrow H^+ + H_3C-HC{=}CH_2 \; H^+ \longrightarrow \underset{\mathbf{B}}{H_3C-\overset{+}{HC}-CH_2H}$$

What is a transition state?

At some point in a reaction, the bond between two atoms, A and B, must begin to form. It is not yet a formal bond, but the bond-making process has begun and is represented by [A-----B] and is known as the *transition state.* A transition state cannot be isolated, or even observed. *A transition state is the logical mid-point of a reaction and it is an energy associated with making and breaking bonds as the reaction proceeds.*

Why is the more stable transition state likely to predict the more stable product in this reaction?

Energy! If the transition state for a reaction is closer in energy to the products than to the starting materials, the more stable transition state of two or more possible transition states will predict the major product.

What is the *Curtin–Hammett principle*?

The *Curtin–Hammett principle* is a principle in chemical kinetics that states: for a reaction that has a pair of reactive intermediates each going irreversibly to a different product, the product ratio will depend on the free energy of the transition state going to each product.

Which is the more stable carbocation, that derived from prop-1-ene or that from 2-methylprop-1-ene? Explain.

The secondary carbocation ***A*** is formed as the major product by the reaction of prop-1-ene and H^+. The reaction of 2-methylprop-1-ene and H^+ gives the tertiary carbocation ***B*** as the major product. Comparing the tertiary carbocation ***B*** and the secondary carbocation ***A***, the more stable tertiary carbocation ***B*** is more stable.

$$(H_3C)(H)C{=}CH_2 \; H^+ \longrightarrow \underset{\mathbf{A}}{H_3C-\overset{+}{HC}-CH_2H} \qquad (H_3C)_2C{=}CH_2 \; H^+ \longrightarrow \underset{\mathbf{B}}{(H_3C)_2\overset{+}{C}-CH_2H}$$

What is a nucleophile?

A nucleophile is an electron rich species that *donates two electrons to a carbon* to form a new covalent bond.

When a carbocation such as *B* from 2-methylprop-1-ene in the preceding question is formed, what can it react with?

The carbocation can react with any reasonable nucleophile. In many cases, the nucleophile is X^-, the counterion of an acid (H—X). The reaction with the positive carbon on the carbocation will form a new C—X bond.

What is the major product when 2-methylprop-1-ene reacts with HCl?

The major product of this reaction is 2-chloro-2-methylpopane.

What is the final product of the reaction of 1-methylprop-1-ene and HCl and what is the structure of the carbocation intermediate?

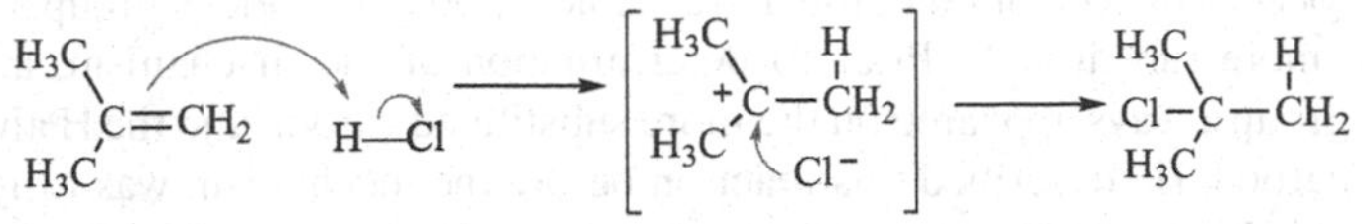

The initial reaction with the alkene generates the tertiary carbocation with the chloride ion as the counterion. The chloride ion is electron rich and reacts as a nucleophile with the carbocation to form a new C—Cl bond in the final product, 2-cloro-2-methylpropane. Note that the carbocation is written within brackets to indicate it is a transient product: an *intermediate.*

What is a mechanism?

A mechanism is the step-by-step pathway for a chemical reaction that includes all products and all intermediates. Both the final product and the intermediate are shown in the answer to the preceding question. Indeed, drawing the starting materials 2-chloro-2-methylpropane and HCl, the product 2-methylprop-1-ene and the tertiary carbocation intermediate constitutes the mechanism of this reaction.

What is the mechanism for the reaction of prop-1-ene with HCl?

The π-bond of the alkene reacts as a Brønsted–Lowry base, donating two electrons to the acidic proton of HCl. This reaction forms a new C—H bond and generates the more stable secondary carbocation. The nucleophilic chloride ion donates electrons to (attacks) the cationic center to form a C—Cl bond and give the final product, 2-chloropropane.

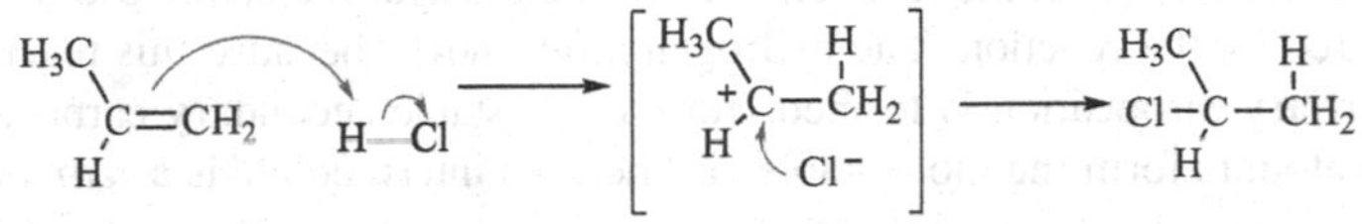

What is the mechanism for the transformation of methylcyclohexene into 1-bromo-1-methylcycloexane by reaction with HBr?

The π-bond the alkene reacts as a base and donates two electrons to the proton of HBr, giving a tertiary carbocation intermediate. The nucleophilic counterion (Br^-) attacks the electrophilic carbon of the carbocation to give the final product, 1-bromo-1-methylcyclohexane.

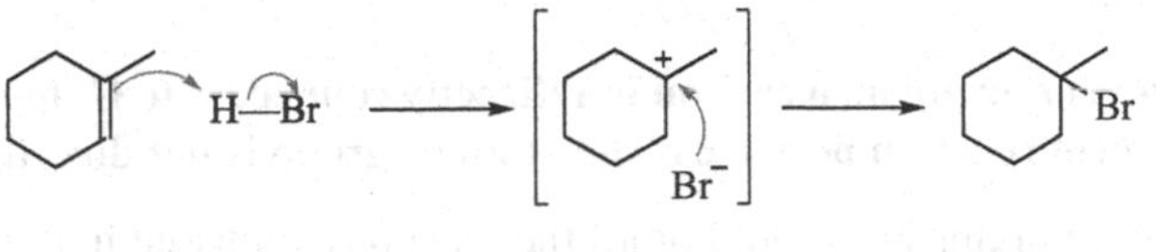

When 2-methylpent-2-ene reacts with HCl, the proton can be transferred to two different carbons. What are both possible cationic intermediates and then the major product?

When 2-methylpent-1-ene reacts with HCl, the two carbocation intermediates are the tertiary carbocation (***B***) and the primary carbocation (***A***), and the tertiary carbocation (***B***) is more stable. Subsequent reaction with nucleophilic chloride ion gives 2-chloro-2-methylpentae as the major isolated product.

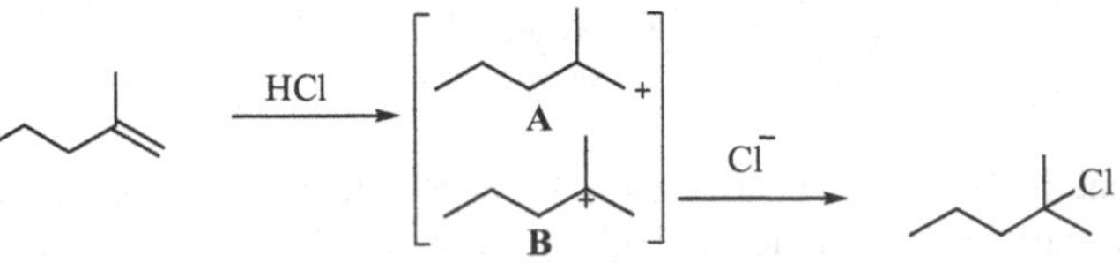

What common name is given to the reaction of alkene with acids of the type HX, where the X group in the major product is always on the more substituted carbon?

Since the reaction proceeds by formation of the more stable carbocation, the X group will always appear on that carbon (the more substituted). Prior to determination of the mechanism, a Russian chemist observed that the X group always appeared on the more substituted carbon and the H always appeared on the less substituted carbon. He described this reaction before the mechanism was fully understood; the reaction is named in his honor. *This type of reaction was then and is now called Markovnikov addition.*

What is the major product isolated when 3-methylpent-1-ene reacts with HBr?

The major product is *not* 2-bromo-3-methylpentane but rather 3-bromo-3-methylpentane.

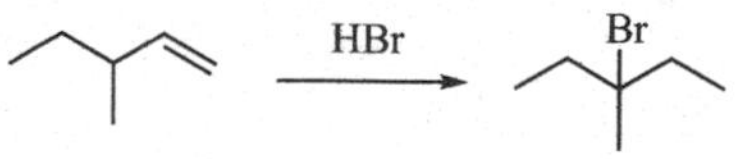

HBr
Br

3-Methylpent-1-ene reacts with HBr to give the secondary carbocation, but if 3-bromo-3-methylpentane is the major product, an atom has moved. What atom has moved?

The hydrogen atom on C3 in the initially formed secondary carbocation has moved to C2, forming a tertiary carbocation *before* the reaction with the bromide ion.

Why should a hydrogen atom move from C3 in the secondary carbocation to C2 in a tertiary carbocation?

The tertiary carbocation is more stable than the initially formed secondary carbocation by 12–15 kcal mol^{-1}. This energy difference makes the reaction that moved the hydrogen atom exothermic, and it is the energetic driving force for the reaction. The hydrogen atom moves because this reaction gives a more stable product: a tertiary carbocation is formed from a less stable secondary carbocation. The movement of a hydrogen atom to form the more stable carbocation intermediate is a *rearrangement* called a *1,2-hydide shift.*

What is the energy difference between a tertiary carbocation and a secondary carbocation? Between a secondary carbocation and a primary carbocation?

A tertiary carbocation is 12–15 kcal mol^{-1} (50.2–62.8 kJ mol^{-1}) more stable than a secondary carbocation. A secondary carbocation is 12–15 kcal mol^{-1} (50.2–62.8 kJ mol^{-1}) more stable than a primary carbocation.

Is it possible for an atom or group on a carbon not directly connected to C^+ to migrate? In other words, is a rearrangement reaction possible if the atom or group is not directly attached to C^+?

For the reactions discussed in this book, no! For all the reactions discussed in this book, only atoms or groups directly attached to C^+ can migrate.

What is the mechanism of the reaction of 3-methylpen-1-ene with HBr?

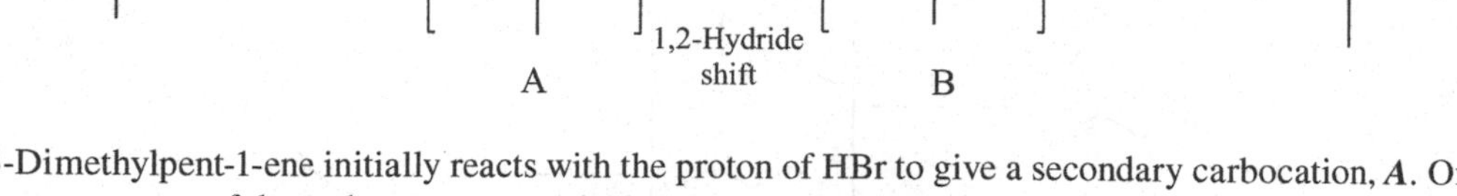

HBr
+
1,2-Hydride shift
A
+
B
Br^-
Br

3,3-Dimethylpent-1-ene initially reacts with the proton of HBr to give a secondary carbocation, ***A***. Only atoms or groups of the carbon atoms attached to C^+ can migrate, leading to a rearrangement. A hydrogen atom is available on the adjacent primary carbon and also on the adjacent tertiary carbon. If the hydrogen atom moves from the primary carbon, a less stable primary carbocation will result, and *such a reaction to give a less stable product will not occur* because it is an endothermic process. However, if the hydrogen atom moves from C3, the tertiary carbon, the product is a more stable tertiary carbocation, ***B***. This reaction of a hydrogen atom moving to an adjacent carbon to give a more stable carbocation is called a *1,2-hydride shift* and represented by the "curly" arrow shown. The mechanism shown involves drawing the starting material, the final product, and all intermediates.

Why does a rearrangement occur before the nucleophile can react with C+?

The rate of the rearrangement reaction is much faster than the rate of the reaction of the nucleophile with C^+. In other words, $k_{\text{rearrangement}} >> k_{\text{substitution}}$.

What is $k_{\text{rearrangement}}$ and what is $k_{\text{substitution}}$?

The term $k_{\text{rearrangement}}$ is the rate of rearrangement of the carbocation and $k_{\text{substitution}}$ is the rate of substitution by the nucleophile.

The mid-point of the 1,2-hyride shift just discussed will be a transition state that cannot be isolated or observed yet must have the moving hydrogen atom between C2 and C3. What is the structure of the transition state?

What is the hydration reaction of an alkene?

When an alkene reacts with a Brønsted–Lowry acid such as HCl, in the presence of water a carbocation intermediate is generated as expected. In the reactions described for HCl and HBr (also HI), the carbocation intermediate reacts with the nucleophilic counterion of the acid to give the final addition product. If, however, the counterion of HX is a weak base and a weak nucleophile (poor reactivity) the reaction with the carbocation is slow. If the water is a stronger nucleophile than the counterion X^-, the water reacts with the carbocation faster and preferentially. The reaction of a carbocation with water gives a new intermediate called an *oxonium ion*, which loses a proton in an acid–base reaction to give an alcohol product. The conversion of an alkene to an alcohol by such a mechanism is called *hydration*.

What is generic structure of an oxonium ion?

oxonium ion

What is the product when 2,4-dimethylhex-1-ene is heated in water?

There is no reaction. Water is not a sufficiently strong acid to react with the weak base (the π-bond of the alkene).

The conjugate base of H_2SO_4 is the hydrogen sulfate anion, HSO_4^-. Is this anion a good nucleophile?

No! The hydrogen sulfate anion is resonance stabilized, so the charge is dispersed over several atoms. Since the charge is not concentrated but rather dispersed, electron donation is very difficult, and the hydrogen sulfate anion is a very weak nucleophile. In other words, it is very unreactive and does not react well with C^+; it is a weak nucleophile.

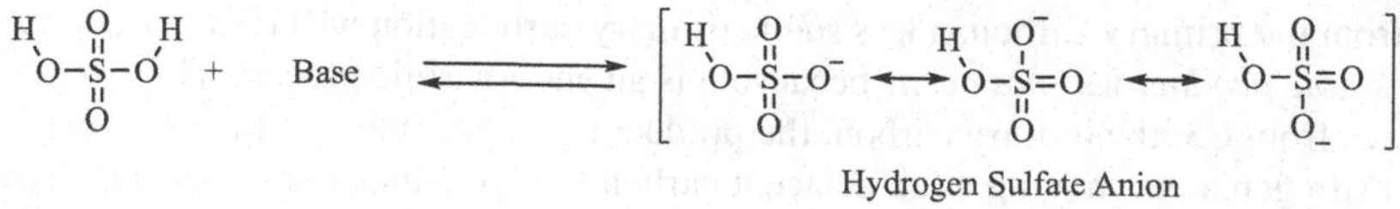

Hydrogen Sulfate Anion

If a catalytic amount of H_2SO_4 is added to the reaction of methylcyclohexene and water, what is the result?

The strong acid catalyst (H_2SO_4) reacts with the alkene moiety of methylcyclohexene to form the more stable tertiary carbocation. Subsequent reaction with water gives an oxonium ion and loss of the proton from the oxonium ion gives 1-methylcyclohexan-1-ol as the final product.

What is the structure of the oxonium ion generated in the preceding question?

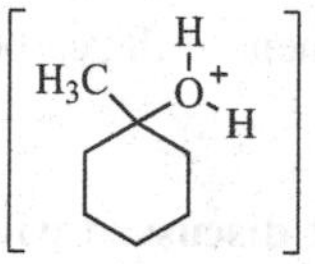

What is the mechanism of the reaction in the preceding question?

The alkene reacts with sulfuric acid to give the tertiary carbocation ***A***. Reaction with the oxygen of water gives oxonium ion ***B***. Subsequent reaction with a base, either water or the alkene starting material, gives the conjugate base of oxonium ion ***B***, which is the final product 1-methylcyclohexan-1-ol.

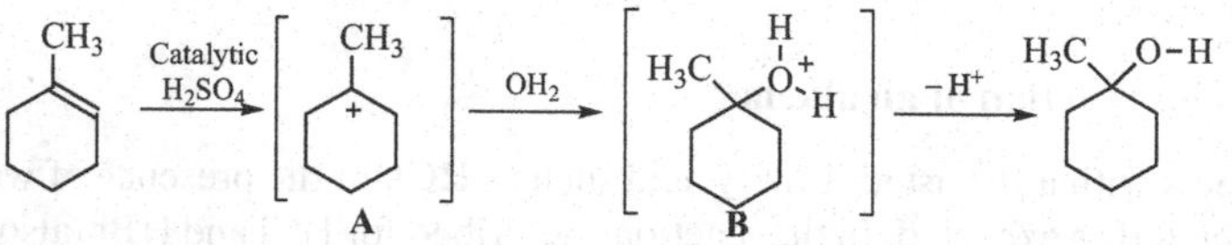

What sort of cation is *B* in the preceding question?

Cation ***B*** in the previous question is the conjugate acid of 1-methylcycloehxanol, where the alcohol reacts as a base with a Brønsted–Lowry acid. The ROH_2^+ species is called an *oxonium ion.*

What sort of reaction is the loss of a proton from intermediate *B* in the preceding question to give the alcohol?

The loss of the proton is an acid–base reaction, where intermediate ***B*** is the acid and the alcohol is the conjugate base.

Why does the alkene react with sulfuric acid?

Sulfuric acid is the strongest acid in the medium. The π-bond of the alkene is electron rich, and functions as a two-electron donor (a base) to the proton of the Brønsted–Lowry acid, sulfuric acid.

Why is only a catalytic amount of sulfuric acid required for this hydration reaction of methylcyclohexene?

It is catalytic because H^+ is released back to the reaction medium in the last step of the reaction, which is the conversion of the oxonium ion to the conjugate base, the alcohol. Sulfuric acid is a catalyst in the reaction, providing the proton that reacts with the alkene to initiate the reaction.

Is the acid in the aqueous acid catalytic or stoichiometric?

The H^+ initially reacts with the alkene to give a carbocation, which reacts with water to give an oxonium ion. Since H^+ is regenerated when the oxonium ion is converted to a product (an alcohol), the reaction is catalytic in H^+.

Why is it difficult to form primary alcohols from primary alkenes ($RCH{=}CH_2$) in aqueous acid?

The addition of an acid catalyst to a monosubstituted alkene will always rearrange to give the more stable secondary or tertiary carbocation as the major product, leading to a secondary or tertiary alcohol in aqueous acid. A primary carbocation is required in order to form a primary alcohol, but such carbocations are too high in energy relative to other possible carbocations to be formed preferentially under these conditions. In other words, primary carbocations are very unstable.

What is the mechanism and major product for the reaction of pent-1-ene with water under the following conditions?

H_2O, THF; Catalytic H_2SO_4

Under these conditions, the alkene reacts with the acid catalyst to form the secondary carbocation. Subsequent reaction with water leads to the oxonium ion and loss of the proton leads to the final product, pentan-2-ol.

H_2O, THF; Catalytic H_2SO_4 → [+] → H_2O → [$\overset{+}{O}H_2$] → $-H^+$ → OH

What type of reaction is the reaction of an alkene with sulfuric acid?

This reaction to form the carbocation is an acid–base reaction, where the alkene is the base and the proton of sulfuric acid is the acid.

What is methanesulfonic acid?

Methanesulfonic acid is CH_3SO_3H, a simple example of a strong organic acid. Sulfonic acids are somewhat stronger acids than carboxylic acids, generally 2–3 pK_a units more acidic. Many sulfonic acids are soluble in organic solvents and do not have some of the deleterious effects of mineral acids, such as sulfuric acid or perchloric acid. This organic acid and other sulfonic acids can be used as an acid catalyst in place of sulfuric acid.

$$H_3C{-}S(=O)_2{-}O{-}H + \text{Base} \rightleftharpoons H_3C{-}S(=O)_2{-}O^-$$

Methanesulfonic acid Methanesulfonate

What is $MeSO_3H$?

This is an abbreviation for methanesulfonic acid, RSO_3H, where R = methyl.

What is the major product for the reactions of *A* and *B*?

A: Aqueous THF; Cataltyic CH_3SO_3H

B: Aqueous THF; Cataltyic CH_3SO_3H

Aqueous (aq.) THF is a solution of the solvent tetrahydrofuran in water. The methanesulfonic acid is the acid catalyst, reacting with ***A*** to give a tertiary carbocation. The reaction of water with ***A*** generates an oxonium ion, which loses a proton to give the product, 2,8-dimethylnonan-2-ol. The second reaction with methanesulfonic acid and alkene ***B*** generates a secondary carbocation, but a 1,2-methyl shift gives the more stable tertiary cation. Subsequent reaction with water to give an oxonium ion and loss of a proton gives the product, 1,2-dimethylcycloheptan-1-ol.

OH OH

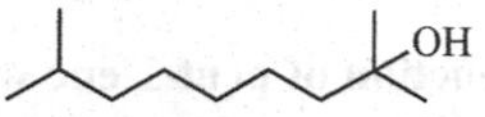

2,8-Dimethylnonan-2-ol 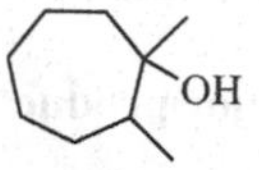 1,2-Dimethylcycloheptan-1-ol

What is THF?

THF is the abbreviation for tetrahydrofuran, the cyclic ether shown. THF is a common organic solvent.

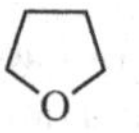

O

What is the structure of the oxonium ion intermediate that precedes the formation of 1,2-dimethylcycloheptan-1-ol?

$\overset{+}{O}H_2$

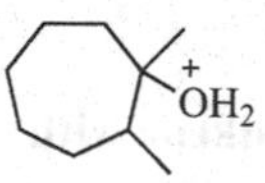

Is it possible for an alkene to give the anti-Markovnikov product, with formation of the less substituted halide?

Yes, if the reaction does *not* proceed by a carbocation intermediate, it is possible. In other words, the *mechanism* between the alkene and HX *must be changed* so that the reaction does not give a carbocation intermediate. If a carbocation is formed, the product will always be the Markovnikov product. Specifically, the anti-Markovnikov product can be formed if the reaction proceeds by a radical mechanism. As a practical matter, the reaction works well only with HBr and a radical initiator to give the radical intermediate. Note that an anti-Markovnikov product will be formed in the discussion of hydroboration of alkenes followed by oxidation to the corresponding alcohol (see Section 7.4).

What is a radical?

A *radical*, sometimes called a *free radical*, is a species with a single unpaired electron, X•.

Which is more stable, a primary radical or a secondary radical?

Alkyl radical can be formed such as R•, where R is primary, such as CH_3CH_2•, secondary, such as $(CH_3)_2CH$•, or tertiary, such as $(CH_3)_3C$•. As with carbocations, the carbon groups are electron releasing and more alkyl groups tend to stabilize the C•. Therefore, a tertiary radical is more stable than a secondary, which is more stable than a primary, which is more stable than a methyl radical, H_3C•.

What is the major radical product formed when but-1-ene reacts with RO•?

The initial product is the more stable secondary radical, formed by the reaction of RO• with a hydrogen atom of butene.

OR

Once formed, what does a carbon radical react with?

Several reactions are possible, but for the time being, attention will be focused on only two: coupling and addition. Carbon radicals, and indeed most radicals react via coupling with other radicals (R• + X• → R—X). Radicals also react with alkenes to give a new radical (RO• + RCH = CH_2 → RCH•—CH_2OR), which can undergo further reactions including reactions with other radicals that give substitution or coupling products.

What is the major product from the reaction of hex-1-ene and HBr, in the presence of di-*tert*-butyl peroxide?

HBr

t-Bu–O–O–*t*-Bu

Di-*tert*-butyl peroxide undergoes O—O cleavage to give two molar equivalents of the oxygen radical, *tert*-butylO•. The reaction of the radical with HBr gives *tert*-butanol and Br•. The alkene then reacts with Br• to give the more stable secondary carbon radical, which has the Br attached to the primary carbon. This carbon radical reacts with more HBr to give the final product, 1-bromohexane and more Br•. If Br• or the carbon radical reacts with another radical, coupling gives a neutral product and formation of 1-bromohexane stops.

HBr OH + Br•

Br• Br HBr Br + Br•

Br• + Br• ⟶ Br—Br

What type of reaction gives product as long as a reaction generates another radical product, but stops if the reaction gives a neutral product?

Such a reaction is termed a *radical reaction* or a *radical chain reaction.*

Why does bromine reside on the less substituted carbon when HBr reacts with hex-1-ene in the presence of a radical.

In the reaction of hex-1-ene, the π-bond of the alkene reacts with Br• rather than with H^+, and the initial product is a carbon radical. The bromine ends up on the less substituted carbon because Br• reacts with the alkene to form the more stable radical, in this case a secondary radical rather than a primary radical.

Do carbon radicals rearrange?

No! An important difference in radical chemistry is the observation that carbon radicals do *not* rearrange as carbocations do. Another important consideration is that the reaction shown for HBr is not general. It works with HBr and a peroxide, but not with HCl or HI.

7.4 REACTION OF ALKENES WITH LEWIS ACID-TYPE REAGENTS

Alkenes react as electron donors with Lewis acids, reagents that have an electrophilic oxygen, or an electrophilic halogen. These reactions will be described as well as the products that are formed.

7.4.1 Hydroxylation

Do alkenes react with molecules other than Brønsted–Lowry acids?

Yes! Alkenes can react with Lewis acid-type reagents, as well as Brønsted–Lowry acids, to form a carbocation. The initially formed carbocation reacts with a nucleophilic counterion or an added nucleophile but a second chemical step is sometimes required to remove an atom or group to give the final product.

What is the structure of mercuric chloride?

The structure of mercuric chloride is $HgCl_2$. The proper name of this compound is mercury (II) chloride.

What does mercuric mean?

This is the term used for divalent mercury, Hg^{+2}.

What is the structure of mercuric acetate?

The structure of mercuric acetate, $Hg(OAc)_2$, is shown. It is the mercury salt derived from acetic acid.

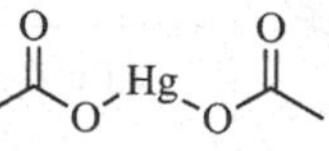

What is acetate?

The term acetate refers to the unit CH_3–C(=O)–O–, derived by replacement of the acidic hydrogen of acetic acid, CH_3COOH, with another group.

How can mercuric acetate be classified as a reagent?

The mercury is electron deficient and behaves as a Lewis acid in its reactions with alkenes. An alkene will donate electrons to mercury, displacing one of the acetate groups.

What is the product of a reaction between 2-methylbut-1-ene and mercuric acetate, assuming this product does not react further?

The initial product of the Lewis acid–Lewis base reaction is the organomercury cation, along with the acetate anion that results from displacement of acetate by the alkene.

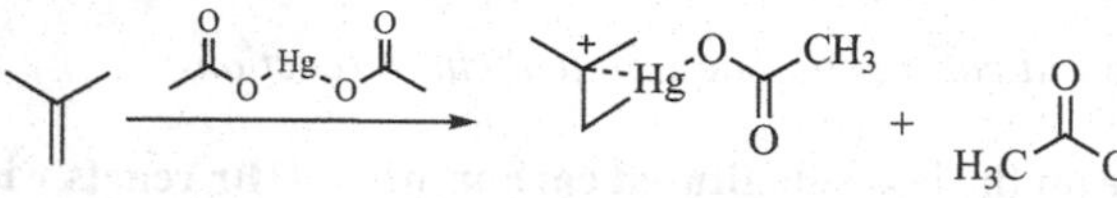

What does the "dashed" line mean in the organomercury cation intermediate in the preceding question?

The mercury stabilizes the cationic center by *"back donation"* of electrons from the d-orbital of mercury, as indicated by the dashed line. The back donation stabilizes the carbocation, but it reacts normally with a nucleophilic species such as water. Subsequent reaction of this carbocation with water gives a hydroxy–mercury product via the usual oxonium ion.

What is back donation?

This concept is also called *π-back bonding*, where electrons from an atomic orbital on one atom coordinate to a π* antibonding orbital on another atom or ligand. In a typical example, electrons from a metal are used to form a coordination bond to the ligand, in this case the cation species.

If the reaction of mercuric acetate and 2-methylpropene is done in an aqueous medium, what is the product?

Except for the stabilization by the mercury, the carbocation intermediate behaves more or less like any other carbocation–water reaction. Organomercury cation ***A*** therefore reacts with water to give an oxonium ion, ***B***. Loss of a proton gives a hydroxy–mercury compound, ***C***. Note that the reaction shown, with the inclusion of structures ***A*** and ***B***, constitutes the mechanism of this reaction.

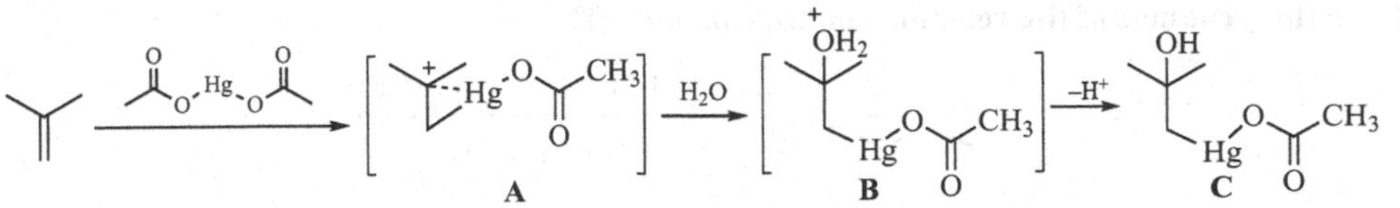

How can the mercury be removed from the hydroxy–mercury compound *C* in the preceding question?

Removal of mercury requires another chemical step, which is cleavage of the C—Hg bond and replacement of Hg with H. This transformation is known as *hydrogenolysis*. This reaction can be done very efficiently by addition of sodium borohydride ($NaBH_4$) followed by aqueous hydrolysis, as shown. The final product is the alcohol that is formed by addition of water to the more substituted carbon. In this reaction, the solvent is shown as EtOH, ethanol. Note the use of 1. and 2. for each reaction. This nomenclature indicates two different reactions. The product of step 1 is followed by treatment with the reagent in step 2.

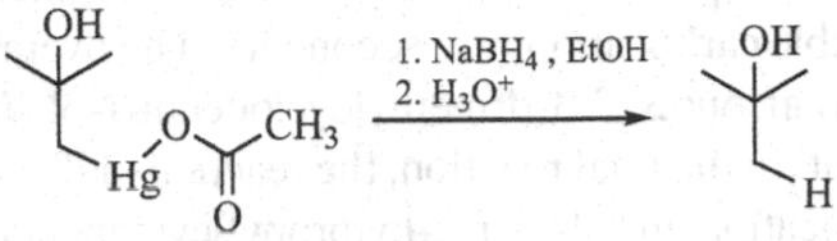

1. $NaBH_4$, EtOH
2. H_3O^+

This overall sequence from alkene to alcohol is called *oxymercuration* or, sometimes, *oxymercuration-demercuration.*

What is sodium borohydride, $NaBH_4$?

Sodium borohydride, $NaBH_4$, also known as sodium tetrahydridoborate, is an inorganic compound, a white solid, and it is a reducing agent used in organic chemistry primarily for the reduction of ketones and aldehydes to alcohols (see Section 14.3).

What is the product when mercuric acetate reacts with 3-methyl-pent-1-ene in the presence of water and then subsequent reaction with sodium borohydride? Is that product the result of a rearrangement? Why or why not?

The product (after treatment with $NaBH_4$) is 3-methylpentan-2-ol and it is formed with *no rearrangement* from the initially formed secondary carbocation to the tertiary carbocation. Note that to form this product, water must react with the initially formed secondary carbocation before a rearrangement can occur. The reason for the faster reaction with the nucleophilic water is that *stabilization by mercury back donation makes rearrangement slower* than the reaction with water. In other words, back donation from the mercury stabilizes the secondary carbocation intermediate and prevents rearrangement but not the reaction with water.

Why is the alcohol formed without rearrangement of the intermediate carbocation?

This question is essentially the same as the preceding question. There is no rearrangement of the intermediate mercuric cation. The mercury stabilizes the secondary cationic center by *back donation* of its d-orbitals. This increased stability diminishes the possibility of rearrangement, and trapping with water is usually faster than the rearrangement. In other words, *there is no rearrangement in oxymercuration reactions.*

What are the products of the reactions of (a), (b), and (c)?

(a) → 1. $Hg(OAc)_2$, Aq. THF; 2. $NaBH_4$, 3. H_3O^+

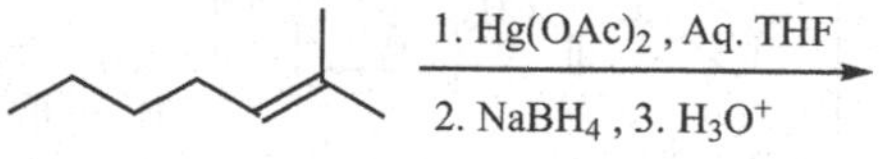

(b) → 1. $Hg(OAc)_2$, Aq. THF; 2. $NaBH_4$, 3. H_3O^+

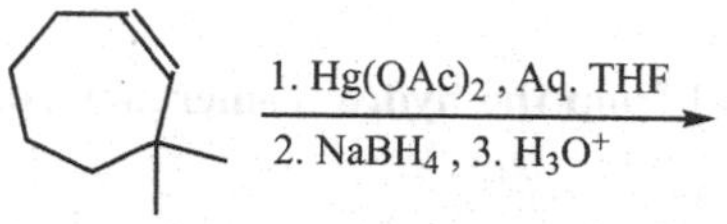

(c) → 1. $Hg(OAc)_2$, Aq. THF; 2. $NaBH_4$, 3. H_3O^+

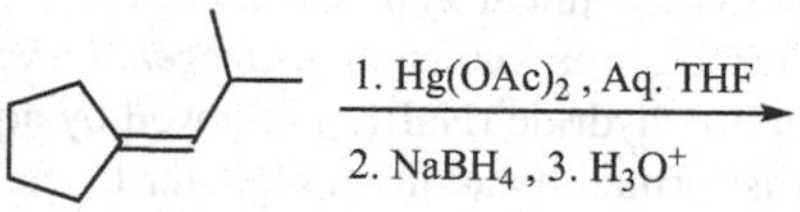

The first reaction converts 2-methylhept-2-ene into the tertiary alcohol, 2-methylheptan-2-ol, ***A***. This hydration reaction proceeds as if it were a normal cation intermediate in an addition reaction. The second reaction with 3,3-dimethylcyclooctene poses a problem. There is no regiochemical preference for addition of the mercury since the two possible carbocations are secondary. The overall sequence will, therefore, produce a roughly 1:1 mixture of two alcohols, 3,3-dimethylcyclooctan-1-ol (***B***) and 2,2-dimethylcyclooctan-1-ol (***C***). There is no rearrangement. In the final reaction, the reaction of (2-methylpropylidene)cyclopentane proceeds to give the tertiary carbocation and, 1-(2-methylpropyl)cyclopentan-1-ol (***D***) is the major product.

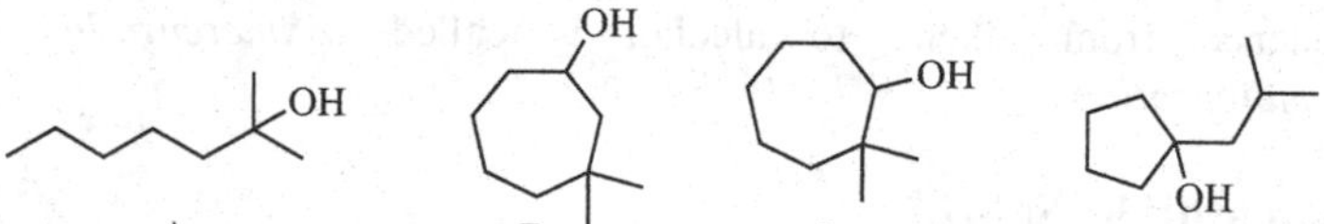

OH OH OH OH

A B C D

What is alkoxymercuration?

Alkoxymercuration is the process by which an alkene is treated with a mercuric salt and an alcohol to give a hydroxy–mercuric compound. Subsequent treatment with sodium borohydride gives the ether.

What is the nature of the intermediate formed by initial reaction of pent-1-ene with mercuric acetate, before reaction with ethanol?

This intermediate is a mercury–carbocation as in oxymercuration. Note that the mercuric acetate unit is on the primary carbon, generating the more stable secondary carbocation. Therefore, the use of mercuric acetate generates the more stable carbocation, as expected. Note also that the initially formed carbocation is stabilized by coordination with the mercury (called back donation), indicated by the dashed line. This is the key intermediate in oxymercuration.

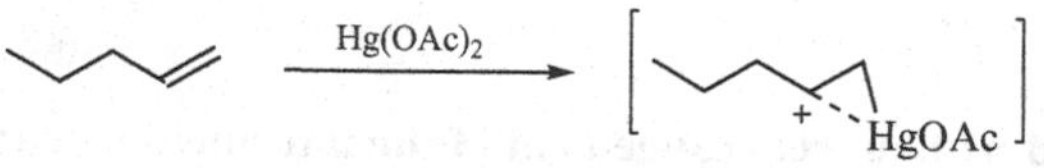

$Hg(OAc)_2$ → [+ HgOAc]

What is the product formed from pent-1-ene, mercuric acetate and ethanol?

The nucleophile in this reaction is ethanol, so the product is the mercuric acetate ether shown.

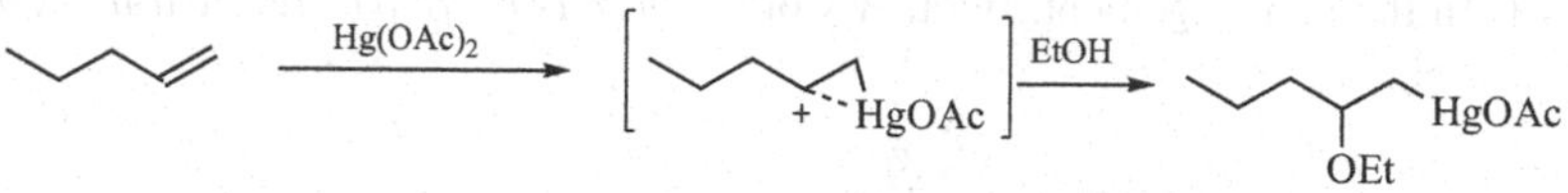

$Hg(OAc)_2$ → [+ HgOAc] EtOH → HgOAc OEt

What is the purpose of treating the ethoxy–mercuric compound with sodium borohydride?

Hydrogenolysis! To remove the mercury (cleave the C—Hg bond) and convert it to a C—H unit.

What is the final product when pent-1-ene is reacted with: 1 $Hg(OAc)_2$, EtOH 2. $NaBH_4$ 3. aq. NH_4Cl?

The product is ethyl 1-methylbutyl ether.

Why does this process lead to an ether rather than an alcohol (as with oxymercuration)?

The only nucleophilic species is the alcohol solvent, leading to the ether.

What is the product of (a) and (b)?

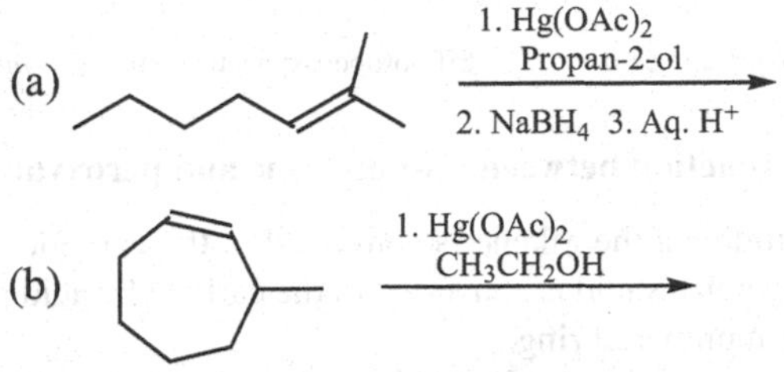

(a) 1. $Hg(OAc)_2$ Propan-2-ol → 2. $NaBH_4$ 3. Aq. H^+

(b) 1. $Hg(OAc)_2$ CH_3CH_2OH →

The more stable cation in (a) is at the tertiary position, and the final product is 2-(1-methylethyl)-2-methylheptane. The reaction in (b) poses two problems. First, both possible cation intermediates are secondary, so there will be a mixture of two products (isomers). In other words, the OEt unit will be incorporated at each carbon of the C=C unit to give two different products. Second, one of the intermediate carbocations is a secondary carbocation but is next to a potential tertiary carbocation site. Remember that in oxymercuration and alkoxymercuration reactions, the mercury stabilizes the cation and rearrangement does not occur. Therefore, the two products are 1-ethoxy-2-methylcycloheptane and 1-ethoxy-3-methylcycloheptane.

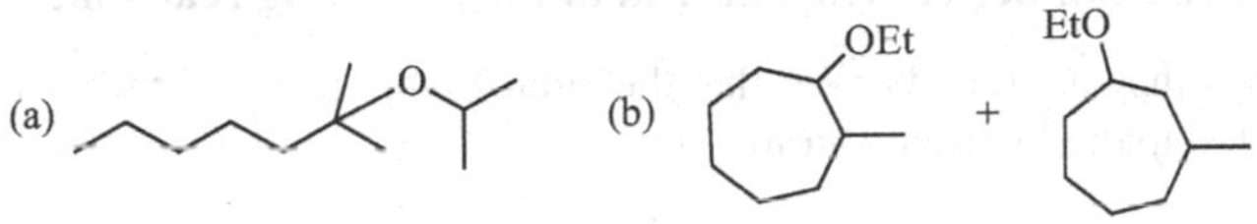

(a) (b) OEt + EtO

7.4.2 Epoxidation

What is an oxirane?

An oxirane is a three-membered ring ether. Oxirane itself is shown in the following structure.

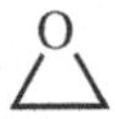

O

Oxirane

What is an epoxide?

An epoxide is the common name for an oxirane. The oxirane shown in the preceding question is commonly named ethylene oxide, taking the alkene the epoxide is derived from, and adding the word oxide.

What is a peroxyacid?

A peroxyacid is a peroxide derivative of a carboxylic acid with the structure RCO_3H.

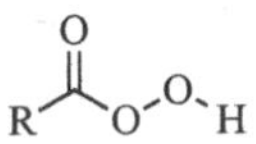

O R O O H

a peroxyacid

What is the structure and name of four common peroxyacids?

Four common peroxyacids are *peroxyformic acid*, derived from formic acid; *peroxyacetic acid*, derived from acetic acid; *trifluoroperoxyacetic acid,* derived from trifluoroacetic acid; and *meta-chloroperoxybenzoic acid*, derived from *meta*-chlorobenzoic acid. Benzene derivatives such as benzoic acid and the term meta- will be described in Section 16.1.

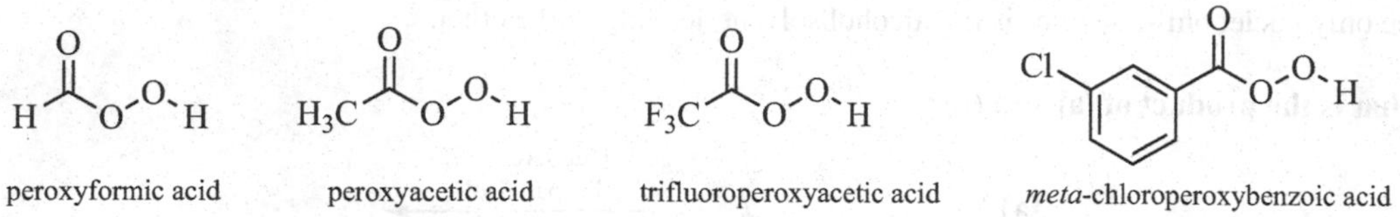

peroxyformic acid   peroxyacetic acid   trifluoroperoxyacetic acid   *meta*-chloroperoxybenzoic acid

What are the products of a reaction between cis-but-2-ene and peroxyacetic acid?

This reaction leads to two products, the alkene is converted to the epoxide, 2,3-dimethyloxirane, with concomitant conversion of the peroxyacid is converted to the carboxylic acid precursor, acetic acid. Note the cis-geometry of the three-membered ring.

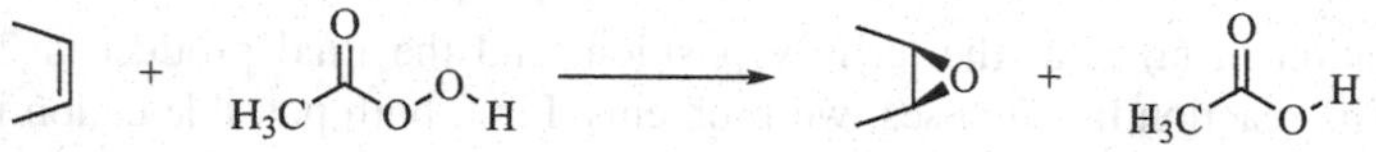

Is there a reactive intermediate in the preceding reaction?

No, there is no observed intermediate. The epoxidation reaction must be described by the transition state for this reaction.

What is the bond polarization in peroxyacetic acid in the preceding reaction?

The bond polarization is shown, and it is clear that the induced dipole of the carbonyl leads to a δ^+ dipole for the oxygen connected to the hydrogen atom.

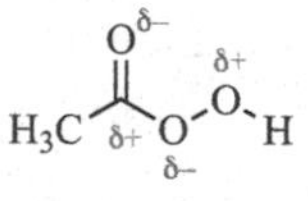

What is the transition state of the reaction with cis-but-2-ene and peroxyformic acid?

The transition state for this reaction is shown.

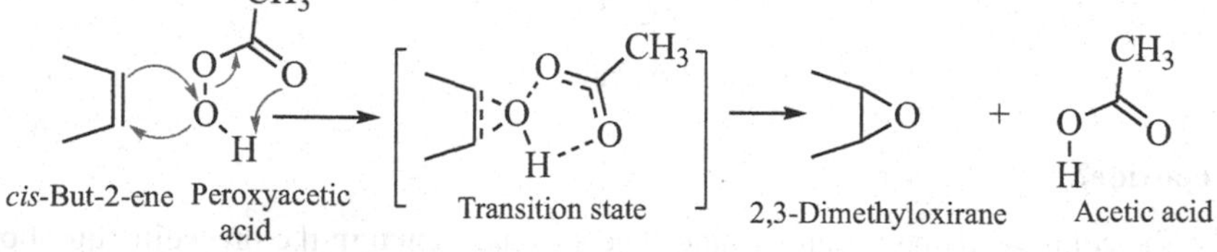

cis-But-2-ene Peroxyacetic acid Transition state 2,3-Dimethyloxirane Acetic acid

What products are formed in the following reactions: (a) 2,3-dimethylpent-2-ene and peroxyacetic acid (b) 1-methylcyclohexene and trifluoroperoxyacetic acid?

(a)

(b)

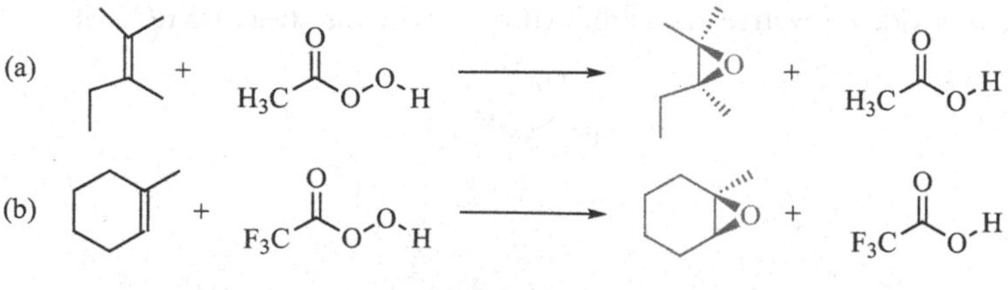

7.4.3 Dihydroxylation

What is a diol?

A diol is a molecule with two hydroxyl units (OH), such as ethanediol (ethylene glycol): $HOCH_2CH_2OH$.

What is the structure of pentane-1,2-diol? Of cyclopentane-1,2-diol?

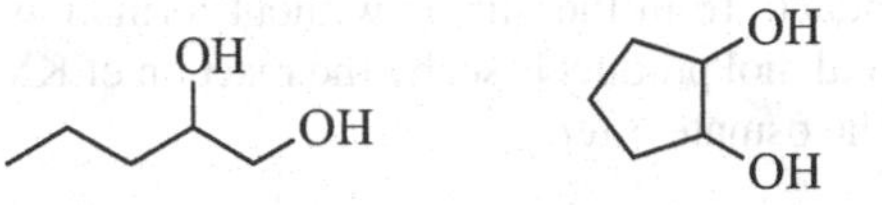

Pentane-1,2-diol   Cyclpentane-1,2-diol

What is the structure of pentane-1,4-diol? Of cyclopentane-1,3-diol?

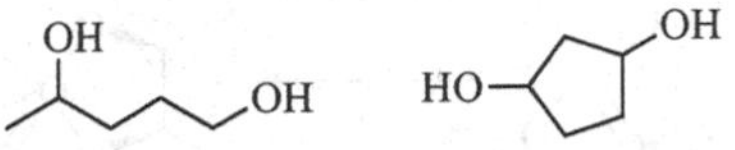

Pentane-1,4-diol   Cyclpentane-1,3-diol

What is a vicinal diol?

A vicinal diol has the two-OH unit on adjacent carbon atoms, as in pentane-1-2-diol.

What is the structure of potassium permanganate? Of osmium tetroxide?

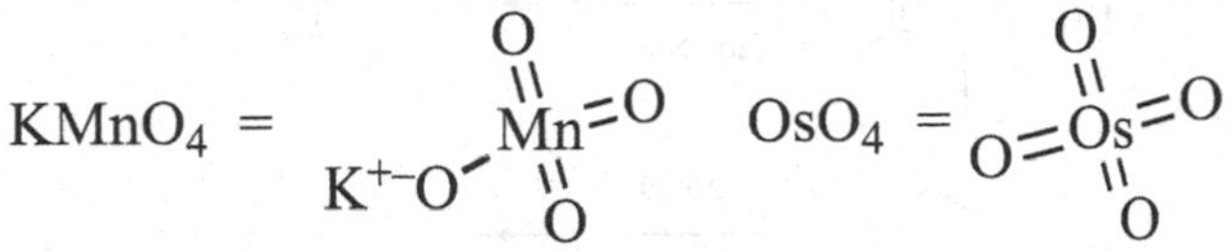

$KMnO_4$ = $K^+{}^-O-Mn(=O)_3$ OsO_4 = $O=Os(=O)_3$

What is the final product of the reaction of cyclopentene and potassium permanganate and aqueous NaOH?

$KMnO_4$, aq. NaOH

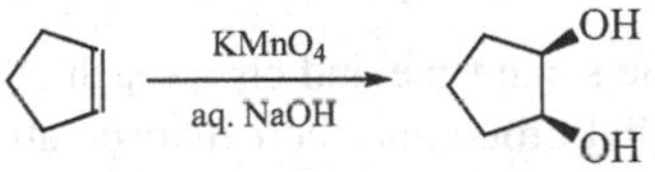

What is the final product of the reaction of hex-1-ene and osmium tetroxide and aqueous *tert*-butyl hydroperoxide?

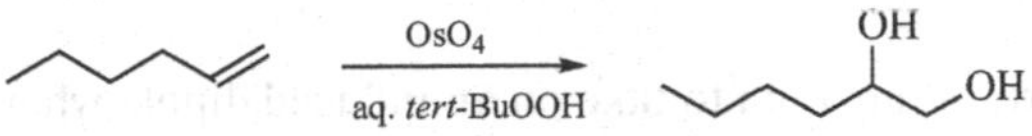

OsO_4, aq. *tert*-BuOOH

What is the intermediate and the name of that intermediate for the reaction of cyclopentene and potassium permanganate and aqueous NaOH?

The intermediate for the reaction of an alkene and $KMnO_4$ is a manganate ester. For comparison, the intermediate for the reaction of an alkene and OsO_4 is an osmate ester (see Section 18.5)

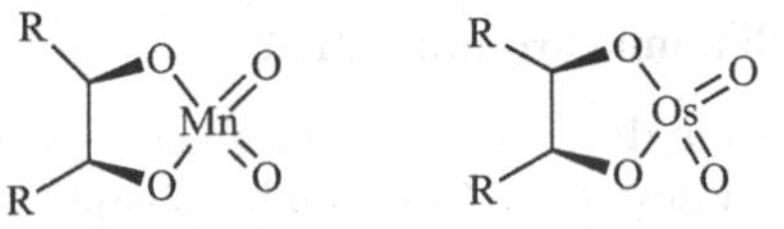

a Manganate ester   an Osmate ester

Why is the product of the reaction of cyclopentene and $KMnO_4$ a cis- diol and not a mixture of cis- and trans- diol?

In the reaction with an alkene, both $KMnO_4$ and OsO_4 react to form two oxygen atoms bonded to both carbon atoms of the alkene. These adjacent oxygen atoms are cis to each other because those bonds are formed at the same time. The reaction to form a manganate ester or the osmate ester proceeds by a cycloaddition reaction (see Section 18.5), as shown in the figure. Such cycloaddition generates the manganate ester or the osmate ester as products from the alkene without formation of an intermediate. In other words, the cis geometry in the final diol product is set by the reaction of $KMnO_4$ or OsO_4 with the alkene to form the manganate ester or the osmate ester.

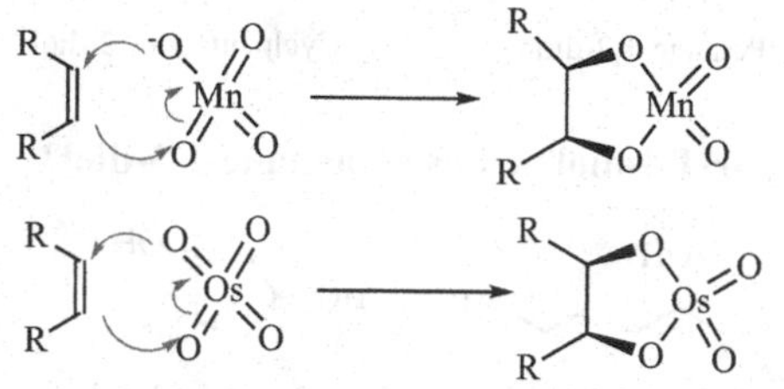

What products are formed in the following reactions: (a) 2,3-dimethylpent-2-ene, potassium permanganate, and NaOH (b) 1-methylcyclohexene, osmium tetroxide, and aqueous *tert*-butyl hydroperoxide?

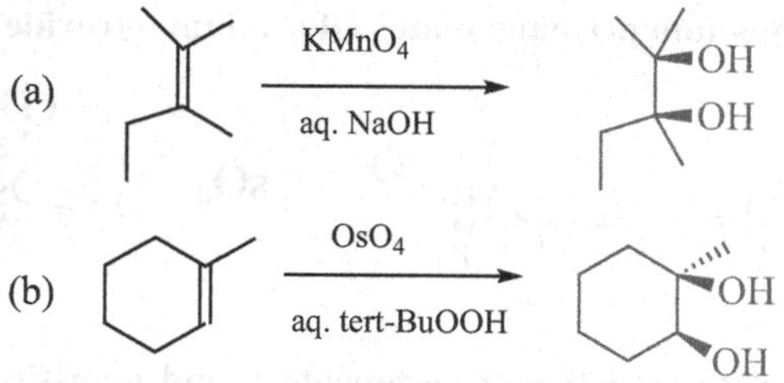

(a) $KMnO_4$, aq. NaOH

(b) OsO_4, aq. tert-BuOOH

Why is the methyl group in reaction (b) of the preceding problem trans to the hydroxyl groups?

Both OH units are incorporated at the same time and cis to each other. The dihydroxylation occurs on the side of the ring opposite the methyl group and their incorporation pushes the methyl group on the opposite of the ring relative to the hydroxyl group; it is trans.

7.4.4 Halogenation

What is polarizability?

Polarizability is the property of an atom to take on an induced dipole when in proximity to another polarized atom. In general, proximity to a positive dipole will induce a negative dipole, and vice-versa.

What are the common molecules that are polarizable?

The halogens, diatomic chlorine, bromine, and iodine are highly polarizable molecules.

Why does an alkene react with diatomic bromine (Br_2)?

The Br—Br bond is polarizable and in the presence of the alkene (the alkene comes into close proximity to one of the bromines), the Br closest to the C=C unit becomes δ^+ by *induced polarization.* In close proximity to the electron rich alkene, therefore, Br—Br becomes $^{\delta+}Br\text{-}Br^{\delta-}$. With this induced dipole, the

π-bond is attracted to the electrophilic bromine and reacts with it by the transfer of two electrons to $Br^{\delta+}$, generating Br^- as a leaving group.

Is the reaction between cyclohexene and diatomic bromine concerted or ionic in nature?

The reaction has a cationic intermediate, so it is ionic in nature.

When diatomic bromine reacts with an alkene, is the reaction spontaneous or is there an intermediate?

There is an intermediate, so it is a stepwise reaction.

What is the intermediate and the final product when cyclohexene reacts with diatomic bromine?

When the π-bond of cyclohexene reacts with Br—Br, a formal carbocation is not formed but rather a three-membered ring intermediate called a *bromonium ion*, ***A***. The bromonium ion is re-drawn to show the proper stereochemical relationship of the ion and the bromide ion it reacts with. The bromide counterion acts as a nucleophile, approaches 180° away from the first bromine atom, opening the three-membered ring to give the trans-dibromide product, trans-1,2-dibromocyclohexane.

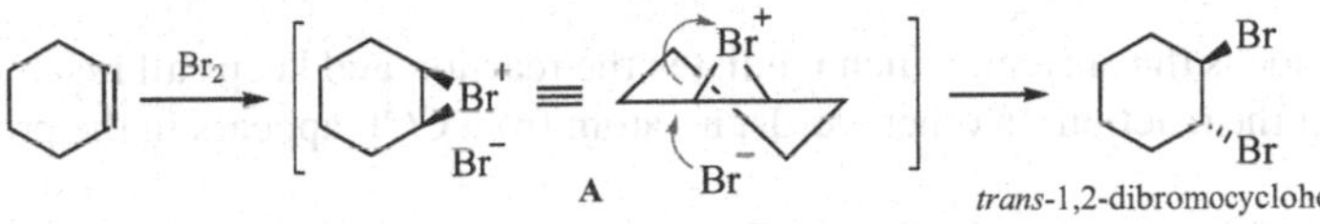

Br_2 → [bromonium ion A, Br^-] → *trans*-1,2-dibromocyclohexane

Why does a bromonium ion form rather than a carbocation?

When the double bond transfers electron density to Br—Br, positive charge "builds up" on the adjacent carbon. The lone electron pairs on the Br form a covalent bond with this positive center, forming the three-membered ring shown. Why does this intermediate form? Because it is more stable than the carbocation intermediate alternative.

When a bromonium ion reacts with bromide (Br^-), from which face will it approach: from the same side as the bromine, or from the opposite side? Justify your answer.

This question is best answered by inspection of the bromonium ion in the previous question. If the nucleophilic bromide ion approaches from the "top," there is both steric and electronic repulsion. This repulsion is minimized by "backside attack," where Br^- approaches the three-membered ring anti- to the Br in the bromonium ion, as shown above. When the new C—Br bond is formed, reaction from the opposite side of the ring dictates that the two bromine atoms will be anti, on opposite sides of the ring. In other words, a trans-dibromide is formed. Such trans- geometry in the product is characteristic of the intermediacy of a bromonium ion (halonium ion is the generic term: chloronium, bromonium, and iodonium for Cl, Br, and I, respectively).

When a cyclic alkene reacts with chlorine, bromine, or iodine, is the cis-dihalide ever observed?

No! The intermediacy of the halonium ion (chloronium, bromonium, iodonium) dictates that subsequent reactions with a nucleophilic halide ion will always lead to the trans product.

What term is used for a reaction that gives one and only one diastereomer of two or more possible diastereomeric products?

The term is *diastereospecific*. Since the reaction of halogens and alkenes gives a single diastereomer, the reaction is diastereospecific.

What does diastereoselective mean?

Diastereoselective means that of two or more possible products, both are formed but one is major, and the other is minor.

What is the product when 4-ethyloct-3*E*-ene reacts with Br_2 in CCl_4?

The reaction of bromine and the alkene proceeds by a bromonium ion intermediate. Anti- attack of the bromide counterion on the three-membered ring is also required which dictates an anti- relationship for the bromines in the product, (3*S*,4*R*)-3,4-dibromo-4-ethyloctane. Since this is an acyclic molecule, cis-/trans-isomers are not possible. Diastereomers are possible, however, since there are two stereocenters. Anti- attack dictates that a single diastereomer is formed, the (3*S*,4*R*) enantiomer shown. Since the bromine can form the bromonium ion on either the "top" or the "bottom" of the alkene, the diastereomer is *racemic.* Formation of a racemic diastereomer is the norm for this reaction, which is diastereospecific but shows no enantioselectivity at all. The bromonium ion can also form with the bromine on the "bottom" rather than the "top." The bromide ion will also attach from the opposite side to give the same diastereomer but the enantiomer: (3*R*,4*S*)-3,4-dibromo-4-ethyloctane. Note that *Br^- attacks the bromonium ion at the less sterically hindered carbon.*

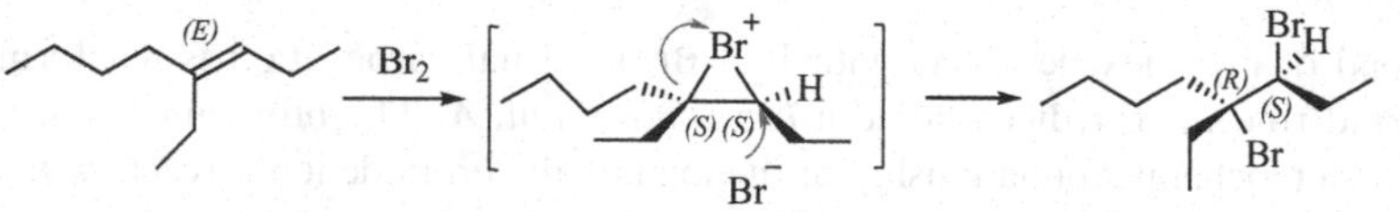

What is the role of CCl_4 in the preceding reaction?

The carbon tetrachloride is the solvent, which mediates the reaction and keeps all reactants soluble, but does not participate in the reaction. In other words, no atom from CCl_4 appears in the product.

What diastereomer is formed when 4-ethyloct-3*Z*-ene reacts with Br_2 in CCl_4?

The diastereomer is a mixture of (3*R*,4*R*)-3,4-dibromo-4-ethyloctane and (3*S*,4*S*)-3,4-dibromo-4-ethyloctane. Formation of the (3*R*,4*R*)-3,4-dibromo-4-ethyloctane enantiomer is shown.

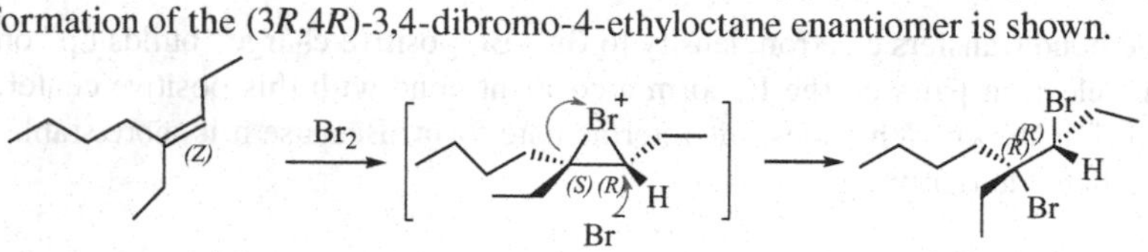

How many stereoisomers are produced when *cis*-but-2-ene reacts with Br_2?

cis-But-2-ene reacts with Br_2 to give a bromonium ion. Anti- attack by Br^- leads to (2*R*,3*R*)-dibromobutane as one enantiomer of the only diastereomer. It is racemic, so (2*S*,3*S*)-dibromobutane is also produced if the bromonium ion is formed with Br on the "bottom" as the ion is drawn. These two stereoisomers are not superimposable and are indeed enantiomers, so two stereoisomers result from this reaction but only one diastereomer.

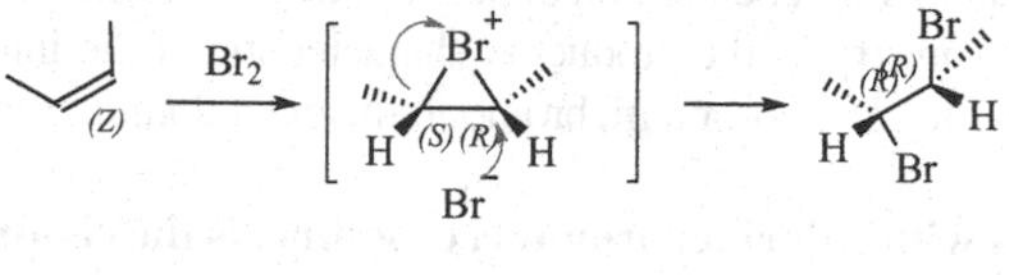

If *trans*-but-2-ene were reacted with Br_2, only one diastereomer would result, meso 2,3-dibromobutane.

What is meso-2,3-dibromobutane?

This diastereomer is (2*R*,3*S*)-2,3-dibromobutane, and note the symmetry in the molecule that leads to its identification as a meso compound.

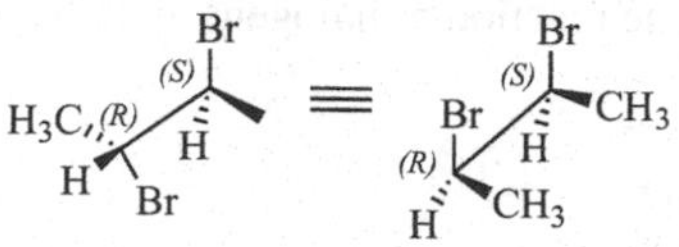

What product is formed when chlorine is dissolved in water?

When chlorine (Cl_2) is dissolved in water, hypochlorous acid (HOCl) is formed. This molecule is polarized as Cl^+ OH^-. Similarly, HOBr is formed when bromine (Br_2) is dissolved in water.

What is the product for the reaction of cyclopentene with HOCl but not in water?

The product is a *vicinal* (on adjacent carbons) chlorohydrin (chlorine and OH in the same molecule), named *trans*-2-chlorocyclopentanol. Initial reaction of cyclopentene with the electrophilic chlorine atom of the HOCl generates a chloronium ion, and the counterion is hydroxide. Remember that no water is present, so the three-membered ring remains largely intact and the nucleophile ($^-$OH) attacks an electrophilic carbon atom from the face opposite the Cl to give the chlorohydrin.

HOCl

Cl^+ $^-$OH

Cl OH

What is the product of the reaction of methylcyclopentene with Cl_2, in H_2O?

Cl^+ $^-$OH

H_2O Cl_2

Cl OH

Cl $^-$OH

Initial reaction of the alkene generates a chloronium ion, but in water some ionization takes place to give the more stable tertiary carbocation, with back donation by the lone electron pairs on chlorine (as shown). The nucleophile ($^-$OH) attacks the less sterically hindered carbon to give the racemic diastereomer, 2-chloro-2-methylcyclopentan-1-ol.

7.4.5 Hydroboration

What is hydroboration?

Alkenes react with borane (BH_3) and its derivatives to give alkylboranes (RBH_2). Treatment of these alkylboranes with various reagents leads to a variety of new functional groups. These reactions are known collectively as *hydroboration*.

What is the structure of diborane?

Diborane (B_2H_6) is a hydride-bridged dimer, ***A***, although it is commonly written as just BH_3.

H H H B B H H H

A

What is the product when borane reacts with cyclopentene?

Diborane reacts with the π-bond of cyclopentene to give a trialkylborane (tricyclopentylborane), which is shown. This reaction is catalyzed by the ether solvent, which is an essential component of the reaction, although it does not appear in the product. More hindered alkenes may stop at the monoalkyl or the dialkylborane. With relatively unhindered alkenes, the trialkylborane is the most common product.

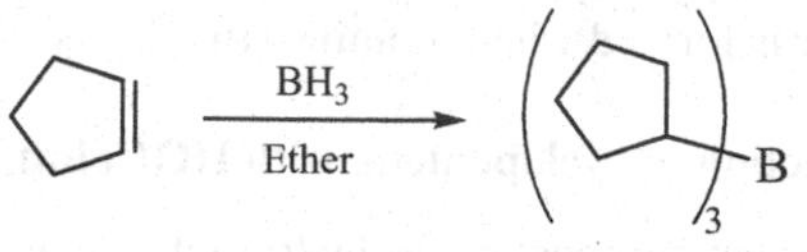

What is ether?

Ether refers to the common solvent, diethyl ether: $CH_3CH_2OCH_2CH_3$.

Why is ether used as a solvent when diborane reacts with alkenes?

Ether solvents catalyze the reaction between borane and alkenes. Without the ether solvent the reaction can require temperatures up to 200–250°C.

What is the nature of the transition state for the reaction of the alkene but-1-ene and diborane?

When borane reacts with an alkene such as but-1-ene, there is no intermediate; no carbocation, carbanion, or radical. The reaction is spontaneous and proceeds by a *four-centered transition state* (***A***). The reaction proceeds with delivery of the boron to one carbon and a hydrogen to the other carbon as in ***B***, with cleavage of a B—H of BH_3. The final product is an *organoborane*, in this case tributylborane, ***C***.

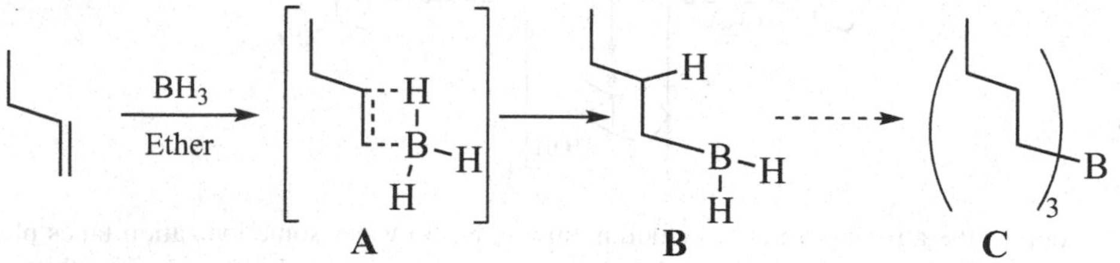

Why is the product of but-1-ene drawn as a trialkylborane?

Monoborane, ***B***, is the initial product for the reaction of but-1-ene and BH_3. In ***B***, there are two more B—H units and each of them can react again with the alkene (here, but-1-ene). The reaction proceeds until there are no additional B—H units, and the final product will be the triborane (***C***), where all three B–H units have reacted with an alkene. In other words, one molar equivalent of borane can react with three molar equivalents of simple alkenes. Note that ***C*** is also drawn as $(CH_3CH_2CH_2CH_2)_3B$.

Why does boron reside on the less substituted carbon (*C*) in the preceding question?

In the transition state, the boron can react at C1 (***A***) or at C2. There is less steric hindrance in ***A*** than the when boron reacts at C2 (***A'***). The final product results from the path that gives the least sterically hindered transition state, which in this case is ***A***, and the final product is ***C***.

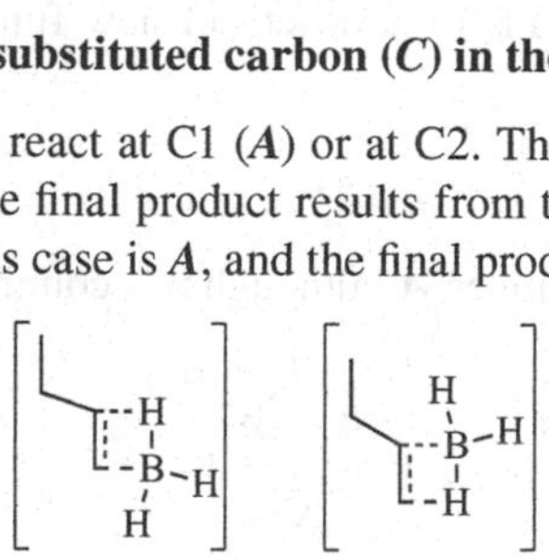

Why does the reaction of 1,2-dimethylcyclohexene lead to a product where the stereochemistry of the methyl groups is cis-?

When 1,2-dimethylcyclohexene reacts with borane, the B and the H of the B—H bond *MUST* add in a cis- manner because the reaction proceeds by a four-centered transition state. Therefore, B and H in the organoborane product are cis- (BR_2 represents the formation of a dialkyl or trialkylborane where R = dimethylcyclohexyl and/or hydrogen). The two methyl groups in the product will be pushed away from the boron in the four-center transition state due to steric repulsion and the two methyl groups will therefore be cis- to each other. As a consequence of the transition state and the B—H bond delivering the two atoms, boron and hydrogen are on the opposite side of the ring relative to the methyl groups.

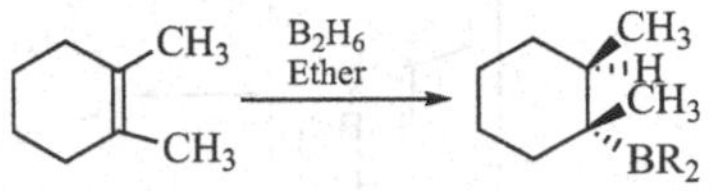

CH_3 CH_3 B_2H_6 Ether CH_3 H CH_3 BR_2

What is the four-center transition state for the conversion of 1,2-dimethylcyclohexene to the organoborane shown in the preceding question?

This stereochemistry in the product arises because the reaction proceeds by a *four-center transition state* such as that shown for addition of borane to the π-bond.

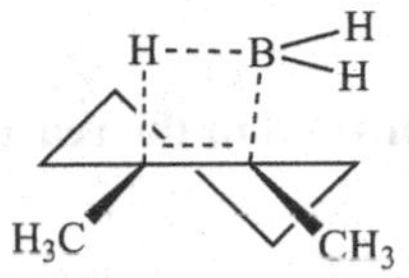

H----B H H H_3C CH_3

What are the two possible products for the reaction of borane and pent-1-ene?

The boron can attach to either the first carbon (path *a*) or the second (path *b*). The two products are ***A*** (via path *a*) and ***B*** (via path *b*). The major product is ***A*** (80–90% yield) and monosubstituted alkenes such as pent-1-ene *always* give attachment at the less sterically hindered carbon as the major product.

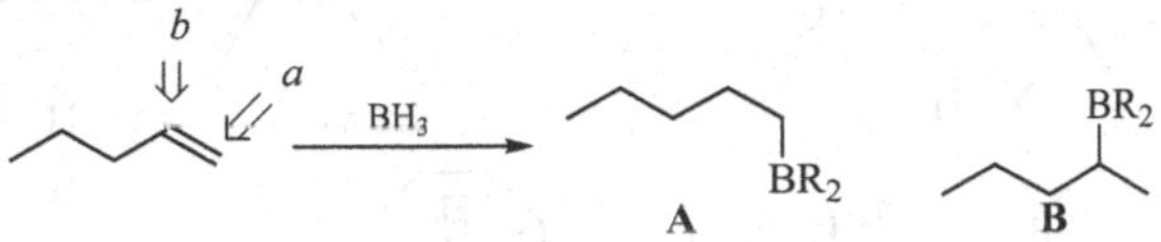

b *a* BH_3 BR_2 **A** BR_2 **B**

What are the transition states for the formation of *A* and *B* from pent-1-ene? Use these drawings to rationalize which is the major product.

Comparison of transition state ***C*** (which leads to ***A*** in the preceding question) with ***D*** (which leads to ***B*** in the preceding question) reveals that the BH_2 moiety interacts sterically with the propyl group in transition state ***D***. In ***C***, however, the bulky BH_2 group interacts only with hydrogens. Since transition state ***C*** is less sterically hindered than ***D***, it is lower in energy and leads to the major product, ***A***.

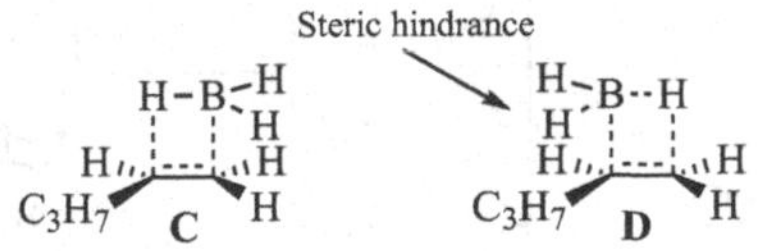

Steric hindrance

H-B H H H H C_3H_7 **C** H   H B H H H H C_3H_7 **D** H

What is the regiochemical preference of the reaction of but-1-ene and diborane?

The major product is the one where boron is attached to the *less* substituted carbon, although about 15% of the other isomer (boron attached to the secondary carbon) is also produced. The products are shown as BR_2 to show general products that put the focus on the regiochemistry.

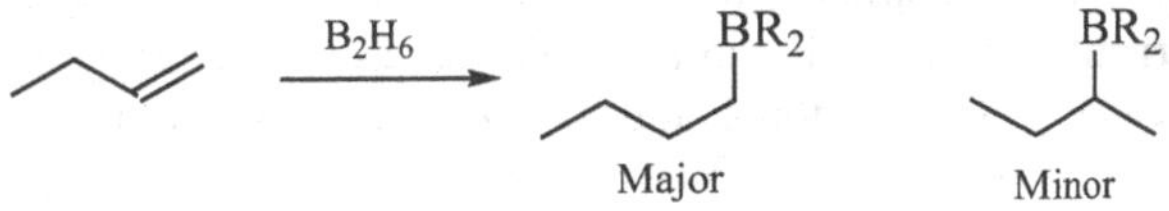

B_2H_6 BR_2 Major BR_2 Minor

Why does one product predominate when diborane reacts with 2-methylbut-1-ene?

The two possible transition states are *A* (which leads to alkylborane *B*) and *C* (which leads to alkylborane *D*). It is clear that the interaction of the ethyl group and methyl group and the BH_2 unit in *C* causes more steric hindrance than the interaction in *A*. This steric interaction drives the reaction to give the major product where boron is attached to the less substituted carbon, *B*.

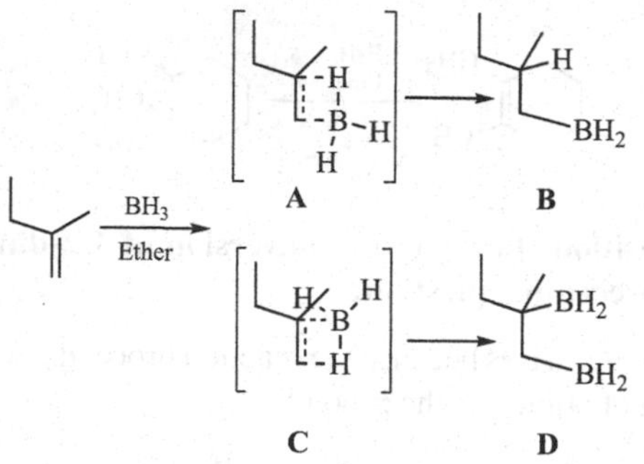

What is the appropriate alkene precursor used in the reaction for the preparation of disiamylborane, thexylborane, and 9-BBN?

When 2-methylbut-2-ene is treated with diborane, a dialkylborane (*A*) is formed. This product is given the common name disiamylborane (siamyl = sec-isoamyl). When 2,3-dimethylbut-2-ene is treated with diborane a monoalkylborane (*B*) is formed. The common name of this product is thexylborane (thexyl = tert-hexyl). When cycloocta-1,5-diene is treated with diborane, boron adds to one alkene to form an alkylborane but then adds intramolecularly to the other alkene unit to give *C*, 9-borabicyclo[4.4.1]nonane (9-BBN).

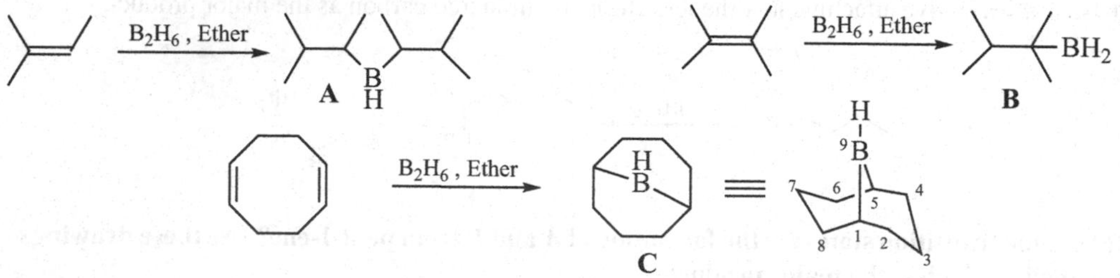

Why does 9-BBN give a higher percentage of the 1-substituted product when compared to diborane in a reaction with but-1-ene?

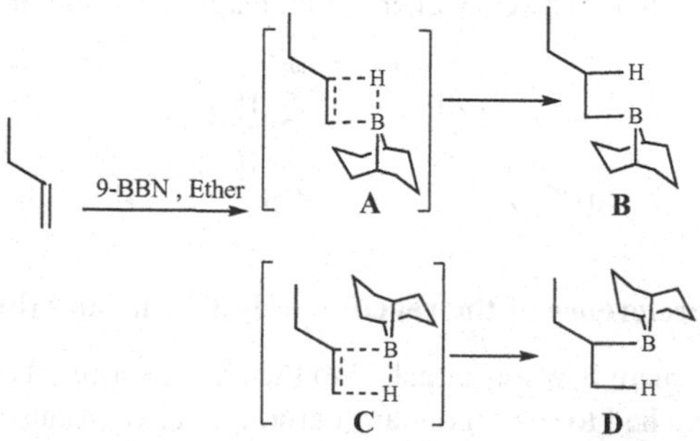

Examination of the two possible transition states (*A* and *C*) for the reaction of 9-BBN and but-1-ene show that *C* is much more sterically hindered due to the bulky nature of the bridged ring system of 9-BBN. This leads to a much greater preference for *A* and formation of *B* as the major product rather than *D* (usually >99:1).

What is the main application of organoboranes?

The main application of hydroboration is the ability to convert the monoalkyl, dialkyl, and trialkylborane products into alcohols by treatment with basic hydrogen peroxide in an oxidation step. Many other transformations of organoboranes are also possible but this section will focus only on the conversion to alcohols.

When the borane product resulting from the reaction of cyclopentene and diborane is treated with sodium hydroxide and hydrogen peroxide, what is the product?

The product is cyclopentanol. Boric acid [$B(OH)_3$] is also formed as a by-product.

What is the active reagent when sodium hydroxide is mixed with hydrogen peroxide?

The initial reaction is between hydrogen peroxide and hydroxide to produce the hydroperoxide anion (HOO^-).

What is the mechanism of the reaction of cyclopentene and diborane?

The hydroperoxide anion (HOO^-) attacks the boron of the tricyclopentylborane generated from cyclopentene, to form ***A***. A B→O carbon shift is accompanied by loss of hydroxide (^-OH) to give a so-called borinate (***B***). Two additional reactions of HOO^- followed by the B→O alkyl shift produces boric acid [$B(OH)_3$] and three equivalents of the alcohol (cyclopentanol). In general, a trialkylborane leads to three equivalents of the alcohol and a dialkylborane leads to two equivalents.

BH_3 HOO⁻ OOH B **A** 3 H_3O^+ B–O **B** 2 OH

What is the major product of reactions *(a)*, *(b)*, and *(c)*?

(a) 1. Thexylborane 2. NaOH , H_2O_2

(b) 1. 9-BBN 2. NaOH , H_2O_2

(c) 1. B_2H_6 2. NaOH , H_2O_2

In the case of (a), the product is the alcohol formed by "delivery" of boron (and thereby OH after the oxidation step) to the less substituted carbon of the alkene. The product is 3,6,7-trimethyloctan-2-ol. In (b) the alkene gives boron at the less hindered carbon of the C=C unit and oxidation gives the secondary alcohol, 1-cyclohexylbutan-1-ol. In (c), 1,2-dimethylcyclohexene is converted to 1,2-dimethylcyclohexan-1-ol, where the "cis" addition leads to the two methyl groups cis to each other but trans to the OH.

OH OH OH

3,6,7-Trimethyloctan-2-ol 1-Cyclohexylbutan-1-ol 1,2-Dimethylcyclohexan-1-ol

7.5 STRUCTURE AND NOMENCLATURE OF ALKYNES

What are alkynes?

Alkynes are organic hydrocarbons that contain a carbon–carbon triple bond, which is composed of two π-bonds that are perpendicular to one another. The chemistry of alkynes is very similar to that of alkenes due to the presence of π-bonds. The proximity of the π-bonds, however, leads to some interesting differences between alkenes and alkynes.

What is the characteristic feature of an alkyne?

Alkynes are characterized by a carbon–carbon triple bond: -C≡C-

What is the structure of acetylene (ethyne)?

Acetylene (ethyne) is a two-carbon molecule with the formula C_2H_2. Its structure is H-C≡C-H, where both hydrogen atoms and both carbons are linear. There is one σ-bond and two π-bonds. The two π-bonds are perpendicular to one another. These bonds are represented in the figure.

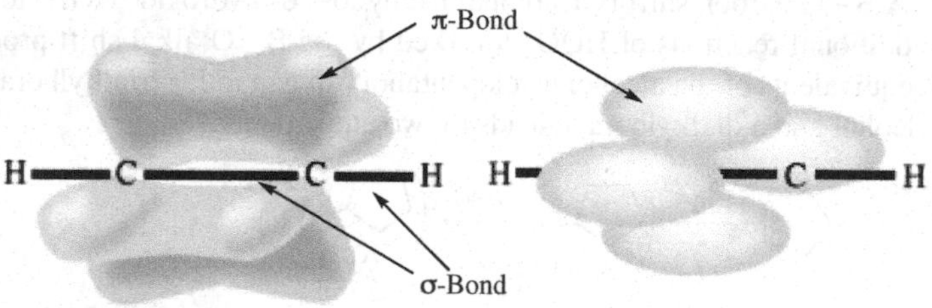

What is the hybridization of each carbon in acetylene?

The carbons are sp hybridized.

What is the spatial relationship of C1 and C4 in the four-carbon alkyne shown?

$$\overset{1}{H_3C}—\overset{2}{C}≡\overset{3}{C}—\overset{4}{CH_3}$$

Alkynes are linear. Since the triple bond is a linear unit, C1 and C4 must be 180° apart.

What is the molecular orbital diagram for the carbon–carbon triple bond of ethyne assuming sp hybridization for the two carbon atoms?

The molecular orbital diagram is shown in the diagram. There are two electrons in sp-hybrid orbitals (for the sp σ-bonds) and two electrons in p-orbitals (for the two π-bonds).

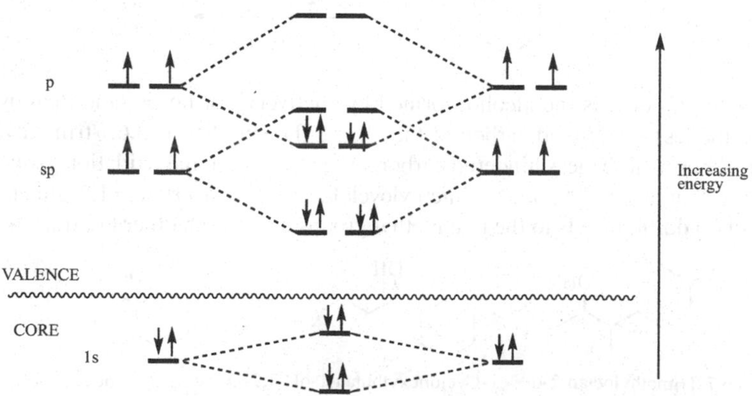

What are the two different structural types of alkynes?

Monosubstituted alkynes and disubstituted alkynes (terminal alkynes and internal alkynes, respectively).

What are the two different isomeric butynes? Provide the IUPAC name for each.

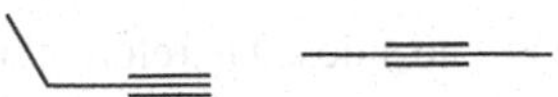

But-1-yne But-2-yne

What is the IUPAC ending for alkyne nomenclature?

The -ane ending of an alkane is dropped and replaced with the alkyne ending, *-yne*. A four-carbon alkyne is, therefore, butyne. The position of the first carbon of the triple bond is given the lowest number and the C≡C unit must be in the longest continuous chain. There are two butynes, and the position of the first alkyne carbon encountered receives the number 1, so the IUPAC names are but-1-yne ($CH_3CH_2C{\equiv}CH$) and but-2-yne ($CH_3C{\equiv}CCH_3$). Another example is the alkyne $CH_3CH_2CH_2C{\equiv}CCH_3$, which is named hex-2-yne.

Are isomers possible for alkynes that do not have substituents attached to the longest continuous chain?

Yes! Monosubstituted (terminal) alkynes have the generic formula R—C≡C—H. Disubstituted (internal) alkynes have the generic formula R—C≡C—R. The triple bond can be between C1–C2, C2–C3, C3–C4, etc. in a longer chain molecule, and each is an isomer.

Draw the structure of each of the isomeric heptynes using the following names: (a) hept-1-yne (b) hept-2-yne (c) hept-3-yne (d) hept-4-yne (e) hept-5-yne (f) help-6-yne.

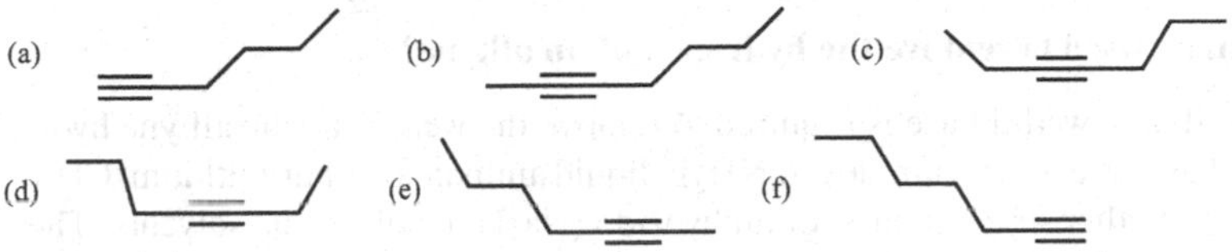

(a) (b) (c)

(d) (e) (f)

In the preceding question, how many different isomers are there?

As shown, there are only three heptynes: hept-1-yne, help-2-yne and hept-3-yne.

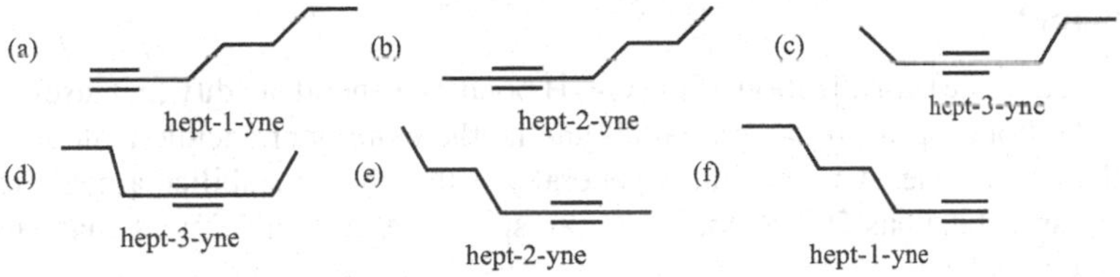

(a) hept-1-yne (b) hept-2-yne (c) hept-3-ync

(d) hept-3-yne (e) hept-2-yne (f) hept-1-yne

What is the correct structure for each of the following: (a) 5-chloro-4-ethylhept-2-yne (b) 5,5-dibromohex-1-yne (c) but-3-ynylcyclohexane (d) octa-2,6-diyne (e) hept-2*E*-en-5-yne (f) 3,3-dimethyloctan-5-yn-2-ol?

The structures are shown for (a)–(f).

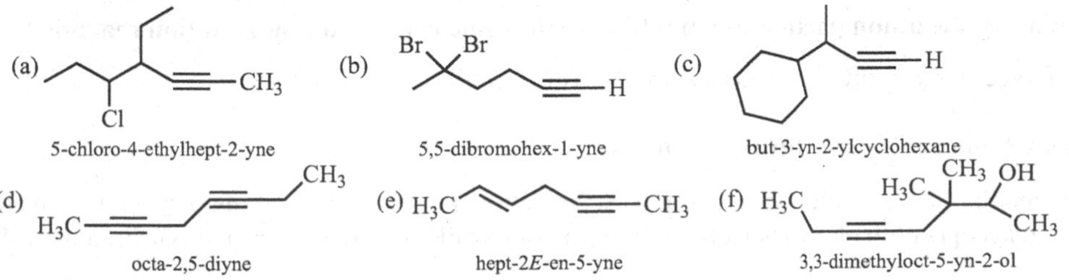

(a) Cl, CH_3 — 5-chloro-4-ethylhept-2-yne

(b) Br Br, H — 5,5-dibromohex-1-yne

(c) H — but-3-yn-2-ylcyclohexane

(d) H_3C, CH_3 — octa-2,5-diyne

(e) H_3C, CH_3 — hept-2*E*-en-5-yne

(f) H_3C, H_3C, CH_3, OH, CH_3 — 3,3-dimethyloct-5-yn-2-ol

Are there stereoisomers for internal alkynes such as but-2-yne?

No! The alkyne unit is linear, and there are no sides. Therefore, there are no stereoisomers.

Can cis/trans or *E*/*Z* nomenclature be used for internal alkynes such as but-2-yne?

No! The alkyne unit is linear, and there are no sides. Therefore, there are no stereoisomers.

7.6 REACTIONS OF ALKYNES

Can alkynes be classified as an acid?

Yes! The hydrogen atom of a terminal alkyne is a weak acid. The terminal hydrogen atom is attached to the sp-hybridized carbon of the triple bond, and this hybridization weakens the C—H bond, which leads to acidity for that hydrogen. Internal alkynes do not have a hydrogen atom attached to the sp-hybridized carbon, and do not have an acidic hydrogen.

What is the pK_a of the C—H bond of acetylene (ethyne)?

The pK_a of the terminal hydrogen on acetylene (H—C≡C—**H**) is about 25. Compared to acetic acid (pK_a of 4.7) and even water (pK_a of 14.0), acetylene is a very weak acid and requires a rather strong base to remove the acidic hydrogen. The product of the acid/base reaction is called an *acetylide* (also known as an *alkyne anion*), with a negative charge residing on carbon:

$$\text{H—C} \equiv \text{C—H} + \text{BASE} \rightarrow \text{H—C} \equiv \text{C:}^-$$

What bases can be used to remove the hydrogen of an alkyne?

As just mentioned, a powerful base is required to remove the weakly acidic alkyne hydrogen. The most commonly used bases are sodium amide ($NaNH_2$ in liquid ammonia), *n*-butyllithium ($CH_3CH_2CH_2CH_2Li$, see Section 10.3) in ether solvents, or sodium hydride (NaH) in anhydrous solvents. The use of sodium hydride is very attractive since the by-product of the acid/base reaction is hydrogen gas (½H_2), which pushes the equilibrium toward the sodium salt of the alkyne (a sodium acetylide, R—C≡C:$^-$$Na^+$).

Why is the hydrogen atom of a terminal alkyne more acidic than the hydrogen atom of an alkene or an alkane?

The acidity is related to the hybridization of the C—H bond. In general, acidity increases with increased "s-character" of the bond: sp > sp^2 > sp^3. An alkyne is, therefore, more acidic than an alkene, which is more acidic than an alkane. An s-orbital is generally better able to stabilize a negative charge than a p-orbital and an sp-orbital has 50% s-character. An sp^3-orbital has only 25% s character and an sp^2-orbital has 33% s-character.

What is the reactivity of an acetylide?

Since the negative charge resides on carbon, acetylides (alkyne anions) are powerful carbon *nucleophiles* and acetylides behave as *carbanions*.

Can an acetylide anion participate in a bimolecular nucleophile in a substitution reaction?

Yes! Bimolecular substitution reactions are described in Sections 8.2 and 8.3.

What is a bimolecular substitution reaction?

A biomolecular nucleophilic substitution, or S_N2 reaction, proceeds by breaking one bond to an atom or group that accepts both electrons from the broken bond while one bond is formed synchronously (in one step). The net result of this reaction is that one group or atom is replaced (substituted) by another. This reaction will be introduced in Section 8.2.

What is the reaction type when the alkyne anion of but-1-yne reacts with iodomethane?

An alkyne anion is nucleophilic and reacts with the δ^+ carbon of an alkyl halide in a bimolecular substitution reaction (Sections 8.2 and 8.3). In this case, the product is pent-2-yne ($CH_3CH_2C{\equiv}C{:}^-Na^+ + CH_3I \rightarrow CH_3CH_2C{\equiv}CCH_3$).

What solvents are appropriate for the reaction of acetylides and alkyl halides?

A polar aprotic solvent should be used such as diethyl ether, tetrahydrofuran (THF), dimethylformamide (DMF), or dimethyl sulfoxide (DMSO).

What is the structure of THF, of DMF, or DMSO?

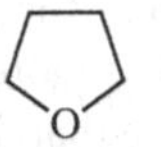

THF 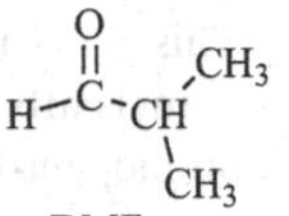 DMF 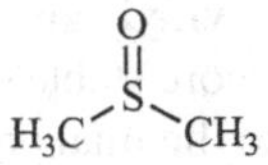 DMSO

What is the major product of reactions (a), (b), and (c)?

(a) 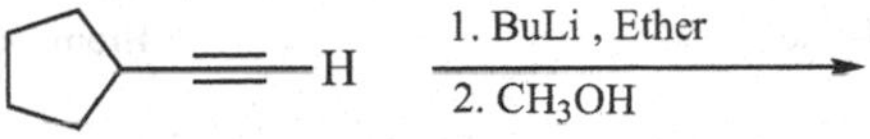 1. BuLi, Ether 2. CH_3OH

(b) 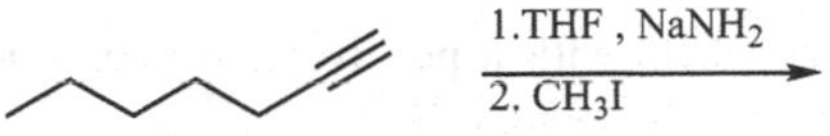 1. THF, $NaNH_2$ 2. CH_3I

(c) 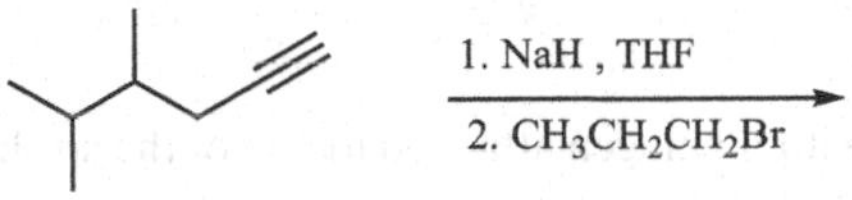 1. NaH, THF 2. $CH_3CH_2CH_2Br$

(d) 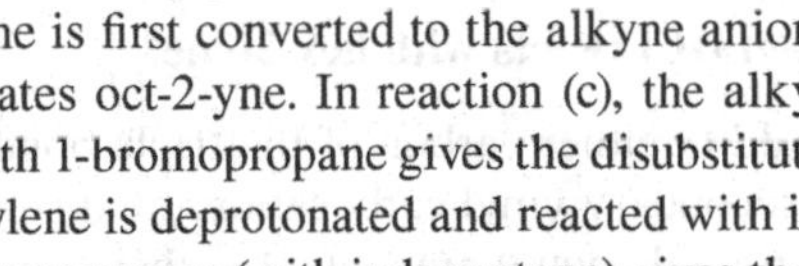 H—≡—H 1. $NaNH_2$, THF 2. CH_3Br 3. $NaNH_2$, Ether 4. 1-iodopentane

In reaction (a), the alkyne reacts with the base to generate the alkyne anion, which is electron rich and can act as a base as well as a nucleophile. Subsequent treatment with methanol, which is an acid in the presence of the basic alkyne anion, leads to protonation to give back the starting material, ethynylcyclopentane. In reaction (b), the alkyne is first converted to the alkyne anion with $NaNH_2$, and subsequent reaction with iodomethane generates oct-2-yne. In reaction (c), the alkyne is converted to the alkyne anion with base, and alkylation with 1-bromopropane gives the disubstituted alkyne product, 7,8-dimethylnon-4-yne. In reaction (d), acetylene is deprotonated and reacted with iodomethane to give 1-propyne. A second deprotonation-alkylation sequence (with iodopentane) gives the final product, oct-2-yne.

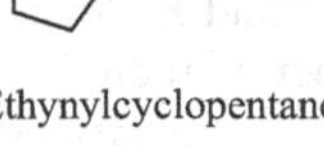

Ethynylcyclopentane 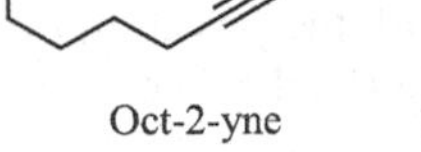 Oct-2-yne 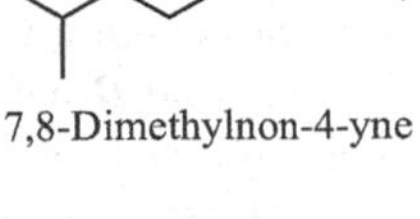 7,8-Dimethylnon-4-yne 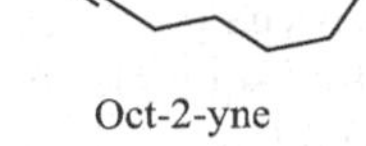 Oct-2-yne

Can alkynes react with Brønsted–Lowry acids (HX)?

Yes! Alkynes react as Brønsted–Lowry bases with acids, HX.

What intermediate is formed when HCl reacts with ethyne (acetylene)?

The intermediate is a vinyl carbocation, with the positive charge on the sp^2-hybridized carbon, as shown.

$$H{-}C{\equiv}C{-}H \longrightarrow \left[\overset{+}{C}H{=}CH_2 \right] Cl^-$$

A vinyl cation

When pent-1-yne reacts with HBr, to which carbon of the triple bond is the bromine attached?

When HBr reacts with pent-1-yne, the hydrogen will add to the less substituted carbon to give the positive charge on the more substituted carbon, which is a secondary vinyl carbocation and more stable than the alternative primary vinyl carbocation. Subsequent reaction with the nucleophilic bromide ion will be attached to the more highly substituted carbon in the final product, 2-bromopent-1-ene.

For the reaction to proceed, one of the two π-bonds of the alkyne donates an electron pair to the acidic proton of HBr to generate a "vinyl carbocation." This acid–base reaction can generate a less stable primary vinyl carbocation or a more stable secondary vinyl carbocation. The more stable carbocation forms and reaction with Br^- leads to the final product, 2-bromopent-1-ene. Note that this sequence that includes the vinyl cation constitutes the mechanism of the reaction.

Pent-1-yne $\xrightarrow{HBr}$ [vinyl cation, Br^-] $\longrightarrow$ 2-Bromopent-1-ene

What is a vinyl carbocation?

A vinyl carbocation is an intermediate with a positive charge on one of the sp^2-hybridized carbons ($C{=}C^+$).

What is a vinyl halide?

A vinyl halide is an alkene with a halogen attached to one of the sp^2-hybridized carbons (C=C—X).

What is the relative stability of a vinyl carbocation?

The presence of a π-bond that is orthogonal to the charge makes a vinyl carbocation highly unstable and therefore very reactive. In general, alkyl carbocations are more stable than vinyl carbocations, and a 2° vinyl carbocation is more stable than a 1° vinyl carbocation. A secondary vinyl carbocation is much less stable than a normal secondary carbocation, but once formed it is more reactive with a nucleophile. Vinyl carbocations do not rearrange and react very quickly.

What products are formed when HCl reacts with hex-2-yne?

The acidic proton of HCl can add to either carbon of the triple bond of hex-2-yne to give two vinyl carbocations, ***A*** or ***B***. Both are secondary vinyl carbocations, and since there is no difference in relative stability, both will form in roughly equal amounts. In other words, there is no energy difference for one carbocation to be formed preferentially over the other. When the nucleophilic chloride ion reacts with ***A*** and ***B***, two vinyl chlorides are formed, 3-chlorohex-2-ene and 2-chlorohex-2-ene. Since the internal alkyne generates a vinyl carbocation with the possibility of *Z*- and *E*-isomers, indicated by the use of a "squiggle" line. Since ***A*** and ***B*** have roughly the same energy, there is no reason to form one in preference to the other, and each of the final alkene products is a mixture of *E*- and *Z*-isomers. A total of four products are formed in this reaction, *E*- and *Z*-chlorohex-2-ene and *E*- and *Z*-2-chlorohex-2-ene.

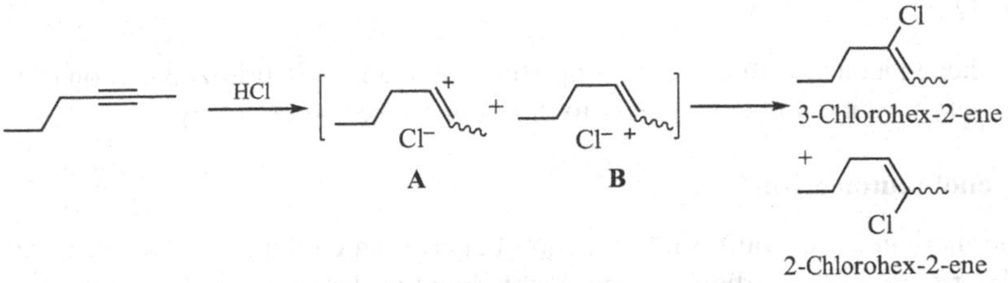

3-Chlorohex-2-ene

2-Chlorohex-2-ene

What is the major product of reactions (a), (b), and (c)?

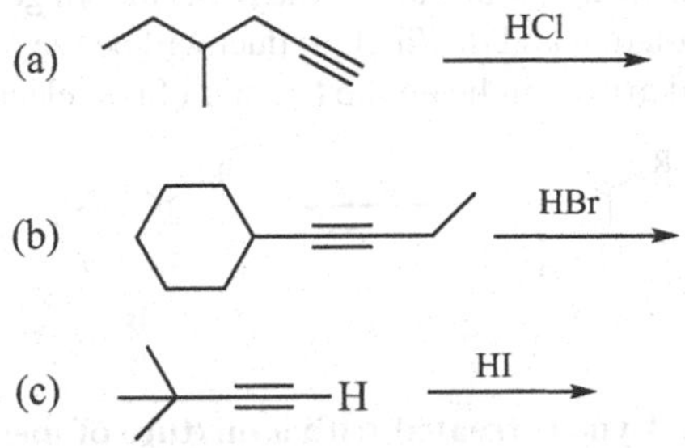

In the reaction of (a), the more stable secondary vinyl carbocation is formed, and the final product is 2-chloro-4-methylhex-1-ene. In the reaction of (b), two secondary vinyl carbocations of essentially equal stability are formed, leading to two products *E*- and *Z*-(1-bromobut-1-en-1-yl)cyclohexane and *E*- and *Z*-(2-bromobut-1-en-1-yl)cyclohexane. Alkyne (c) is a terminal alkyne, and formation of the secondary vinyl carbocation leads to the major product, 2-iodo-3,3-dimethylbut-1-ene.

2-Chloro-4-methyl-hex-1-ene (1-Bromobut-1-en-1-yl)-cyclohexane (2-Bromobut-1-en-1-yl)-cyclohexane 2-Iodo-3,3-dimethyl-but-1-ene

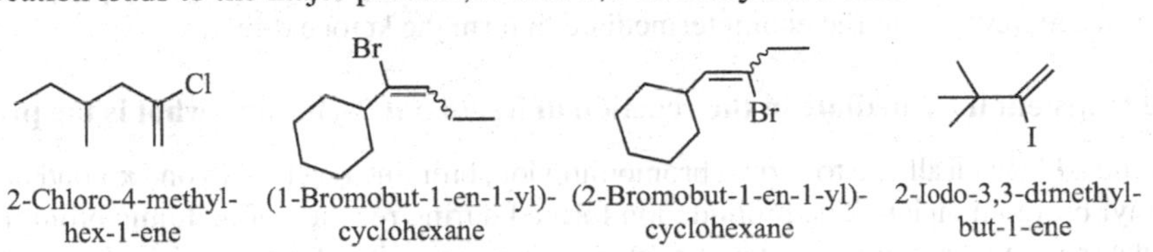

Does pent-1-yne react with water when no other reagent is present?

No! Water is too weak of an acid to react with the very weakly basic π-bonds of an alkyne. A reaction can only occur if a strong acid is added to the alkyne, to generate a vinyl carbocation, allowing water to react as a nucleophile.

What is the initial product when pent-1-yne reacts with aqueous acid? What is the fate of that initial product?

The initial reaction of pent-1-yne and H^+ generates vinyl carbocation ***A***. Water is a nucleophile in this system, and it attacks the vinyl carbocation to form an oxonium ion (***B***), which loses a proton to form an *enol* (***C***), which is named pent-1-en-2-ol. Enols are relatively unstable and internal transfer a hydrogen (from the O—H) to the adjacent carbon of the carbon–carbon double bond to generate a carbonyl, in this case ketone, pentan-2-one. The *initial product* is, however, enol ***C***. Enols are discussed in more detail in Section 17.1.

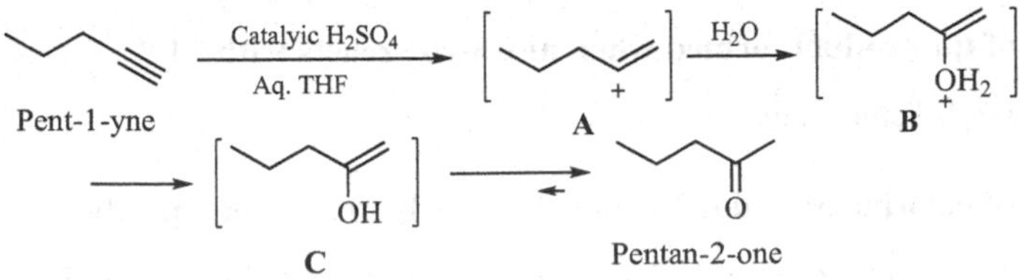

Pent-1-yne → (Catalytic H_2SO_4, Aq. THF) → A → (H_2O) → B → C ⇌ Pentan-2-one

What is an enol?

An enol is an alkene alcohol, with the OH group attached to an sp^2-hybridized carbon of the C=C unit. Most enols are very unstable and tautomerize to the isomeric ketone or aldehyde.

What is keto–enol tautomerism?

Keto–enol tautomerism is the equilibrium reaction between an enol and its carbonyl partner (as with ***A*** and ***B***). If the π-bond of the carbon–carbon double bond in the enol (see ***A***) donates electrons to the acidic O—H bond, a new C—H bond is formed and a new π-bond is formed between carbon and oxygen (the keto form, a carbonyl – see ***B***). This equilibrium almost always favors the keto form over the enol form unless other electron-withdrawing groups are in the molecule. In general, assume that if an enol is formed, it will not be stable to isolation and the final product will be the carbonyl (ketone or aldehyde in these cases). Note that the curved arrows indicate the transfer of two electrons.

R O–H A ⇌ R CH$_2$ H O B

What is the product when pent-1-yne is treated with a mixture of mercuric acetate and mercuric sulfate in aqueous media?

A π-bond on the alkyne reacts with the mercury to give the mercury–vinyl cation. Just as in oxymercuration reaction of alkenes, the mercuric salts stabilize the vinyl carbocation (the more stable secondary vinyl carbocation), and addition of water leads to an enol that tautomerizes to pentan-2-one as the major product. The difference between alkynes and alkenes is that the vinyl–mercury compound is unstable and rapidly loses mercury from the enol intermediate to form the ketone directly.

What is the transient intermediate in the reaction of Br_2 to but-2-yne, and what is the product?

Just as bromine adds to an alkene to form a bromonium ion, bromine reacts with one π-bond of but-2-yne to form a vinyl bromonium ion. The bromide ion formed during reaction of diatomic bromine with the alkyne attacks the vinyl bromonium ion as a nucleophile, opening it to form the vicinal vinyl dibromide, in this case 2,3-dibromobut-2-ene. In general, the trans isomer predominates since the ring opening requires anti attack, as with reactions of alkenes.

H$_3$C–≡–CH$_3$ + Br–Br → [H$_3$C, Br$^+$, CH$_3$, Br$^-$] A → Br, CH$_3$, H$_3$C, Br

(*E*)-2,3-dibromobut-2-ene

Why do the bromine atoms in the product of a reaction between hex-3-yne and bromine have a trans relationship?

As noted in the formation of the trans product *trans*-2,3-dibromobut-2-ene, a "vinyl bromonium ion" is formed and the nucleophilic bromide ion that opens this intermediate will attack on the face opposite the bromine (anti- attack) due to steric and electronic repulsive forces.

What is the name of the product formed when hex-3-yne reacts with Cl_2?

The product is *trans*-3,4-dichlorohex-3-ene.

If two equivalents of chlorine are added to hex-3-yne, what is the final product?

The product is 3,3,4,4-tetrachlorohexane. The C=C unit of the initially formed 3,4-dibromo-3-hexene reacts with additional bromine (Section 7.4.4) to give the product.

What is the major product when 5,6-dimethyl-1-cyclohexyl-oct-3-yne is treated with Br_2 in CCl_4?

The major product is (*E*)-(3,4-dibromo-5,6-dimethylhept-3-en-1-yl)cyclohexane.

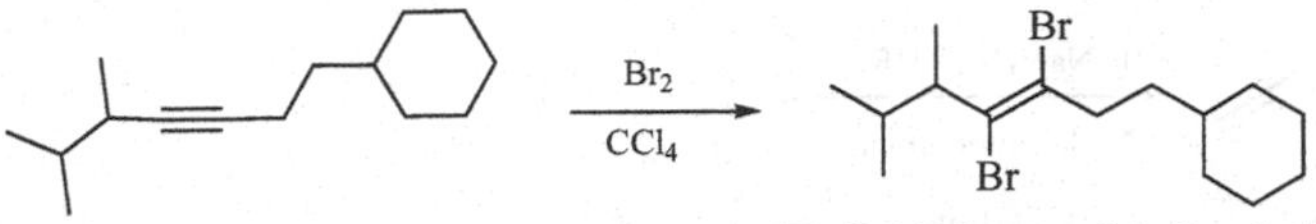

Br_2 / CCl_4

(*E*)-(3,4-Dibromo-5,6-dimethylhept-3-en-1-yl)cyclohexane

Why does (*E*)-(3,4-dibromo-5,6-dimethylhept-3-en-1-yl)cyclohexane in the preceding problem not have a chlorine atom in it, when carbon tetrachloride was used?

Carbon tetrachloride is the solvent in this reaction, does not react with the alkyne, and does not participate in the reaction other than the properties of a solvent.

END OF CHAPTER PROBLEMS

1. What is the geometry of the atoms in 2,3-dimethylbut-2-ene?
2. Name $CH_3CH_2CH_2C{=}C(Br)Cl$.
3. Discuss why alkene ***A*** is more stable than alkene ***B***.

A B

4. Give the IUPAC name for each of the following:

(a) (b) (c)

(d) (e) (f)

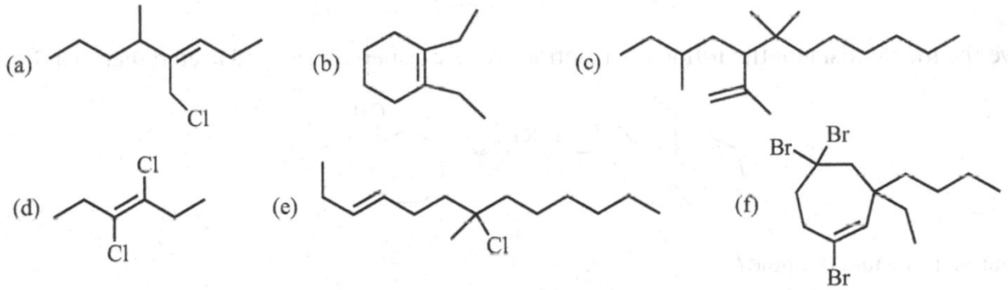

5. Explain how 3-chlorohex-3Z-ene is also properly labeled as a trans-alkene (i.e., why does *Z not* translate directly to cis).
6. Give the correct IUPAC names for each of the following:

(a) (b)

(c) (d)

(e)

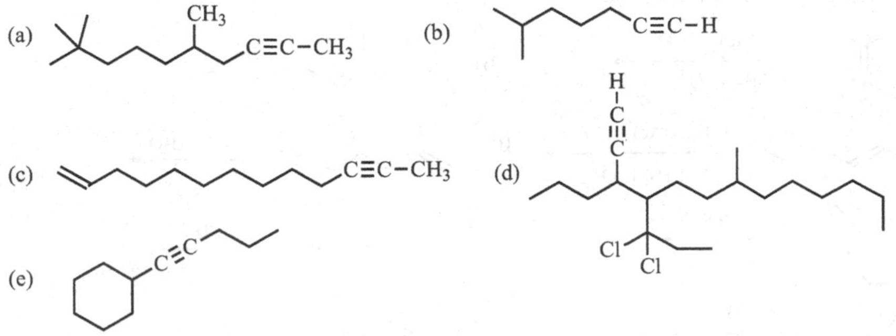

7. Which hydrogen is removed first when H—C≡C—CO_2H is treated with one equivalent of *n*-butyllithium? Explain.
8. In each case give the major product of the reaction. Remember stereochemistry and if there is no reaction, indicate by N.R.:

(a) 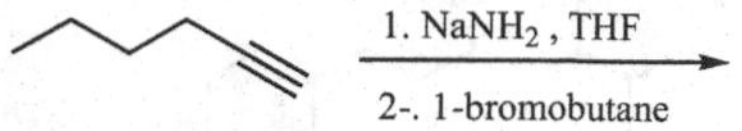 1. $NaNH_2$, THF; 2-. 1-bromobutane

(b) 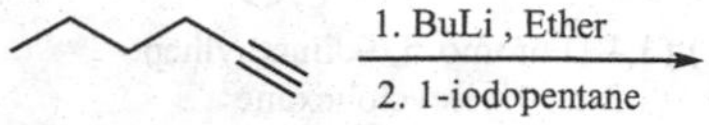 1. BuLi, Ether; 2. 1-iodopentane

(c) 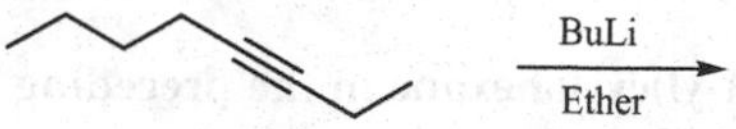 BuLi; Ether

(d) 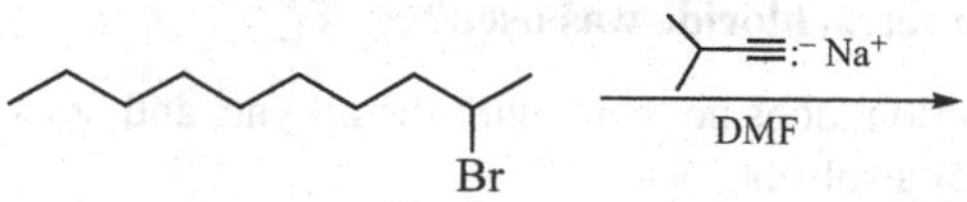 ≡:⁻ Na^+; DMF; Br

9. Give the mechanism for the following reaction:

HCl; Cl

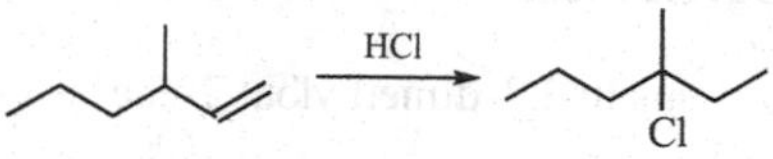

10. Why does 2-methylbut-2-ene react faster with HCl than does but-1-ene?
11. Explain why the H^+ of HBr adds to C1 rather than C2 to give the major product.

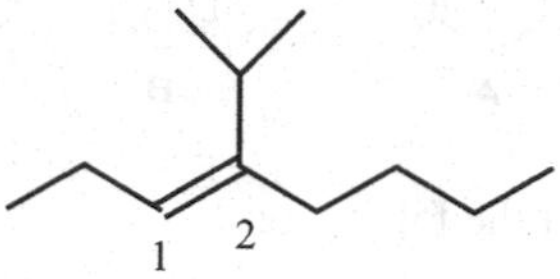

1 2

12. Give the mechanism for the following reaction. Why was perchloric acid used rather than HCl?

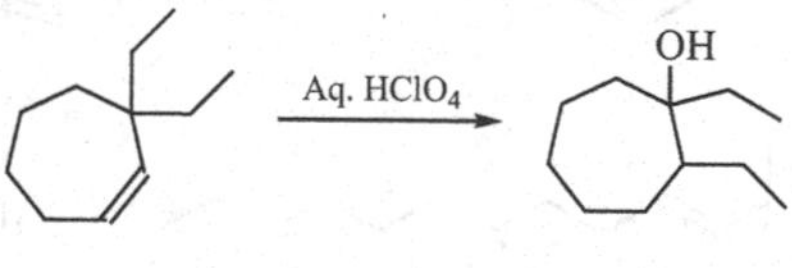

Aq. $HClO_4$; OH

13. What is an induced dipole?
14. Does trans-but-2-ene react with iodine to give a meso compound or the d,l pair?
15. In the reaction of 2-methylpent-1-ene and bromine, which carbon is attacked by the bromide ion? Explain.
16. In each of the following reactions give the major product. Remember stereochemistry and if there is no reaction, indicate by N.R.:

(a) 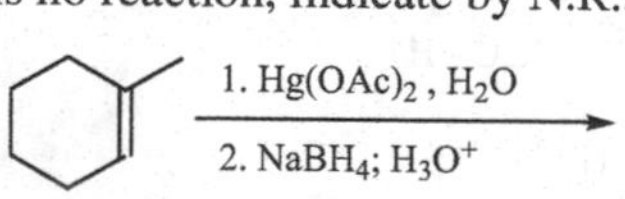 1. $Hg(OAc)_2$, H_2O; 2. $NaBH_4$; H_3O^+

(b) 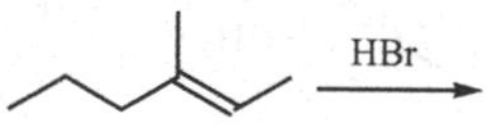 HBr

(c) 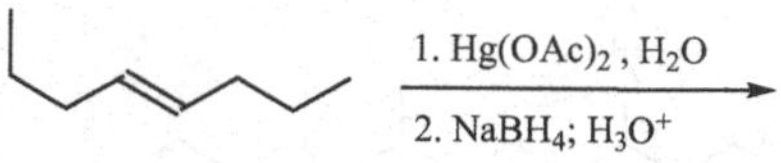 1. $Hg(OAc)_2$, H_2O; 2. $NaBH_4$; H_3O^+

(d) 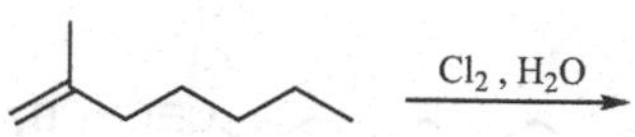 Cl_2, H_2O

(e) 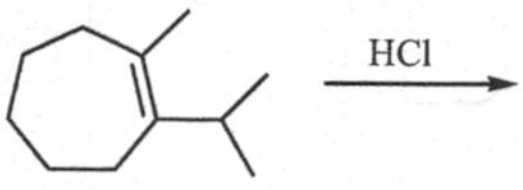 HCl

(f) 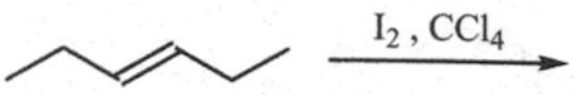 I_2, CCl_4

(g) 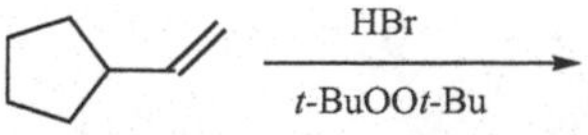 HBr; *t*-BuOO*t*-Bu

(h) Br_2; CCl_4

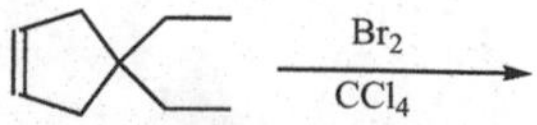

17. In each case give the major product of the reaction. Remember stereochemistry and if there is no reaction, indicate by N.R.:

(a) 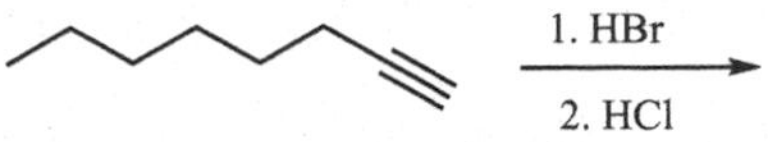 1. HBr; 2. HCl

(b) 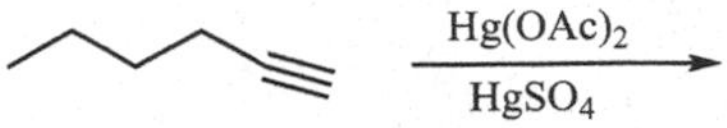 $Hg(OAc)_2$, $HgSO_4$

(c) 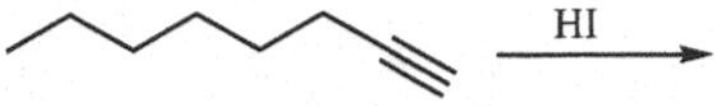 HI

(d) 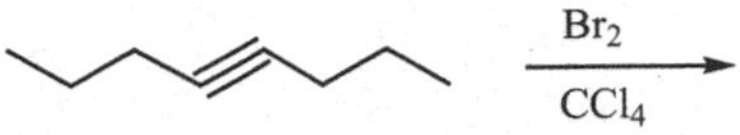 Br_2, CCl_4

(e) 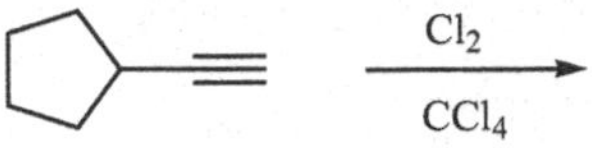 Cl_2, CCl_4

(f) 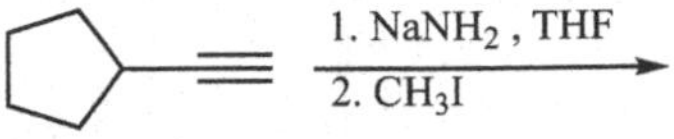 1. $NaNH_2$, THF; 2. CH_3I

(g) 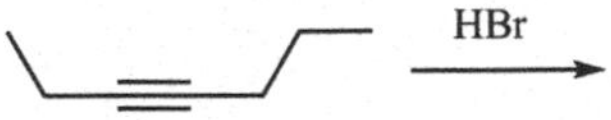 HBr

18. For each of the following reactions give the major product. Remember stereochemistry where appropriate and if there is no reaction, indicate by N.R.:

(a) 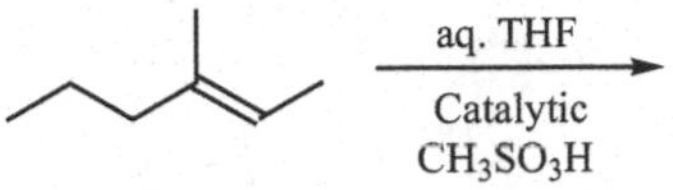 aq. THF, Catalytic CH_3SO_3H

(b) 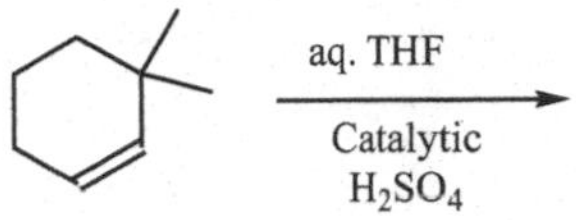 aq. THF, Catalytic H_2SO_4

(c) 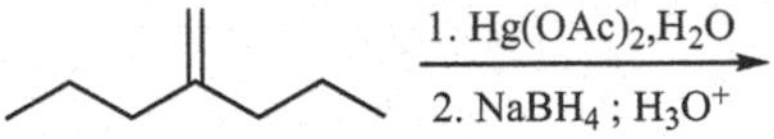 1. $Hg(OAc)_2$,H_2O; 2. $NaBH_4$; H_3O^+

(d) 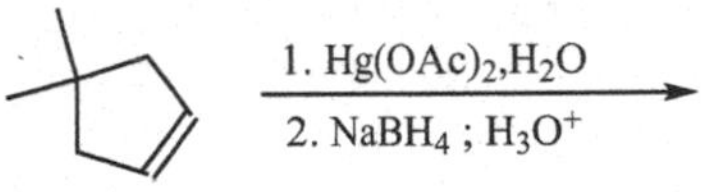 1. $Hg(OAc)_2$,H_2O; 2. $NaBH_4$; H_3O^+

(e) 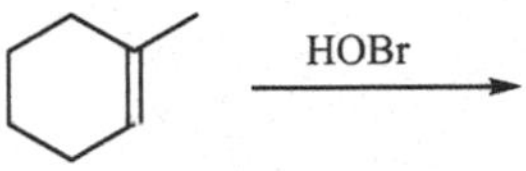 HOBr

(f) 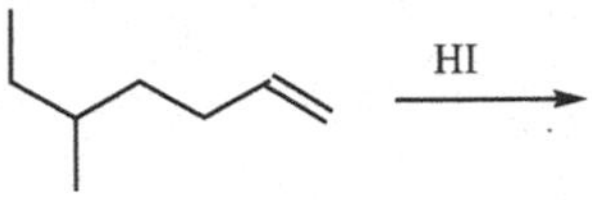 HI

19. Give the complete mechanism for the following reaction:

$Hg(OAc)_2$, EtOH

OEt

HgOAc

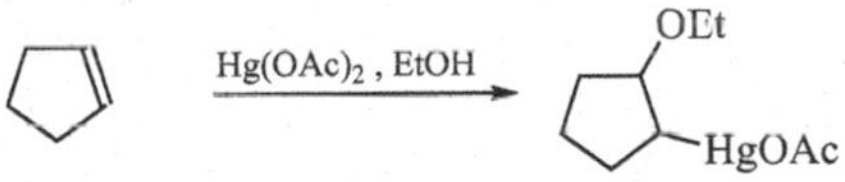

8

Alkyl Halides and Substitution Reactions

Alkyl halides are molecules with one or more F (alkyl fluorides), Cl (alkyl chlorides), Br (alkyl bromides), or I (alkyl iodides) atoms attached to a carbon. Each C–halogen bond (C—X) is polarized C^{+}–$X^{\delta-}$, and a variety of reagents (called nucleophiles) can react with $C^{\delta+}$ to generate other types of functional groups. The reaction just described is known as a substitution reaction, where one atom or group attaches to carbon and replaces the X group of the C—X bond. Reactions that generate halides will be discussed as well as the reactions of halides to form other compounds.

8.1 STRUCTURE, PROPERTIES, AND NOMENCLATURE OF ALKYL HALIDES

What is an alkyl halide?

An alkyl halide is any molecule that contains one or more halogen atoms attached to a carbon atom. In most cases, the carbon atom will be sp^3-hybridized, but halogens can be attached to sp^2- and also sp-hybridized carbon, so alkene halides and alkyne halides are known.

Why is the C—X bond of an alkyl halide polarized?

Alkyl halides are characterized by a C—X bond, where X = F, Cl, Br, or I. Since all halogen atoms are more electronegative than carbon, the C—X bond must be polarized. Indeed, the C—X bond is highly polarized with a δ^+ carbon and a δ^- halogen. Fluorine is the most electronegative element and the C—F bond is the most polarized. Fluorine is a small atom, however, and that bond is relatively strong. Although less polarized, the C—I bond is relatively weak due to the long bond length dictated by the large iodine atom when bonded to carbon.

What are the generalized physical properties of alkyl halides?

Despite the polarized C—X bond, alkyl halides are not considered to be polar compounds when compared to water or an alcohol. Alkyl halides are more polar than alkanes but tend to be insoluble in water. The carbon that bears the halogen has a δ^+ dipole and that carbon can react with certain molecules containing atoms that can donate electrons. The electron-donating molecules that react at carbon are known as *nucleophiles*.

Is the halogen in an alkyl halide considered to be a functional group?

No! In an alkyl halide, the halogen is considered to be a substituent.

What is the IUPAC nomenclature rule for naming alkyl halides?

Determine the longest continuous chain of carbon atoms and assign the appropriate prefix and suffix. Each halogen is treated as a *substituent* and assigned a number to designate its position on the carbon chain. Drop the *-ine* from fluorine, chlorine, bromine, or iodine and replace that suffix with *-o*. Fluorine becomes fluoro, chlorine becomes chloro, bromine becomes bromo, and iodine becomes iodo. Also see Section 4.4.

What is the IUPAC name of the compound shown?

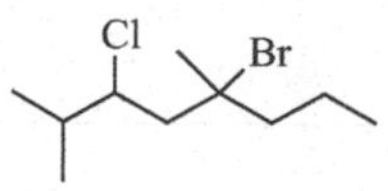

This compound is named 5-bromo-3-chloro-2,5-dimethyloctane.

What is the nomenclature rule if the halogen atom is part of a substituent rather than attached to the longest continuous chain?

Name the halogen as a substituent on the substituent. Determine the longest chain of the substituent from the point of attachment to the longest continuous chain, and then assign the halogen the appropriate number on the substituent chain. For example, $-CH_2Cl$ is chloromethyl and $-CH(Br)CH_2CH_3$ is 1-bromopropyl.

What is the name of the compound shown?

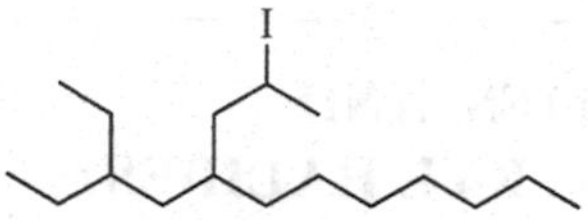

This compound is named 3-ethyl-5-(2-iodopropyl)dodecane.

8.2 SECOND-ORDER NUCLEOPHILIC SUBSTITUTION (S_N2) REACTIONS

What type of reaction is typified by displacement of halogen in an alkyl halide?

When an atom or group replaces another atom or group, at carbon, the process is known as a substitution reaction. When the substitution proceeds without an intermediate, but rather via a concerted process, it is known as nucleophilic biomolecular substitution, and given the designator S_N2.

What is a substitution reaction?

A substitution reaction is characterized by one atom or group replacing another atom or group at an sp^3-atom (usually carbon). This transformation is made possible by the presence of a polarized bond in an alkyl halide (C—Cl, C—Br, or C—I), where the carbon is electron deficient and has a polarity of δ^+. That carbon is most likely to react with an electron donating species.

What is a nucleophile?

If an electron rich species donates its electrons to a *carbon*, it is called a *nucleophile.* This definition is used to distinguish reactions at carbon from reactions at other atoms. When an electron rich species donates electrons to an atom other than C or H, it is known as a *Lewis base*. An electron rich species that donates two electrons to hydrogen is a *Brønsted–Lowry base.*

What is an electrophilic carbon?

The carbon that bears the halogen is an electrophilic carbon with δ^+ polarization. This electrophilic carbon reacts with a nucleophile, forming a new bond to the nucleophile.

What is nucleophilic substitution?

The replacement of one atom or group by a nucleophile.

What is a S_N2 reaction?

A S_N2 reaction is a second-order bimolecular nucleophilic substitution reaction. This reaction is a collision process where a nucleophile collides with an electrophilic carbon and such a reaction follows second-order kinetics. The rate constant depends on the concentration changes for both reactants.

What are the characteristics of a $S_N2$reaction?

A S_N2 reaction is bimolecular, which means that a collision occurs between the nucleophile and the molecule that bears the leaving group. The reaction follows second-order kinetics. The nucleophile approaches the carbon bearing the leaving group from 180° opposite the leaving group (backside attack).

What is a simple example of a nucleophilic substitution that involved molecules with no more than one carbon?

A simple example of a substitution is the reaction of a nucleophile (iodide) with bromomethane (the electrophile) to give iodomethane and the bromide ion. The positive counterion is omitted so the focus can be on the substitution reaction. Note the use of the *curved arrows,* indicating that *iodide ion donates two electrons* to the electrophilic carbon, forming a new C—I bond, and the C—Br bond is broken and the electrons in that bond are transferred to bromine to form the bromide ion.

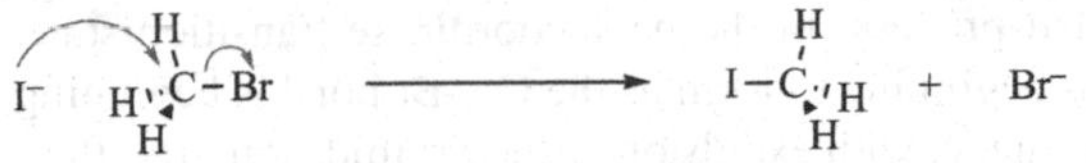

$$I^- \quad H_3C{-}Br \longrightarrow I{-}CH_3 + Br^-$$

What does a curved arrow indicate in a chemical reaction?

The so-called *curved arrow formalism* indicates electron flow. The curved arrow in a reaction is used to indicate the transfer of two electrons form a bond between two atoms or from an electron pair to another atom to form a new covalent bond.

What is a leaving group?

A leaving group is the group that "leaves" in a substitution reaction. Actually, the leaving group (Br in the preceding question) does not spontaneously leave but is "kicked out" (displaced) by the nucleophile as the nucleophile collides with the electrophilic carbon in this substitution reaction.

What is a reactive intermediate?

A reactive intermediate is the product of a reaction that is high in energy, and reacts further to give a stable, isolable product. The most common reactive intermediates that will be seen in this book involve carbon atoms including carbocations (also known as carbenium ions, such as those seen in the reactions of alkenes and alkynes with mineral acids in Section 7.3). Other intermediates include carbanions and carbon radicals.

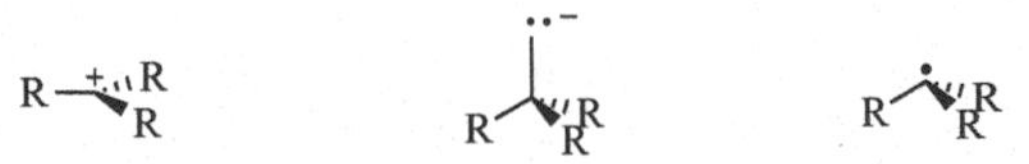

$$R_3C^+ \qquad R_3C^{:-} \qquad R_3C\cdot$$

Carbocation Carbanion Carbon Radical

Has a reactive intermediate ever been observed in bimolecular substitution reactions; e.g., the conversion of bromomethane to iodomethane?

No! This transformation is believed to be a synchronous process (no intermediate).

What is a synchronous reaction?

A synchronous reaction is one that occurs without a reactive intermediate. In other words, bond breaking and bond making occur in a synchronous manner, once the activation energy for bond breaking/making has been attained, and the result is the product. There are no reactive intermediate products along the way.

What is a concerted reaction?

For all reactions presented in this book, a concerted reaction will be considered the same as a synchronous reaction are the same.

What is the activation energy?

Activation energy is the energy required to initiate a chemical reaction (see Section 3.2). In other words, the energy required to initiate bond making and bond breaking in a chemical reaction.

What is a transition state?

A transition state is the logical mid-point of a reaction in which bonds are beginning to be broken and other bonds beginning to be formed. *A transition state cannot be isolated or even detected.* The transition state for the conversion of bromomethane to iodomethane should be the *pentacoordinate species* shown if this is a concerted process. In the pentacoordinate transition state, there are not really five bonds but the C—I bond is beginning to form as the C—Br bond is beginning to break. As the reaction proceeds, the C—I bond is made, with expulsion of the bromide ion after the C—Br bond is completely broken. Note the use of dashed lines in the transition state to indicate bonds being broken or formed, and the use of the bracket to indicate a transient entity.

Transition State

Can a transition state be isolated?

No! A transition state is the midpoint of bond breaking–bond making, but is not an intermediate or a product and cannot be isolated (see Section 3.2).

Given that bromomethane is three-dimensional (tetrahedral), from what angle will the bromide ion be most likely to approach the carbon atom to minimize steric and electronic repulsions?

There will be significant electronic repulsion as the electron rich iodide approaches over the electron rich bromine atom, as well as steric repulsion. If iodide approaches near any of the hydrogen atoms, there will be steric repulsion. If the iodide approaches from 180° relative to the bromine (*backside attack*), as shown, electronic and steric repulsion will be minimized, and backside attack is the preferred trajectory for this reaction.

What is the transition state for nucleophilic bimolecular substitution at carbon?

The incoming nucleophile (such as the iodide ion) must *collide* with the electrophile (the δ^+ carbon of CH_3Br) for the substitution reaction to occur. The iodide is negatively charged and will be repelled by the δ^- bromine of bromomethane. If iodide approaches the tetrahedral carbon over one of the hydrogen atoms, the iodide and hydrogen repel (*steric repulsion*) as they attempt to occupy the same space. The path of least resistance that also minimizes electronic repulsion is, therefore, *backside attack*, where iodide approaches the carbon 180° away from the bromine. As iodide approaches carbon, the hydrogen atoms are pushed away until a five-coordinate (pentacoordinate) *transition state* is formed (see above) where the three hydrogens and the carbon are coplanar, the C—I bond is beginning to form, and the C—Br bond is beginning to break. This transition state is the logical mid-point of the reaction and is *not* a product that can be isolated or even observed. As the C—I bond is formed, the hydrogens are pushed further away and the C—Br bond is broken, to form iodomethane. The net result of this collision via backside attack is *inversion of configuration at the electrophilic carbon.* To observe such an inversion, the molecule must have a stereogenic center at the carbon bearing the halogen. This inversion of configuration has been called *Walden inversion*, which is the logical consequence of a reaction that proceeds via a pentacoordinate transition state.

How can the conversion of bromomethane to iodomethane be classified when there is no intermediate?

The conversion of bromomethane to iodomethane is a collision process (involves two molecules), so the reaction follows second-order kinetics, which makes it a *bimolecular reaction.* It is a second-order bimolecular substitution reaction that is termed a *S_N2 reaction.* The rate of the reaction is the disappearance of the starting material in mol sec^{-1} or appearance of product in mole sec^{-1}, usually measured as disappearance of starting material. The reaction rate is given by the expression: rate = k [nucleophile] [halide], where [ ] represents the concentration in moles/liter of each molecule. For a S_N2 reaction, increasing the concentration of either nucleophile or halide will increase the rate of the reaction. The parameter (k) is called the rate constant. Larger rate constants are associated with faster reactions.

Can other alkyl halides react by a S_N2 reaction?

Yes! Methyl halides, primary alkyl halides, and secondary alkyl halides react with nucleophiles by a S_N2 reaction. Tertiary halides do not react due to steric hindrance around the electrophilic carbon

What nucleophiles are used in the S_N2 reaction?

Initially, the nucleophiles to be discussed are the halide ions, iodide bromide and chloride ion. Iodide will displace bromide and chloride, and bromide will displace chloride in a S_N2 reaction. The chloride ion will not displace either bromide or iodide, and the bromide ion will not displace iodide. Other nucleophiles include alkoxide ions (RO^-), amines (RNH_2 or R_2NH), cyanide ion (^-CN), and the azide ion (N_3^-).

What is steric hindrance?

Two objects cannot occupy the same space. When two atoms or groups come close to each other and attempt to occupy the same space intermolecularly or intramolecularly there is a large energy barrier and those atoms or groups repel. The larger the bulk of the atom or group, the greater the steric interaction, the greater the steric hindrance, and the greater the energy barrier.

Why does bromomethane react with sodium iodide much faster than 2-bromopropane?

For S_N2 reactions, primary halides react much faster than secondary halides with the same nucleophile, via a pentacoordinate transition state. Tertiary halides are essentially unreactive under the same conditions. The S_N2 reaction with methyl, primary, and secondary halides is useful with a variety of nucleophiles, but S_N2 reactions with tertiary halides give no substitution. The reason is *steric hindrance in the pentacoordinate transition state.* The *relative rate constants* are: CH_3X = 1.0; primary (such as CH_3CH_2X = 0.033; secondary (such as $Me_2CHX = 8.3 \times 10^{-4}$; and, 3° (such as Me_3CX) = 5.5×10^{-5}.

As seen in the transition state, when the alkyl group (R) is small, the four coplanar atoms (C,R,R,R) are easily accommodated in the five-center transition state. When the R groups are large (R=R=R=methyl) the steric crowding is too great, leading to a very high activation energy for formation of that transition state. For primary and secondary systems, the activation energy is low enough that a reasonable rate is observed.

How can the difference in rate be explained using reaction curves and activation energy?

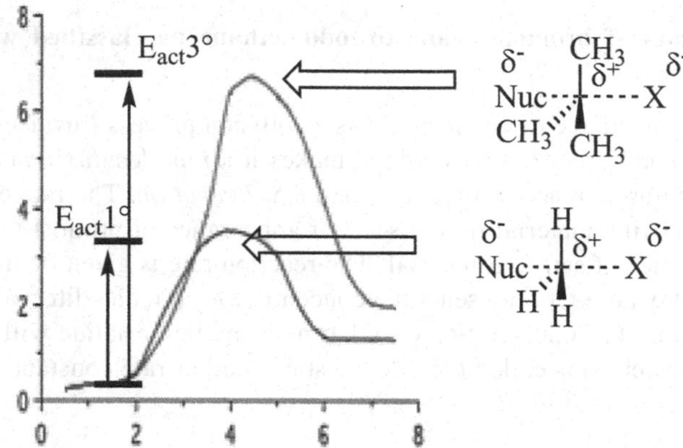

Reaction curves for the S_N2 reaction are used to show the activation energy (E_{act}), which is the energy required to initiate bond breaking. The peak of the curve is the transition state energy. Comparison of the curves for methyl halide with a tertiary halide shows that the activation energy for the tertiary (3°) is much higher, so the transition state energy is much higher. Indeed, the activation energy is so high that the reaction does not occur under normal conditions, even with heating. For a methyl, primary (1°), or secondary (2°) halide, the activation energy is low enough that the reaction can proceed, but as the steric hindrance in the pentacoordinate transition state increases, the activation energy increases. All of this discussion indicates that the steric hindrance for a tertiary halide is so great that the transition state activation energy is too high for the reaction to proceed. Due to steric hindrance in the transition state, a secondary halide reacts slower than a primary halide and a methyl halide reacts fastest of all.

What is the highest point in a reaction curve?

This point is the transition state for the reaction and energetically corresponds to the activation energy.

What is the term used for the energy difference between the starting material and the transition state?

This energy corresponds to the activation energy (E_{act}) for that reaction (see Section 3.2). The higher the transition state energy, the more energy required to begin bond making/breaking, and the reaction will be slower.

What nucleophiles are commonly found in S_N2 reactions?

Apart from iodide and bromide, and occasionally chloride, common nucleophiles used to prepare new functional groups by S_N2 reactions include NaCN or KCN, where the cyanide ion is the nucleophile and nitriles (RCN) are prepared. Sodium azide, NaN_3, where the azide ion is the nucleophile and nitrogen is introduced into a molecule (RN_3). Alkoxide ions, RO^-, are common nucleophiles to introduce oxygen into a molecule (R′OR).

What is the product formed for reactions (a), (b), and (c)?

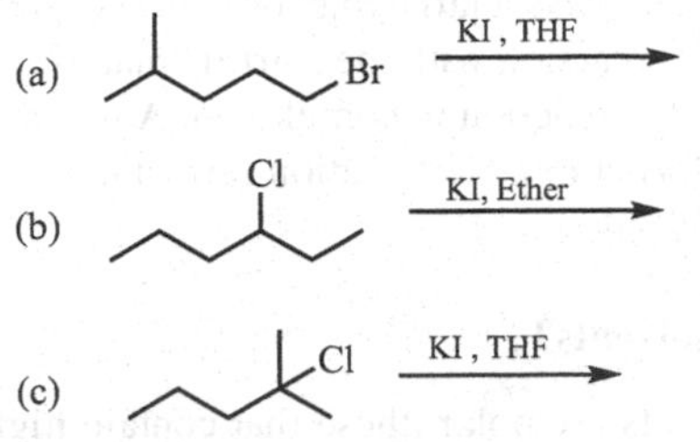

(a) Br —KI, THF→

(b) Cl —KI, Ether→

(c) Cl —KI, THF→

Reaction (a) gives 1-iodo-4-methylpentane by a S_N2 reaction with a primary bromide, and reaction (b) also gives a S_N2 reaction with a secondary chloride to give 3-iodohexane. Reaction (c) would be a S_N2 reaction, but since this a tertiary halide there is no reaction.

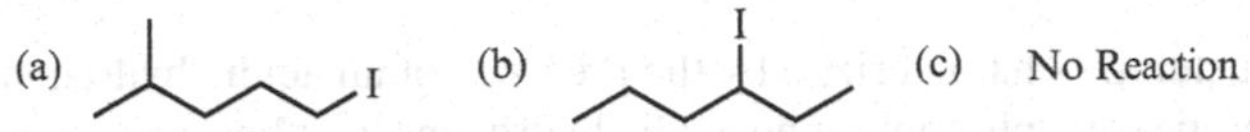

(a) I (b) I (c) No Reaction

Noting that iodomethane does not have a stereogenic center, how can inversion of configuration be detected?

If the S_N2 reaction is done with an alkyl halide such as (2*R*)-bromobutane, inversion of configuration must give (2*S*)-iodobutane via the pentacoordinate transition state. This change in absolute configuration demonstrates the inversion of configuration and also backside attack of the nucleophile. Indeed, the inversion of configuration is characteristic of this type of nucleophilic substitution (replacement of one atom or group by another atom or group) and it is used to substantiate and predict the pentacoordinate transition state and backside attack.

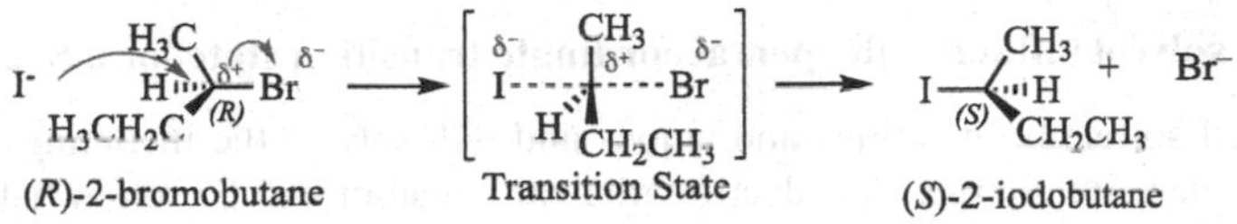

I^- H_3C H $\delta+$ $\delta-$ Br H_3CH_2C (*R*) → [$\delta-$ CH_3 $\delta+$ $\delta-$ I----C----Br H CH_2CH_3] → I—(*S*) CH_3 H CH_2CH_3 + Br^-

(*R*)-2-bromobutane Transition State (*S*)-2-iodobutane

What is the product and the (*R*)- or (*S*)-configuration of that product for (a) and (b)?

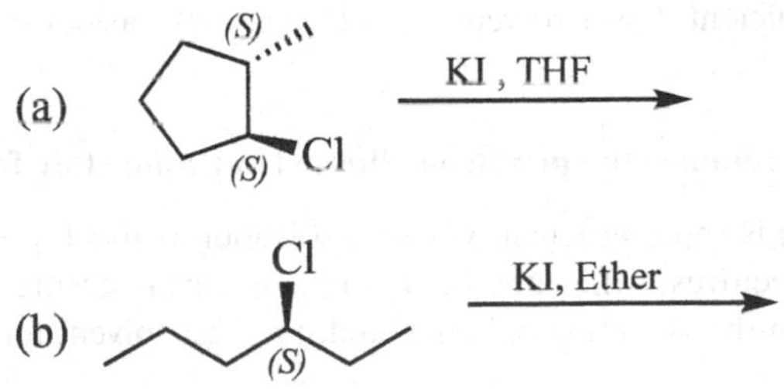

(a) (*S*) (*S*) Cl —KI, THF→

(b) Cl (*S*) —KI, Ether→

Both reactions (a) and (b) are S_N2 reactions, proceed by backside attack, and therefore proceed with *inversion of configuration*. Therefore, the (*S*)-stereogenic center is inverted to give the (*R*)-center in the product, (1*R*,2*S*)-1-iodo-2-methylcyclopentane. The (*S*)-stereogenic center in (b) is also inverted to give the (*R*)-center in the product, (*R*)-3-iodohexane.

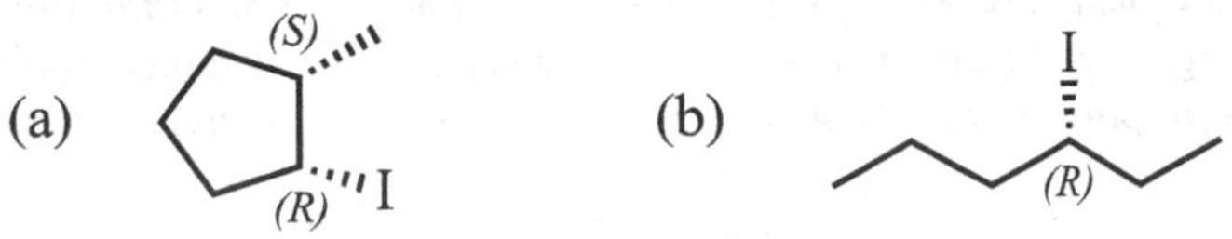

(a) (*S*) (*R*) I (b) I (*R*)

Why is the solvent important?

For substitution reactions, the solvent plays a large role, both in stabilizing or destabilizing the transition state, but also in assisting the initial reaction with the starting materials. The solvent can also help stabilize the products, helping to drive the reaction to completion. A protic solvent will solvate and stabilize carbocations, which assists their formation. Carbocation formation is difficult in an aprotic solvent that cannot solvate and stabilize ions (Section 8.4).

What are polar and non-polar solvents?

Two major classifications for solvents are polar (these that contain highly polarizable atoms and bonds and usually have a high dipole moment) and non-polar (they have a low or zero dipole moment and generally contain no heteroatoms or heteroatoms whose individual bond moments cancel).

What are protic and aprotic solvents?

Protic solvents are structurally characterized by the presence of an acidic hydrogen (X—H), where X is usually O, S or N). Aprotic solvents contain no acidic hydrogens or at best weakly acidic hydrogens such as C—H. Common *protic solvents* are: H_2O, CH_3OH (MeOH), CH_3CH_2OH (EtOH), NH_3, CH_3COOH.

An aprotic solvent does not have an acidic hydrogen atom. Common *aprotic solvents* are pentane, diethyl ether, tetrahydrofuran (THF), dichloromethane, dimethyl sulfoxide (DMSO), and dimethylformamide (DMF).

Water is the most polar of the protic solvents listed. DMSO followed by DMF are the most polar of the aprotic solvents listed. Pentane (a hydrocarbon with no heteroatoms) is the least polar of the aprotic solvents listed. In general, polar protic solvents are water soluble and non-polar aprotic solvents are water insoluble. The S_N2 reaction proceeds best in aprotic solvents and is slowest in protic solvents. The S_N1 reaction proceeds best in protic solvents and is slowest in aprotic solvents (Section 8.4).

How does a protic solvent influence the pentacoordinate transition state for a S_N2 reaction?

A protic solvent will solvate both cations and anions and will solvate the incoming nucleophile when that species bears a negative charge. The electrophilic carbon atom will be somewhat solvated as well, requiring that the solvent be "moved aside" before collision can occur. Such solvation will slow down the S_N2 reaction.

If an aprotic solvent is used, the nucleophile will be poorly solvated, and collision with the carbon substrate should be more efficient (fewer solvent molecules to move aside), and the S_N2 reaction should be faster.

How does a polar solvent influence the pentacoordinate transition state for a S_N2 reaction?

In a polar solvent, solvation is more efficient, whereas solvation is much poorer in an aprotic solvent. Typically, the S_N2 reaction requires sufficient polarity in the solvent to ensure solubility and stabilization of the transition state. Given the solvation effects noted, the best solvent for a S_N2 reaction is a polar, aprotic solvent.

What is the rate of a reaction?

As a practical matter, the rate of a reaction is how rapidly the starting materials react to form the isolated product. Formally, rate is the change in concentration of reactants or products as a function of time. The rate of a reaction is a dynamic property of *changes in the concentration of the starting materials as a function of time* during the course of the reaction. The rate is therefore obtained from a differential equation; *reaction rate is proportional to the molar concentration of the starting materials and also time.*

$$\text{rate} \propto \left[\text{starting materials}\right]\left[\text{time}\right]$$

When these parameters are plotted the slope of the resulting line is the proportionality constant, k, which is the rate constant for the reaction. In other words, the proportionality constant (k) is the rate constant for a reaction.

$$\text{rate} = k\left[\text{starting materials}\right]\left[\text{time}\right]$$

What is a first-order reaction?

A first-order reaction is one that obeys first-order kinetics such as the conversion of a reactant A to a product. In effect, the rate of the reaction depends only on the concentration of one molecule, A. The first-order rate equation is the change in concentration as a function of time, which is a differential equation that describes the reaction: rate $= \frac{-d[\mathrm{A}]}{dt}$ where the rate is proportional to both concentration of A and time. The rate is obtained from the differential equation: rate $= -\int_{[\mathrm{A}]_0}^{[\mathrm{A}]_t} \frac{d[\mathrm{A}]}{\mathrm{A}} = k\int_0^t dt$ where the concentration of A changes during the course of the reaction: $[\mathrm{A}]_0$ is the concentration of A at time = 0, and $[\mathrm{A}]_t$ is the concentration of A at any specified time. The reaction takes time to proceed, so time changes from $t = 0$ to t = end time. When this differential equation is integrated such that [A] is $[\mathrm{A}]_0$ at $t = 0$ and is $[\mathrm{A}]_t$ at t = "end time," the expression obtained is: $\ln\frac{[\mathrm{A}]_0}{[\mathrm{A}]_t} = k\left(t_{\text{end time}} - t_0\right)$ and if $t_0 = 0$ (as defined),

$$\text{then} \quad \ln\frac{[\mathrm{A}]_0}{[\mathrm{A}]_t} = kt$$

How can the rate constant from the differential equation in the preceding question be determined?

In a reaction, the concentration can be determined at different times. A plot of ln [A] versus time will result in a straight-line plot, and the slope of this line is k, the rate constant for that reaction. Since the rate depends only on the concentration of A, it is a first-order reaction.

What is the rate constant for a first-order reaction?

A plot of the concentration of the starting material A as a function of time (1 mole of A at time = 0; 0.9 moles of A at $t = 40$ min; 0.8 moles of A at t = 0/68 min, etc.) a curve is obtained. If the time is plotted against the ln [A], however, a straight line is obtained, and the slope is the first-order rate constant, k.

What is a second-order reaction?

A second-order reaction is one that obeys second-order kinetics where the rate of the reaction depends on two molecules (A + B) reacting to form a different molecule. To calculate the rate constant, first recognize that *both* reactants are important for reaction to occur, so the rate expression is

$$-\frac{d[\mathrm{A}]}{dt} = k[\mathrm{A}][\mathrm{B}] \text{ or,} \qquad \text{rate} = k[\mathrm{A}][\mathrm{B}]$$

The differential equation for this reaction is solved to give a complex expression:

$$\frac{1}{[\mathrm{A}]_0 - [\mathrm{B}]_0}\ln\frac{[\mathrm{B}]_0[\mathrm{A}]_t}{[\mathrm{A}]_0[\mathrm{B}]_t} = kt$$

where the $[\ ]_0$ terms denote the initial concentrations of A or B (at time = 0), and the $[\ ]_t$ terms indicate the concentrations of A and B at a specified time.

How can the rate constant for a second-order reaction be determined?

Normally, a plot similar to $\ln\frac{[A]_t}{[B]_t}$ versus time gives a straight-line plot, and the slope of this line is the second-order rate constant, k.

How can a reaction be identified as first-order or second-order?

The rate data (concentration vs. time) is obtained experimentally and that data is plotted. If the data gives a straight-line plot for ln [A] versus time, k can be determined, and it is a first-order reaction. If the data gives a straight-line plot with $\frac{1}{[A]_o - [B]_o}\ln\frac{[B]_o[A]_t}{[A]_o[B]_t} = kt$, it is a second-order reaction.

What is the half-life of a reaction?

The first half-life of a reaction is the time required for half of the remaining starting material to be consumed.

What is the half-life of a first-order reaction?

The *half-life for a first-order reaction* is given the symbol $t_{1/2}$ and is calculated from the simple formula:

$$\text{half-life } = t_{1/2} = k/\ln 2 = k/0.693$$

What is the half-life if the rate constant (k) for a first-order reaction is 12 M min^{-1} (moles per liter per minute)?

In this case, $t_{1/2}$ is 12/0.693 = 17.3 minutes.

What is the half-life is the rate constant (k) for a first-order reaction is 1.4×10^{-5} M sec^{-1} (moles per liter per second)?

In this case, $t_{1/2}$ is 1.4×10^{-5} /0.693 = 2.02×10^{-5} seconds and the reaction will rapidly be completed.

How many half-lives are usually required for a reaction to be complete?

The reaction begins with 1 mol of starting material, 0.5 mol will remain after one half-life – i.e., 50% of the starting material has reacted. After another half-life, 0.5 (0.5) will remain, = 0.25. In other words, 75% of the starting material has reacted. After five half-lives, $1 \times 0.5 \times 0.5 \times 0.5 \times 0.5 \times 0.5 \times 0.5 =$ 0.031 mol of starting material remain – so 99.97% of the starting material has reacted. Therefore, *it takes about five to six half-lives for a reaction to be considered as complete.*

How long will it take for five half-lives for the reaction with a rate constant (k) of 12 M min^{-1}?

In this case, $t_{1/2}$ is 12/0.693 = 17.3 minutes. Five half-lives = 17.3×5 = 86.5 minutes.

How long will it take for five half-lives for a reaction with a rate constant (k) of 1.4×10^{-5} M sec^{-1}?

In this case, $t_{1/2}$ is 1.4×10^{-5} 0.693 = 2.02×10^{-5} seconds. Five half-lives = 2.02×10^{-5} seconds $\times 5 = 10.1 \times 10^{-5}$ seconds = 0.000101 seconds. This example is a very fast reaction.

Given the bond polarity of the C—Br bond in an alkyl bromide, what type of charged intermediate might be expected for carbon, if bromine the C—Br bond were broken before the reaction with the nucleophile?

The bond polarity of the C—Br bond is such that bromine has a negative dipole and carbon has a positive dipole. Therefore, cleavage of the C—Br bond might occur in some cases to give a positive carbon, which is a carbocation.

8.3 OTHER NUCLEOPHILES IN S_N2 REACTIONS

What is the distinguishing feature of an alcohol?

An alcohol is characterized by a C—O—H unit, with an acidic hydrogen atom (pK_a about 16–18).

What is the distinguishing feature of a thiol?

A thiol is the sulfur analog of an alcohol and is characterized by a C—S—H bond where the hydrogen atom is acidic (pK_a about 10–11).

What is the bond polarization for an O—H group?

Since the oxygen is more electronegative than hydrogen, the oxygen is the negative pole and the hydrogen is the positive pole ($^{\delta-}$O—H$^{\delta+}$). Therefore, the hydrogen is slightly acidic (pK_a, 16–18).

Name some common bases that will deprotonate an alcohol in an acid–base reaction.

Relatively strong bases are required for this reaction, specifically those that give a conjugate acid that is significantly weaker than an alcohol. Typical bases include sodium hydride, organolithium reagents such as methyllithium or butyllithium, sodium amide, or even sodium metal.

What is the conjugate base when an alcohol (ROH) loses its acidic proton?

The conjugate base of an alcohol (ROH) is the alkoxide, RO^-. Clearly, the positive counterion will be that associated with the base used to deprotonate the alcohol, typically sodium, lithium, or potassium.

What is the geometry of an alcohol if attention is focused upon the oxygen?

The lone electron pairs cannot be "seen." If the methyl group and hydrogen of methanol are included with the lone pairs in a VSEPR model (see Section 2.2), however, the geometry around the oxygen is "tetrahedral." With a focus on the atoms one can see, the geometry is angular (bent) around the oxygen as shown.

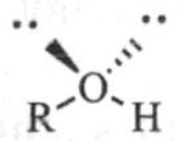

R–Ö–H

What is the suffix for an alcohol using the IUPAC rules of nomenclature?

The IUPAC ending for an alcohol is -ol, where the -e of the alk*ane* is dropped (or -e in alkene or -e in alkyne) and replaced with -ol, as in ethane to ethanol.

Why is the C6 alcohol with the formula $C_6H_{14}O$ called hexanol rather than hexol?

There are more than one possibility since a six-carbon alcohol could have an alkane backbone ($CH_3CH_2CH_2CH_2CH_2CH_2OH$, ***A***), an alkene backbone ($CH_3CH{=}CH_2CH_2OH$, ***B***) or an alkyne backbone ($CH_3C{\equiv}CCH_2CH_2CH_2OH$, ***C5***). In order to specify the one being considered, either the alkan-, alken-, or alkyn- prefix is retained, as in hexan-1-ol for ***A***, hex-4-en-1-ol for ***B***, and hex-4-yn-1-ol for ***C***.

If a C=C or C≡C unit is in the molecule with an OH, is the suffix for the molecule -ene, -yne, or -ol?

The OH has the highest priority (O > C), so molecules are named as an -enol or an -ynol.

What is the name of (a), (b), and (c)?

(a) 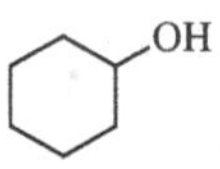 [cyclohexyl–OH] (b) 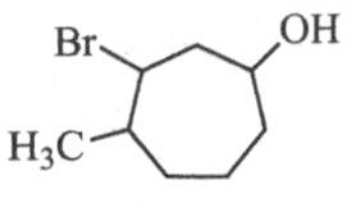 [cycloheptane with OH, Br, H_3C] (c) 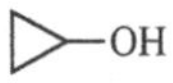 [cyclopropyl–OH]

The usual rules apply, with the -ol suffix to indicate an alcohol and the carbon bearing the OH should receive the lowest number so it is always C1. Therefore, (a) is cyclohexanol, (b) is 3-bromo-4-methylcycloheptan-1-ol, and (c) is cyclopropanol. Note that the 1- for the position of the C—OH unit is omitted from the name since it is obvious.

What is the IUPAC name for (a)–(f)?

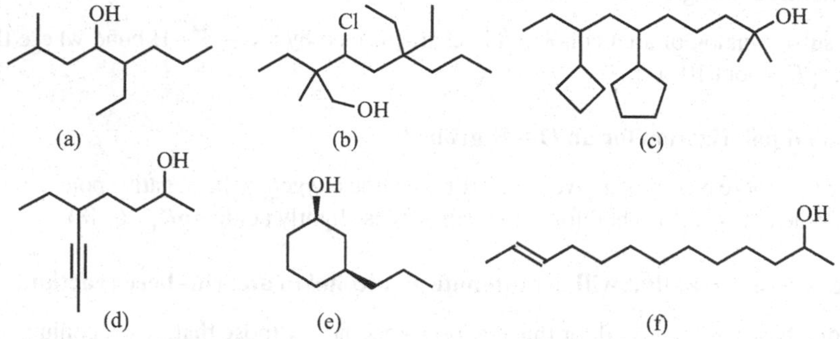

(a) (b) (c)

(d) (e) (f)

The names are: (a) 5-ethyl-2-methyloctan-4-ol, (b) 3-chloro-2,5,5-triethyl-2-methyloctan-1-ol, (c) 8-cyclobutyl-6-cyclopentyl-2-methyldecan-2-ol, (d) 5-ethyloct-6-yn-2-ol, (e) (1*R*,3*S*)-3-propylcyclohexan-1-ol, (f) (*E*)-tridec-11-en-2-ol.

What is the common name for (a)–(d).

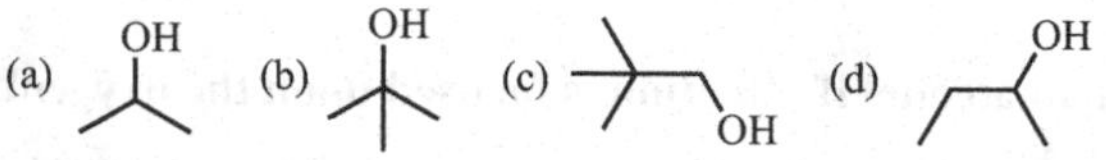

(a) (b) (c) (d)

There are several, usually lower molecular weight alcohols that have common names. The common name of (a) is isopropyl alcohol (rubbing alcohol); (b) is *tert*-butyl alcohol or *tert*-butanol or *t*-butyl alcohol; (c) is neopentyl alcohol; and (d) is *sec*-butyl alcohol.

Is the S_N2 reaction possible for organic molecules other than alkyl halides?

Yes!

What is the product when an alcohol reacts with a Brønsted–Lowry acid such as HCl?

The oxygen of an alcohol reacts with HCl as a Brønsted–Lowry base to give an oxonium ion, ROH_2^+.

Primary alcohols are converted to halides upon treatment with HX. Is the mechanism of this reaction the same as observed with tertiary alcohols?

No! The difference in energy between primary and tertiary carbocations is evident in the reaction of the primary alcohol butan-1-ol with HCl. The initial acid–base reaction forms an oxonium salt. Loss of water to form a primary carbocation, however, requires too much in energy and does not occur (see Sections 7.3, 7.4, and 8.4). The chloride will instead attack the *carbon* connected to the $^+OH_2$ species to form a new C—Cl bond and breaking the C—O bond in an S_N2 reaction. The carbon of the C—O bond is *electrophilic* (literally "electron loving") and so reacts with a nucleophile (an electron-donating species). Displacement by chloride leads to the product, 1-chlorobutane. Both HBr and HI react by a similar mechanism to give alkyl bromides and alkyl iodides. The reaction with HI is not as efficient, however.

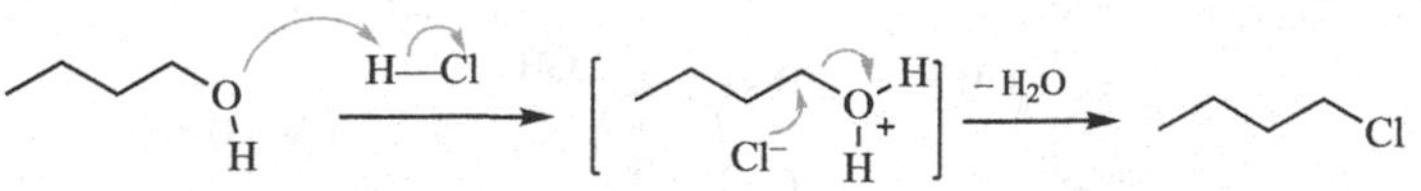

H—Cl; Cl⁻; $-H_2O$; Cl

What is the product when alcohols react with sulfur and phosphorus halides?

Alcohols are converted to alkyl chlorides or alkyl bromides by reaction with these reagents.

What is the structure of thionyl chloride, thionyl bromide, phosphorus trichloride, phosphorus pentachloride, and phosphorus tribromide?

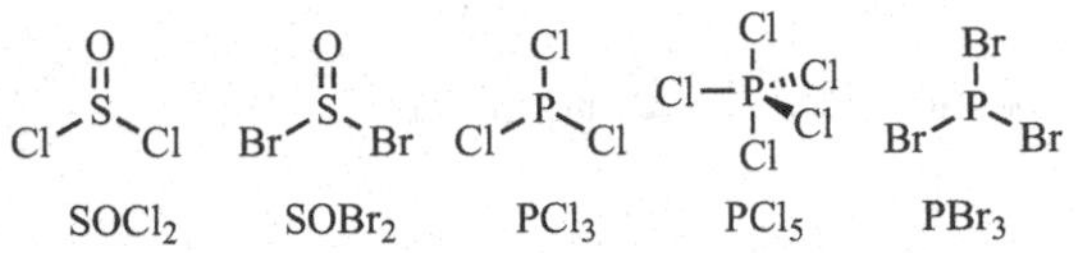

$SOCl_2$ $SOBr_2$ PCl_3 PCl_5 PBr_3

What is the product of a reaction between cyclopentanol and thionyl chloride?

Thionyl chloride reacts with cyclopentanol to give chlorocyclopentane.

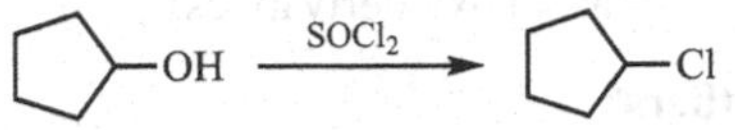

What is the product of a reaction between 2-methylpentan-2-ol and phosphorus tribromide?

Phosphorus tribromide reacts with 2-methylpentan-2-ol to give 2-bromo-2-methylpentane.

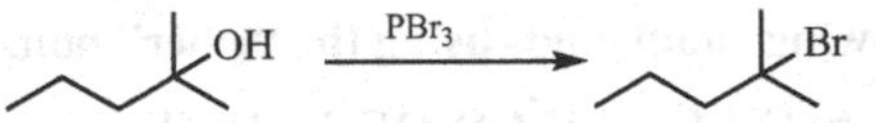

How does thionyl chloride convert pentan-(2*S*)-ol into (2*S*)-chloropentane, with net retention of configuration?

Thionyl chloride ($SOCl_2$) reacts with primary, secondary, and tertiary alcohols to give the corresponding chloride. Thionyl bromide ($SOBr_2$) reacts similarly to give the primary, secondary, or tertiary bromide. There are two versions of the reaction with thionyl chloride (but *not* with thionyl bromide), with and without base. When an amine (such as triethylamine) is added, it functions as the base and the mechanism is different from the reaction without a base. When pentan-(2*S*)-ol reacts with thionyl chloride, the oxygen attacks the sulfur, displacing a chloride to form a sulfinate ester and HCl. Intramolecular decomposition of this molecule leads to loss of SO_2 (sulfur dioxide) and a chlorine atom is delivered to the carbon bearing the oxygen to give (2*S*)-chloropentane, with retention of configuration. This reaction is known as *a* $S_N{}^i$ *reaction (nucleophilic substitution, intramolecular)*.

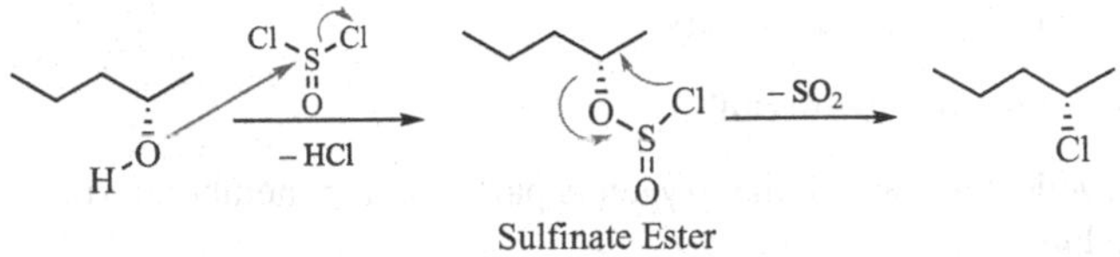

Sulfinate Ester

When triethylamine is added to the reaction of pentan-(2*S*)-ol and thionyl chloride, the product is (2*R*)-chloropentane. Why?

When an amine base (triethylamine, NEt_3) is added to this reaction, pentan-2*S*-ol reacts with thionyl chloride to give a sulfinate ester and HCl. In this reaction, the added amine, which is a base, reacts with HCl to form triethylammonium hydrochloride, so there is a nucleophilic chloride in the reaction medium. Rather than an intramolecular decomposition leading to (2*S*)-chloropentane, the sulfinate ester reacts with the chloride ion *intermolecularly* to give (2*R*)-chloropentane by a S_N2 reaction. The product is (2*R*)-chloropentane, which is the result of backside attack of the chloride ion and inversion of configuration.

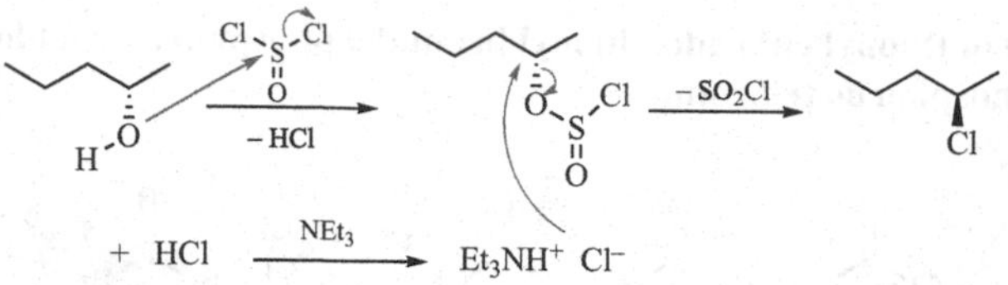

$+ HCl \xrightarrow{NEt_3} Et_3NH^+ Cl^-$

What is an ether?

An ether is a molecule that contains an oxygen and is characterized by a C—O—C unit.

What is the IUPAC suffix associated with naming an ether?

Ethers are usually named as "ethers" or as alkoxy derivatives.

What are the rules for naming ethers?

Ethers are named in two ways. In the first method, the two alkyl units that are connected to the oxygen are named, followed by the word ether. In the second method, one RO unit is named as an alkoxy group, attached to the longest chain alkane, alkene, or alkyne unit (the "other" R group).

What is the name of the following compounds using the "ether" nomenclature system?

(a) $CH_3CH_2CH_2OC(CH_3)_3$? (b) $CH_3CH_2CH_2CH_2OCH_2CH(CH_3)_2$ (c) $CH_3CH_2CH_2OCH_2CH_3$

Ether (a) is named *n*-propyl 1,1-dimethylethyl ether and the common name is propyl *tert*-butyl ether. Ether (b) is butyl 1-methylethyl ether. Ether (c) is ethyl propyl ether.

What is the name of the following compounds using the alkoxy nomenclature system?

(a) $CH_3CH_2CH_2OC(CH_3)_3$ (b) $CH_3CH_2CH_2CH_2OCH_2CH(CH_3)_2$ (c) $CH_3CH_2CH_2OCH_2CH_3$

Ether (a) is named 1-[(1,1-dimethyl)ethoxy]propane. Ether (b) is 1-(2-methylpropyl)butane. Ether (c) is 1-ethoxypropane.

Give two different examples of alkyl ethers.

Two examples are ethyl methyl ether ($CH_3CH_2OCH_3$) and diethyl ether ($CH_3CH_2OCH_2CH_3$).

Is it possible for the oxygen of an ether to be part of a ring?

Yes! There are many examples of cyclic ethers.

What is the structure of tetrahydrofuran?

Tetrahydrofuran is a cyclic ether where the oxygen is part of a five-membered ring. The IUPAC name of tetrahydrofuran is oxolane.

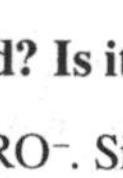

What is the conjugate base of an alcohol called? Is it a strong base or a weak base?

The conjugate base of an alcohol is an alkoxide, RO^-. Since alcohols are relatively weak acids, alkoxides are relatively strong bases. Alkoxides are somewhat stronger bases than hydroxide but much weaker than carbon, such as organolithium reagents.

How can sodium methoxide be classified as a reagent?

Sodium methoxide is an alkoxide, the conjugate base of methanol. The oxygen in sodium methoxide is classified both as a base and a nucleophile.

What is the product when sodium methoxide reacts with 1-iodoethane?

In reactions with alkyl halides such as iodoethane, methoxide is a nucleophile (Na is the positive counterion) and will react at the electropositive carbon that bears the iodine. The product of this reaction is an ether, ethyl methyl ether: $CH_3CH_2OCH_3$.

What type of reaction is the reaction of sodium methoxide and a primary alkyl iodide?

The reaction is a bimolecular substitution reaction, S_N2.

What is the common name of this reaction?

The *Williamson ether synthesis.*

What is the product when potassium *t*-butoxide reacts with 1-iodoethane?

The product of the nucleophilic *t*-butoxide and iodoethane is ethyl *t*-butyl ether: $(CH_3)_3COCH_2CH_3$

What is the product when sodium ethoxide in diethyl ether reacts with 2-bromo-2-methylbutane?

The nucleophile is ethoxide, but the electrophilic center is a tertiary halide. *The S_N2 reaction will not occur at a tertiary center.* Since ethoxide is also a base, removal of a β-hydrogen from 2-bromo-2-methylbutane will lead to an E2 reaction and the final product will be 2-methylbut-2-ene (Section 9.1).

If the reaction of an alkoxide with an alkyl halide is S_N2, will an alkyl halide with a stereogenic center give the ether with inversion of configuration?

Yes!

What is the stereochemistry of the product formed with $CH_3CH_2O^-$ reacts with (2*R*)-iodopentane? With (2*S*)-bromo-4-methylpentane?

The reaction of ethoxide with (2*R*)-iodopentane gives (2*S*)-ethoxypentane and the reaction with (2*S*)-bromo-4-methylpentane gives (2*R*)-ethoxy-4-methylpentane.

OCH₂CH₃ (*S*) OCH₂CH₃ (*R*)

(*S*)-2-Ethoxypentane (*R*)-2-Ethoxy-4-methylpentane

What is the major product of reactions (a) and (b)?

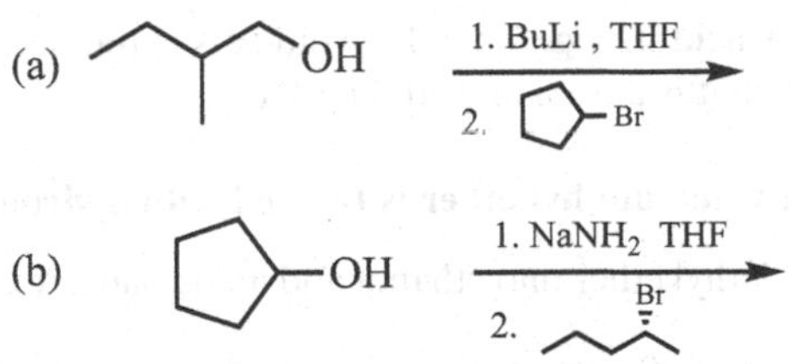

(a) 2-methylbutan-1-ol OH → 1. BuLi, THF; 2. cyclopentyl–Br

(b) cyclopentyl–OH → 1. $NaNH_2$ THF; 2. Br (2-bromopentane)

In reaction (a), the alcohol reacts with the base to give the alkoxide, which is a nucleophile, in a S_N2 reaction to give the ether, (2-methylbutoxy)cyclopentane. In reaction (b), the alkoxide is formed and reacts as a nucleophile to give the ether, (*S*)-(pentan-2-yloxy)cyclopentane, with inversion of the stereocenter.

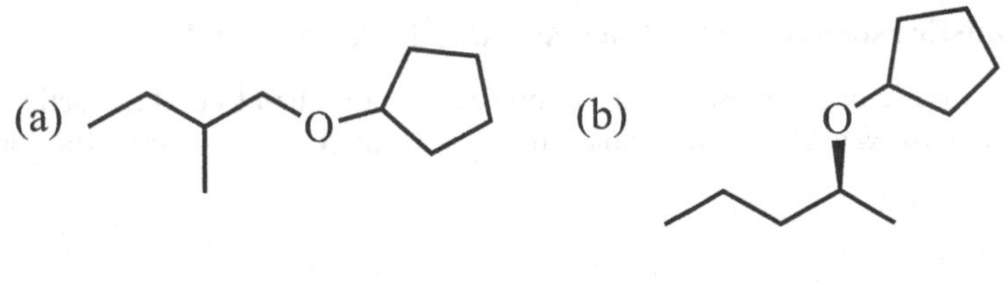

(a) O (b) O

Why are ethers important as a class of molecules?

Ethers are an important class of molecules for two reasons. Simple ethers are used as solvents in many organic reactions. Ethers are also found as structural components of many naturally occurring molecules as well as those molecules used in medicine and industrial applications.

What is synthesis?

Chemical synthesis is a series of chemical steps to convert one compound into another by reaction with other molecules and/or reaction with regents that modify the functional group.

What is a synthetic route to ethyl *tert*-butyl ether from molecules containing four carbons or less?

The synthesis requires the use of *tert*-butanol as the starting material and its conversion to an alkoxide (with $NaNH_2$ in THF). Subsequent reaction with bromoethane or iodoethane, which is more reactive, gives the ether product, *tert*-butyl ethyl ether. It is not possible to use sodium ethoxide (from ethanol) as the starting material since the subsequent reaction with the tertiary halide that will give no reaction in a S_N2 reaction.

1. $NaNH_2$, THF
2. CH_3CH_2Br, THF
CH_2CH_3

What is the product when 4-bromobutan-1-ol is treated with NaH in ether?

The reaction of 4-bromobutan-1-ol with NaH will form the alkoxide, ***A***. This initially formed alkoxide will react with the bromide at the end of the molecule in an intramolecular Williamson ether synthesis to give tetrahydrofuran.

NaH
THF
A

Is an alkyl ether a strong base or a weak base?

Ethers are very weak Brønsted–Lowry bases and relatively weak Lewis bases, requiring very strong Brønsted–Lowry acids or strong Lewis acids for a reasonable reaction.

What Brønsted–Lowry acids would be strong enough to protonate an ether and lead to further reaction?

HI is the most common and any acid stronger than HI would also protonate an ether. Note that HBr also protonates many ethers, although it is a weaker acid than HI.

What is the reaction product when diethyl ether is treated with hydroiodic acid (HI)?

The powerful acid HI cleaves diethyl ether into ethanol and iodoethane. It is known that HBr also reacts.

What is the product when diethyl ether is treated with hydrochloric acid (HCl)?

In general, HCl is too weak to induce cleavage of the ether, and we should recover the ether without any reaction.

What is a mechanistic rationale for how an alkyl ether is cleaved by HI?

The ether oxygen is basic in the presence of the powerful acid. Therefore, the reaction occurs by protonation of the ether oxygen to give an oxonium ion such as ***A***. The nucleophilic iodide counterion attacks the less sterically hindered carbon in a S_N2 reaction, displacing ethanol as a leaving group to give iodoethane.

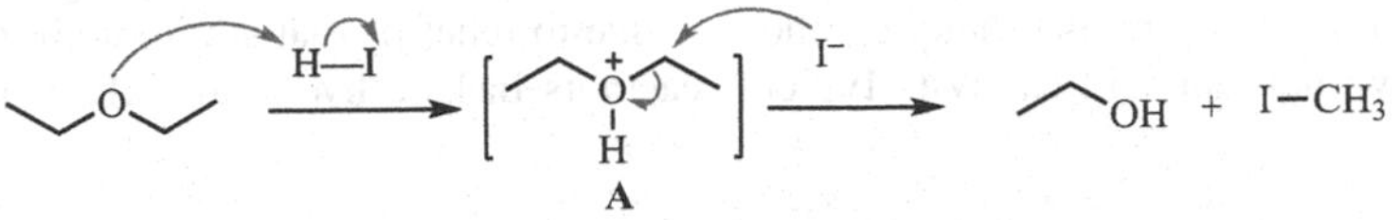

What is the product when methyl isopropyl ether is treated with HI?

The products are isopropanol and iodomethane. The oxygen of the ether is protonated to give an oxonium ion. The nucleophilic iodide ion attacks the less sterically hindered methyl carbon in an S_N2 to give iodomethane and propan-2-ol. Very little attack at the secondary carbon is observed.

What is an oxirane (also known as an epoxide)?

An oxirane is a three-membered ring ether derived by the oxidation of alkenes (see Section 13.2). The strain inherent to a three-membered ring makes oxiranes very reactive, in contrast to other ethers.

How are oxiranes named?

The oxygen in an oxirane is assigned 1 and substituents are named as attached to C2 or C3.

What is the name of the following oxiranes, (a), (b), and (c)?

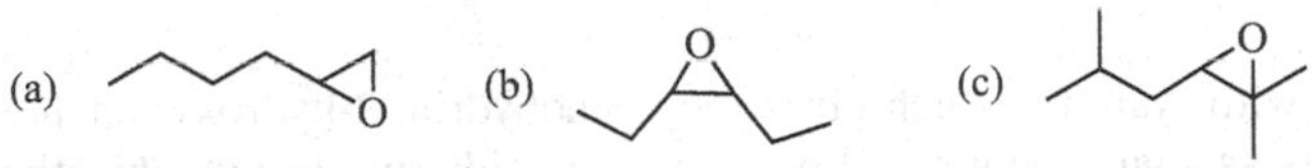

Oxirane (a) is named 2-butyloxirane. Oxirane (b) is named 2,3-dieethylocirane, and oxirane (c) is named 3-isobutyl-2,2-dimethyloxirane. Note that an alternative method for naming oxiranes is to name the alkene, followed by the word oxide. Therefore (a) can be named hex-1-ene oxide, (b) is hex-3-ene oxide, and (c) is 2,5-dimethylhex-2-ene oxide.

Oxiranes react with Brønsted-Lowry acids. How are oxiranes classified in reactions with an acid?

The oxygen of an oxirane reacts as a Brønsted–Lowry base.

What is the initial product when 2-methyloxirane reacts with HCl?

As with any other ether, an oxirane reacts with HCl to form an oxonium ion, in this case *A*.

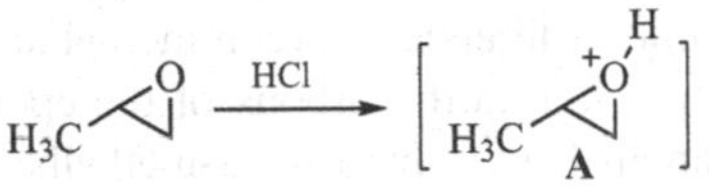

What is the final product of the reaction of 1-methyloxirane and HCl?

Once the oxonium ion (*A*) is formed, the three-membered ring will be opened by the nucleophilic chloride ion, which is the counterion formed by the reaction of the oxirane with HCl. Ring opening leads to formation of a so-called chlorohydrin, 1-chloroproan-2-ol. Note that the nucleophilic chloride ion attacks *A* at the least sterically hindered carbon, analogous to a S_N2-type reaction.

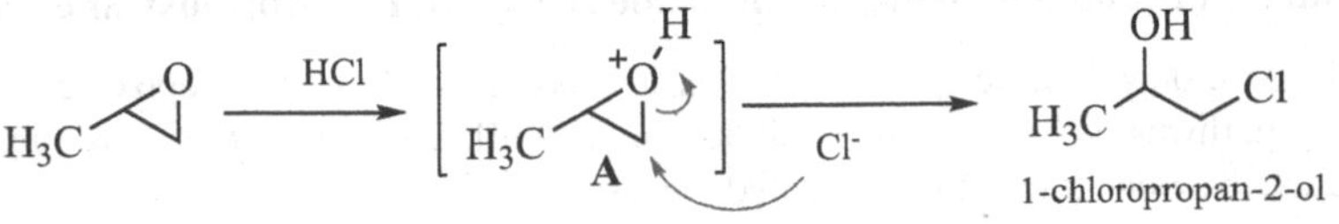

1-chloropropan-2-ol

Is it possible for an oxirane to react with a nucleophile in the absence of an acid catalyst?

Yes! The three-membered ring ether is under the strain inherent to such a small ring and reaction with a nucleophile to open that ring is usually exothermic due to relief of that strain. Oxiranes are reactive to nucleophiles without an acid catalyst. Typical reactants include hydroxide, alkoxides, and carbon nucleophiles.

What is the product when 1-methyloxirane reacts with sodium hydroxide and then dilute acid?

As noted, it is not necessary to first protonate the ether oxygen to induce ring opening. Epoxides are sufficiently strained that reaction with good nucleophiles give the ring opened product. In this case, 1-methyloxirane is opened by hydroxide to give the diol, propane-1,2-diol, after hydrolysis. The nucleophile attacks the least sterically hindered carbon in what is essentially an S_N2-like process.

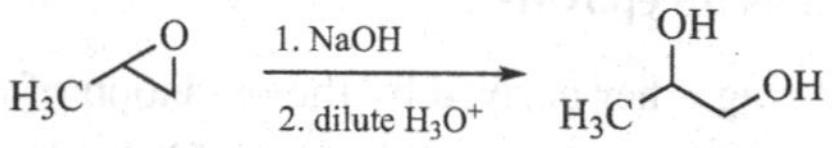

1. NaOH
2. dilute H_3O^+

Why the reaction is highly regioselective for the less substituted carbon of the epoxide?

If this reaction is an S_N2 process, the transition state for the less sterically hindered carbon is lower in energy than that for the more highly substituted carbon.

What is the product when cyclohexene oxide reacts (a) with NaCN (b) with $NaOCH_3$ (c) with sodium acetylide?

The first reaction is with cyanide, which gives the cyanohydrin, 2-hydroxycyclohexane-1-carbonitrile. The methoxide reacts as a nucleophile and opens the epoxide ring to give the ether, 2-methoxycyclohexan-1-ol. Acetylide is a powerful nucleophile and the anion derived from acetylide gives 2-ethynylcyclohexan-1-ol. Note that acetylide (alkyne anion) nucleophiles are discussed in Section 7.6.

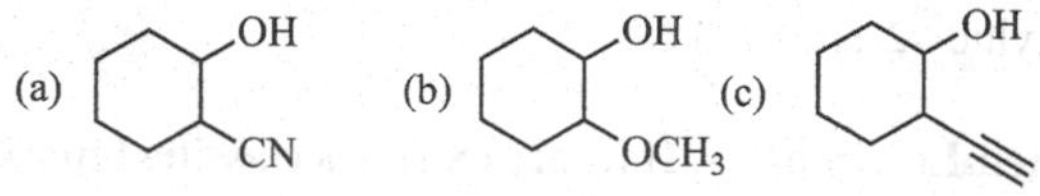

(a) (b) (c)

What is the product or products when sodium cyanide reacts with 2-methyl-3-propyloxirane? Explain!

The nucleophilic cyanide will attack the less sterically hindered carbon of the epoxide since that will be the lowest energy pathway. In this case, however, the oxirane has a similar substitution pattern at each carbon, and energetically there is little difference between methyl and propyl. In such cases, a mixture of two products is expected from attack at both carbons of the epoxide. In this reaction after hydrolysis, the two products are the cyanohydrins 3-hydroxy-2-methylhexanenitrile and 2-(1-hydroxyethyl) pentanenitrile.

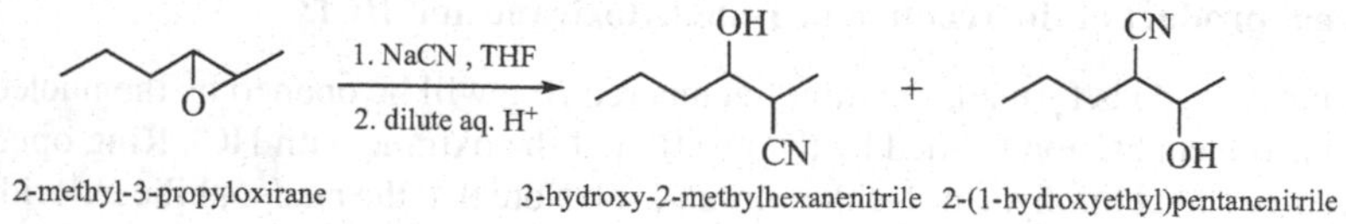

1. NaCN, THF
2. dilute aq. H^+

2-methyl-3-propyloxirane 3-hydroxy-2-methylhexanenitrile 2-(1-hydroxyethyl)pentanenitrile

What is the product or products when sodium azide reacts with 2- propyloxirane? Explain!

The nucleophilic cyanide will attack the less sterically hindered carbon of the epoxide since that will be the lowest-energy pathway. Therefore, the azide ion nucleophile will react at the less-substituted carbon to give the product, 1-azidopentan-2-ol, after hydrolysis.

2-propyloxirane $\xrightarrow[\text{2. dilute aq. } H^+]{\text{1. } NaN_3\text{ , THF}}$ 1-azidopentan-2-ol

What solvents are most favored for nucleophilic ring opening reactions with epoxides?

Since this is considered to be an S_N2-like process, polar aprotic solvents such as ether or THF are most commonly used.

8.4 FIRST-ORDER SUBSTITUTION (S_N1) REACTIONS

Do substitution reactions occur in highly polar solvents such as water?

Yes, but in water, ionization can be facile and the substitution reaction often follows a different mechanism that the S_N2 reaction. In water, the substitution reaction occurs after ionization to a carbocation intermediate. Substitution reactions can occur with tertiary halides in highly polar, protic media such as water via ionization, for example, and the reaction follows first-order kinetics. Such first-order nucleophilic substitution reactions are termed S_N1.

What is a S_N1 reaction?

A S_N1 reaction is a first-order bimolecular nucleophilic substitution reaction. This reaction is an ionization process to generate a carbocation intermediate. Subsequent reaction with a nucleophile and the overall reaction follows first-order kinetics. In other words, first-order kinetics means that the rate constant depends on the concentration changes for only one reactant. The overall rate of substitution can be first-order if the ionization step has a slower rate constant than the reaction of the nucleophile with the intermediate (see Section 7.3).

When 3-bromo-3-methylpentane is heated with KI in aqueous ethanol, is there a substitution product for this tertiary alkyl halide?

Yes! The product is 3-iodo-3-methylpentane.

Does the reaction in the preceding question proceed by a S_N2 pathway?

No! A S_N2 reaction with a tertiary halide does not occur due to a very high activation energy.

Why does 3-bromo-3-methylpentane react with KI in aqueous ethanol to give 3-methyl-3-iodopentane, when the same reaction in anhydrous THF gave no reaction?

In aqueous media, the carbon–bromine bond of 3-bromo-3-methylpentane can ionize, and the bromine atom is "pulled off" as the bromide ion by interaction with the water in the solvent. The water "pulls" the bromine atom from the carbon by hydrogen bonding (O----H----Br). As the bond begins to weaken, the charge increases, and water begins to solvate the developing charges until the ionic intermediates (carbocation *A* and bromide ion). These ions are assumed to be separated due to complete solvation by the water. Therefore, water not only assists in pulling off the bromine but also solvates the charges as they form. This carbocation is quickly attacked by the nucleophilic iodide to give the product, 3-iodo-3-methylpentane. Note that iodide can attack the planar carbocation from both the "top" or the "bottom." This process constitutes a completely different mechanism than the S_N2 reaction.

Br —(Aq. EtOH, KI)→ [A]$^+$ —(I^-)→ I

In the two-step process shown in the preceding question, is one step slower than another?

The first step, ionization of the alkyl bromide to the carbocation, is much slower than the rapid reaction of the highly reactive carbocation with the nucleophilic iodide ion.

Does the transformation of 3-bromo-3-methylpentane to 3-iodo-3-methylpentane follow first-order or second-order kinetics?

The reaction follows first-order kinetics (Section 8.2). The rate of the reaction depends on the slow step, ionization of the halide to give the carbocation.

What is the rate expression for this reaction?

The rate = k [3-bromo-3-methylpentane], where k is the rate constant. Remember that [ ] indicates the molar concentration of the substrate, which in this case in the alkyl halide.

Should this reaction be identified as first-order by simply looking at it, before studying the reaction?

No! This fact is determined by plotting the concentration of the starting halide as a function of time, and the outcome of that analysis identifies the reaction as first-order.

If the overall reaction is first-order, the rate depends only on the concentration of the halide starting material, but the iodide product can only be formed if there is a reaction with iodide. How can this be?

Mechanistically, this reaction is a two-step process. The first reaction is the slow ionization of the tertiary bromide to give the carbocation intermediate. The second reaction of the iodide with the carbocation is very fast and gives the iodide product. For the first-order kinetic data to be consistent, the first reaction must be very slow and the second very fast. Indeed, rapid collision of the iodide and the carbocation leads to product, but the rate is so fast that this reaction does not have a significant influence on the overall rate of reaction. In other words, ionization of the halide starting material to the carbocation may have a half-life of 4.5 seconds, whereas the reaction of the carbocation with iodide to give the iodide product may have a half-life of 0.00005 seconds. Note that these numbers are meant to be illustrative and are not experimentally determined. In this example, the overall rate of the transformation is dictated by the slower ionization: $k = 4.5$ sec + 0.00005 sec = 4.50005. The second term can be ignored since it does not introduce a significant error, and there is little or no effect on the overall rate.

What type of reaction is the conversion of a tertiary bromide to a tertiary iodide in aqueous media?

The reaction is a nucleophilic substitution that follows first-order kinetics, S_N1.

What are the characteristics of a S_N1 reaction?

A S_N1 reaction involves the relatively slow ionization of a substrate, so it is unimolecular. The reaction requires water or a highly polar, protic solvent to facilitate ionization to ions. Since the reaction involves a planar carbocation intermediate, the product is racemic, so that a chiral halide substrate will give a racemic product, which is a 50:50 mixture of the (R)- and (S)-products.

Which is the more stable carbocation: that derived from ionization of 2-bromo-2-methylpropane, or that from ionization of bromoethane?

A tertiary halide ionizes (reacts) faster than the primary. This is correlated with the relative stability of the intermediate cations. The tertiary carbocation is more stable than the secondary, which is more stable than the primary: i.e.,

$$3° > 2° > 1° > {}^{+}CH_3.$$

Why is a tertiary carbocation more stable than a secondary, etc.?

The reason for this order of stability is the presence of carbon groups on the cationic carbon. Carbon groups are *electron releasing.* If electron density is pushed toward the empty p-orbital (the cationic center), the net formal charge of the cation is diminished. Lower charge is associated with greater stability and the more carbon groups attached to the cationic center, the more stable will be that cation. The tertiary carbocation has three carbon groups, the secondary has two, and the primary has one (methyl has no carbon groups).

Which halide reacts faster with KI in aqueous ethanol, 2-bromo-2-methylpropane or 2-bromopropane?

The tertiary halide reacts much faster under S_N1 conditions. The intermediate is a carbocation and a tertiary carbocation is more stable than a secondary, so it is formed faster. Therefore, formation of the intermediate in the rate-determining step makes the reaction of the tertiary halide faster than the secondary halide. The relative rate of reaction for tertiary, secondary, and primary halides that react with KI in aqueous acetone is: $CH_3Br = 1.0$; $CH_3CH_2Br = 1.0$; $(CH_3)_2CHBr = 11.6$; $(CH_3)_3CBr = 1.2 \times 10^6$. Therefore, the general reaction rate for halides in the S_N1 reaction is: $3° > 2° >> 1° >>> X\text{–}CH_3$.

Why does 2-bromo-2-methylpropane ionize to a carbocation when it is a perfectly stable molecule?

The bromine (called a *leaving group*) does not "fly off" the molecule as the bromide ion does. First, there must be something to help "pull" it off, which in these reactions is the protic solvent water ($^{\delta+}H\text{—}O^{\delta-}\text{—}H^{\delta+}$) where the electropositive hydrogen coordinates to the electronegative bromine atom and "pulls." This pulling lengthens the C—Br bond, making that bond weaker, which increases the δ^+ charge on the C2-carbon of 2-bromo-2-methylpropane. The water therefore assists removal of the leaving group, which is essential for a S_N^1 reaction.

The second important consideration is stability of the ion being formed. Tertiary carbocations are stable and relatively easy to form whereas primary carbocations are relatively unstable and difficult to form. The carbocation product is stabilized by the aqueous solvent where the $^{\delta-}O$ of water donates electron density to the positive center of the carbocation, further stabilizing it by *solvation.* A solvent that can solvate the carbocation product is essential.

Solvation of the carbocation and the anion counterion is important for another reason. Water solvates both cations and anions, solvent separating them (as with NaCl). Coordination of water to the δ^+ carbon of the halide and to the $Br^{\delta-}$ will help separate them by solvation. Solvation accelerates the rate of ionization.

Why does the reaction of 3-bromo-2-methylpentane with KI in aqueous ethanol lead to 2-iodo-2-methylpentane, where the iodine atom is on a different carbon?

Br —KI / Aq. EtOH→ I

Comparing the starting material and the product clearly reveals that there has been a *skeletal rearrangement,* since the bromine in the starting material is in on C3 and the iodide of the product in on C2. This reaction is S_N1, so initial ionization generates a secondary carbocation as the intermediate. However, there is rotation about the C—C single bonds, and in one rotamer, the adjacent C—H bond on the tertiary carbon can be parallel to the p-orbital on the cationic center, and the electron density of that bond can migrate toward the electron deficient center. If the bond carrying the hydrogen moves to that carbon (C3 from C2) via a 1,2-hydride shift (Section 7.3), a more stable tertiary carbocation will be formed. The tertiary carbocation is lower in energy, so the rearrangement is *exothermic* by about 12–15 kcal mol^{-1} (50.2–62.8 kJ mol^{-1}), which is the driving force for the reaction. As the hydrogen atom migrates from C2 to C3, the positively charged structure ***A*** represents the mid-point of this rearrangement. At the mid-point, the hydrogen atom bridges C2 and C3 and formation of the more stable tertiary carbon cation drives the rearrangement of hydrogen from C2 to C3. As noted, this hydrogen migration is called a *1,2-hydride shift.*

H
H_3C
H_3C
H
H
H_3C
H_3C
H
A
H
H_3C
H_3C
H

Can a tertiary carbocation undergo a 1,2-hydride shift to give a secondary carbocation?

No! The tertiary carbocation is more stable than the secondary, so a shift would be endothermic (require energy) and would not occur. Rearrangement always occurs from a less stable carbocation into a more stable carbocation.

Why does rearrangement take place in a carbocation?

The migration of the atom or group occurs only if the carbocation formed after the rearrangement is more stable than the initially formed carbocation.

What is the order of carbocation stability?

A tertiary carbocation is more stable than a secondary, which is more stable than a primary.

What is the energy-driving force for a carbocation rearrangement?

The difference in energy between the starting carbocation and the rearranged carbocation is the energetic driving force for the reaction if the reaction is exothermic. Since a tertiary carbocation is 12–15 kcal mol^{-1} (50.2–62.8 kJ mol^{-1}) more stable than a secondary, which is 12–15 kcal mol^{-1} (50.2–62.8 kJ mol^{-1}) more stable than a primary, the rearrangement of a secondary to a tertiary carbocation is exothermic by 12–15 kcal mol^{-1} (50.2–62.8 kJ mol^{-1}), and the rearrangement is spontaneous. A similar comment can be made for a primary to a secondary rearrangement or a primary to a tertiary rearrangement.

Can groups other than hydrogen migrate in this type of cationic rearrangement?

Yes! A methyl or ethyl group can migrate if the migration leads to a more stable carbocation, and other groups as well. In general, the smaller group will migrate if there are different groups, and a hydrogen atom will usually migrate in preference to an alkyl group. The reason is simply that it takes less energy to migrate a smaller group or atom.

What is the product when 3-bromo-2,2,-dimethylpentane is heated with KI in aqueous ethanol?

The product is 2-iodo-2,3-dimethylpentane. In aqueous ethanol, ionization gives a secondary carbocation ***B*** but migration of the adjacent methyl group (a 1,2-methyl shift) occurs to give the more stable tertiary carbocation, ***C***. Subsequent reaction with iodide gives the final product, 2-iodo-2,3-dimethylpentane.

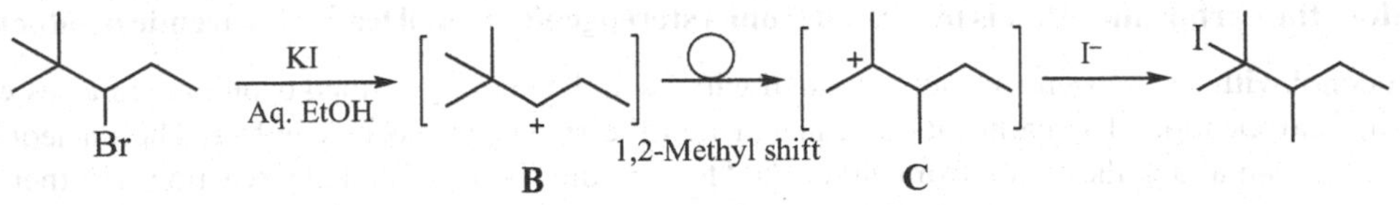

KI / Aq. EtOH → B → 1,2-Methyl shift → C → I^-

In the reaction of 2-bromo-2-methylpepntane, why does the hydrogen atom migrate and not one of the methyl groups, when there are two methyl groups and only one hydrogen atom?

The hydrogen is smaller than a methyl group and requires less energy to migrate via a transition state such as ***A*** in the question above. In general, the smaller group will migrate unless there are special electronic or steric effects.

What is the major product for reactions (a), (b), and (c)?

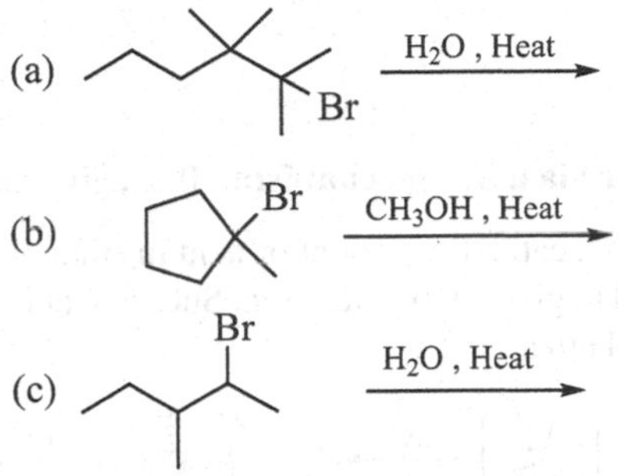

(a) H_2O, Heat →

(b) CH_3OH, Heat →

(c) H_2O, Heat →

The solvolysis product of (a) is the alcohol 2,3,3-trimethylhexan-2-ol. Solvolysis of (b) in methanol gives the ether, 1-methoxy-1-methylcyclopentane. Solvolysis of the secondary halide in (c) initially gives a secondary carbocation, but rearrangement to a more stable tertiary carbocation allows reaction with water and formation of 3-methylpentan-3-ol as the final product.

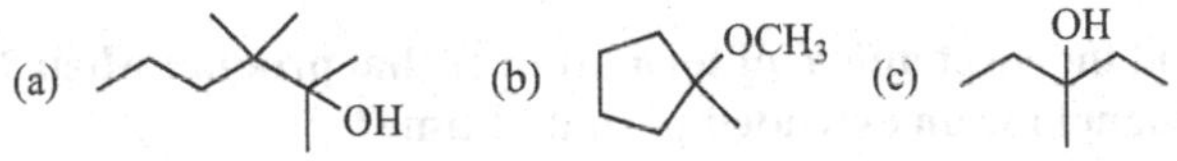

(a) (b) (c)

Can a secondary or tertiary alcohol react with a mineral acid such as HCl, HBr, or HI?

Yes! Secondary or tertiary alcohols react with HX to give a carbocation that can react with the nucleophilic counterion.

What is the product of the reaction between 3-methylpentan-3-ol and HCl?

The products are 3-chloro-3-methylpentane and water.

What is the mechanism for the reaction of 2-methylpentan-2-ol and HCl to give 2-chloro-2-methylpentane?

The oxygen of an alcohol reacts as a *base* in the presence of strong acids such as HCl or HBr. The alcohol (2-methylpentan-2-ol) is protonated by HCl to form an oxonium salt. This oxonium ion ionizes by loss of water (H_2O) to form a tertiary carbocation. In this solution, both the water and chloride ion (Cl^-) can react as a nucleophile with the carbon. In this case, the chloride counterion is the best nucleophile and reaction with the carbocation gives 2-chloro-2-methylpentane.

HCl → $-H_2O$ → Cl^- →

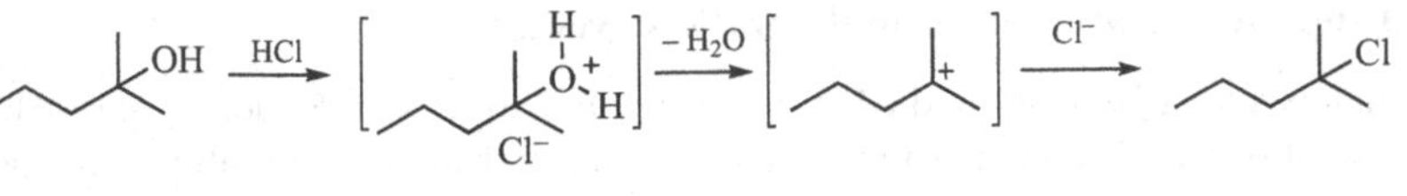

Why does the carbocation that is produced from a stereogenic alcohol lead to a racemic product?

If an alcohol with a stereogenic center is treated with HCl, the initially formed oxonium ion loses water to form a carbocation. The carbocation is planar and the stereogenic center is lost. The nucleophilic chloride ion can attack the cation from either the "top" or the "bottom" and any reaction will therefore produce a mixture of two chlorides as racemic mixture.

What is the solvolysis reaction of alkyl halides?

Most commonly, solvolysis is by defined as the nucleophilic displacement of a leaving group by the electron rich atom of a solvent such as the oxygen atom in water or an alcohol. As a practical matter and in the presence of water, tertiary alkyl halides slowly ionize to an intermediate carbocation, which reacts with water to give an alcohol.

What is the product when 2-methyl-2-bromopentane is heated in water for an extended period of time, say a week?

The product is 2-methylpentan-2-ol.

Is it possible to prepare an ether via a S_N1 mechanism? If so, give an example.

Yes! If *tert*-butanol is treated with a catalytic amount of acid in ethanol solvent, the initially formed tertiary cation can react with ethanol to give an oxonium ion. Subsequent loss of a proton from this oxonium intermediate gives ethyl *tert*-butyl ether.

Br —Aq. EtOH→ [+] —EtOH→ [H O+ Et] —−H⁺→ O

What is the product when an alkyl halide is heated with an alcohol such as ethanol?

Solvolysis can occur in alcohol solvents, and the product is an ether.

What is the product and the mechanism of formation of that product when 2-bromo-2-methylpentane is heated in ethanol for an extended period of time?

Ionization of the bromide gives a tertiary carbocation as before. The only nucleophilic species is ethanol, or specifically the oxygen of the alcohol. Subsequent reaction of ethanol with the carbocation gives an oxonium ion and loss of a proton gives the ether, 2-ethoxy-2-methylpentane.

Br —Aq. EtOH→ [+] —EtOH→ [H O+ Et] —−H⁺→ O

8.5 COMPETITION BETWEEN S_N2 vs. S_N1 REACTIONS

Can the S_N2 and S_N1 reactions compete?

Yes! Both require the reaction of a substrate with a nucleophile and there are many reactions where the S_N2 (direct reaction and no intermediate) and S_N1 (ionization and carbocation intermediate) reactions compete with each other, resulting in mixtures of products.

What is the difference between protic and aprotic solvents?

A protic solvent has a polarized and acidic hydrogen attached to O, N, or S such as in HOH, ROH, RNH_2, or RSH. Because of the X—H unit, a protic solvent solvates both anions and cations and therefore, facilitates both ionization of appropriate compounds and solvation of the resulting ionic products. An aprotic solvent does not have an X—H unit and is non-polar in that only cations are solvated, not anions, and aprotic solvents do not facilitate ionization or the separation of charge.

Is the reaction of bromomethane with KI faster in aqueous ethanol or in tetrahydrofuran?

In general, protic solvents such as water and ethanol solvate both cations and anions, separating those charges. The more polar solvent (water) efficiently separates and solvates ions. Aprotic solvents solvate cations, but anions are poorly solvated, making separation of ions difficult if not impossible, and nucleophilic reactions are more favorable. If the nucleophile and/or halide is solvated, the solvent molecules "get in the way" of the collision, slowing it down. Aprotic solvents only solvate cations, so the nucleophile (which is usually anionic) is not solvated and can approach the electrophilic center of the halide much easier, facilitating collision and reaction. For this reason, bromoethane reacts with KI by a S_N2 process faster in tetrahydrofuran (an aprotic solvent) than in the protic solvent, aqueous ethanol.

Why does 2-bromo-2-methylpentane not give the S_N2 product when heated with KI in ether?

The activation energy for this tertiary halide is too high to allow a S_N2 reaction. In other words, collision of iodide with the tertiary carbon does not provide enough energy to overcome the activation energy barrier necessary to achieve the S_N2 transition state.

Why does 2-bromo-2-methypentane give 2-iodo-2-methylpentane when the reaction with KI is done in a mixture of ether and water?

In the presence of water and given that the S_N2 reaction is so slow, for all practical purposes it does not occur. In the presence of water, slow ionization of the bromide gives an intermediate carbocation that reacts with the strongest nucleophile to give the product. In other words, the water facilitates a S_N1 reaction and iodide is the strongest nucleophile in this reaction mixture, which leads to 2-iodo-2-methylpentane.

Why does bromomethane react with KI to give iodomethane via a S_N2 mechanism in aqueous tetrahydrofuran?

Tertiary halides give essentially no reaction under S_N2 conditions but react efficiently under S_N1 conditions. Primary halides react rapidly under S_N2 conditions but give no reaction under S_N1 conditions. Secondary halides such as 2-iodobutane are midway in reactivity and secondary cations are midway in stability. In other words, both S_N1 and S_N2 reactions are possible for secondary substrates. Primary carbocations are very difficult to form due to their instability, and high activation energy for formation. The conditions described in this question are S_N1 conditions but given the difficulty in ionization to form a primary carbocation, the S_N2 process competes and "wins" and the reaction proceeds via S_N2, even in the presence of water.

In general, primary halides give exclusively S_N2 reactions in protic and aprotic solvents, including water. Tertiary halides give no reaction under S_N2 conditions and ionization followed by substitution under S_N1 conditions. The product formed from secondary halides depends upon the nucleophile and the reaction conditions. In polar, aprotic solvents, S_N2 reactions dominate but in water, the S_N1 reaction competes with the S_N2 reaction. In polar, protic solvents, elimination dominates if the nucleophile is also a base (Sections 9.1 and 9.2).

Why is the reaction in the preceding question done in aqueous THF rather than just in water?

The alkyl halides are generally insoluble in water so the THF is there to solubilize the starting material(s). However, the water is necessary for the S_N1 reaction, and since THF and water are miscible, the aqueous THF is the choice for the solvent.

Can a reaction be identified as S_N2 or S_N1 in the absence of kinetic data?

If an alkyl halide has a configurationally pure stereogenic center (*R*) or (*S*), then an S_N2 process will show inversion of configuration, and the specific rotation of the product can be measured and compared with the theoretical amount. However, ionization that accompanies a S_N1 reaction gives a carbocation that leads to a racemic product. Therefore, measuring the extent of asymmetric induction will allow a determination of how much S_N2 occurred and how much S_N1.

If a pure enantiomer is subjected to a S_N1 reaction, will the product be enantiopure or racemic?

The initially formed intermediate in a S_N1 reaction is a carbocation. Carbocations are planar, and an incoming nucleophile can react from either face, giving both enantiomers in equal amounts (a racemic mixture). Therefore, in the reaction described in the question, it is anticipated that the pure enantiomer starting material will be converted to a racemic product.

What is the product when (2*S*)-iodoheptane reacts with KCN in THF? Explain the stereochemistry!

The product of the reaction of (2*S*)-iodoheptane and potassium cyanide is (2*R*)-cyanoheptane. This S_N2 reaction proceeds with complete inversion of configuration at the stereogenic center.

I (S) —KCN, THF→ CN (R)

What is the product when (2*S*)-iodopheptane reacts with KCN in aqueous ethanol? Explain the stereochemistry!

Ionization of an alkyl halide is too slow to be of value in any protic solvent except water. The water can be the only solvent, although with organic halides, a cosolvent is usually necessary in addition to the water. The presence of water makes the S_N1 reaction competitive, and the reaction is assumed to proceed with formation of a *planar*, achiral carbocation intermediate. This cationic carbon can be attacked by cyanide from either face to give racemic 2-cyanoheptane. Attack from one face generates the (2*S*)-enantiomer with net inversion of configuration, but attack from the other face generates the (2*R*)-enantiomer with net retention of configuration.

I (S) —KCN, EtOH/H_2O→ CN (R) + CN (S)

A reaction of (2*S*)-bromopentane and potassium iodide gives only (2*R*-)-iodopentane. Does this reaction proceed by S_N2 or by a mixture of S_N2 and S_N1?

The fact that 100% inversion of configuration occurs (note that the solvent was omitted from the question), indicates that the reaction was a clean S_N2 process.

8.6 RADICAL HALOGENATION OF ALKANES

Is it possible for alkyl halides to react without formation of a cation or anion?

Yes! When exposed to peroxides or to light, chlorine and bromine can break apart to form chlorine or bromine radicals. Such radicals react with alkanes by removing a hydrogen atom, form HCl or HBr and a carbon radical. The carbon radical then reacts with more chlorine or bromine to give an alkyl chloride or an alkyl bromide.

What is the term for breaking a bond such that each atom receives one electron? What is the name of the resulting intermediate?

Certain molecules are characterized by breaking a bond in a homolytic manner (*homolytic cleavage*, where each atom of the covalent bond receives one electron) and the resulting products have a single electron. These intermediates are called *free radicals* and are capable of reacting with alkanes (and other molecules) to remove a hydrogen, generating a carbon radical.

What is the normal reactivity of a radical once formed?

Radicals are highly reactive intermediates and among several other possible reactions, they react with other atoms to remove that atom and generate a new radical. Such a reaction is known as an *atom-transfer reaction.* In another common reaction, radicals react with other radicals to give a *coupling reaction,* where a new bond is formed between the radical atoms (e.g., X• + Y• → X–Y), where each radical donates one electron to the new two-electron covalent bond.

When a radical removes a hydrogen atom from a carbon, the resulting carbon radical reacts with another molecule of halogen, and the overall process replaces a hydrogen of the alkane precursor with a halogen atom. This transformation is often called a *radical substitution reaction.* In general, radical substitution is not a selective reaction unless the radical reacts faster with one type of hydrogen rather than another. This statement means that the rate of reaction of the radical with a primary hydrogen may be slower than the rate of reaction for a tertiary hydrogen.

What is the product when diatomic chlorine or bromine is heated to 300°C or exposed to light?

When diatomic chlorine (Cl_2) or bromine (Br_2) is heated to 300°C or greater, they fragment by homolytic cleavage to give chlorine radicals (Cl•) or bromine radicals (Br•). It is also known that exposure of chlorine or bromine to light (usually ultraviolet, UV) will generate the corresponding radical. Radicals are highly reactive molecules and are intermediates (not isolated) that initiate reactions with alkanes.

What wavelengths are associated with UV light?

The wavelengths of light associated with UV are 10–400 nm (100–4000 Å).

What is the product when methane reacts with chlorine gas in the presence of UV light?

Formation of chlorine radicals, removal of a hydrogen atom from methane, and reaction of the methyl radical with more chlorine leads to chloromethane and HCl as the products.

What is the mechanism for the transformation of 2-methylpropane to 2-chloro-2-methylpropane in the presence of UV light?

The chlorination of 2-methylpropane is a radical chain process. The process begins by exposure of Cl—Cl to UV light, which initiates homolytic cleavage and formation of two chlorine radicals in what is called a *chain initiation step.* The chlorine radical reacts with 2-methylpropane to give HCl (one product) and the carbon radical. A reaction that produces a neutral molecule and a new radical is a chain-carrier step or a *chain propagation step.* The chain carrier radical reacts with another molecule of Cl—Cl to produce the 2-chloro-2-methylpropane product and a chain-carrying chlorine radical in another *chain propagation step.* If two of the radicals collide, either a chlorine radical or a carbon radical as shown (a coupling reaction), they form a neutral molecule but do not produce a new radical chain carrier. Such a reaction stops the radical process and is called a *chain termination step.* To begin the process again, a new chain initiation step is necessary.

Cl—Cl —hv (UV)→ 2 Cl• Initiation Step

(2-methylpropane)–H —Cl•→ HCl + [tert-butyl radical] —Cl—Cl→ (2-methylpropane)–Cl + Cl• Propagation Steps

Cl• + Cl• → Cl—Cl

[tert-butyl radical] + [tert-butyl radical] → (2,2,3,3-tetramethylbutane) Termination Steps

[tert-butyl radical] —Cl•→ (2-methylpropane)–Cl

How many different chlorinated products are formed by the reaction of 2-methylpropane chlorine at 300°C?

In reactions with alkanes, halogen radicals abstract one of the hydrogens from the alkane to produce H—X and a carbon radical such as $(CH_3)_3C\bullet$ from 2-methylpropane. That radical then reacts with additional halogen to produce 2-chloro-2-methylpropane. However, there are nine primary hydrogen atoms and removal of one of these gives $\bullet CH_2CH(CH_3)_2$, which reacts with Cl• to give $ClCH_2CH(CH_3)_2$. Therefore, *there are two different products from this reaction.* The important lesson of this answer is the knowledge that *every* hydrogen atom in the alkane can be removed and replaced with a halogen.

Why does 2,4-dimethylpentane react with chlorine to give three different chlorinated products?

2,4-Dimethylpentane can react with chlorine gas at 300°C to give three different products, ***A***, ***B***, and ***C***. These three products arise by removal of three different kinds of hydrogen, H_a, H_b, and H_c. Replacement of H_a (there are 12 H_a since all four methyl groups are chemically identical) gives ***A***; replacement of H_b (there are two H_b) gives ***B***; and replacement of H_c (there are two H_c) gives ***C***.

It is important to reiterate that *every* hydrogen atom in 2,4-dimethylpentane is replaced by a chlorine atom. Replacement of some hydrogen atoms leads to the same product and so they are chemically identical. In 2,4-dimethylpentane there are only three *different* kinds of hydrogen atom, so there are three different products. In other words, if all 16 hydrogen atoms are replaced with chlorine, and those 16 structures are compared, some structures will be identical and only 3 different isomers can be found, ***A***, ***B***, and ***C***.

Can the relative ratio of products *A*, *B*, and *C* in the preceding question be predicted?

If each hydrogen is replaced at a given rate (see the next question), then the relative amounts of ***A***, ***B***, and ***C*** can be predicted based on the number of each kind of hydrogen and the different rates of reaction for each kind of hydrogen.

What are the relative percentages of *A*, *B*, and *C* from the chlorination of 2,4-dimethylpentane via reaction of H_a, H_b, and H_c?

To answer this question, the rate of reaction for each type of hydrogen atom must be known, as well as the number of each different kinds of hydrogen atom. For alkanes, a chlorine radical removes primary hydrogens with a relative rate of 1, secondary hydrogens with a relative rate of 3.9, and tertiary hydrogens with a relative rate of 5.2 [3°:2°:1° = 5.2:3.9:1]. For 2,4-dimethlpentane, there are 12 primary H_as (all identical hydrogens), 2 tertiary H_bs, and 2 secondary H_cs. The relative amount is then:

$$\text{Relative } \%A = \frac{(12\text{H}_a \times 1)}{(12\text{H}_a \times 1) + (2\text{H}_b \times 5.2) + (2\text{H}_c \times 3.9)} = \frac{12}{30.2} \times 100$$

$$\text{Relative } \%\boldsymbol{A} = 0.397 \times 100 = 39.7\%.$$

Similarly, the relative % ***B*** $= \dfrac{10.4}{30.2} \times 100 = 34.5\%$ and the relative % ***C*** $= \dfrac{7.8}{30.2} \times 100 = 25.8\%$.

The generic formula to calculate the percentage of each different type of hydrogen is

$$\text{Relative } \% = \frac{\text{Number of hydrogen atoms of a particular type}}{\text{Total number of hydrogen atoms in the molecule}} \times 100$$

Bromination of 2,4-dimethylpentane leads to nearly 95% of a single isomer, in contrast to the chlorination reaction when reaction occurs at H_a, H_b, and H_c (see previous question). What is this product and what is the selectivity?

Bromine and chlorine react at different rates since the midpoint of the reaction for chlorine comes earlier than the midpoint of bromine. The factors that influence the stability of the radical intermediate are, therefore, more important for the bromine reaction, and the relative rates for bromination of a hydrogen are: 1°:2°:3° = 1:82:1640. Therefore, in a reaction with 2,2-dimethylpentane and bromine, there will be a preponderance of one product. Using the same calculations as above, replacement of H_a (see the preceding question) will give 1-bromo-2,4,4-trimethylpentane, $\frac{(12\times 1)}{(12\times 1)+(2\times 82)+(2\times 1640)} - \frac{12}{3456} = 0.35\%$.

Likewise, there will be 4.75% of 2-bromo-2,4,4-trimethylpentane via replacement of H_b but 94.91% of 3-bromo-2,4-dimethylpentane via replacement of H_c.

Why does prop-1-ene react so rapidly with chlorine radicals?

If prop-1-ene is reacted with the chlorine radical (Cl•), the product is the so-called allyl radical, ***A***. When the alkane hydrogen is on a carbon adjacent to a π-bond, that hydrogen is removed by radicals at a faster rate than removal of hydrogen atoms that are not connected to a C=C unit. The reason for this rate difference is because the resulting allylic radical is more stable than the other possible radical that can be formed; it is *resonance stabilized.* In other words, the radical is *delocalized* over several atoms rather than localized on a single atom. The radical is in a p-orbital, as shown in ***B***, which is parallel to the p-orbitals of the π-bond. These orbitals can overlap in a manner that delocalizes the radical over all the carbons, and *both* resonance structures shown for ***A*** or ***B*** are necessary to represent the actual structure. A resonance-stabilized structure is more stable and lower in energy. In the radical reaction, this extra stability means the radical is formed *faster*, allowing reaction with more chlorine to give the allyl chloride (3-chloroprop-1-ene).

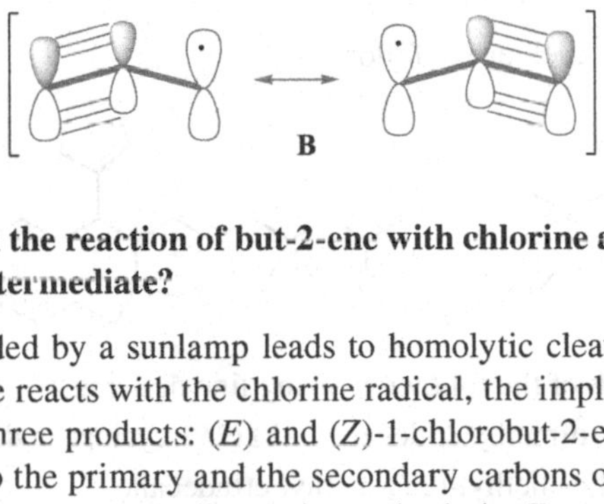

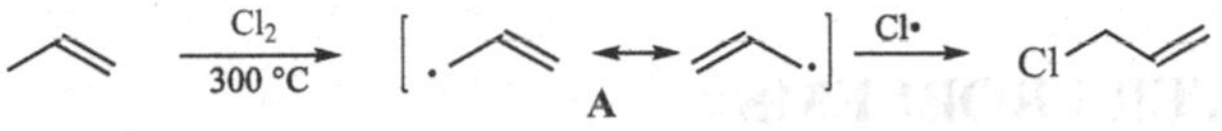

Cl_2, 300 °C; Cl•; Cl

A

B

What are the products from the reaction of but-2-ene with chlorine and what are all resonance structures for the radical intermediate?

Photochemical energy provided by a sunlamp leads to homolytic cleavage of diatomic chlorine into chlorine radicals. If but-2-ene reacts with the chlorine radical, the implications of the resonance intermediate can be seen in the three products: (*E*) and (*Z*)-1-chlorobut-2-ene and also 3-chlorobut-1-ene. A chlorine radical attaches to the primary and the secondary carbons of the radical sites in the allylic intermediate. The C=C unit in the intermediate exists as both the *E*- and the *Z*- radicals and both react to give the corresponding product. This phenomenon can also be explained by examination of the resonance stability of this radical. One contributor has the radical on a secondary carbon and there are two contributors (*E*- and *Z*-) with the radial on a primary carbon. There are, therefore, three products. Note that 1-chlorobut-2-ene is a mixture of (*E*) and (*Z*) isomers since the stereochemistry is lost due to resonance.

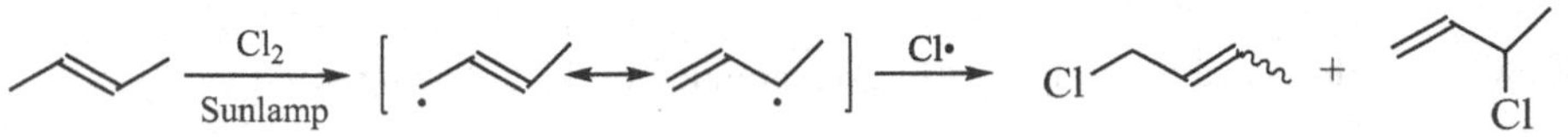

Cl_2, Sunlamp; Cl•; Cl; +; Cl

What is the structure of *N*-chlorosuccinimide (abbreviated NCS) and *N*-bromosuccinimide (abbreviated NBS)?

N-Chlorosuccinimide and *N*-bromosuccinimide are cyclic derivatives of succinic acid (see Section 15.3).

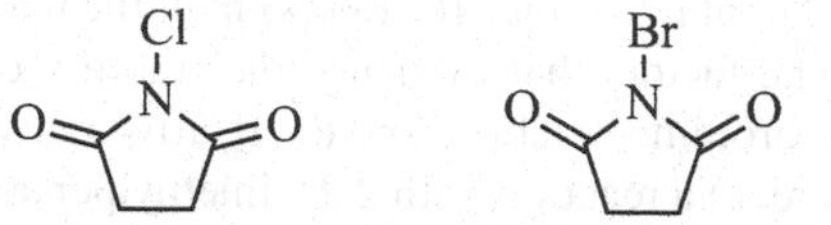

N-Chlorosuccinimide (NCS) N-Bromosuccinimide (NBS)

How are NCS and NBS used in radical halogenation reactions?

Chlorine is a toxic and corrosive gas and bromine is a red, viscous, and corrosive liquid. To avoid deleterious effects of these reagents, NCS is used as a surrogate for chlorine and NBS as a surrogate for bromine. Both are solids, easily handled, and in the presence of a radical source or upon exposure to UV light, are converted to chlorine radicals or bromine radicals. Therefore, NCS and NBS can be used in the radical chlorination or radical bromination reactions described in this section.

What is the product when NCS reacts with 2,2-dimethylpropane? When NBS reacts?

When heated in a solvent such as carbon tetrachloride in the presence of photochemical energy (a sunlamp) 2,2-dimethylpropane reacts with the chlorine radicals generated by the light reaction with NCS to give 1-chloro-2,2-dimethylpropane. Since 2,2-dimethylpropane has only one kind of hydrogen atom, there is only one product. Similarly, NBS is a source of bromine and bromine radicals. Therefore, when NBS reacts with 2,2-dimethylpropane to give 1-bromo-2,2-dimethylpropane. Again, there is only one product.

NBS, Sunlamp / CCl_4 ; NCS, Sunlamp / CCl_4

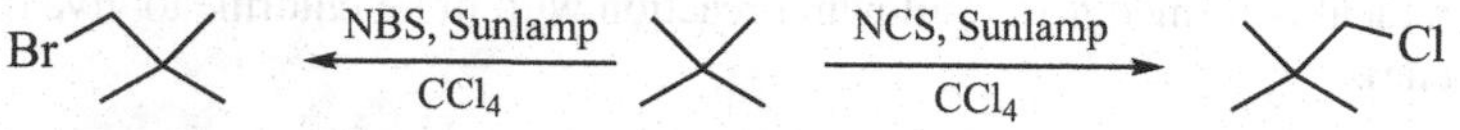

END OF CHAPTER PROBLEMS

1. Give the IUPAC name for each of the following:

(a) (b) (c)

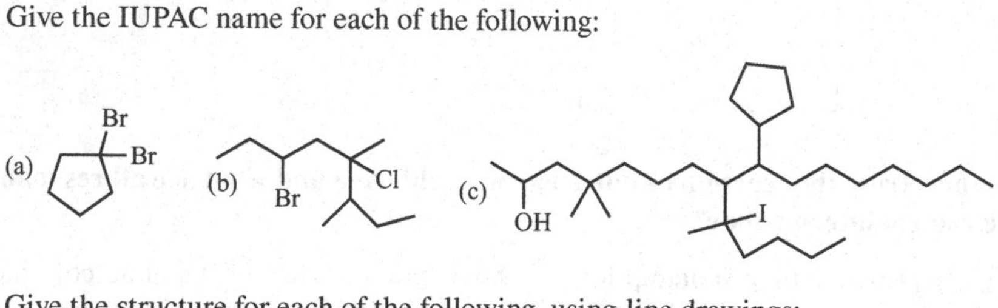

2. Give the structure for each of the following, using line drawings:
   (a) 5-(2-fluoropropyl)- 4,4-dimethyldodecane (b) (2*R*)-cyclopropyl-(3*S*)-iodohexane
   (c) 1-bromo-(8*S*)-chloro-4,4-diethyl-(2*S*)-methyltetradecane
3. Explain why cation ***A*** is less stable than cation ***B***.

A **B**

4. Show all products and the relative % of each product for the following reaction:

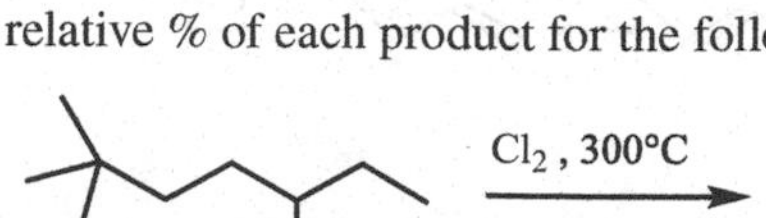

Cl_2 , 300°C

5. If the concentration of KI in the reaction of KI and 1-bromopentane is increased to 10 equivalents, what is the effect on the rate of that reaction? Explain.

6. Explain why the rate of reaction of 1-bromo-2,2-dimethylpropane in a S_N2 reaction is 3.3×10^{-7} when compared to the rate of reaction of bromomethane, which is one (1) under the same conditions, although both are primary halides.
7. Explain why the rate of reaction of allyl bromide in an S_N2 reaction is 1.3 times faster than the rate of reaction of bromomethane, under the same conditions.
8. Write the rate expression for a S_N1 reaction. What is the effect on the rate if 10 equivalents of 2-bromo-2-methylpropane are added to 1 equivalent of KI when compared to the reaction when 1 equivalent of both reagents are used?
9. Explain why the hydrogen migrates in this reaction rather than the methyl.

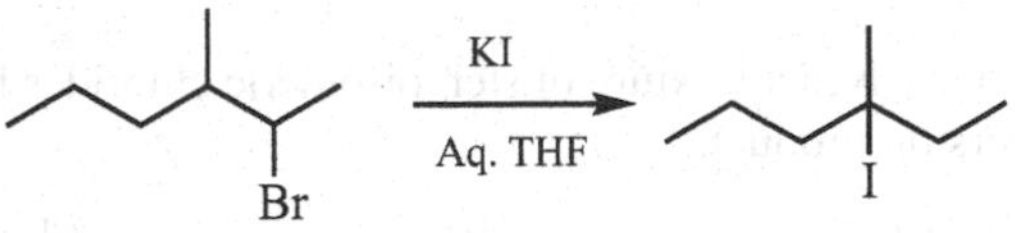

Br —KI / Aq. THF→ I

10. Explain why this reaction gives a mixture of enantiomeric chlorides but there is a slight preponderance of the inversion product.

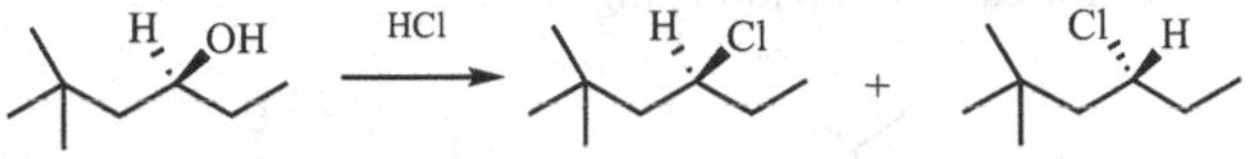

H OH —HCl→ H Cl + Cl H

11. In each case give the major product of the reaction. Remember stereochemistry and if there is no reaction, indicate that by N.R.

(a) 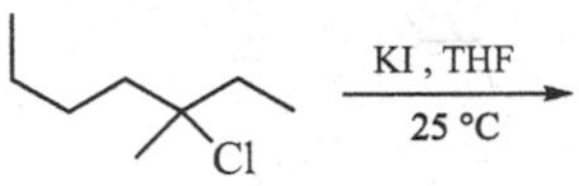 Cl —KI, THF / 25 °C→ (b) 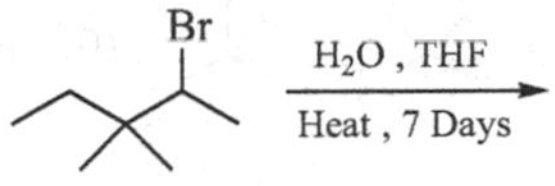 Br —H_2O, THF / Heat, 7 Days→

(c) 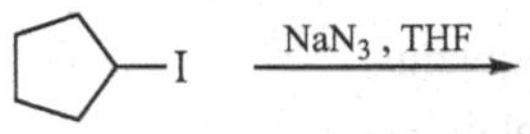 I —NaN_3, THF→ (d) 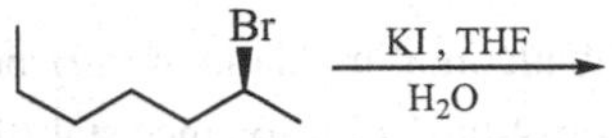 Br —KI, THF / H_2O→

(e) 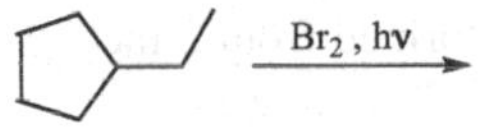 —Br_2, hv→ (f) 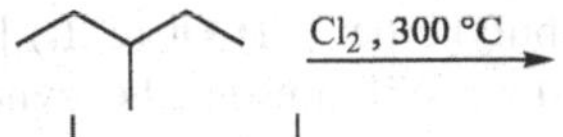 —Cl_2, 300 °C→

(g) 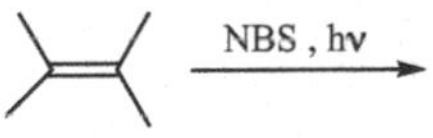 —NBS, hv→ (h) 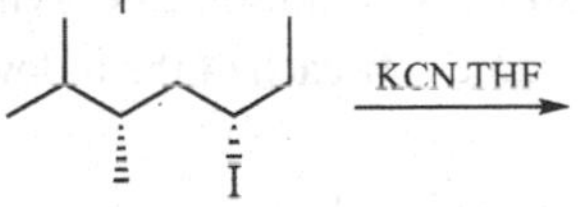 I —KCN THF→

(i) 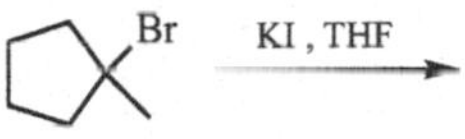 Br —KI, THF→ (j) 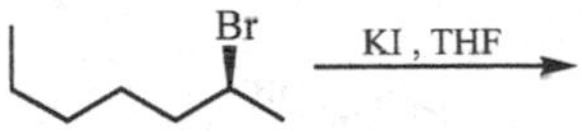 Br —KI, THF→

(k) C_5H_{11}—≡:⁻ Na^+ —1-Iodobutane / THF→ (l) 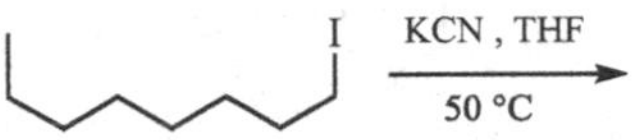 I —KCN, THF / 50 °C→

(m) 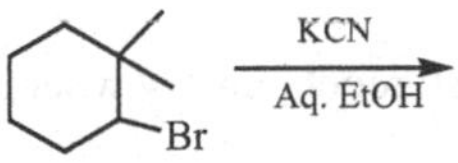 Br —KCN / Aq. EtOH→ (n) 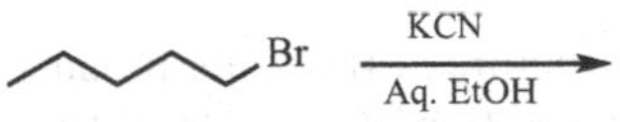 Br —KCN / Aq. EtOH→

12. Give the complete mechanism for each of the following:

(a) 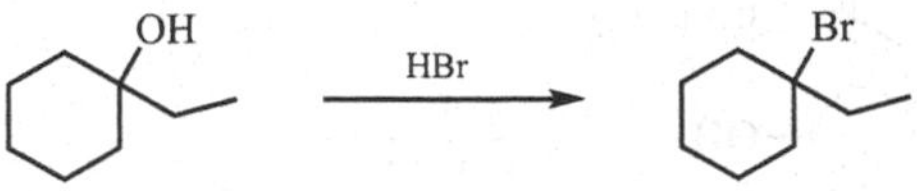 OH —HBr→ Br

(b) 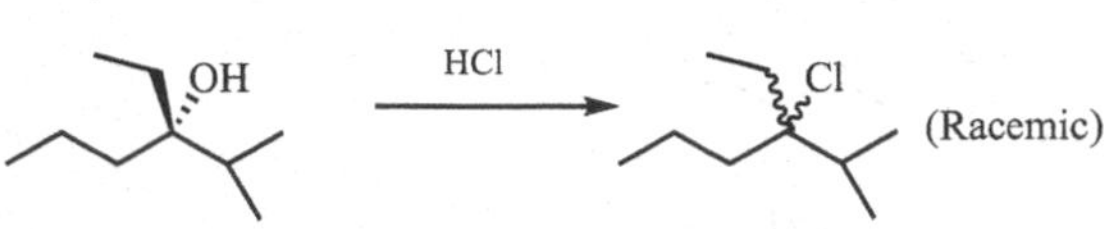 OH —HCl→ Cl (Racemic)

13. What is the intermediate, if any, when pentan-1-ol is treated with HCl under anhydrous conditions? What is the product, if any?

14. Give the major product for the following reactions:

(a) 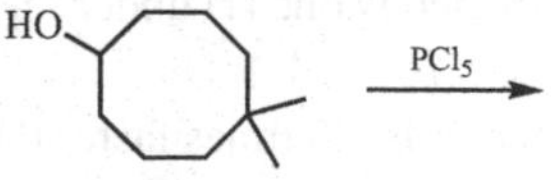 $\xrightarrow{PCl_5}$ (b) 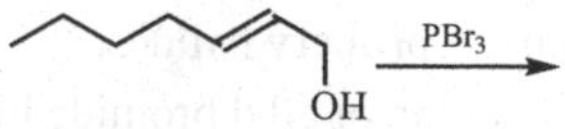 $\xrightarrow{PBr_3}$

(c) 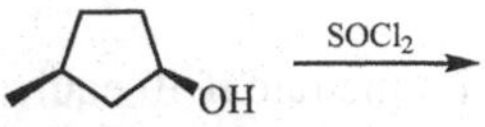 $\xrightarrow{SOCl_2}$ (d) 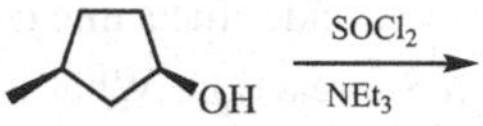 $\xrightarrow[NEt_3]{SOCl_2}$

(e) 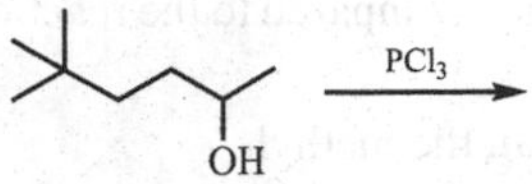 $\xrightarrow{PCl_3}$

15. Explain why this reaction gives a mixture of stereoisomeric chlorides but there is a slight preponderance of the inversion product.

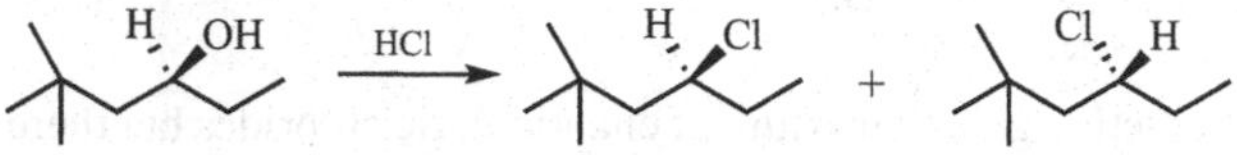

$\xrightarrow{HCl}$ +

16. Give the IUPAC name for each of the following:

(a) 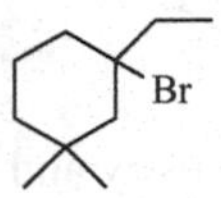 (b) 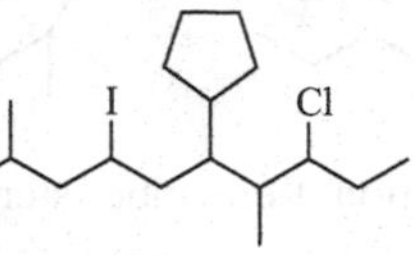 (c)

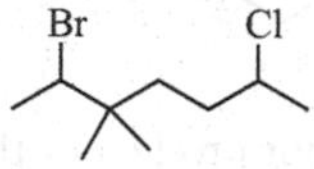

(d) 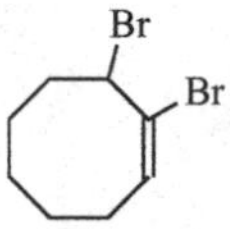 (e) 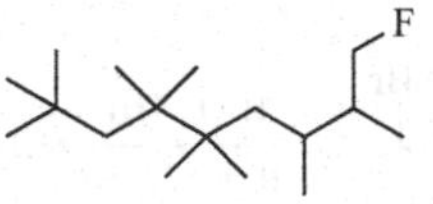 (f)

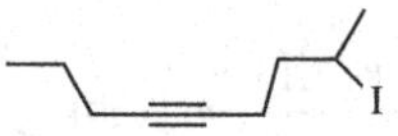

17. Which is the most acidic alcohol: methanol or *tert*-butanol? Explain.
18. Is the sodium salt of prop-2-en-1-ol resonance stabilized? Explain.
19. Explain why methyl *tert*-butyl ether [$CH_3OC(CH_3)_3$] cannot be formed from 2-methyl-2-iodopropane and methanol using a Williamson ether synthesis.
20. Give the correct IUPAC names for each of the following:

(a) 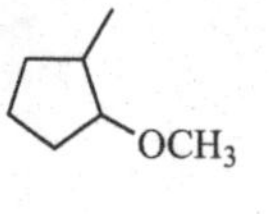 (b) 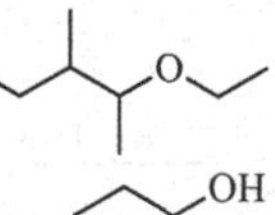 (c)

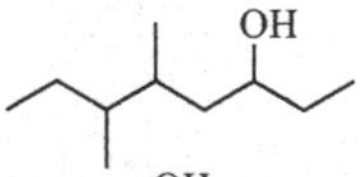

d) 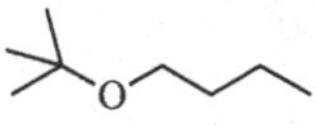 (e) 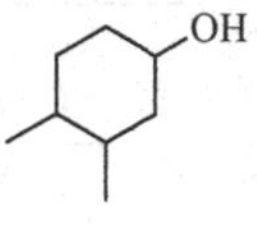 (f)

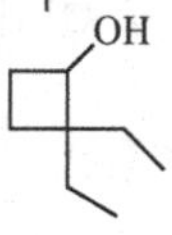

21. In each case give the structure of the major product. Remember stereochemistry where appropriate and if there is no reaction, indicate by N.R.

(a) 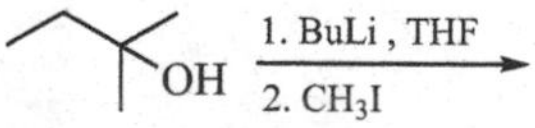 1. BuLi, THF 2. CH_3I (b) 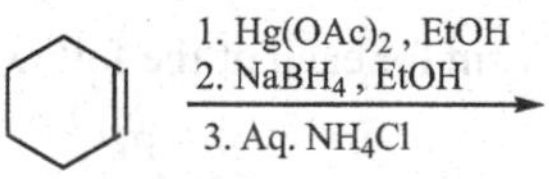 1. $Hg(OAc)_2$, EtOH 2. $NaBH_4$, EtOH 3. Aq. NH_4Cl

(c) 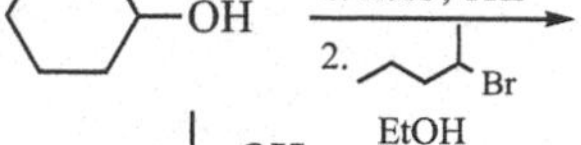 1. NaH, THF 2. (d) 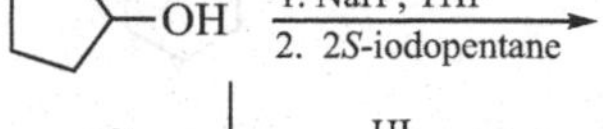 1. NaH, THF 2. 2*S*-iodopentane

(e) 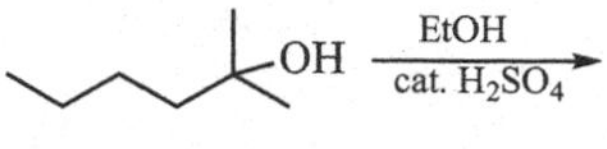 EtOH cat. H_2SO_4 (f) 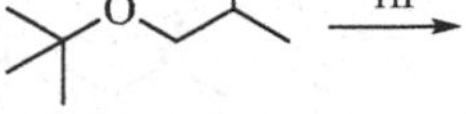 HI

(g) 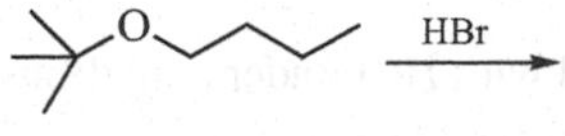 HBr (h) 1. PBr_3 2. $CH_3CH_2O^-Na^+$ EtOH

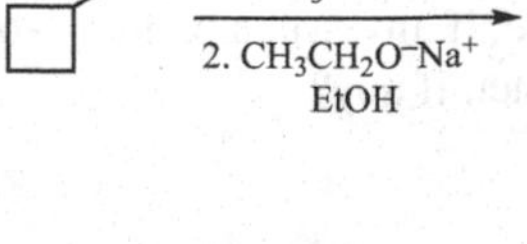

9

Elimination Reactions

There are several important methods for the preparation of alkenes and alkynes. The most prevalent reactions are acid–base reactions, where the presence of a leaving group renders a β-hydrogen atom acidic, and reaction with a suitable base induces an elimination reaction to form an alkene or an alkyne. This chapter will focus on what are arguably the most important methods, bimolecular and unimolecular elimination from alkyl halides. The syn elimination reaction will also be discussed.

9.1 THE E2 REACTION

If the carbon bearing the bromine atom in 2-bromo-2-methylpropane is called the α-carbon, what is the β-carbon?

The carbon atoms of the three identical methyl groups of 2-bromo-2-methylpropane could be considered β-carbons – i.e., they are attached to the α-carbon. In general, all carbon atoms attached to the α-carbon are β-carbons.

```
                 β-carbon
                   H ↓H
                   H-C'          α-carbon
  β-carbon ↘  H       \  ↙
            H-C——C——Br
              H       /
                   H-C-H
                     H  ↖ β-carbon
```

Where is a β-hydrogen in 2-bromo-2-methylpropane?

A β-hydrogen must be attached to one of the β-carbon atoms. Therefore, any of the hydrogen atoms of the three equivalent methyl groups in 2-bromo-2 methylpropane is a β-hydrogen. In general, all hydrogen atoms attached to a β-carbon are β-hydrogen atoms.

```
                 H  H ←—— β-hydrogen
                 H-C'
              H       \
β-hydrogen ——→H-C——C——Br
              H       /
                 H-C-H ←— β-hydrogen
                   H
```

When 2-bromo-2-methylpropane is mixed with a nucleophile, a S_N2 reaction is not possible. Why not?

2-Bromo-2-methylpropane is a tertiary halide, and the activation energy for a S_N2 reaction at a tertiary carbon is so high that for all practical purposes, the reaction cannot proceed.

When 2-bromo-2-methylpropane is mixed with KOH in ethanol, a S_N2 reaction is not possible, but a rapid reaction takes place giving methylprop-2-ene as the product. What reaction is most important for this molecule?

The hydroxide (^-OH) reagent is nucleophilic and will be attracted to the carbon bearing the bromine. The energy required for this S_N2 reaction is too high (see Section 8.2) so for all practical purposes a S_N2 reaction will not occur. Bond polarization makes the β-hydrogen (the hydrogen attached to the second carbon away from the bromine, the β-carbon) electropositive. The hydroxide attacks the β-hydrogen in an acid–base reaction, as shown. Removal of this hydrogen leads to an E2 transition state where a β-hydrogen atom that is anti- to the bromine leaving group is acidic and attached by the basic hydroxide. The other product is water (H—OH), formed as the bromine is displaced and a carbon–carbon double bond is beginning to form. The final product is methylprop-2-ene.

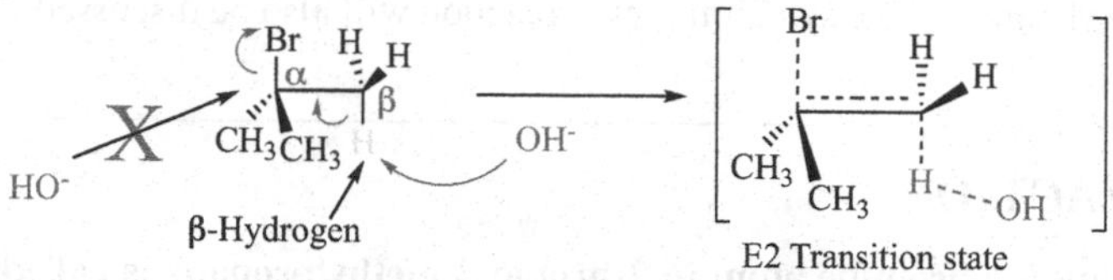

Br H H α β CH_3CH_3 H HO⁻ OH⁻ β-Hydrogen

Br H H CH_3 CH_3 H---OH

E2 Transition state

Is the reaction that converts 2-bromo-2-methylpropane to methylprop-2-ene concerted (one step) or does it have an ionic intermediate?

There is no intermediate, and it is a concerted reaction that proceeds via an E2 transition state, as shown in the preceding question.

Does the reaction that converts 2-bromo-2-methylpropane to methylprop-2-ene follow first-order or second-order kinetics?

The reaction is bimolecular (it requires a collision of OH and the β-hydrogen) and is, therefore, second order in its kinetics [rate = k (RX) (^-OH)].

What is the orientation of the bromine and the β-hydrogen in 2-bromo-2-methylpropane when the reaction with the hydroxide ion occurs to generate transition state?

The β-hydrogen atom in 2-bromo-2-methylpropane is removed by hydroxide in an acid–base reaction. Since the hydrogen atom is removed as a proton, the electrons in that C—H bond stay with the substrate (the two electrons in the new H—OH bond come from hydroxide). In effect, the two electrons from the C—H bond expel the bromide to generate the new π-bond in methylprop-2-ene. Since the bromine in 2-bromo-2-methylpropane is displaced by the electrons in the C—H_β moiety, those electrons should displace Br from the rear (backside attack). This requires that the β-hydrogen be oriented at an angle of close to 180° relative to the leaving group (Br). This reaction therefore requires an anti- orientation of the β-hydrogen and the bromine. In general, attack of the base (^-OH) on the β-hydrogen to initiate this reaction occurs *only* in the rotamer where the leaving group and β-hydrogen have an anti-relationship. This transformation is an *elimination reaction* since the elements of Br and H are *eliminated* from 2-bromo-2-methylpropane. This bimolecular elimination is termed *E2*.

This reaction is called an elimination reaction, but is it possible to use another reaction description to describe it?

It is a Brønsted–Lowry acid–base reaction. The conversion of 2-bromo-2-methylpropane to methylprop-2-ene involves the attack of a base on the β-hydrogen, with concomitant displacement of the leaving group.

Why doesn't the E2 reaction occur when 2-bromo-2-methylpropane reacts with potassium iodide in ethanol?

Potassium iodide is a very poor base (the conjugate acid is HI; a strong acid will generate a weak conjugate base and the iodide ion is considered to be a weak base). The iodide ion is not a sufficiently strong base to remove the β-hydrogen from 2-bromo-2-methylpropane. If there is no base to remove this hydrogen, there is no acid–base reaction and the E2 reaction is not possible.

What is standard free energy?

Standard free energy is the free energy change associated with the formation of a substance from the elements in their most stable forms as they exist under standard conditions (see Section 3.2). The standard free energy is calculated by combining standard enthalpy of formation and the standard entropy of a substance. *Standard free energy* ($\Delta G°$) *assumes that the reaction is done in a standard state*: in solution with a concentration of 1 mol/liter (1 Molar), and at one atmosphere of pressure for gases. The standard free energy can be calculated from enthalpy ($H°$) and entropy ($S°$) by the equation:

$$\Delta G° = \Delta H° - T\Delta S°$$

What constitutes an exothermic reaction?

An exothermic reaction releases energy, so it is one where more energy is released by the reaction than is required to initiate the reaction, so the products are lower in energy than the starting materials. In the diagram, energy is generated by the reaction and this diagram represents an exothermic reaction.

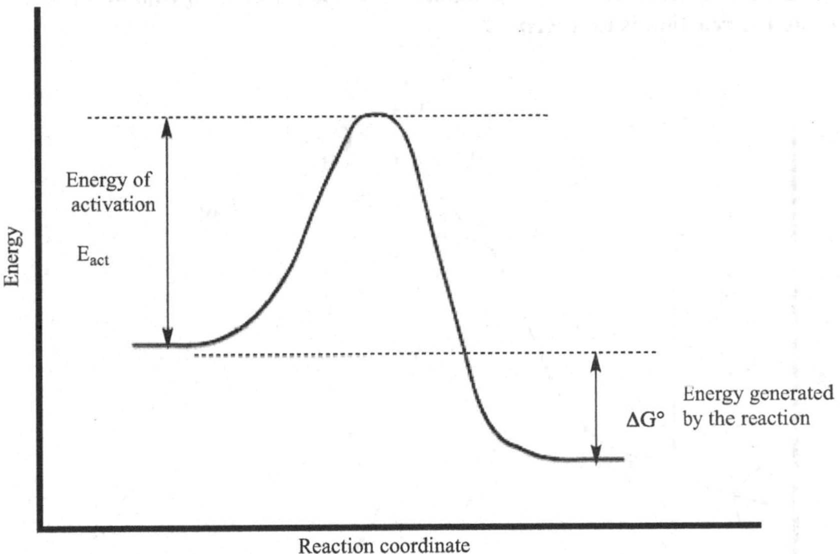

What is the term for the amount of energy required to initiate bond making/bond breaking?

This amount of energy is the activation energy, and it is marked on the diagram.

At what point in the energy diagram is the transition state energy in a reaction found?

The transition state is the midpoint of the reaction and it occurs at the highest point of the energy barrier as marked in the diagram. The amount of energy required to initiate the reaction to achieve the transition state is the activation energy.

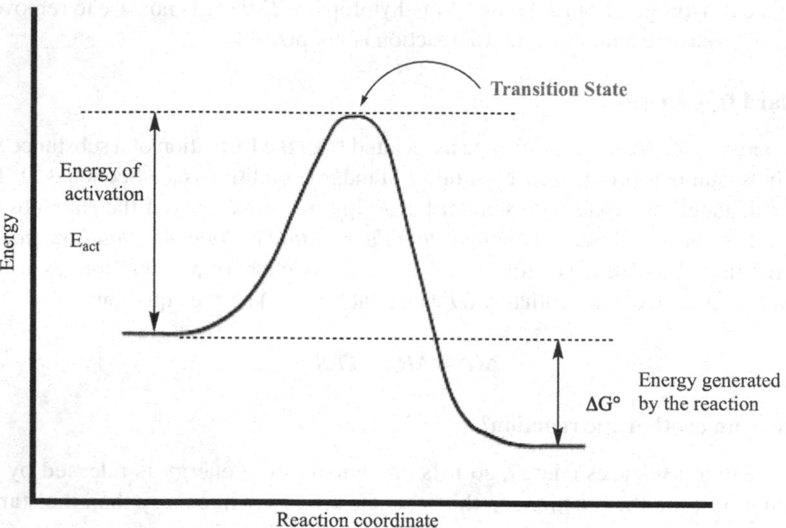

What is the reaction diagram for the conversion of 2-bromo-2-methylpropane to methylprop-2-ene, assuming the reaction is exothermic?

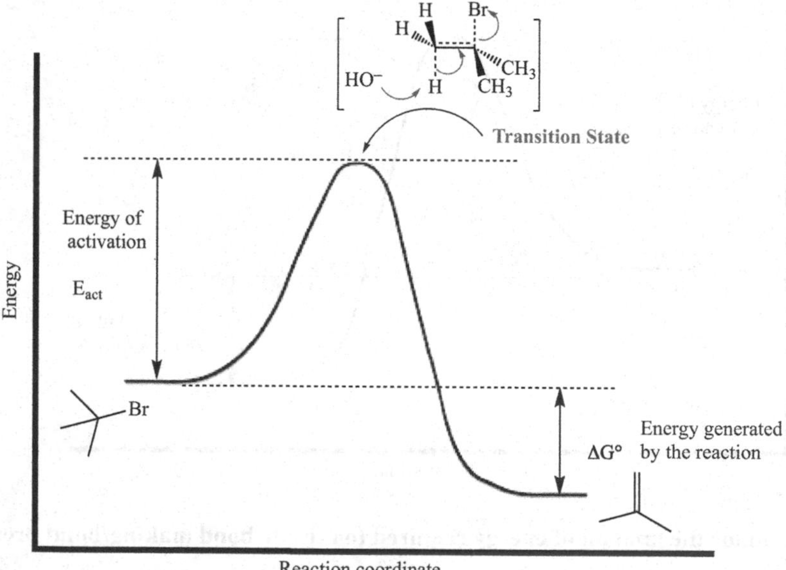

The diagram shows the reaction coordinate, with the assumption that the reaction is exothermic, with 2-bromo-2-methylpropane marked as the starting material, 2-methylpropene marked as the product, and the transition state for this E2 reaction shown at the appropriate place on the reaction curve.

On the diagram from the previous question, what is the position of the transition state?

The transition state position and structure are indicated in the diagram for the preceding question.

What is the Hammond postulate?

The *Hammond postulate* states that the transition state of a reaction resembles either the reactants or the products, whichever is closer in energy.

What is the general name for the reaction in which H and a halogen are eliminated from an alkyl halide?

Dehydrohalogenation.

What is a late transition state?

A late transition state is one that is closer in free energy to the products than the starting material.

How many different β-hydrogen atoms are there in 2-bromo-3-methylhexane?

There are two structurally different β-hydrogen atoms, H_a and H_b.

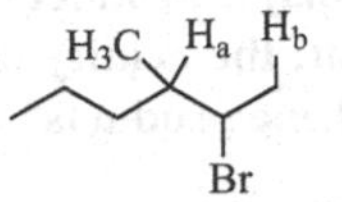

H_3C H_a H_b

Br

Removal of two different β-hydrogen atoms will lead to two different alkenes from 2-bromo-3-methylhexane. What are they?

The two possible alkenes are 3-methylhex-2-ene if H_a is removed by the base, and 3-methylhex-1-ene if H_b is removed by the base.

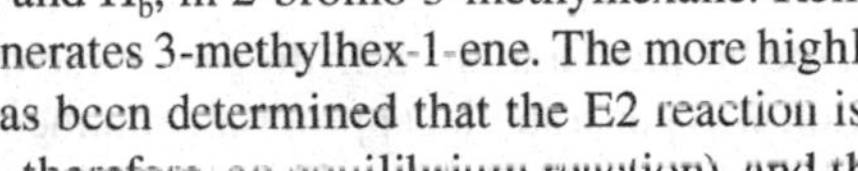

CH_3 H_b H_3C H_a

3-Methylhex-2-ene 3-Methylhex-1-ene

Why does the E2 reaction of (2*S*,3*S*)-2-bromo-3-methylhexane give 3-methylhex-2-ene as the major product rather than 3-methylhex-1-ene?

There are two β-hydrogens, H_a and H_b, in 2-bromo-3-methylhexane. Removal of H_a generates 3-methylhex-2-ene and removal of H_b generates 3-methylhex-1-ene. The more highly substituted alkene is the more thermodynamically stable. It has been determined that the E2 reaction is under thermodynamic control (it is an acid–base reaction and, therefore, an equilibrium reaction), and the major product will always be the more thermodynamically stable alkene, in this case 3-methylhex-2-ene. The more thermodynamically stable alkene, and the major product of the E2 reaction, will *always be the most highly substituted alkene.*

What is the transition state for the conversion of (2*S*,3*S*)-2-bromo-3-methylhexane to (*E*)-3-methylhex-2-ene, and also the transition state for the conversion of 2-bromo-2-methylpentane to 2-methylpent-1-ene?

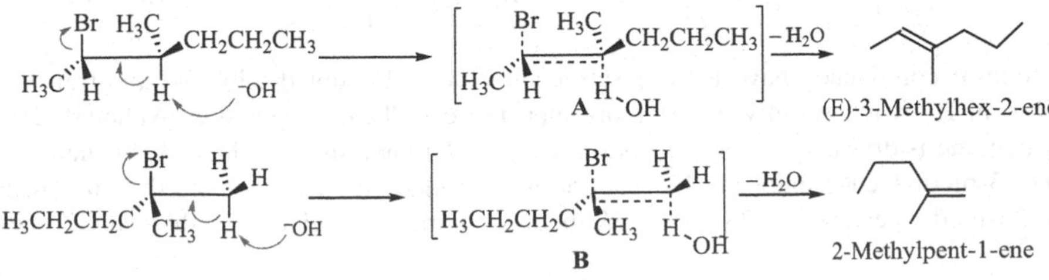

Br H_3C $CH_2CH_2CH_3$ H_3C H H ^-OH → [Br H_3C $CH_2CH_2CH_3$ H_3C H H OH] **A** $-H_2O$ → (E)-3-Methylhex-2-ene

Br H H $H_3CH_2CH_2C$ CH_3 H ^-OH → [Br H H $H_3CH_2CH_2C$ CH_3 H OH] **B** $-H_2O$ → 2-Methylpent-1-ene

The transition state for the formation of (*E*)-3-methylhex-2-ene, is ***A***; the transition state for formation of 2-methylpent-1-ene is ***B***.

What are the two possible products for an E2 reaction of (2*S*,3*S*)-2-bromo-3-methylhexane?

Removal of the β-hydrogen from the more substituted β-carbon gives (*E*)-3-methylhex-2-ene, as shown in the preceding question. Removal of the β-hydrogen from the less substituted carbon, the methyl group, leads to (3*S*)-methylhex-1-ene.

Which is more acidic, H_a in (2*S*,3*S*)-2-bromo-3-methylhexane or H_b?

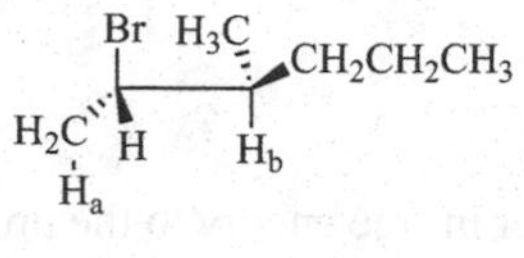

Br H_3C $CH_2CH_2CH_3$ H_2C H H_b H_a

The hydrogen on the less substituted carbon is more acidic than a hydrogen atom on a less substituted carbon. Since H_a is attached to the less substituted carbon, H_a is more acidic than H_b.

If (*E*)-3-methylhex-2-ene is the observed major product for an E2 reaction of (2*S*,3*S*)-2-bromo-3-methylhexane, which is more important, the acidity of the β-hydrogen atom in the starting material or the relative stability of the alkene products?

If the more stable product 3-methylhex-2*E*-ene is the major product, the transition state for that product is more important since in a late transition state, the stability of the product determines the outcome of the reaction. Removal of the more acidic H_a would give (3*S*)-methylhex-1-ene, but the major product is 3-methylhex-2*E*-ene by removal of H_b. Therefore, it is logical to assume that the stability of the final product via a late transition state is more important for E2 reactions.

What is Zaitsev (also called Saytzeff) elimination?

A rule formulated in 1875 by Alexander Zaitsev, who observed that in dehydrohalogenation reactions the alkene formed in greatest amount is the one that corresponds to the removal of the hydrogen from the β-carbon having the fewest hydrogens. Formation of the more substituted and therefore the more stable alkene via an E2 reaction is now termed *Zaitsev elimination.*

The E2 reaction of 2*R*-bromo-3*R*-methylpentane gives exclusively one isomer, 3-methylpent-2*E*-ene. Explain why the other stereoisomer is not formed.

In 2*R*-bromo-3*R*-methylpentane, the bromine and the β-hydrogen on the more substituted carbon are *not* anti in the rotamer drawn. Rotation will generate the appropriate rotamer (shown in the transition state). When the hydroxide attacks the β-hydrogen, as shown, all of the substituents in the resulting transition state are "locked" in the same position as a result of the two stereogenic centers. The two methyl groups are on the same side (cis- to each other) in the E2 transition state, and they *will be cis- to each other in the final product, 3-methylpent-2E-ene.*

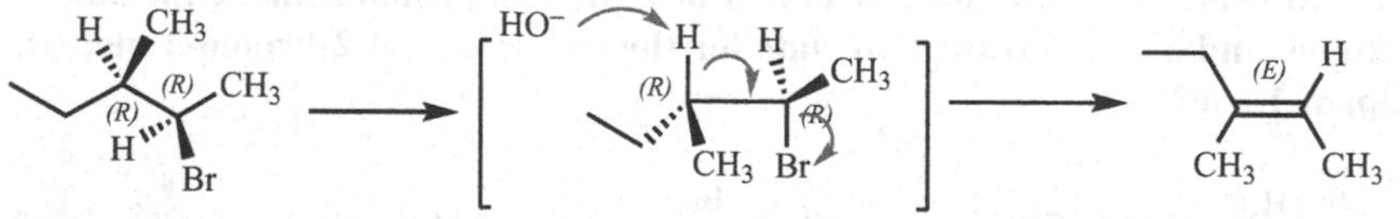

H CH_3 (R) CH_3 (R) H Br → [HO^- H H (R) CH_3 (R) CH_3 Br] → (E) H CH_3 CH_3

The enantiopure compounds have a fixed sterochemistry and coupled with the anti-transition state required for an E2 reaction, only one stereoisomer, the cis alkene, is possible. Although 2*R*-bromo-3*R*-methylpentane is drawn as a single enantiomer, a similar analysis with the (2*S*,3*S*) enantiomer also leads to *(E)*-3-methylpent-2-ene. The E2 reaction is termed *stereospecific*. Note that the enantiomers 2*R*-bromo-3*S*-methylpentane or 2*S*-bromo-3*R*-methylpentane both give 3-methylpent-2*Z*-ene as the product.

A secondary alkyl halide can undergo a S_N2 reaction or an E2 reaction. What solvents are used to promote an E2 reaction? A S_N2 reaction?

A protic solvent such as ethanol or water promotes an E2 reaction whereas an aprotic solvent such as diethyl ether or tetrahydrofuran (THF) promotes a S_N2 reaction.

An E2 reaction is promoted in a protic solvent such as alcohol or water whereas substitution is promoted by an aprotic solvent such as diethyl ether or tetrahydrofuran (THF). Why?

Common solvents may be organized into two categories: *polar* or *nonpolar*, and then *protic* or *aprotic*. Apart from being protic or aprotic, an important property of a solvent is polarity, which helps determine the ability of the solvent to solvate and separate ions (solvation). A polar solvent usually has a substantial dipole and a nonpolar solvent tends to have a small dipole, or none at all. A protic solvent is one that contains an acidic hydrogen (O—H, N—H, S—H, essentially a weak Brønsted–Lowry acid), whereas an aprotic solvent does not contain an acidic hydrogen. *The essential difference between protic and aprotic solvents is the ability of protic solvents to solvate both cations and anions, whereas aprotic solvents efficiently solvate only cations. Ionization is favored only when both ions are solvated, allowing them to be separated.*

If the solvent is water, or if it contains water, the bimolecular (collision) processes between a neutral substrate and a charged nucleophile (e.g., nucleophilic acyl addition reactions and nucleophilic displacement with alkyl halides) are slower due to solvation effects. On the other hand, water is an excellent solvent for the solvation and separation of ions, so unimolecular processes, which involve ionization to carbocations may be competitive.

Substitution is generally a faster process relative to elimination. If the solvent is aprotic, only a cationic species can be solvated – not anions. Since nucleophiles are typically negatively charged or have a negative dipole, an aprotic solvent facilitates approach of a nucleophile to an electrophilic center. Therefore, an aprotic solvent will generally favor substitution.

What does stereospecific mean?

The term stereospecific means that of two or more possible products, one stereoisomer gives one and only one product, whereas the other stereoisomer will give a different product. In the preceding example, stereoisomers 2*R*-bromo-3*R*-methylpentane or 2*S*-bromo-3*S*-methylpentane gives the *E*-alkene and whereas the diastereomeric 2*R*-bromo-3*S*-methylpentane or 2*S*-bromo-3*R*-methylpentane enantiomers will give the *Z*-alkene.

The cyclohexane derivative 2*S*-bromo-1*S*-ethyl-3*S*-methylcyclohexane gives 3*S*-ethyl-1-methylcyclohex-1-ene as the alkene product of an E2 reaction. Why?

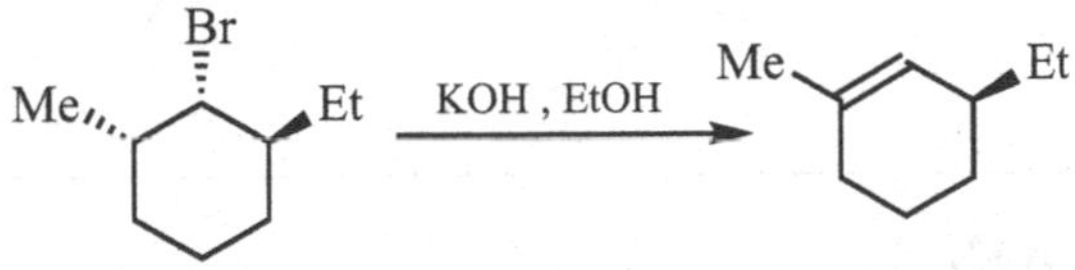

Remember that for an E2 reaction the β-hydrogen and the leaving group must assume an anti- conformation. Such an anti- conformation is only possible if the β-hydrogen atom and the leaving group are trans-diaxial.

This question cannot be answered using the "flat" drawing shown. Cyclohexane derivatives exist primarily as the two equilibrating chair conformations shown (see Section 5.2). There are two β-hydrogens, but in only one is the β-hydrogen atom and the Br anti- (they have a trans-diaxial relationship). The other β-hydrogen is equatorial, and essentially at right angles to the equatorial Br. In other words, only the trans-diaxial H:Br pair can give an E2 reaction. In the other chair conformation, the β-hydrogen in light gray is equatorial, but the bromine atom is also equatorial and there is no possibility of an E2 reaction. The blue β-hydrogen atom is axial, but since the Br is equatorial an E2 is not possible. Only removal of H_a can give the E2 product. Because of this phenomenon, the alkene is formed *only* toward the methyl (Me) and not towards the ethyl (Et), so the product is 3*S*-ethyl-1-methylcyclohex-1-ene. The bromine-bearing carbon is probably too sterically hindered to give a S_N2 reaction.

β-Hydrogen is anti, or trans diaxial to Br

β-Hydrogen is equatorial. but not anti to Br so an E2 is not possible

KOH, EtOH

This β-hydrogen is axial but the Br is equatorial, so an E2 is not possible

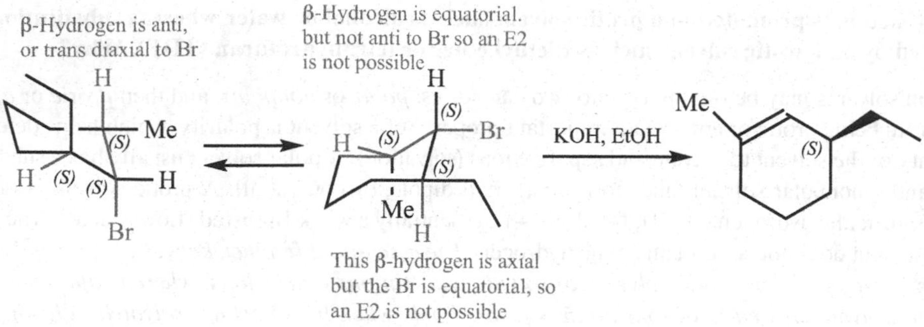

The cyclohexane derivative 2*S*-bromo-1*S*-ethyl-3*R*-methylcyclohexane gives no elimination products at all under E2 reaction conditions. Why?

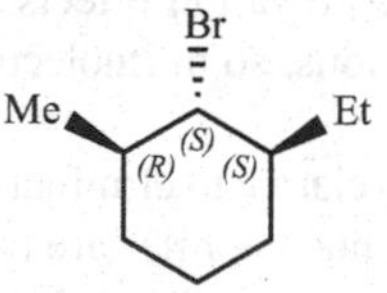

The equilibrating chair conformations for 2*S*-bromo-1*S*-ethyl-3*R*-methylcyclohexane are shown. For an E2 reaction, there must be a β-hydrogen atom with a trans-diaxial relationship to the bromine. The Br is axial in only one conformation and it is equatorial in the other. Both β-hydrogens are equatorial in the conformation that has an axial Br, but the Br is equatorial when both hydrogen atoms are axial in the other conformation. An E2 reaction is *not* possible from either conformation by treatment with hydroxide. The bromine-bearing carbon is probably too sterically hindered to give a S_N2 reaction.

No β-Hydrogen is anti, or trans diaxial to the axial Br s E2 is not possible

Both β-hydrogens are axial. but Br is equatorial, so an E2 is not possible

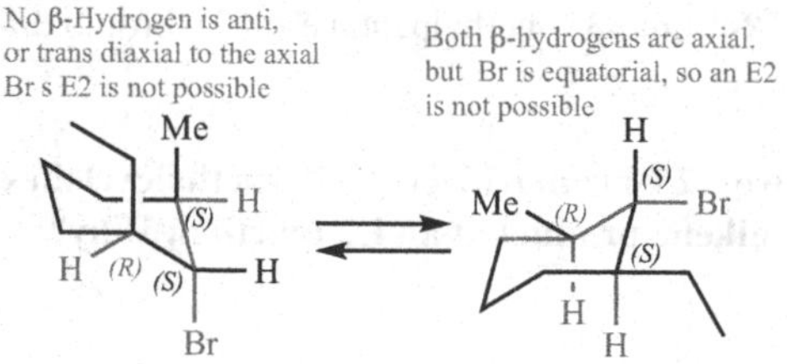

9.2 THE E1 REACTION

Can a reaction that generates a carbocation intermediate lead to an elimination?

When a highly ionizing medium such as water is present and substitution is slow, elimination can occur via a carbocation intermediate. Typically, E2 reactions are faster in protic solvents, but a first-order elimination reaction, termed E1, can occur under certain conditions.

When 2-bromo-2-methylpropane reacts with KOH in dry ethanol, is carbocation formation possible?

Yes, but the reaction is extremely slow! Since ethanol is a polar protic solvent, ionization is possible. However, ionization in pure ethanol is *very* slow. For example, NaCl essentially is insoluble in pure ethanol. In other words, the halide does not ionize in 100% ethanol and ionization is a slow process, particularly when compared with water.

Why is the 2-methylpropyl carbocation planar?

A positively charged carbon is essentially an empty unhybridized p-orbital and the attached atoms will distribute to a trigonal planar array. The planar geometry of the carbocation is due to electronic repulsion of the bonds and steric repulsion of the groups, which is the lowest energy distribution of those groups about the positively charged carbon.

When 2-bromo-2-methylpropane reacts with KOH in aqueous ethanol, is carbocation formation possible?

Yes! The presence of water makes ionization much more facile since the protic solvent can solvate both cations and anions and assists in "pulling" off the bromine atom. Ionization leads to the planar, tertiary 2-methylpropyl carbocation as the positive ion, with the bromide ion as the negative ion.

$$\text{(CH}_3)_3\text{C–Br} \xrightarrow[\text{Aqueous ethanol}]{-\text{Br}^-} [(\text{CH}_3)_3\text{C}^+]\ [\text{Br}^-]$$

How many atoms are electrophilic in the 2-methylpropyl carbocation?

The β-hydrogen atoms have a δ^+ charge due to their proximity to the positively charged carbon and are electrophilic. However, the positively charged carbon is more electron deficient since it has a formal charge of +1 and is clearly electrophilic.

Which site in the 2-methylpropyl carbocation is more attractive to hydroxide, the carbocation carbon or a β-hydrogen atom?

The carbon has a formal positive charge whereas the β-hydrogen atoms have a δ^+ dipole, so the hydroxide ion should be most strongly attracted to the carbon with a formal charge of +1.

If hydroxide reacts with the carbon in the 2-methylpropyl carbocation rather than a β-hydrogen, what type of reaction does this represent?

Collision with carbon makes hydroxide a nucleophile, and such a reaction is essentially like a S_N1 reaction. The product is an alcohol, 2-methylpropan-2-ol.

If hydroxide reacts with a β-hydrogen in the 2-methylpropyl carbocation rather than the carbon atom, what type of reaction does this represent?

Such a reaction is an elimination reaction to form an alkene, 2-methylprop-2-ene. The reaction proceeds via an intermediate carbocation, follows first-order kinetics, and is termed a first-order elimination reaction, E1. The hydroxide reacts with the β-hydrogen to form water, and the double bond in the alkene product.

$$\text{(CH}_3)_3\text{C–Br} \xrightarrow[\text{Aqueous ethanol, KOH}]{-\text{Br}^-} [\text{H–CH}_2\text{–C}^+(\text{CH}_3)_2]\ [\text{Br}^-] \xrightarrow{^-\text{OH}} \text{CH}_2\text{=C(CH}_3)_2$$

What is the product when cyclohexanol reacts with an acid, H^+?

When cyclohexanol reacts with H^+, the oxygen atom behaves as a base, and the product is the oxonium ion, cyclohexyloxonium. Note that this acid–base reaction is reversible.

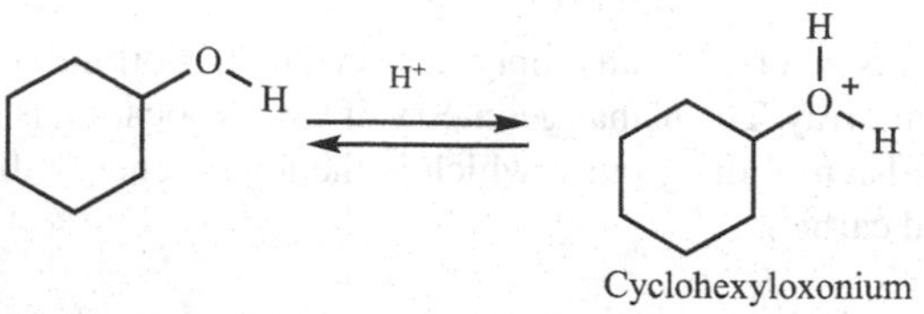

Cyclohexyloxonium

What are the possible reactions of the cyclohexyloxonium intermediate, formed by the reaction of cyclohexanol and sulfuric acid?

In cyclohexyloxonium, the HOH unit (water) is a good leaving group. The possible reactions are loss of water by removal of a β-hydrogen to give the alkene directly (E2), ionization to a carbocation by loss of water, or reaction with a nucleophile with direct displacement of water (S_N2) to give the product. Note that loss of a β-hydrogen from the carbocation will give cyclohexene by an E1 mechanism and that collision of the carbocation with the very weak nucleophile bisulfate anion will give cyclohexyl hydrogen sulfate by a S_N1 mechanism. It is important to know that this hydrogen sulfate derivative is very unstable and when the solvent is aqueous (contains water), loss of the hydrogen sulfate anion is facile, and the equilibrium is shifted toward the carbocation.

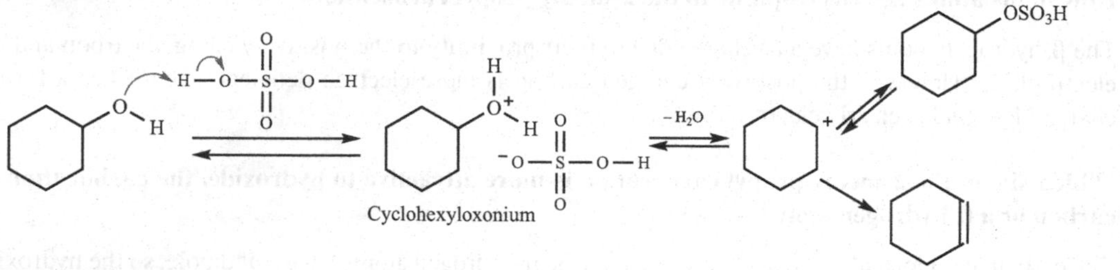

Cyclohexyloxonium

In the reaction of cyclohexanol with concentrated sulfuric acid (little water), is there a nucleophilic species present?

In concentrated sulfuric acid, water is not considered to be present in sufficient quantity to be a nucleophilic species. The only other nucleophile is the hydrogen sulfate anion, which is resonance stabilized and is a very weak nucleophile. Under these conditions, cyclohexanol does not react with the carbocation to form an ether, presumably because any alcohol is protonated and not available for a substitution reaction.

What are all resonance forms of the hydrogen sulfate anion?

The three resonance forms are shown, where the negative charge is delocalized and upon reaction with a carbon atom, somewhat sterically hindered. Therefore, electrons cannot be readily donated, and the hydrogen sulfate anion is a weak nucleophile.

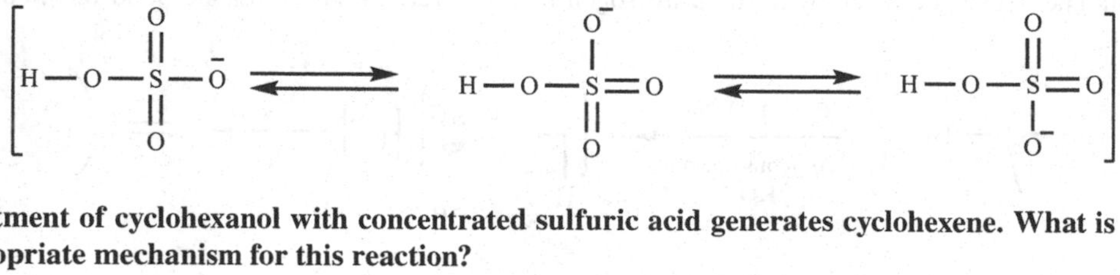

Treatment of cyclohexanol with concentrated sulfuric acid generates cyclohexene. What is an appropriate mechanism for this reaction?

The oxygen of cyclohexanol reacts with the acidic hydrogen of sulfuric acid to form an oxonium salt. The by-product of losing H^+ from H_2SO_4 is the hydrogen sulfate anion, HSO_4^-, which is a very poor nucleophile due to the resonance stability. This fact makes an S_N2 displacement or a S_N1 reaction very slow. In concentrated sulfuric acid, which is a good dehydrating agent, the carbocation readily loses water to form the cyclohexyl carbocation. The hydrogen sulfate anion is a weak base and the β-hydrogen in the carbocation is acidic due to its proximity to the cation center. This hydrogen atom is removed, via an acid–base reaction, to generate the alkene, cyclohexene. This is a unimolecular process via ionization to the carbocation, and the overall process is an elimination, therefore it is an El reaction.

H_2SO_4 ; HSO_4^- ; $- H_2O$; HSO_4^- ; $- H^+$

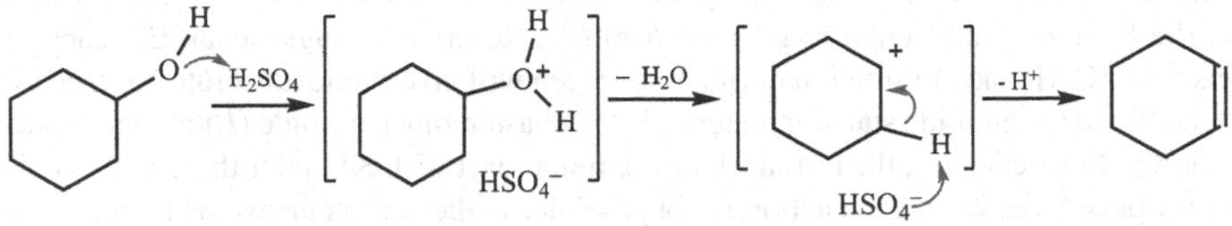

When does the E1 reaction compete with E2, S_N2, and S_N1?

The El reaction is the major process *only* when a cation is formed in the presence of a base, and there is no nucleophile in the medium to react via a S_N1 process to compete with elimination. For ionization to a carbocation to be competitive, the S_N2 process must be very slow, as is the case with tertiary alkyl halides.

When cyclohexanol is treated with aqueous sulfuric acid, a significant amount of cyclohexanol is recovered. Why?

The oxonium ion from cyclohexanol is formed and ionization to the carbocation follows. In aqueous media, however, water is present, which can function as a nucleophile. If water attacks the carbocation, the oxonium ion is formed, and, in the presence of water loss of a proton, regenerates the starting alcohol. The El reaction occurs as the major process only when there is no good nucleophile is present. If water were added to this reaction, it would function as a nucleophile making the S_N1 process more likely than the El reaction.

What are the requirements (structure of the halide or alcohol and reaction conditions) for an E1 reaction?

In general, a tertiary halide or alcohol precursor must be used since a relatively stable tertiary carbocation will be generated. Primary substrates do not give the cation, and secondary substrates give relatively stable secondary cations. The secondary cation may give some El product, but other reactions often compete. With alkyl halides, water is usually necessary to help form and stabilize the cation, but water will be a nucleophile and can give the S_N1 reaction as the major process. In such cases, El is usually a minor process. With alcohols, anhydrous acids can be used to generate the cation, but the conjugate base of that acid must not be nucleophilic. Therefore, the acids used include sulfuric acid (H_2SO_4), perchloric acid ($HClO_4$), and tetrafluoroboric acid (HBF_4).

What is (are) the major product(s) for the reactions of (a)–(d)? Offer an explanation for each choice.

(a) OH — aq. EtOH , cat. H^+ / KI →

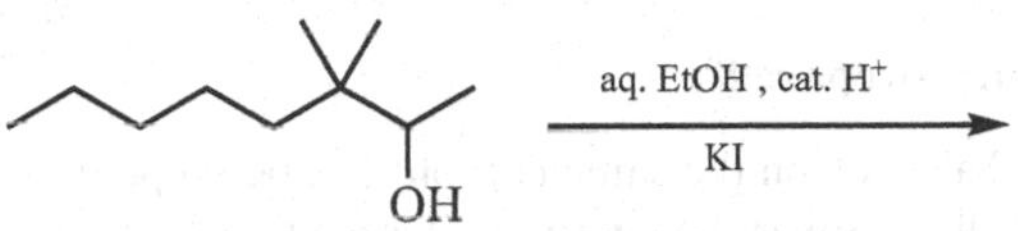

(b) CH_3 H I — KCN , DMF , heat →

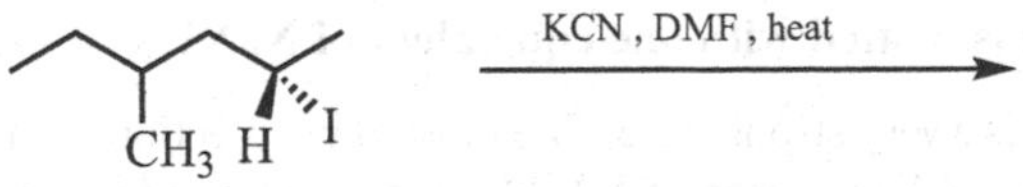

(c) H_3C H Br CH_3 — KOH , EtOH →

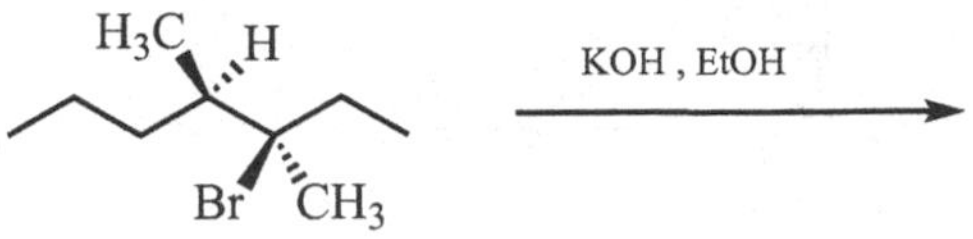

(d) Br CH_3 — KI , THF , heat →

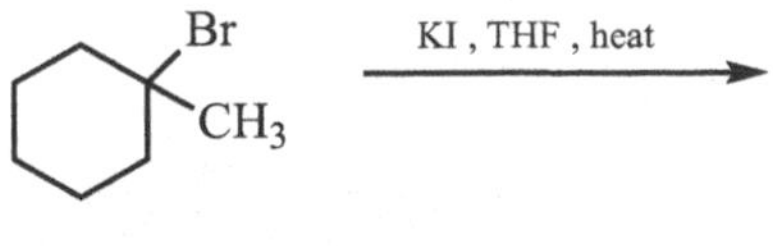

In reaction (a), the aqueous solvent and acid catalyst suggest an S_N1 reaction. Ionization to a cation is followed by rearrangement (the methyl group migrates to give a more stable tertiary cation) and iodide attacks the cation to give the tertiary iodide product. Reaction (b) is an S_N2 reaction and proceeds with 100% inversion of configuration at the stereogenic center. The nucleophile ($^-$CN) displaces the leaving group (I) at the *S*- stereogenic center to give the *R*-nitrile. Reaction (c) suggests an E2 reaction (tertiary halide reacts with KOH) and elimination of the β-hydrogen will give a tetrasubstituted alkene as the more stable product. Since the bromide starting material is one diastereomer, a single (*E*)-alkene product will be formed as shown. In reaction (d), the tertiary halide cannot react with KI under these S_N2 conditions, and iodide is a very poor base, so an E2 reaction is not possible, so the correct answer is no reaction.

(a) 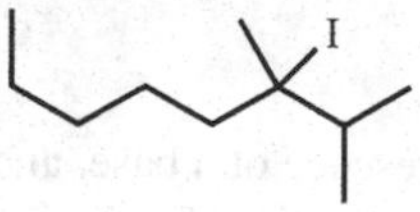 I (b) 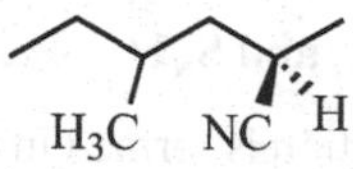 H_3C NC H (c) 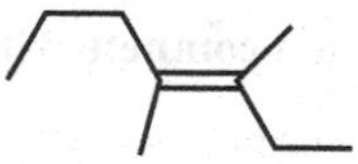 (d) No Reaction

9.3 PREPARATION OF ALKYNES

Is it possible to use elimination reactions to prepare alkynes?

Yes! Most alkynes are prepared in one of two ways: elimination of geminal dihalides with strong base or by alkylation of acetylene or monosubstituted alkynes, as seen in Sections 8.2 and 8.3. This section will focus on the preparation of alkynes, as well as vinyl halides, by elimination reactions.

What is a geminal dihalide?

A geminal dihalide has both halogen atoms on the same carbon, as in 2,2-dibromobutane.

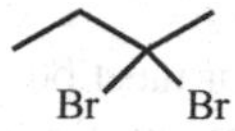

Br Br

What is a vicinal dihalide?

A vicinal dihalide has the two halogen atoms on adjacent carbon atoms, as in 2,3-dibromobutane.

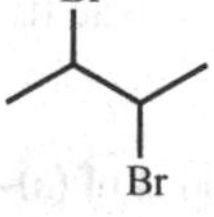

Br Br

How are geminal dihalides prepared?

Geminal dihalides (both halogens on the same carbon) can be prepared from alkynes. Sequential addition of HBr or HCl to an alkyne gives the geminal dihalide (see Section 7.6)

If 1,2-dibromopentane is treated with one equivalent of $NaNH_2$, what is the product?

Sodium amide ($NaNH_2$) is a very strong base. The most likely reaction is an E2, but there are two bromine atoms. The initial product of the reaction of 1,2-dibromopentane and sodium amide in ammonia is a *vinyl halide*, 1-bromopent-1-ene, which is derived from an E2 reaction to produce the more stable alkene.

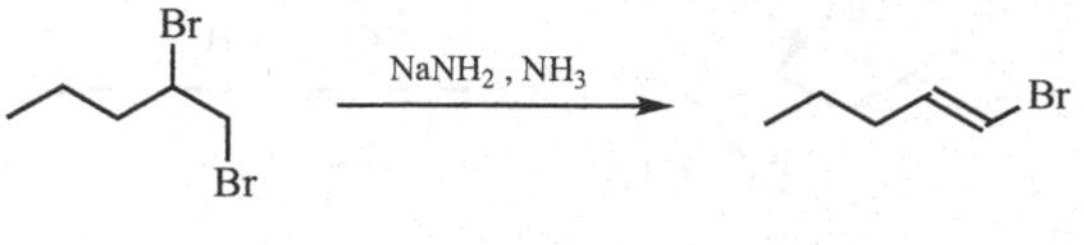

Br Br $\xrightarrow{NaNH_2, NH_3}$ Br

What is a vinyl halide?

A vinyl halide is an alkene where a halogen atom is directly attached to one of the sp^2-hybridized carbon atoms of the C=C unit.

Another alkene product is possible in the elimination reaction of 1,2-dibromopentane, via loss of the hydrogen atom β- to the bromine on C2. What is this product and what is an explanation as to why 1-bromopent-1-ene is formed preferentially?

The alternative product is 2-bromopent-1-ene, a disubstituted alkene where the bromine atom and the propyl group are on the same carbon. The E2 reaction is under thermodynamic control, and gives the more substituted alkene, which is more stable. In this case 1-bromopent-1-ene is more stable than 2-bromopent-1-ene. The hydrogen atom on C1 is also more acidic than the hydrogen atoms on C2 since C1 is less substituted. This property also leads to preferential elimination to 1-bromopent-1-ene.

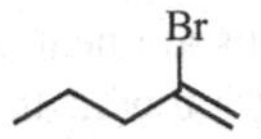

Br

What is the product when 1,2-dibromopentane is treated with an excess of sodium amide in liquid ammonia?

In the presence of at least two equivalents of sodium amide ($NaNH_2$), 1,2-dibromopentane is first converted to 1-bromopent-1-ene. However, sodium amide is a sufficiently strong base to remove the hydrogen on the carbon–carbon double bond, and in the presence of an excess of sodium amide, 1-bromopent-1-ene gives a second E2 reaction to give the alkyne, pent-1-yne.

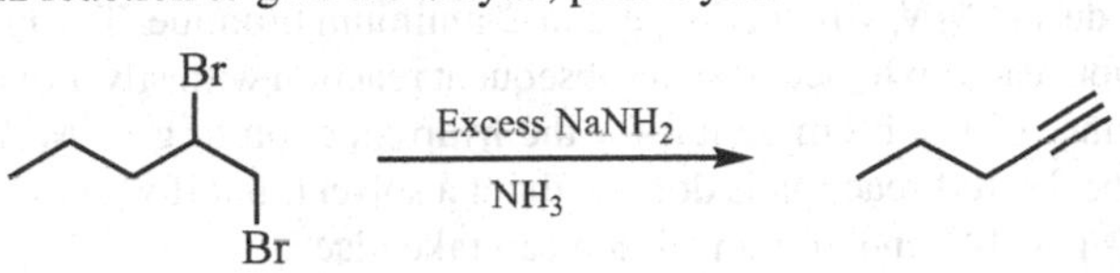

Br Br —Excess $NaNH_2$ / NH_3→

What is the product when the geminal dibromide 2,2-dibromopentane reacts with one equivalent of sodium amide?

The reaction of 2,2-dibromopentane with the strong base will give an E2 reaction. Removal of a hydrogen atom from the methyl group leads to a disubstituted alkene, whereas removal of a hydrogen atom from C3 leads to the more stable trisubstituted alkene, 2-bromopent-2-ene. However, there is no stereocenter in 2,2-dibromopentane so there are two different β-hydrogen atoms, which will give both the *E*- and *Z*-isomers. In other words, there is no stereochemical bias in 2,2-dibromopentane, so this reaction produces two products, 2-bromopent-2*Z*-ene and 2-bromopent-2*E*-ene.

Br Br —$NaNH_2$ / NH_3→ Br + Br

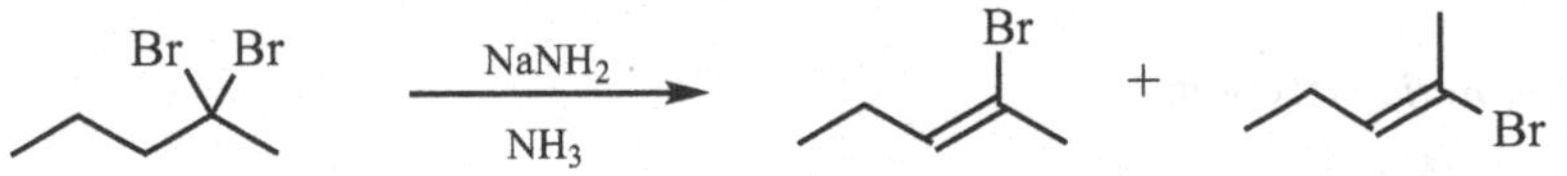

(*Z*)-2-Bromopent-2-ene (*E*)-2-Bromopent-2-ene

What product is formed when 2,2-dibromopentane reacts with an excess of sodium amide?

The initial reaction with sodium amide, gives 2-bromopent-2*Z*-ene and 2-bromopent-2*E*-ene, but with an excess of the base, another E2 reaction with either vinyl halide gives pent-2-yne.

9.4 SYN ELIMINATION

What is syn elimination?

The term syn elimination refers to removal of a β-hydrogen atom by base to give an alkene, but an eclipsed (syn) conformation is required to remove than hydrogen atom since the base is tethered to the molecule, so it is an intramolecular reaction.

What does the term "tethered base" mean?

A basic atom or group is part of the molecule rather than a separate entity so that the only hydrogen atoms readily available for an acid–base reaction are within the same molecule.

What is an example of a molecule that has a "tethered base"?

An example is *N,N,N*-trimethylpentan-2-aminium hydroxide. However, the hydroxide can only be "tethered" to the molecule if the reaction conditions are neat (no solvent) such that the ions are not solvent separated. Such a "tethering" is called a tight ion pair. In other words, the hydroxide remains in close proximity to the positively charged ammonium unit.

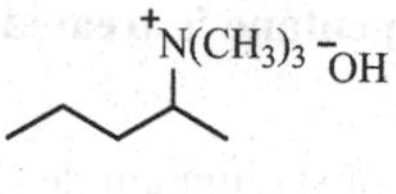

$\overset{+}{N}(CH_3)_3\ {}^{-}OH$

How can *N,N,N*-trimethylpentan-2-aminium hydroxide be prepared?

The reaction of 2-bromopentane and trimethylamine gives a S_N2 reaction if an aprotic solvent such as THF is used, so the product is *N,N,N*-trimethylpentan-2-aminium bromide. The bromide ion is not basic enough for an elimination reaction to occur, so a subsequent reaction with silver oxide and one equivalent of water leads to exchange of the bromide ion for the hydroxide ion to give *N,N,N*-trimethylpentan-2-aminium hydroxide. The desired reaction is done without a solvent, but if water is used as a solvent then separation of the ions is possible and an E2 reaction can take place.

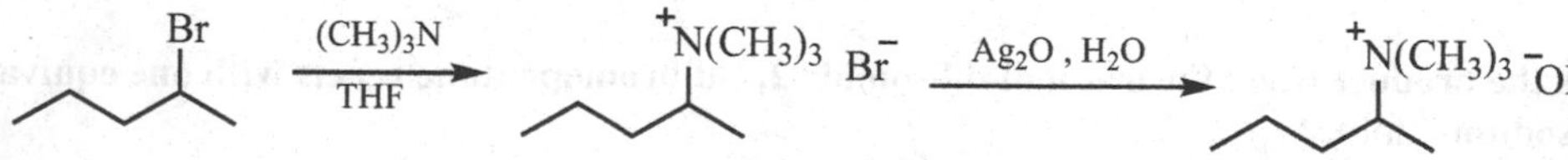

Br $\xrightarrow[\text{THF}]{(CH_3)_3N}$ $\overset{+}{N}(CH_3)_3\ Br^-$ $\xrightarrow{Ag_2O\ ,\ H_2O}$ $\overset{+}{N}(CH_3)_3\ {}^{-}OH$

When *N,N,N*-trimethylpentan-2-aminium hydroxide is heated to about 200°C, the product is an alkene. What is the major product of this reaction?

Pent-1-ene.

The reaction scheme that converts 2-bromopentane to pent-1-ene is a named reaction. What is that name?

The *Hofmann elimination* reaction.

How does heating *N,N,N*-trimethylpentan-2-aminium hydroxide lead to pent-1-ene?

The hydroxide unit is a base and is tethered to the molecule as a tight ion pair. For the hydroxide to react with a β-hydrogen atom in the tight ion pair, an eclipsed or syn conformation is required. The hydroxide can react with the β-hydrogen atom H_a via an intramolecular reaction, as shown in the figure, to generate water, pent-1-ene, and the neutral molecule trimethylamine, which functions as a leaving group in this reaction. The β-hydrogen atom H_b is less available than H_a, so removal of H_a leads to the major product.

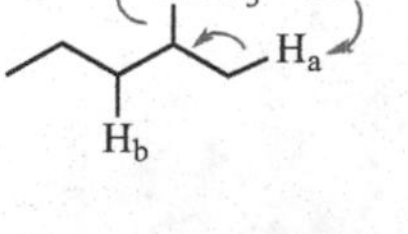

$NMe_3^+\ OH^-$ H_a H_b

Why is the Hofmann elimination referred to as a syn elimination?

The internal acid–base reaction that leads to elimination cannot occur unless the β-hydrogen atom that is removed and the ammonium unit are eclipsed, or in a syn conformation.

Why is H_a removed in preference to H_b in the Hofmann elimination?

Examination of the two eclipsed rotamers of *N,N,N*-trimethylpentan-2-aminium hydroxide ***A*** and ***B*** show the two available β-hydrogen atoms H_a and H_b to an intramolecular reaction with hydroxide. Inspection of these rotamers shows that ***A*** is less sterically hindered than ***B***, and so it is lower in energy. Therefore, rotamer ***A*** has a higher percentage in the rotamer population of the molecule than rotamer ***B***. For this reason, hydroxide is more likely to remove H_a to give pent-1-ene, which is the major product.

NMe_3^+ OH^- H_a H H CHH_bEt **A**

H_b NMe_3^+ OH^- H H CH_2H_a Et **B**

Why is heating to 200°C necessary for this reaction when an E2 reaction occurs at a significantly lower temperature?

An eclipsed rotamer is higher in energy than an anti rotamer, and higher energy is required for there to be a significant working population of the rotamer required for the intramolecular acid–base reaction.

Why does Hofmann elimination give the less substituted alkene?

Since a syn (eclipsed) rotamer is required for the internal acid–base reaction, the less sterically hindered eclipsed rotamer will be lower in energy, the preferred conformation, and will lead to the major product. The less sterically hindered eclipsed rotamer will form at the less sterically hindered carbon (see ***A*** in the preceding question), and removal of the hydrogen atom from the less substituted carbon (H_a in the preceding question) will lead to the less substituted alkene as the major product.

What is the major product formed when *N,N,N*-triethylpentan-2-aminium hydroxide is heated to 200°C?

There are two products, ethylene (ethene) and *N,N*-diethylpentan-2-amine. *The Hofmann elimination will always give the least substituted alkene* for the reasons explained in the previous question. Here, the least substituted alkene is ethylene, which is the product because all four of the groups attached to nitrogen have β-hydrogen atoms, including the three ethyl groups. The reaction with hydroxide will therefore preferentially remove a β-hydrogen atom from an ethyl group to give ethylene and the second product is *N,N*-diethylpentan-2-amine.

N^+ ^-OH —200°C→ N + $CH_2{=}CH_2$

What is the major product formed when *N,N,N*-triethylpentan-2-aminium hydroxide is heated in aqueous ethanol?

N^+ ^-OH —aq. EtOH, Heat→ N^+ H ^-OH → + N + H_2O

In the aqueous solvent the ammonium cation and the hydroxide anion are solvent-separated, so an intramolecular reaction is not possible. However, the triethylamine unit is a good leaving group and hydroxide is a base, so an E2 intermolecular reaction of the ammonium salt leads to but-2-ene and triethylamine as products, along with water. If the trimethylammonium salt is used rather than the triethylammonium salt, an E2 reaction will be preferred under these conditions and the products will be but-2-rne and trimethylamine.

What is Cope elimination?

The *Cope elimination* is the reaction of trialkylamine N-oxide, which is heated, and syn elimination leads to the less substituted alkene and a hydroxylamine.

What is the structure of trimethylamine *N*-oxide?

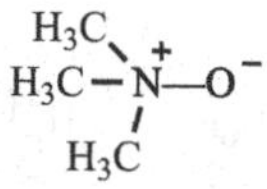

$(H_3C)_3N^+–O^-$

How are amine *N*-oxides prepared from amines?

The reaction of an amine with an oxidizing agent (also see Chapter 13) such as hydrogen peroxide leads to the amine *N*-oxide. An example is the reaction of *N*,*N*-dimethylhexan-2-amine with hydrogen peroxide, which gives *N*,*N*-dimethylhexan-2-amine oxide as the product.

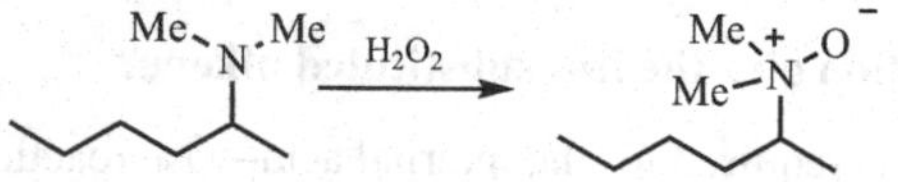

Me, Me, N — H_2O_2 → Me, Me–N⁺–O⁻

What is the product formed when *N*,*N*-dimethylhexan-2-amine oxide is heated to 200°C?

The product is pent-1-ene via syn elimination of *N*,*N*-dimethylhydroxylamine. As with the Hofmann elimination, the product is the less substituted alkene since the reaction proceeds via an eclipsed rotamer for the intramolecular reaction.

Me, Me–N⁺–O⁻, H — 150°C, - Me_2N-OH →

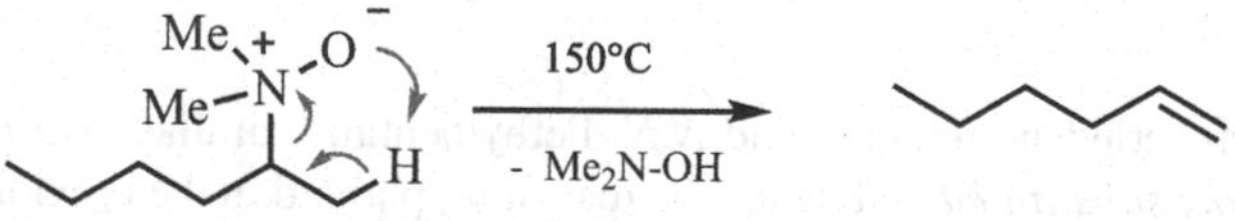

What is the "tethered base" in the example shown in the preceding question?

The base is the negatively charged oxygen of the amine N-oxide.

END OF CHAPTER PROBLEMS

1. Draw the transition state leading to the major product for the reaction of 2-bromo-3-methylbutane with KOH in ethanol and draw that product.
2. Briefly explain why 3-bromo-2,2,4,4-tetramethylpentane does not give an E2 product when heated with KOH in ethanol.

3. In each of the following reactions give the major product. Remember stereochemistry and if there is no reaction, indicate by N.R.:

(a) 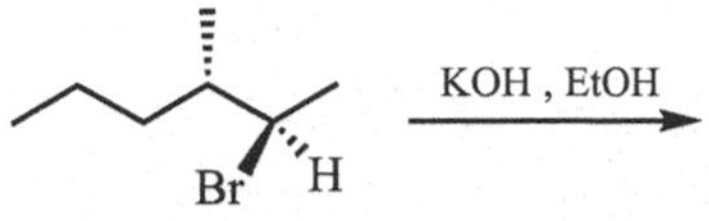
Br
H
KOH , EtOH

(b) 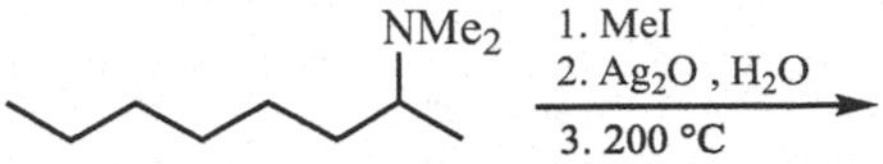
NMe2
1. MeI
2. Ag2O , H2O
3. 200 °C

(c) 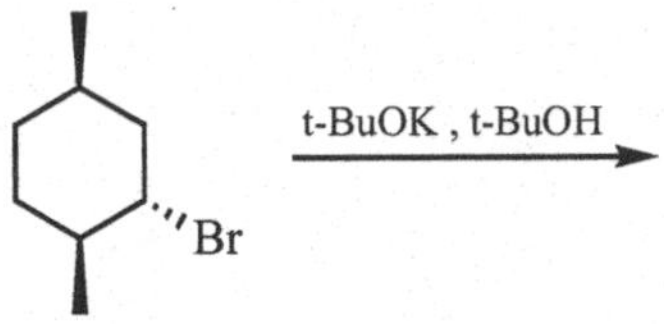
Br
t-BuOK , t-BuOH

(d) 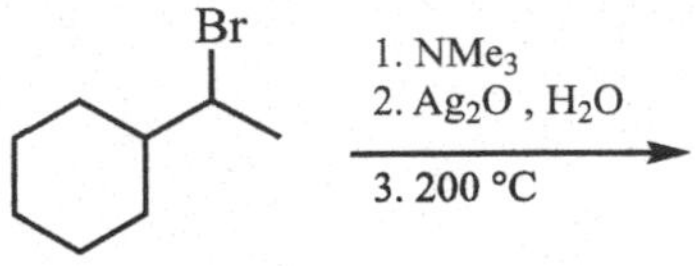
Br
1. NMe3
2. Ag2O , H2O
3. 200 °C

(e) 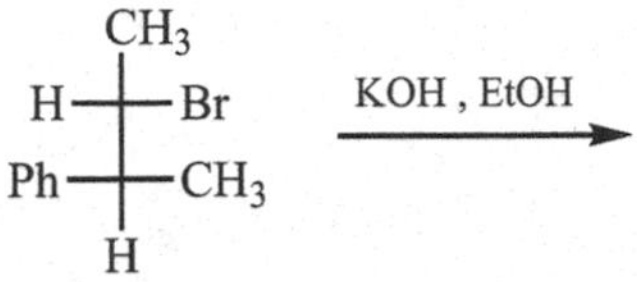
CH3
H
Br
Ph
CH3
H
KOH , EtOH

(f) 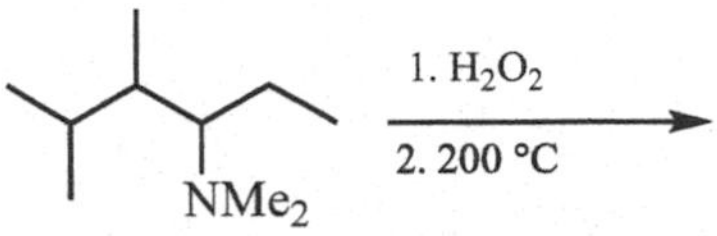
NMe2
1. H2O2
2. 200 °C

(g) 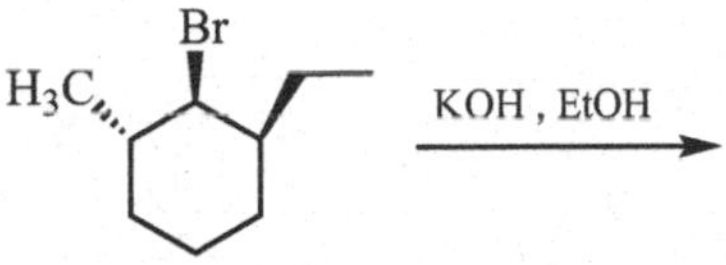
Br
H3C
KOH , EtOH

(h) 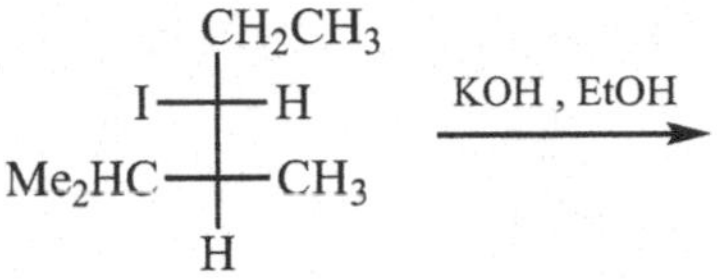
CH2CH3
I
H
Me2HC
CH3
H
KOH , EtOH

(i) 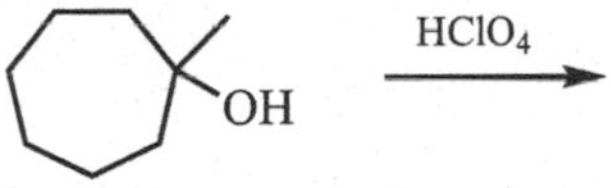
OH
HClO4

(j) 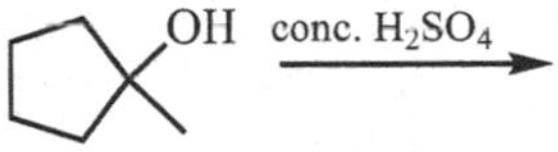
OH
conc. H2SO4

(k) 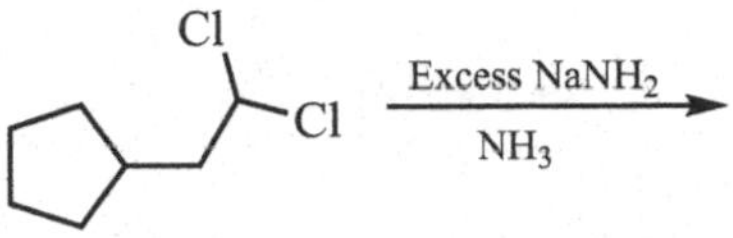
Cl
Cl
Excess NaNH2
NH3

(l) 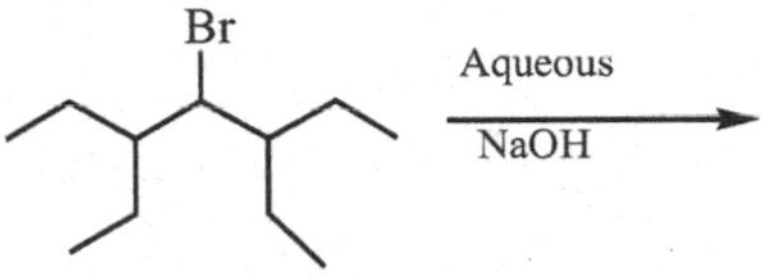
Br
Aqueous
NaOH

4. Draw the mechanism for the E1 conversion of cyclohexanol to cyclohexene in concentrated sulfuric acid.

10

Organometallic Compounds

Carbon can form covalent bonds to many elements found in the periodic table. When carbon forms covalent bonds to certain metals, an interesting and highly useful class of compounds is formed that are known as *organometallic compounds.*

10.1 ORGANOMETALLICS

What is an organometallic?

An organometallic is a compound that contains at least one carbon–metal bond.

What is the valence of group 1 metals such as lithium or sodium?

Both lithium and sodium have a valence of 1. Therefore, such metals should form a C—Li or C—Na bond.

What is the valence of group 2 metals such as magnesium?

Magnesium has a valence of 2. Therefore, such metals should form a C—Mg—X bond, where X is another group or atom. In most cases, X is a halogen atom such as chlorine or bromine.

Is the C—Li bond polarized? If so, indicate the bond polarization.

Yes! The C—Li bond is polarized because carbon is more electronegative than lithium. Therefore, the bond polarization is $C^{\delta-}$–$Li^{\delta+}$.

Is the C—Br bond polarized? If so, indicate the bond polarization.

Yes! The C—Br bond is polarized because carbon is less electronegative than bromine. Therefore, the bond polarization is $C^{\delta+}$—$Br^{\delta-}$. This bond polarization is the normal dipole as seen in previous chapters.

Is the C—Mg bond polarized? If so, indicate the bond polarization.

Yes! The C—Mg bond is polarized because carbon is more electronegative than magnesium. Therefore, the bond polarization is $C^{\delta-}$–$Mg^{\delta+}$.

Focusing on the carbon atom, would a Li—C unit react as a nucleophile or an electrophile with a positively polarized carbon atom?

Carbon is more electronegative than lithium, so the polarization is $C^{\delta-}$–$Li^{\delta+}$. Since the lithium has a negative dipole, it should react as a nucleophile in the presence of a positively polarized carbon atom.

10.2 ORGANOMAGNESIUM COMPOUNDS

Does magnesium metal react with an alkyl halide?

Magnesium metal reacts with alkyl halides to form an organic molecule that contains magnesium, an organometallic compound. This type of reaction was first discovered by Philippe Barbier, but his student,

Victor Grignard, discovered the organomagnesium intermediate and exploited the most useful version of this reaction in the early 1900s. This type of organomagnesium compound is therefore known as a *Grignard reagent* and its reactions with ketones and aldehydes, initially discovered by Barbier, are now known as Grignard reactions (see Section 12.3).

What is the product when iodomethane reacts with magnesium metal in diethyl ether?

The product is H_3C—Mg—I (methylmagnesium iodide). In ether, magnesium inserts between the C—I bond. This is a highly reactive molecule and the ether is necessary to stabilize it sufficiently by coordination of ether (via the oxygen) with the magnesium, for use in a chemical reaction.

What is the nomenclature system for compounds such as RMgX?

If CH_3MgI is taken as an example, the name is methylmagnesium iodide. Use the nomenclature term for the alkyl group followed by magnesium as one word, and then the name of the halide. Likewise, $(CH_3)_2CH_2CH_2MgCl$ is 2-methylpropylmagnesium chloride.

What is the role of the diethyl ether solvent?

The oxygen of the diethyl ether is a Lewis base, and Mg is a Lewis acid. The diethyl ether donates an electron to (a) assist in the insertion of the magnesium between the C–X bond, and (b) to stabilize the Grignard reagent via coordination with the magnesium.

What is a *Grignard reagent*?

A *Grignard reagent* is the product of the reaction between an alkyl halide and magnesium metal. A Grignard reagent has the generic structure R–Mg—X, where R is an alkyl group, and X = Cl, Br, I.

What is the bond polarization of the C—Mg bond?

Since Mg lies to the left of carbon in the periodic table, carbon is the most electronegative atom. The bond polarity is: $^{\delta-}$C—Mg$^{\delta+}$ and the carbon of the Grignard reagent behaves as a *carbanion* (nucleophilic carbon) in most of its reactions.

Is it possible to form the Grignard reagent from vinyl halides?

Yes! Vinyl halides (C=C—X) react with magnesium to form C=C—MgX, but the reaction is sluggish compared to alkyl halides.

What is the product formed when vinyl halide, (*E*)-1-bromobut-1-ene, reacts with magnesium in THF?

The product is but-1*E*-en-1-ylmagnesium bromide.

Br —(Mg°, THF)→ MgBr

Why was THF used in the preparation of but-1*E*-en-1-ylmagnesium bromide rather than diethyl ether?

Formation of the vinyl Grignard reagent, but-1*E*-en-1-ylmagnesium bromide, is slow, requiring the use of THF. The solvent THF is more basic than diethyl ether, providing assistance for the formation of the Grignard reagent and also extra stabilization of the Mg after the reagent is formed.

Is it possible to form the Grignard reagent from aryl halides such as bromobenzene (PhBr)?

Yes! Aryl halide (derivatives of benzene; see Section 16.1; Ar–X) react with magnesium to form Ar-MgX, but the reaction is sluggish compared to alkyl halides. In this case, the product is phenylmagnesium bromide, PhMgBr.

What does the symbol Ph mean?

The symbol Ph is short for phenyl, which is used to indicate a benzene ring as a substituent. Therefore, $PhCH_2CH_2OH$ is 2-phenylethan-1-ol and PhBr is bromobenzene. The structures for both molecules are shown.

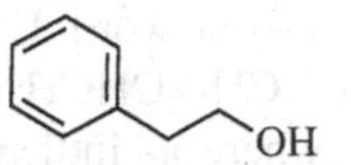

2-Phenylethan-1-ol 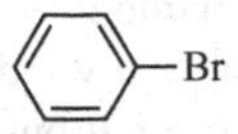 Bromobenzene

What is the product when bromobenzene reacts with magnesium in THF?

In the example shown, bromobenzene reacts with magnesium to form phenylmagnesium bromide. Formation of aryl Grignard reagents is slow, again requiring the assistance of the better Lewis base, THF, relative to diethyl ether.

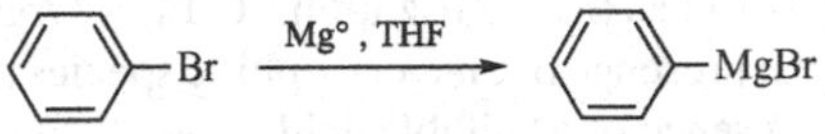

What are the major products of the reactions of (a), (b), and (c)?

(a) 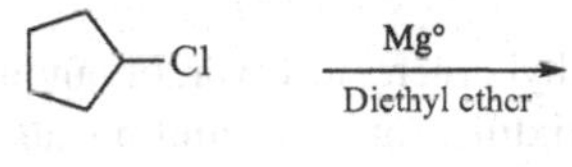 Mg°, Diethyl ether

(b) 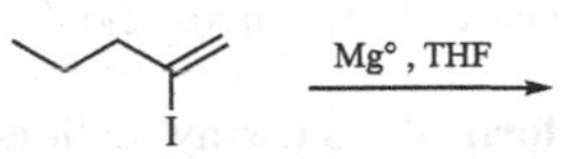 Mg°, THF

(c) 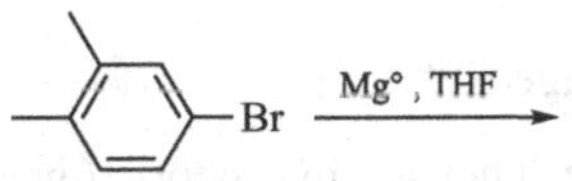 Mg°, THF

In all three cases, the product is the corresponding Grignard reagent. In (a) chlorocyclopentane gives cyclopentylmagnesium chlorides; in (b) the product is pent-2-enylmagnesium iodide; and in (c) the product is 3,4-dimethylphenylmagnesium bromide. In the latter two cases (the vinyl halide and the benzene derivative), THF is used rather than diethyl ether. THF is a stronger Lewis base than diethyl ether and the extra coordination with Mg is required to stabilize these Grignard reagents.

(a) 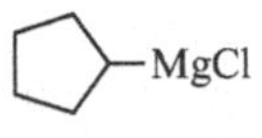 —MgCl (b) 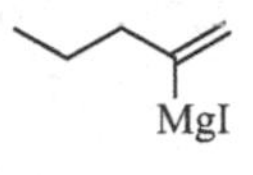 MgI (c) 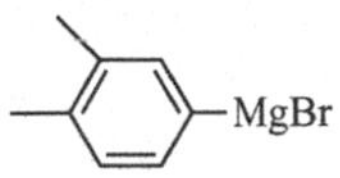 —MgBr

10.3 ORGANOLITHIUM COMPOUNDS

Does lithium metal react with alkyl halides?

Just as magnesium reacts with alkyl halides to form Grignard reagents, lithium reacts with alkyl halides to form organolithium reagents. This is another example of an organometallic compound.

What is the reaction product when lithium metal reacts with 1-bromobutane?

This reaction produces *n*-butyllithium ($CH_3CH_2CH_2CH_2Li$). Unlike Grignard reagents, lithium is monovalent, but two molar equivalents of lithium are required, forming C—Li and Li—X. The generic reaction is:

$$\text{R—X} + \text{Li—Li} \xrightarrow{\text{Diethyl ether}} \text{R—Li} + \text{Li—X}$$

Why are two equivalents of lithium required in the preceding question?

Lithium usually exists as Li—Li and both equivalents of Li are used in the reaction.

What is the nomenclature system for compounds such as RLi?

Taking CH_3Li as an example, the name is methyllithium – one word. Use the nomenclature term for the alkyl group followed by lithium as one word. Likewise, $(CH_3)_2CHCH_2Li$ is 2-methylpropyllithium and $CH_3CH_2CH_2CH_3Li$ is butyllithium or *n*-butyllithium, where *n*- indicates *normal* for a straight-chain butane. These compounds can also be named where lithium is a substituent, indicated by lithio and the number of the carbon to which it is attached. In other words, CH_3Li is 1-lithiomethane, $(CH_3)_2CHCH_2Li$ is 1-lithio-3-methylpropane, and $CH_3CH_2CH_2CH_3Li$ is 1-lithiobutane.

What is the predicted reactivity of an organolithium reagent such as butyllithium?

Organolithium reagents are characterized by a C—Li bond, which is polarized similarly to the C—Mg bond of a Grignard reagent (the C—Li has the polarization $^{\delta-}$C-Li$^{\delta+}$). Organolithium reagents will, therefore, function as nucleophiles in the presence of an electrophilic species such as acetone or other ketones and aldehydes or as bases in the presence of a suitable acid.

What solvent is used to form organolithium reagents?

Typically, the reaction is done in diethyl ether. However, organolithium reagents are decomposed in ether solvents, and it is common to see mixtures of ether and hexane used, or even pure hexane (sometimes other alkanes) to prolong the life of the organolithium reagent. Note that protic solvents such as alcohols or water, which have an acidic proton, react with RLi in an acid–base reaction and are therefore unsuitable.

Can organolithium compounds be formed from vinyl halides and aryl halides?

Yes! Both are known to form vinyllithium and aryllithium reagents, respectively.

How reactive are organolithium reagents?

These reagents are extremely reactive. They are pyrophoric (they react with moisture and air) and they are powerful bases. Extreme caution should be used when handling organolithium reagents, especially tertiary organolithium reagents such as *tert*-butyllithium.

What are the major products of the reactions of (a), (b), and (c)?

(a) 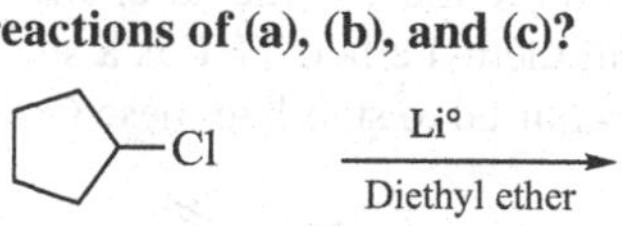 —Cl —Li°, Diethyl ether→

(b) 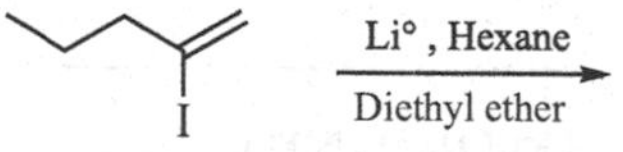 I —Li°, Hexane, Diethyl ether→

(c) 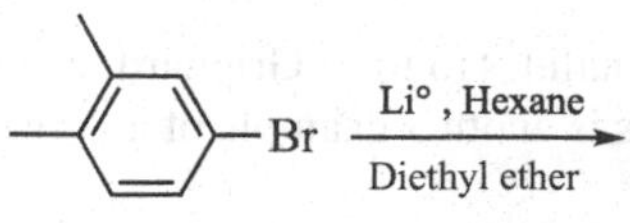 —Br —Li°, Hexane, Diethyl ether→

In all three cases, the product is the corresponding organolithium reagent: (a) lithiocyclopentane, (b) 2-lithiopent-2-ene, and (c) 3,4-dimethylphenylithium.

(a) 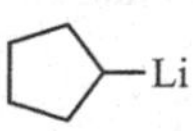 —Li (b) 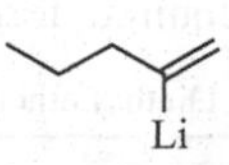 Li (c) 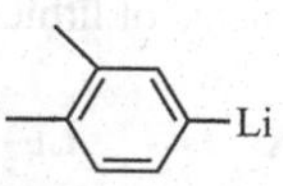 —Li

10.4 BASICITY

Is the carbon of C—Mg or C—Li basic?

Yes! The negatively polarized carbon atom of a Grignard reagent or an organolithium reagent can function as a nucleophile in the presence of a positively polarized carbon atom. Such negatively polarized carbon atoms are also powerful bases, in the presence of compounds having a hydrogen atom. Such bases are so powerful that they react with some compounds that have not heretofore been considered to be acids.

Why is methyllithium considered to be a base?

The carbon bearing the lithium atom is polarized with a negative dipole. A negative dipole is strongly attracted to an acidic hydrogen (which has a strong positive dipole). In an acid–base reaction, methyllithium reacts with an acid (H^+) to give a conjugate acid CH_3–H (methane). Using the old axiom, strong acids give weak conjugate bases and weak acids give strong conjugate bases, if methane is a very weak conjugate acid, methyllithium must be a very strong base.

What is the pK_a of methane?

Methane is an extremely weak acid (p$K_a > 40$).

What is the conjugate base of the reaction between methyllithium and water?

Methyllithium lithium reacts violently with water to give methane and lithium hydroxide. In this reaction, lithium hydroxide is the conjugate base.

Can methylmagnesium bromide react with ethanol? If so, what are the products?

Yes! Just as methyllithium is a very strong base, methylmagnesium bromide is a strong base. Ethanol has an acidic hydrogen, with a pK_a of about 17. The reaction gives methane as the conjugate acid and $EtO^{-}\,^{+}MgBr$ as the conjugate base.

Can butyllithium react with ammonia? If so, what are the products?

Yes! If the conjugate acid of butyllithium is methane, with pK_a > 40, butyllithium should react with compounds that have pK_a values of <35-40. With these parameters, ammonia has a pK_a of about 25 and so it reacts as an acid with butyllithium. The reaction gives butane as the conjugate acid and $Li^{+}\,^{-}NH_2$ as the conjugate base.

Which is more polarized, C—Li or C—Mg?

C—Li.

Which is the stronger base, an organolithium reagent or a Grignard reagent?

The C—Li bond is more polarized than the C—Mg bond and organolithium reagents are generally more reactive than Grignard reagents. Indeed, organolithium reagents are much stronger bases than the corresponding Grignard reagent.

Can propylmagnesium iodide or butyllithium react with but-1-yne? If so, what are the products?

Yes! Although organolithium reagents are stronger bases relative to the corresponding Grignard reagent, the conjugate acid of both reagents is an alkane, which is a very weak acid. Propylmagnesium iodide is a strong base and reacts rapidly with but-1-yne, which has a pK_a of about 25. The reaction gives propane as the conjugate acid and $IMg^{+}\,^{-}C{\equiv}CEt$ as the conjugate base. Likewise, butyllithium reacts with the terminal alkyne to give the same product, except the positive counterion is Li^+.

What is the major product of the reactions of (a), (b), and (c)?

(a) pentyllithium $\xrightarrow{(CH_3)_2NH}$

(b) cyclohexylmagnesium bromide (MgBr) $\xrightarrow{HOH}$

(c) phenyllithium (Li) $\xrightarrow{CH_3CH_2OH}$

Each of these reactions is an acid–base reaction where the organolithium is the base. The reaction product of (a) is pentane, (b) cyclohexane, and (c) benzene.

(a) pentane (b) cyclohexane (c) benzene

10.5 REACTION WITH EPOXIDES

Why should a Grignard reagent react with an epoxide?

A Grignard reagent is a source of nucleophilic carbon and the oxygen of the epoxide polarizes adjacent carbon atoms with a δ^+ dipole. This nucleophilic carbon will attack the electropositive carbon of an epoxide, generally at the less sterically hindered site, and cleave the C—O bond. Remember that an oxirane is a three-membered ring ether, and therefore the ring is strained and highly susceptible to attack by nucleophiles.

What is the initial product of the reaction of ethylmagnesium bromide and 2-butyloxirane? What is the product after aqueous hydrolysis?

The reaction proceeds as with any other nucleophile, with the nucleophilic carbon of the Grignard reagent attacking the less sterically hindered carbon of the oxirane to give an alkoxide, ***A***. Hydrolysis gives octan-4-ol.

2-butyloxirane $\xrightarrow{EtMgBr,\ THF}$ **A** ($O^-\ MgBr^+$) $\xrightarrow{H_3O^+}$ octan-4-ol (OH)

10.6 OTHER METALS

Are metals other than lithium or magnesium used in organic chemistry?

Yes! A complete description of the use of metals in organic chemistry is beyond the scope of this book. Indeed, organometallic chemistry is a vast and extremely useful area. However, copper is a particularly useful metal in organic chemical reactions.

How is copper used in organic chemistry in a way that is related to organomagnesium and organolithium reagents?

The formation of the organocopper reagents known as organocuprates is well known and these reagents are extremely useful in organic chemistry.

Carbon forms bonds to copper in several ways. One of the more useful ways is to form an organocuprate, which has the structure R_2CuLi. In various reactions the carbon atom in organocuprates functions as a nucleophile.

What is an organocuprate?

An organocuprate has the generic structure R_2CuLi, where R is the generic term for an alkyl group.

$$\begin{matrix} R \\ & \diagdown \\ & & Cu-Li \\ & \diagup \\ R' \end{matrix}$$

What is a Gilman reagent?

To honor the work of Henry Gilman, the organocuprate reagent R_2CuLi is commonly referred to as a *Gilman reagent*.

How are organocuprates named?

Such reagents are named by identifying the metal (lithium), followed by the two alkyl groups attached to copper (dialkyl), and finally cuprate, to indicate the oxidation state of the copper. Therefore, Me_2CuLi is lithium dimethylcuprate and $(CH_3CH_2CH_2)_2CuLi$ is lithium dipropylcuprate.

What is the structure of lithium di-*n*-butylcuprate?

When two equivalents of 1-lithiobutane (butyllithium) react with cuprous iodide (CuI), which is Cu(I), the copper forms an "*-ate*" *complex*, which occurs when a metal expands its valence and assume a negative charge. In this case, R_2Cu^- forms, with Li^+ as the counterion. Dibutylcuprate is, therefore, $[Bu–Cu–Bu]^-$ and lithium di-*n*-butylcuprate is $LiBu_2Cu$ or Bu_2CuLi.

What is the product formed when iodoethane reacts with lithium dibutylcuprate?

The reaction is the rapid and high yield coupling to give hexane, as shown.

$$Bu_2CuLi \quad + \quad CH_3CH_2I \xrightarrow[-10\ °C]{\text{Diethyl ether}} CH_3CH_2—Bu$$

How does an organocuprate react with alkyl halides?

The primary reaction is the rapid and high yield coupling with alkyl halides. In this reaction, one of the alkyl groups displaces the halogen of the alkyl halide to give the substitution product (a coupling product). 1-iodoethane, for example, reacts with lithium dibutylcuprate to give hexane, $CH_3CH_2—Bu$, as shown in the preceding question.

What is the product when a Grignard reagent or an organolithium reagent reacts with 1-bromopentane?

Grignard reagents and organolithium reagents give very poor yields of substitution products when they react with alkyl halides. *n*-Butyllithium, for example, reacts with 1-bromobutane but very little, or no, octane (Bu–Bu, the substitution product) is produced. Elimination (see Chapter 9) and *disproportionation* (self-oxidation reduction) products predominate. In this case, disproportionation leads to pentene and pentane as the major products.

Do Grignard reagents or organolithium reagents react with simple alkyl halides?

Not usually! In general, alkyl halides do not give good yields of substitution products with Grignard reagents or organolithium reagents, *unless a transition metal is added to the reaction*. However, both RMgX or RLi can react with "activated" alkyl halides, which means that the halide is conjugated to a C=C unit or a benzene ring (allylic or benzyl halides).

END OF CHAPTER PROBLEMS

1. Explain why ethanol cannot be used as a solvent for reactions of ethylmagnesium bromide.
2. Explain why butyllithium is a good reagent to convert pent-1-yne to the alkyne anion, 1-lithiopentyne.
3. Draw the structure of the Grignard reagent formed form each of the following and name each product:

(a) 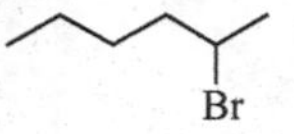 Br (b) I (c) 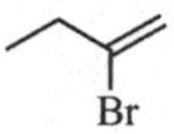 Br

(d) 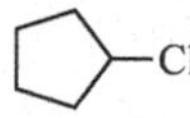 Cl (e) 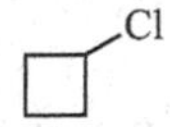 Cl (f) 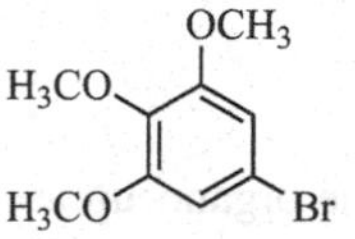 OCH_3, H_3CO, H_3CO, Br (g) 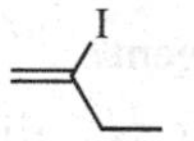 I

4. Draw the Gilman reagent formed for each of the following reactions:

(a) 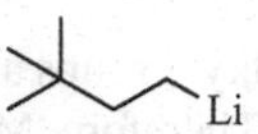 Li (b) 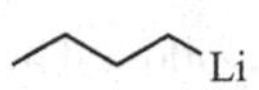 Li (c) 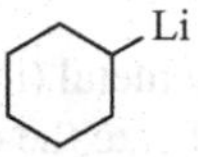 Li (d) 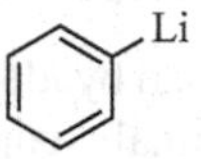 Li

5. Amines (R_2NH) are usually viewed as bases due to the presence of the lone electron pair. Explain why Et_2NH (diethylamine) behaves as an acid in the presence of butyllithium.
6. In each case give the major product of the reaction:

(a) 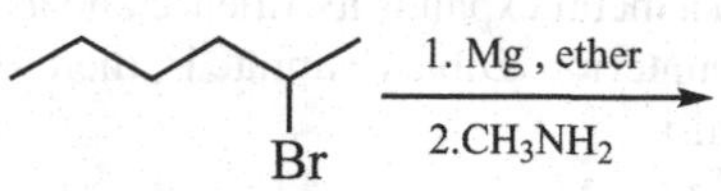 Br → 1. Mg, ether 2. CH_3NH_2 (b) 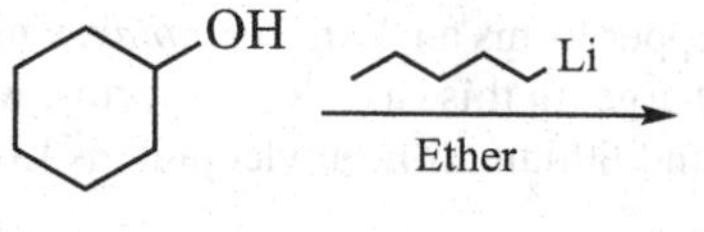 OH → Li, Ether

(c) 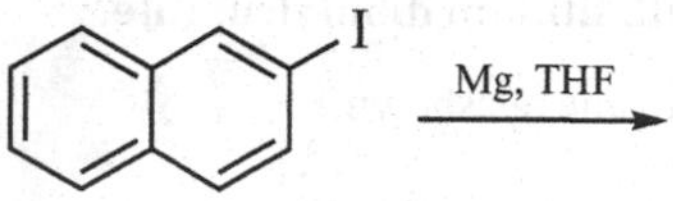 I → Mg, THF (e) 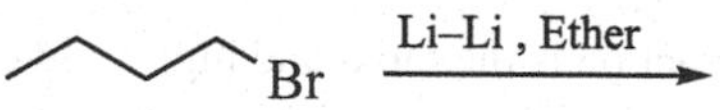 Br → Li–Li, Ether

(e) 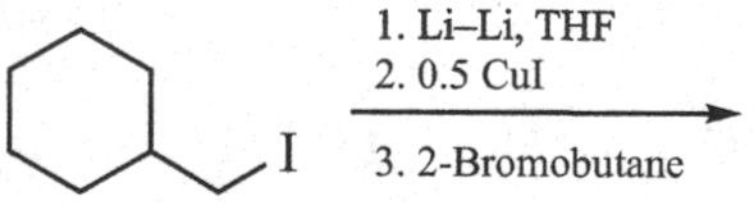 I → 1. Li–Li, THF 2. 0.5 CuI 3. 2-Bromobutane (f) 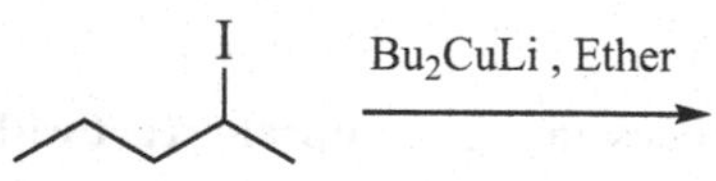 I → Bu_2CuLi, Ether

11

Spectroscopy

How do organic chemists identify organic molecules? The answer involves the observation of how organic functional groups interact with various forms of energy. Three techniques are commonly used to give structural information for most organic molecules. The first technique is mass spectrometry, and in the simplest form organic molecules are bombarded with 70 electron volts of energy and the fragmentation of the resulting high-energy ionic particles is monitored. When infrared light is absorbed by an organic molecule, the bonds in the molecule dissipate that energy by vibrational and rotational motion. The frequency of vibration is different for different bonds within functional groups, which is the basis for identifying functional groups. When an organic molecule is placed in a strong magnetic field, each hydrogen in the molecule behaves as a tiny electromagnet. When irradiated with electromagnetic energy in the radio frequency range, the hydrogen atoms absorb the energy and change their spin state (with or against the large external magnetic field). The frequency of this absorption depends on the magnetic and chemical environment of each hydrogen and can be used to identify different types of hydrogens. The three techniques just described can be used to identify the structure of an organic molecule.

11.1 THE ELECTROMAGNETIC SPECTRUM

What is the electromagnetic spectrum?

The electromagnetic spectrum is simply the range of energies associated with various forms of "light." The electromagnetic spectrum not only includes ultraviolet, visible, and infrared light but also low energy microwaves and high energy x-rays and cosmic rays. A simplified version of the electromagnetic spectrum is shown in both wavelength (in meters, m) and frequency (in hertz, ν).

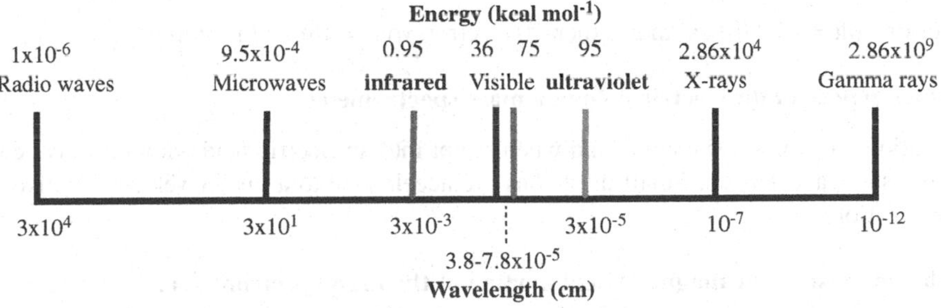

What is the relationship between wavelength (λ) and frequency (ν)?

These two parameters are inversely proportional, by the equation $c = \nu\lambda$, where c is the speed of light (3×10^8 m/sec). In general, a high frequency is related to a small wavelength.

Which is higher in energy, infrared light or ultraviolet light?

High energy is associated with a high frequency (low wavelength) and low energy is associated with low frequency (high wavelength). Since ultraviolet light has a higher frequency than infrared light, UV light is higher in energy. Similarly, X-rays are very high energy radiation and radio-waves are very low energy radiation.

At what wavelengths do molecules absorb infrared light?

The general absorption frequency range for organic molecules is 2.5×10^{-6} m to 16×10^{-6} m. Since an angstrom (Å) is 1×10^{-8} meters, infrared light absorbs in the range 2500–1600 Å.

11.2 MASS SPECTROMETRY

What is a mass spectrometer?

A mass spectrometer is an instrument that bombards an organic molecule (or any other molecule) with high energy electrons to ionize the molecule. Such bombardment usually generates a radical cation although other ions can also be produced under the proper conditions. Usually, an initially formed high-energy radical cation fragments into other (smaller) mass radical cations. An electric field accelerates and focuses the ions toward a large magnet, which separates the radical cations that are produced according to their mass and charge. The ions then pass into a detector, where they are recorded. The recorded collection of ions arranged by their mass is known as the mass spectrum for a molecule.

How many kilocalories (kcal) correlate with one electron volt (eV)?

One electron volt is equivalent to 23.061 kcal mol^{-1} of energy.

How many kilojoules (kJ) correlate with one electron volt (eV)?

One electron volt is equivalent to 96.487 kJ mol^{-1} of energy.

What is the energy used to bombard a molecule in a mass spectrometer?

A focused, high energy beam of electrons is directed toward an organic molecule. A typical electron beam will bombard the molecule with at least 70 electron volts (eV) of energy, although this is adjustable. Such energy is usually enough energy to cause ionization to radical cations and subsequent fragmentation.

How many kcal mol^{-1} are there in 70 eV??

If one electron volt = 23.061 kcal mol^{-1}, then 70 electron volts = 1614.27 kcal mol^{-1}.

What is the purpose of the electric field in a mass spectrometer?

A radical cation has a positive charge, and when swept into an electric field with a positive charge, the radical cations are accelerated. Small mass ions are accelerated to a higher velocity relative to higher mass radical cations.

What is the purpose of the magnetic field portion of the mass spectrometer?

The radical cations produced by electron bombardment are accelerated by the applied voltage and pass into a strong magnetic field. The magnetic field deflects the flight path of the radical cations. "Heavy" radical cations are deflected most for a given magnetic field strength and a given velocity, whereas "light" ions are deflected least. Ions that are too heavy or too light will not traverse the instrument but will "crash" into its sides and be lost (not detected). By adjusting both the magnetic field and accelerating voltage, this separation of "heavy" and "light" can be refined to separate ions differing by fractions of a mass unit.

What is a molecular ion (the arcane term is parent ion)?

When a molecule is bombarded with electrons, an electron is ejected from the molecule to form a radial cation. This initial product has the same mass as the parent molecule that was introduced into the mass spectrometer and is called the *molecular ion*, or the *parent ion*. In other words, the molecular ion has the mass of the original molecule minus one electron.

What is the significance of the molecular ion?

The molecular ion has the same mass as the neutral molecule and the charge of this radical cation is +1. It is a radical cation. The unit used for the mass is actually m/z (m = mass, z = charge), so if the charge is +1, the m/z of the radical cation is the actual mass. Mass spectrometry and identification of the parent ion therefore allow determination of the molecular weight of the original molecule, as well as the mass of all fragment radical cations.

What is the general result of a molecule being bombarded with high energy electrons?

Bombardment of a molecule with a high energy electron will expel an electron from the molecule, forming a radical cation. In the example shown, propan-2-one (acetone) is bombarded with an electron beam, expelling one electron (probably from oxygen) and leaving a positively charged oxygen atom that also has an unshared electron (this ion is a radical cation). This radical cation has a mass of 58, the mass of neutral acetone, minus a single electron. Therefore, the mass of the radical cation is essentially the mass of the molecule and can be measured. The exact electron removed from a molecule is not known exactly, so the radical cation is represented by showing the structure of the molecule with a bracket showing a •+.

e⁻ (70 eV)

Mass = 58 | Mass = 58 - 1e⁻ | m/z = 58 Molecular ion

What are product ions?

The *product ion* is a radical cation that results from a cleavage reaction of the molecular ion or another product ion. A product ion is always of a lesser mass relative to the molecular ion. Note that the arcane term for product ion is *daughter ion*.

What are two logical product ions that are formed by fragmentation of the molecular ion of acetone?

Fragmentation of the molecular ion will largely correlate with known chemical processes, so weaker bonds are likely to be cleaved relative to stronger bonds. Cleavage of the C—C bond that connects a methyl group to the carbonyl carbon leads to two product ions: the acyl radical cation with m/z 43 and the methyl radical cation with m/z 15. Other fragmentations are possible, but this cleavage illustrates how product ions are formed.

e⁻ (70 eV)

Mass = 58 | m/z 58 | m/z 43 | m/z 15

What is a mass spectrum?

The mass spectrum of a molecule is a graph of the molecular ion and all radical cation fragments, arranged by their increasing mass. Formally, it is a plot of intensity versus m/z (mass to charge ratio) where each m/z value correlates with the molecular ion and all product ions.

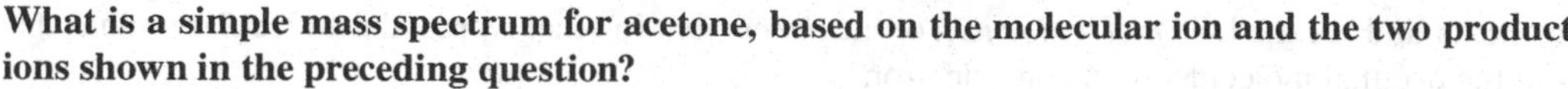

What is a simple mass spectrum for acetone, based on the molecular ion and the two product ions shown in the preceding question?

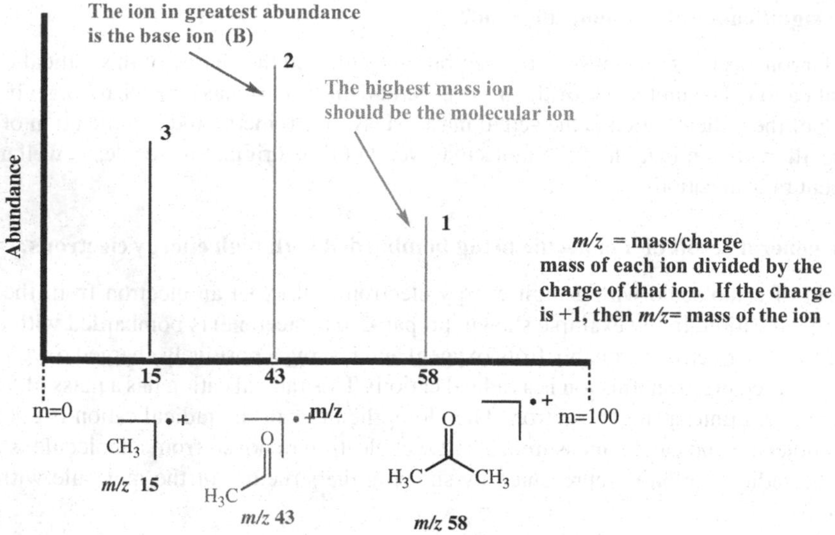

What is the base ion?

The base ion (B) has the greatest abundance in a mass spectrum. All other ions are reported as a percentage of the base ion, where B is assumed to be 100%.

What are the natural abundance isotopic ratios of ^{2}H, ^{13}C, ^{34}S, ^{18}O, ^{37}Cl, ^{15}N, and ^{81}Br?

For deuterium (^{2}H) the natural abundance is 0.015%; ^{13}C is 1.11%; ^{34}S is 4.22%; ^{18}O is 0.204%; ^{37}Cl is 24.47%; and ^{81}Br is 49.46%.

For a given organic molecule, what is the natural percentage of deuterium and ^{13}C in the molecule?

In organic molecules composed of carbon and hydrogen, the "hydrogen" atoms in that molecule are actually a mixture of 99.985% ^{1}H and 0.015% of ^{2}H. Similarly, the carbon atoms are a mixture of 98.89% ^{12}C and 1.11% of ^{13}C.

If the molecular ion represents the molecular weight of the molecule, why are there higher mass fragments that show peaks of +1 and +2 mass units greater than the parent?

These are the isotope peaks that arise from small amounts of ^{13}C, ^{15}N, and ^{2}H. All three of these isotopes contribute to the molecular ion + 1. The isotope of oxygen (^{18}O) will contribute to the molecular ion + 2.

What is the significance of the M+1 fragment?

Since the isotopic ratios of $^{12}C/^{13}C$, $^{2}H/^{1}H$, and $^{15}N/^{14}N$ are fixed, the ratio of the M+1 to the M (molecular) ion allows the calculation of the number of carbon atoms and nitrogen atoms in the molecular ion. The isotopic ratio of deuterium is so small that calculation of the number of hydrogens is not useful using this method.

What is the significance of the M+2 fragment?

Since the isotopic ratios of $^{18}O/^{16}O$, $^{34}S/^{32}S$, $^{37}Cl/^{35}Cl$, and $^{81}Br/^{79}Br$ are fixed, the M+2 ion can be used to calculate the number of oxygen, sulfur, chlorine, and bromine atoms in the molecular ion.

Based on the isotopic ratios of atoms, how can the M+1 fragment be used to calculate the number of carbon and nitrogen atoms in the molecule?

The ratio %M+1 to %M can be used to determine the formula: M+1 = [Number of C/1.11] + 0.36 (#N). If the ratio of M/M+1 is 6.66%, this ratio implies a total of six carbons (6.66/1.11 = 6C). Important in this calculation is an estimation of the number of nitrogen atoms. If the molecular weight is *odd*, assume that the molecule will contain an *odd* number of nitrogen atoms (1, 3, 5, 7…) and the first assumption is the presence of one nitrogen rather than three or more. If the molecular weight is *even*, assume that the molecule must contain an *even* number of nitrogen atoms (0, 2, 4, 6, 8…). The first assumption is that there are zero nitrogen atoms rather than two or more. If the molecular weight is 100 (M = 100), one assumes #N = 0, and if the M+1 is 6.66% of M, there are six carbons in the molecule.

In these calculations, the ratio is based on the intensity of the molecular ion not the intensity of the base ion. In other words, the molecular ion is assumed to be 100% and the M+1 is some percentage of M.

How can the M+2 fragment be used to calculate the number of oxygens in the molecule?

The isotopic ratios lead to the formula M+2 = [(Number of carbon atom/1.11)^2/200] + 0.20 (#O). The first term is the contribution of naturally occurring tritium (^3H) and the second term is due to isotopic oxygen. Note that it is assumed there are no S, Cl, or Br atoms in the molecule. If these atoms, all with significant M+2 isotopes, are in the molecule, the formula shown *cannot be used*. In other words, the formula could be extended to include: + 4.22 (#S) + 24.47 (#Cl) + 100 (#Br). These isotope terms are so large that they would overwhelm the relatively small oxygen term and so are omitted. With these isotopes omitted, the calculation is straightforward once the number of carbon atoms and nitrogen atoms is known from the M+1 calculation.

For a molecule with a molecular weight of 100, the M+1 term indicates six carbons and the M+2 term is measured to be 0.42. For six carbons, the first term is 0.22 and solving for #O leads to one (1) oxygen. The formula will therefore be C_6O.

How is the number of hydrogen atoms in an empirical formula calculated from mass spectral data?

The isotope ratio for a hydrogen atom is too small to be of value in a calculation using the M+1 or M+2 formulas. The hydrogen atoms must be calculated by difference with the molecular ion. If the molecular ion (M) has a *m/z* of 100, the mass is 100. The mass of C_6O, determined by the M+1 and M+2 calculations, is 88 and 100 – 88 = 12. It is therefore assumed that there are 12 hydrogen atoms and the formula will be $C_6H_{12}O$.

If the M+1 peak is 13.69% of the molecular ion and the M+2 peak is 1.09% of the molecular ion, what is the empirical formula of a molecule with a molecular ion *m/z* = 191?

The odd mass suggests one (1) nitrogen, and the isotope ratio for one N is 0.37. Using the M+1 formula [M+1 = (#C/1.11) + #N so M+1 = (#C/1.11)] + 0.37, one nitrogen leads to M+1 = (13.69 – 0.37)/1.11 = 12 C, or (M+1) – 0.37 = #C/1.11. Therefore, [(M+1) – 0.37]/1.11 = #C. In this case, (13.69–0.37)/1.11 = #C, so #C = 13.32/1.11 = 12. Assuming there are no S, Cl, or Br atoms, using the M+2 formula for C_{12}, M+2 = (1.09–0.89)/0.2 = 1 O. The partial formula is, therefore, $C_{12}NO$ (mass = 174). The number of hydrogens is calculated by 191–174 = 17H, and the final formula is $C_{12}H_{17}NO$.

Given the appropriate M+1 and M+2 ratios, what is the empirical formula for each of the following?

(a) M+1 = 9.99, M+2 = 0.50; (b) M+1 = 7.77, M+2 = 0.50; (c) M+1 = 9.25, M+2 = 0.39; (d) M+1 = 10.36, M+2 = 0.70.

The formula for (a) is C_9H_{20}; (b) is $C_7H_{14}O$; (c) is $C_8H_{19}N$; (d) is $C_9H_{11}NO$.

What is the significance of a M+2 peak that is 25–33% of the molecular ion?

This is a clear indication that there is one chlorine in the molecule. The ^{37}Cl isotope is about 25–33% of the ^{35}Cl peak.

What is the significance of a M+2 peak that is 100% of the molecular ion?

This is a clear indication that there is one bromine in the molecule. The ^{79}Br and ^{81}Br isotopes have about the same abundance.

What is the significance of a M+2 peak that is about 4–5% of the molecular ion?

This is consistent with one sulfur in the molecule where the ^{34}S is about 4% of the ^{32}S.

What fragment is associated with a M-15 peak? M-29? M-43?

A M-15 fragment is usually associated with loss of methyl ($-CH_3$), M-29 with loss of ethyl ($-CH_2CH_3$), and M-43 is loss of C_3H_7 which could be isopropyl or *n*-propyl. Loss of acetyl ($CH_3CO^{+\bullet}$) also correlates with a mass of 43.

What is α-cleavage?

The fragmentation of a radical cation at the bond between a carbon and a carbon bearing a heteroatom (C-x-C—O, C-x-C—S, C-x-C—N) or between a carbon and a functional group (C-x-C=O, C-x-C≡N, C-x-CO_2R, etc.) is called α-cleavage.

What functional groups undergo α-cleavage?

Ethers, amines, alcohols, acid derivatives, ketones and aldehydes and nitriles all undergo α-cleavage. Examples are the α-cleavage of the molecular ion of diethyl ether and the α-cleavage of the molecular ion of butanal.

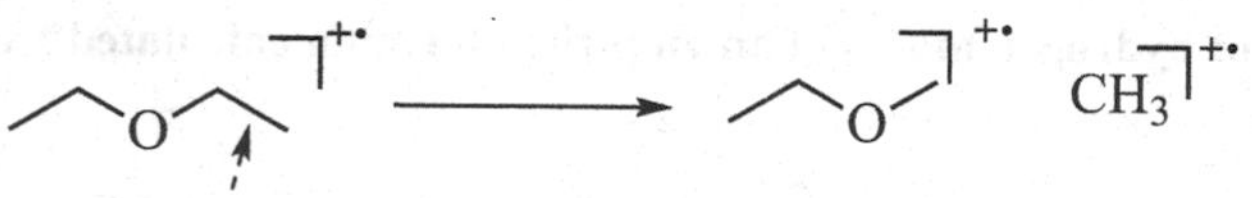

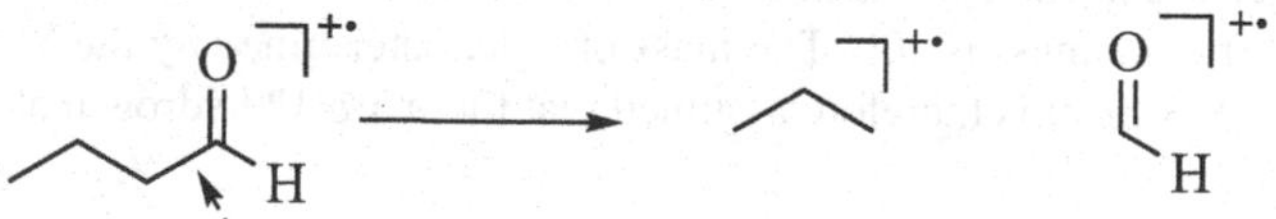

Why does an alcohol usually exhibit a M-18 fragment?

A *m/z* of 18 corresponds to water and M-18 is characteristic of a molecule that loses a molecule of water (dehydration). Under ion bombardment, most alcohols readily lose water from the parent ion. Usually, the molecular ion is not observed at all, and the first ion actually observed in significant concentration is the M-18 product ion.

11.3 INFRARED SPECTROSCOPY (IR)

What is the wavelength range for infrared light in the electromagnetic spectrum?

Infrared radiation appears at 7.8×10^{-7}–1×10^{-4} m (78Å to 10,000Å), which can be converted to 7.8×10^{-5}–1×10^{-2} cm (in wavelength), or 0.78–100 μm (where a μm is 10^{-4} cm or 10^{-6} meters – usually abbreviated as μ, or microns). The wavelength (λ) unit is, therefore, measured in μm. This energy range can also be expressed in frequency ($\tilde{v}$) where the unit is cm^{-1} (reciprocal centimeters or wavenumbers).

What wavelength range is used in infrared spectroscopy for organic molecules?

In most infrared spectrophotometers, the infrared radiation is measured between 4000–666.7 cm^{-1} or 2.5–15 μ. Most organic molecules absorb infrared radiation in this energy range.

How does an infrared spectrophotometer work?

Infrared light is directed toward a prism and split into two equal parts. These two beams are focused by a mirror system, one passing through the sample and the other through a reference cell. The beams are refocused with mirrors and another prism and the two are compared. If an organic molecule in the sample beam absorbed infrared light, the sample beam will be less intense than the reference beam. The spectrophotometer scans through a range of wavelengths (2.5–16 μ) and those regions of the spectrum that were absorbed by the organic molecule appear as peaks. This series of peaks is the infrared spectrum.

Why is it necessary to have a reference cell?

It is essential to compare the amount of light directed at the sample (incident radiation) with the amount of infrared radiation after absorption by the sample. Comparison of the two signals allows the instrument to determine how much infrared light was absorbed.

What materials are used to make the infrared cells that contain the organic sample?

The material must be transparent to infrared light (not absorb infrared light). Pressed plates of NaCl or KBr are the most common materials.

When an organic molecule absorbs infrared light, what happens to the molecule?

If a molecule absorbs infrared light, this excess energy is dissipated by molecular vibrations. Bending and stretching vibrations are the most common. There are symmetric and asymmetric stretching vibrations as well as symmetric and asymmetric bending vibrations (both "in plane" and "out of plane"). These vibrations occur at different infrared frequencies (also measured in wavelength) and lead to the various "peaks" in the infrared spectrum.

How does a change in dipole moment for a bond influence infrared absorption?

If the dipole moment of a bond changes during a bending or stretching vibration, that absorption is particularly strong. The larger the change in dipole moment, the stronger the absorption. If the vibration is not accompanied by a change in dipole moment, it is usually a very weak absorption. When a symmetrical bond (such as C—C) vibrates, the change in dipole is small and an infrared absorption is usually very weak. Indeed, the C—C signal in the infrared is very weak (it is virtually non-existent).

What types of bonds are expected to give strong infrared signals? Weak infrared signals?

Bonds with significant dipole moments will give strong signals in the infrared. Examples are O—H, C—O, C=O, N—H, Cl—C=O, and N—C=O. Bonds that give weak signals have symmetrical bonds, including C—C, O—O, and N—N. Interestingly, the C—H signal is strong although C and H have similar dipole moments and the C—H bond is not considered to be polarized vis-à-vis chemical reactions.

As a bond gets stronger, is the wavelength of infrared absorption expected to increase or decrease?

A stronger bond absorbs infrared light at a lower frequency (higher wavelength). A comparison of the C≡C bond with the C=C bond reveals that C≡C absorbs at 2100–2260 cm^{-1} (4.76–4.42 μ), at higher frequency (higher energy) than the absorption for C=C at 1650–1670 cm^{-1} (6.06–5.99 μ)

Which is associated with higher energy, high infrared wavelength or lower infrared wavelength?

Since short wavelengths are generally of higher energy, a low infrared wavelength (2.0–4.0 μ for example as compared to 11–14 μ) will be of higher energy. Analysis of the triple bond vs. the double bond shows this to be true. It takes more energy to make the stronger C≡C bond vibrate than it does for the weaker C=C bond.

What is an infrared spectrum?

An infrared spectrum is the plot of either *absorbance* or *percent transmittance* as a function of wavelength and/or frequency, or both. When an organic molecule absorbs infrared energy of a particular wavelength, it will appear as a "peak." If the signal absorbs a large amount of infrared radiation, it will show as a strong absorption (weak percent transmittance) and if little energy is absorbed the peak will show a small absorption (large percent transmittance). The infrared spectrum for hexane is shown as an example.

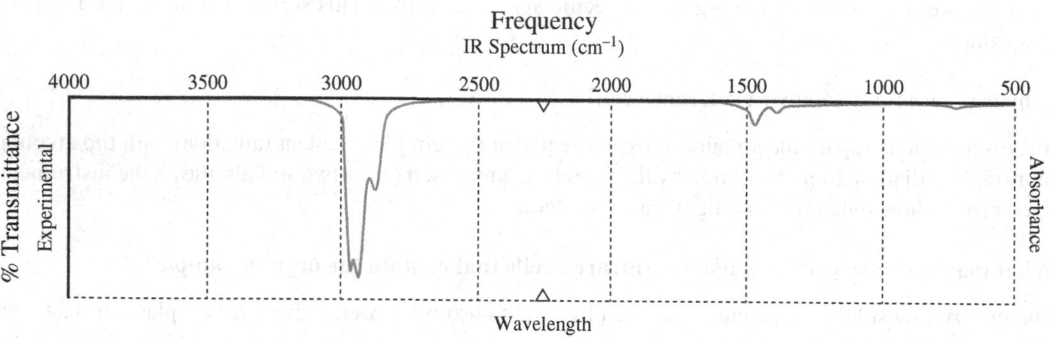

What labels are pertinent to an infrared spectrum?

The parameters are marked on an infrared spectrum of hexane. Most infrared spectrophotometers are calibrated in "% Transmittance" and "Absorbance" with the scale linear in frequency (cm^{-1}). The wavelength scale (in μ) is sometimes also shown. High energy signals appear to the left of the spectrum whereas low energy signals appear to the right of the spectrum. A strong absorbance peak is marked as well as a weak absorbance peak.

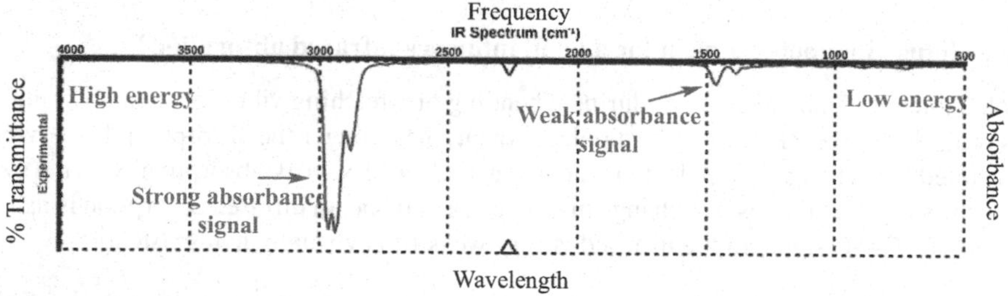

Is 90%T associated with a strong signal or a weak signal?

If 90% of the light is transmitted, only 10% was absorbed, so 90%T is a weak signal.

Is 70%A associated with a strong signal or a weak signal?

If 70% of the light was absorbed, 70%A is a strong signal.

What is the relationship between wavelength and frequency?

They are inversely proportional: ν (cm^{-1}) = 1000/λ (μ)

What units are used for wavelength in infrared spectroscopy?

Wavelength (λ) uses microns as the basic unit ($1\ \mu = 1 \times 10^{-4}$ cm).

What units are used for frequency in infrared spectroscopy?

Frequency (ν) uses reciprocal centimeters as the unit (cm^{-1}).

Is 700 cm^{-1} associated with high energy or lower energy?

An infrared absorption at 700 cm^{-1} is at the low energy end of the spectrum and would be associated with a weaker bond.

Is 3.45 μ associated with high energy or low energy?

This wavelength is a short wavelength absorption and is, therefore, higher in energy.

Which is the lower energy absorption, 10.57 μ or 2335 cm^{-1}?

An absorption at 10.57 μ is equivalent to 946 cm^{-1}. This signal is much lower in energy than the signal at 2335 cm^{-1}.

Why is an O—H group expected to absorb in generally the same region of the infrared, regardless of what else is in the molecule?

Infrared spectroscopy focuses on the vibrations of individual bonds. The O—H bond will give stretching and bending vibrations characteristic of the strength of that bond and the masses of O and H. Electronic effects will clearly play a role, but the fundamental absorption frequency will be generally the same for all molecules containing an OH group. This absorption appears at 3400–3640 cm^{-1} (or at 2.94–2.75 μ as a strong, broad signal).

Which is expected to absorb at higher energy, an O—H group or a C—H group? Explain.

The bond dissociation energy for O—H (from methanol) is 102 kcal mol^{-1} and the bond dissociation energy for C—H (from methane) is 104 kcal/mole. They are obviously rather close and bond dissociation energy calculations do not provide an answer. The O—H unit absorbs at 3400–3640 cm^{-1} and the C—H unit generally absorbs at 2850–2960 cm^{-1} (3.51–3.38 μ), making the O—H signal the higher energy.

The O—H bond is significantly more polarized than the C—H bond and should, therefore, give a much stronger absorption. In fact, the O—H absorption is very strong (usually 0–10%T) and quite broad. Hydrogen bonding will increase the relative bond polarity of the O—H and the more extensive the hydrogen bonding, the broader the signal (broad = larger range of infrared absorption frequencies).

Which group gives the lowest energy infrared absorption, C—C, C=C or C≡C? Explain!

It takes less energy for the single covalent bond in C—C and it is expected to have the lowest energy absorption. The symmetrical C—C bond has no dipole and is expected to be a weak signal, and it is usually not reported, perhaps appearing at 1000–1100 cm^{-1} [10–9 μ]. The two bonds in the C=C unit indicate that it takes energy to separate the C=C unit and is considered to be stronger. The C=C unit absorbs at 1650–1670 cm^{-1} [6.06–5.99 μ] and the three bonds of the C≡C bond are expected to lead to the strongest of all bonds, and this unit absorbs at 2100–2260 cm^{-1} [4.76–4.42 μ].

What is the fingerprint region of the infrared?

The low energy portion of the infrared spectrum between 1400–625 cm^{-1} (7.0–16 μ) contains the majority of the common functional group absorptions (C=C, C—O, C–halogen, C–aromatic and aromatic carbons) and it is usually the region where low energy bending and stretching vibrations absorb. Each individual molecule will have its own peculiar set of bending, stretching, rocking, twisting, and wagging vibrations due to the carbon "backbone" of the molecule as well as the functional group bonds.

The combination of these vibrations leads to a "fingerprint" of the molecule that can often be used to identify a specific molecule by "matching fingerprints," if a library of known compounds is available. This region of the infrared spectrum is generally called the *fingerprint region.*

What is the use of the fingerprint region?

If there is an unknown organic molecule and a "library" of prerecorded infrared spectra exists, the fingerprint region can be used to find the proper "match." Fingerprinting the molecule in the library allows its identification. Obviously, if a molecule is not in the library, this technique cannot be used to identify it.

What are the generic infrared absorptions for the following major functional groups: (a) alcohols (b) ketones (c) aldehydes (d) carboxylic acids (e) amines (f) esters (g) amides (h) nitriles (i) alkenes (j) alkynes (k) benzene derivatives (l) ethers (m) acid chlorides (n) acid anhydrides (o) alkyl halides?

(a) **alcohols:** O—H [3400–3610 cm^{-1}, 2.94–2.77 μ] and C—O [1050–1150 cm^{-1}, 9.52–8.70 μ]

(b) **ketones:** C=O [1725–1680 cm^{-1}, 5.80–5.95 μ]

(c) **aldehydes:** C=O [1740–1695 cm^{-1}, 5.75–5.90 μ] and O=C-H [2816 cm^{-1}, 3.55 μ]

(d) **carboxylic acids**: O=C—O—H [3300–2500 cm^{-1}, 3.03–4.0 μ], O=C–OH [1725–1680 cm^{-1}, 5.80–5.95 μ]

(e) **amines**: 1° amines N—H [3550–3300 cm^{-1} – a doublet of peaks for each N—H, 2.82–3.03 μ] 2° amines N—H [3550–3400 cm^{-1} a single peak for the only N-H, 2.82–2.94 μ]

(f) **esters:** O=C—O—C [1780–1715 cm^{-1}, 5.61–5.83 μ], O=C-O-C [1050–1100 cm^{-1}, 9.52–9.09 μ]

(g) **amides:** O=C—N— Amide I – 1° [1690 cm^{-1}, 5.92 μ] 2° [1700–1670 cm^{-1}, 5.88–6.00 μ]. The Amide II band is – 1° [1600 cm^{-1}, 6.25 μ] 2° [1550–1510 cm^{-1}, 6.45–6.62 μ]. amide N—H – 1° [3500 cm^{-1}, 2.86 μ], 2° [3460–3400 cm^{-1}, 2.89–2.94 μ]

(h) **nitriles:** C≡N [2260–2200 cm^{-1}, 4.42–4.56 μ]

(i) **alkenes**: C=C—H [3040–3010 cm^{-1}, 3.29–3.32 μ]; C=C [there is a relatively weak to moderate signal at 1680–1620 cm^{-1} [5.95–6.17 μ];

(j) **alkynes:** C≡C—H [3300 cm^{-1}, 3.03 μ], C≡C [terminal, 2140–2100 cm^{-1}, 4.67–4.76 μ; non-terminal, 2260–2150 cm^{-1}, 4.42–4.65 μ];

(k) **benzene derivatives**: Ar–H [3040–3010 cm^{-1}, 3.29–3.32 μ], Ar C=C [about 1600 and 1510 cm^{-1}, 6.25 and 6.63 μ]

(l) **ethers:** C—O [1150–1060 and 1140–900 cm^{-1}, 8.70–9.43 and 8.77–11.11 μ];

(m) **acid chlorides:** O=C—Cl [1815–1750 cm^{-1}, 5.51–5.71 μ], C-Cl [730–580 cm^{-1}, 13.70–17.24 μ];

(n) **acid anhydrides:** $(O{=}C)_2O$ [1850–1780 and 1790–1710 cm^{-1}, 5.41–5.62 and 5.59–5.85 μ];

(o) **alkyl halides**: C—Cl [730–605 cm^{-1}, 13.70–16.53], C—Br [645–605 cm^{-1}, 15.50–16.53 μ], C—I [600–560 cm^{-1}, 16.67–17.86 μ].

Does the C—H signal in the infrared generally provide useful information?

Most organic molecules have carbons and hydrogen atoms, and therefore will have C—H signals in the infrared. This strong absorption for C—H appears at 2850 cm^{-1} (3.50 μ). If there are C—H units in a molecule, this absorption will always appear but is not considered to be a functional group. Because it is ubiquitous, the presence of C—H absorption does not always give useful information about structure, although there are exceptions to this statement, including the hydrogen atoms attached to a double or triple bond, or an aldehyde hydrogen, but other examples will not be discussed here. If this signal is absent, there are no C—H units in the molecules, which is a significant structural indicator.

What is the effect of conjugation on the absorption of a carbonyl (compare cyclohexanone with cyclohexenone)?

In general, conjugation shifts the absorption to longer wavelengths (shorter frequencies): lower energy. The C=O group of cyclohexanone, for example, absorbs at 1725–1705 cm^{-1} [5.80–5.87 μ] but the conjugated C=O group of cyclohexenone will absorb at 1685–1665 cm^{-1} [5.93–6.01 μ]. *The absorption was shifted to lower energy (longer wavelength) by conjugation.*

How can each of the following functional groups be identified based entirely on the provided molecular formula and the infrared spectrum: (a) $C_4H_{10}O$ and a strong, broad absorption signal at 3400–3610 cm^{-1}; (b) $C_6H_{12}O_2$ and a strong, broad signal at 3300–2500 cm^{-1},with another strong signal at 1725–1680 cm^{-1}; (c) $C_5H_{13}N$ and two moderate bands at 3550–3300 cm^{-1}?

In infrared (a), the molecule has only one oxygen, and there is an O—H absorption so this molecule is, therefore, likely to be an alcohol such as butan-1-ol or butan-2-ol. Infrared (b) has two oxygens, expanding the possible choices to include carboxylic acids and esters. The molecule has a strong C=O absorption that could be an aldehyde, ketone acid, or ester. The strong, broad signal at 3300–2500 cm^{-1}, coupled with the strong signal at 1725–1680 cm^{-1} indicates that the molecule is a carboxylic acid. There are several possible structures with six carbon atoms. In (c), the molecule contains one nitrogen and could be an amine or a nitrile. There is no CN absorption, so the molecule cannot be a nitrile. It is an amine and there are two peaks in the N—H region, suggesting a primary amine such as 1-aminopentane.

11.4 NUCLEAR MAGNETIC RESONANCE SPECTROSCOPY (nmr)

Why is a proton considered to be a small electromagnet?

A hydrogen atom or indeed any atom is a positive nucleus surrounded by negative electrons. Since it has the property of spin, a spinning charge will generate a small magnetic field and, therefore, act as an electromagnet when in the presence of a larger magnetic field. The key principle to remember is that a spinning charge generates a magnetic field, and the proton is a spinning charge.

What quantum number is important in nmr?

The spin quantum number (I) is important to nuclear magnetic resonance.

Which common atoms have a spin = ½?

The most commonly examined nuclei with $I = ½$ are ^{1}H, ^{13}C, ^{19}F, ^{15}N (spin = −½), and ^{31}P.

Which common atoms have a spin = 1?

The most commonly examined nuclei with $I = 1$ are ^{2}H and ^{6}Li.

Which common atoms have no spin ($I = 0$)?

Many nuclei commonly found in organic molecules have no spin ($I = 0$) and *cannot* be used in a nmr experiment. The most common are ^{12}C, ^{14}N, ^{16}O, and ^{32}S.

What effect does a large external magnet have on the small magnetic proton?

The spin of the small magnet (the proton) can be aligned in parallel with the external magnetic field or can be opposed to it. When the proton field is aligned opposite the external field, it requires more energy than when it is aligned with the field. This creates an energy gap (ΔE). This energy difference is usually of about the same frequency as radio waves ($\nu = 3 \times 10^6$–3×10^8 Hz).

Modern magnetic field strength is measure in Tesla. How many Tesla (T) equal 14,100 gauss?

One gauss = 1×10^{-4} Tesla, so one Tesla = 10,000 gauss. Therefore, 14,100 gauss = 1.4 T.

What is the magnetic field strength for a 60 MHz, a 100 MHz, a 300 MHz, a 500 MHz, a 600 MHz, and a 900 MHz nmr instrument?

A 60 MHz instrument uses a 1.4 T (14,100 gauss) magnet; a 100 MHz instrument uses a 2.35 T (23,500 gauss) magnet; a 300 MHz instrument uses a 7.05 T (70,500 gauss) magnet; a 500 MHz instrument uses a 11.7 T (117,000 gauss) magnet; a 600 MHz instrument uses a 14.1 T (141,000 gauss magnet); and, a 900 MHz instrument uses a 21.1 T (215,000 gauss) magnet.

What is the influence of a 14,100 gauss magnet when compared to a 63,450 gauss magnet on a proton in proton nmr?

When the magnetic field is 14,100 gauss, the ΔE for the proton being examined will be about 60 MHz (5.7×10^{-6} kcal mol^{-1}). When the magnet field strength is increased to 63,450 gauss, ΔE for the proton being examined will increase to 270 MHz (25.7×10^{-6} kcal mol^{-1})

What is the magnitude of the energy gap (ΔE) for a hydrogen atom?

This energy gap is in the radio signal range, which typically spans the range 4–600 MHz

What energy source can cause the proton to absorb energy equal to ΔE?

A radio signal of controlled frequency is directed toward the sample inside the strong magnetic field.

What radio wave frequencies are used in nmr?

For nmr experiments, radio signals in the range 60–1000 MHz are typically used.

What is the energy range of the ΔE imposed by introduction of a proton into a magnetic field?

This ΔE is in the range of radio waves (1000×10^{-4}–100000×10^{-4} cm [1000–100,000 λ]) = 10–0.1 cm^{-1}.

How are the applied radio frequency signal and the magnetic field strength related?

The radio signal frequency used to irradiate the sample is in Megahertz. At a certain magnetic field strength (the flux density or field intensity), usually measured in Tesla or gauss, the proton will come into resonance and absorb the energy. The consequence of this resonance can be measured as an absorption signal.

For a given radio signal, what magnetic field strength is required for a nmr signal?

Resonance between the field strength of the instrument and the magnet field strength leads to the following data: at a *magnet strength* of 1.41, Tesla protons resonate at a *frequency* of 60 MHz; 2.35 Tesla at 100 MHz; 7.05 Tesla at 300 MHz; 9.4 Tesla at 400 MHz; 11.7 Tesla at 500 MHz; 14.1 Tesla at 600 MHz; and, 21.1 Tesla at 900 MHz. Since 1 Tesla = 10,000 gauss: 14,100 gauss protons resonate at a *frequency* of 60 MHz; 23,500 gauss at 100 MHz; 70,500 gauss at 300 MHz; 94,000 gauss at 400 MHz; 117,000 gauss at 500 MHz; 141,000 gauss at 600 MHz; and, 215,000 gauss at 900 MHz.

What happens when a proton in a magnetic field is bombarded with energy equal to ΔE?

A proton with spin not equal to zero will *absorb* ΔE, and the nuclei will change its spin state (flips its spin state) as illustrated in the figure. As shown, the energy gap ΔE increases with a larger magnetic field since they must be in resonance for absorption to occur.

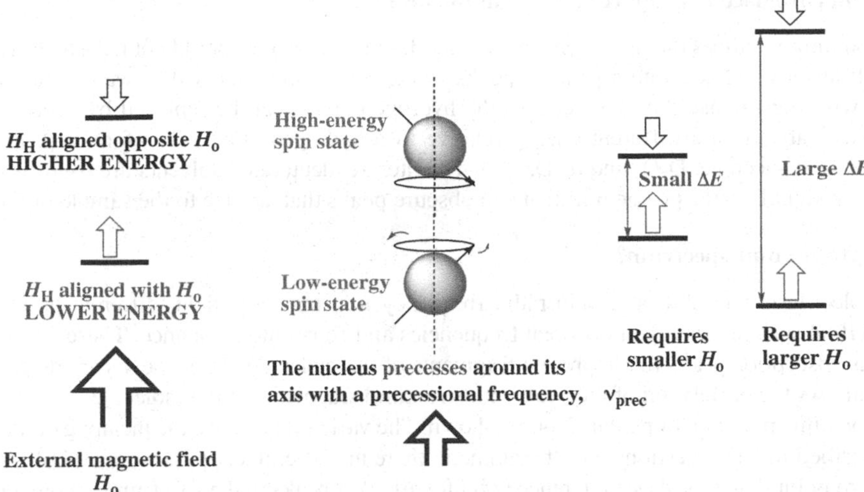

Is this phenomenon an absorption or emission process?

The proton absorbs energy; it is an absorption process.

Is ΔE larger or smaller as the magnetic field strength increases?

As suggested in the diagram in the preceding question, as the magnetic field strength increases, ΔE will become larger for a given nuclei. IMPORTANT: *If the ΔE is kept constant, say at 60 MHz, then the magnetic field strength due to different nuclei (also protons in different magnetic environments) will change slightly and these differences can be measured.*

How does a nmr spectrometer work?

A sample is dissolved in an appropriate solvent and placed in a thin glass tube. This tube is lowered into a magnetic field and spun (to average out inhomogeneous areas in the magnetic field). A radio signal (linked to the magnetic field strength – a 14,100 gauss magnet requires a 60 MHz radio signal for protons to absorb the energy) is applied to the sample. The holder into which the sample tube is lowered is surrounded by a radio generating coil. The radio signal is kept constant and the magnetic field is varied slightly. Those protons that absorb the radio signal at the various magnetic field strengths will be recorded as absorption "peaks." The collection of these absorption peaks is the nmr spectrum.

What process is examined in the nmr?

The absorption of energy by a nucleus with spin, in a magnetic field. The most commonly examined nuclei are the proton (^{1}H) and ^{13}C. Other nuclei can also be examined, including ^{2}H, ^{6}Li, ^{15}N, and ^{19}F.

Why do different nuclei require different magnetic field strengths?

Each nucleus will absorb different amounts of energy for a given magnetic field strength (different ΔE). For a ^{1}H in a 14,100-gauss magnetic field, ΔE is 60 MHz but ΔE for ^{13}C is 15 MHz at 14,100 gauss.

Why is a solvent necessary for most nmr experiments?

Although modern techniques are available for examining solid materials, for nmr analysis of compounds by most nmr techniques, the organic chemical, solid, or liquid must be dissolved in a solvent, allowing for homogeneity of the sample solution.

What solvents are used to prepare samples in the nmr?

Since proton nmr examines the hydrogen atoms in a sample, the solvent should not have hydrogen atoms as they will absorb and generate a peak or peaks in the proton nmr that will "swamp out" all signal associated with the sample. Alternatively, all the hydrogen atoms can be replaced by deuterium since deuterium will absorb at a different energy relative to a hydrogen atom. Therefore, typical solvents include $CDCl_3$, d_6-acetone, D_2O, and d_6-DMSO. To reiterate, deuterated solvents are used so they will not contribute signals to the proton nmr that can obscure peaks that are due to the sample of interest.

What is a proton nmr spectrum?

When a molecule is pulsed at a certain radio frequency in a magnetic field, different protons in the molecule will absorb the energy at different frequencies and come into resonance. These signals can be displayed as absorption peaks that represent fragments of the molecule. These peaks are displayed on a graph that allows the correlation of the peak with structural fragments of the molecule.

The proton nmr spectrum for pentan-2-one is shown. The various peaks and the meaning of those peaks will be described in later questions. For the moment, there are several key parameters. First is the presence of a zero point that is used as a reference point for all other peaks in the spectrum. A compound used for the zero point will be discussed below. There is also the ppm scale that defines the position of each peak relative to the zero point, and this scale must be discussed. Molecules that have protons that require a larger magnetic field to come into resonance are marked as high field and those protons that require less of a magnetic field are marked as low field. The reasons for this effect must be discussed and how the absorption of protons at high field or low field can be correlated with structure will also be discussed.

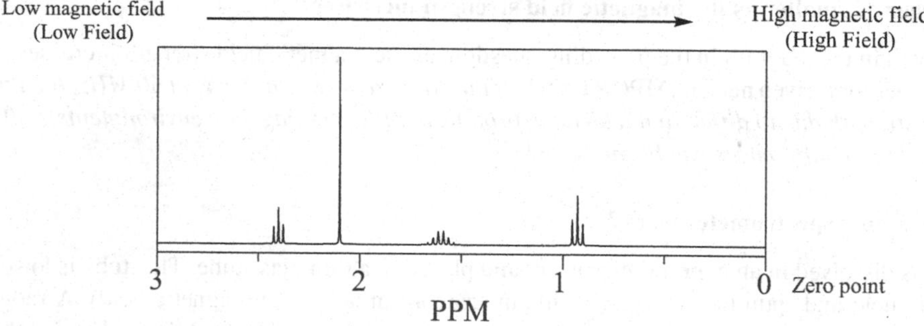

What is the ppm scale?

A given proton absorbs ΔE, but different protons have different magnetic field strength, requiring a different ΔE. For the nmr experiment where ΔE is held constant, the fact that different types of protons have different magnetic field strength means that they will absorb at different energies.

A convenient method for measuring the position of an absorption signal is in Hz. The differences in field strength vary by <1–1200 Hz in a 60 MHz field. Since 1 MHz is 1×10^6 Hz, the changes in field in Hz represent millionths of the total field strength of 60 MHz. In general, differences of a signal position in hertz is small relative to a field strength in MHz. There is a problem, however, since a signal that appears at 60 Hz in a 60 MHz instrument will appear at 300 Hz in a 300 MHz instrument. To consolidate these data, the ppm scale was created.

In this scale, the absorption signal (in Hz) is divided by the field strength (in MHz). A signal at 60 Hz in a 60 MHz field will then be calculated to be (60 Hz/60 × 10^6 Hz) = 1×10^{-6} or one part-per-million (1 ppm). The same signal at 300 MHz will be (300 Hz/300 × 10^6 Hz) = 1×10^{-6} = 1 ppm. In this way, absorption signals at different field strengths can be identified as the same signal. This system generates the *ppm scale*.

Why is an internal standard used in nmr?

There has to be a "zero point" in order to provide a well-defined position in the nmr for a given molecule that can be repeated and identified. A scale makes no sense unless there is a peak that all other peaks in the spectrum can be related to. Such a peak is due to an added compound that can be used as a reference standard. This standard must be taken as the zero point in all samples under all conditions. All absorption peaks are therefore reported with reference to this standard. The most common standard in nmr is the chemical tetramethylsilane (TMS), which is added to the sample.

Where is the "zero point" in nmr?

The zero point in nmr is the absorption signal for TMS, which is added to the sample. The instrument is adjusted so that the TMS signal is set to zero. Almost all signals in the nmr are reported as positive peak positions to the left of the zero point, or at lower field relative to the zero point. The peaks associated with the sample are said to be "downfield" relative to the zero point.

What is the structure of tetramethylsilane?

Tetramethylsilane has the structure $(Me_3)_4Si$. At all field strengths and all radio frequencies, TMS is set to 0 ppm. In other words, the instrument is adjusted to make the signal for TMS appear at 0 ppm.

Why is tetramethylsilane an ideal internal standard?

Tetramethylsilane absorbs at a position in most magnetic fields at higher energy (higher local field strength) than most protons in most organic molecules. In the nmr spectrum for pentan-2-one, the absorption peaks of the sample resonate at lower energy and appear further to the left side of the spectrum further away from TMS, while signals of higher field strength appear closer to TMS. Indeed, the TMS reference signal (assigned 0 ppm) will appear to the far right (high field) and all signals due to the organic sample will appear at lower energy, to its left (lower field). The signal at about 2.1 ppm is further downfield and requires a lower magnetic field strength than the three signals at about 1.05 ppm, which is upfield and at higher energy.

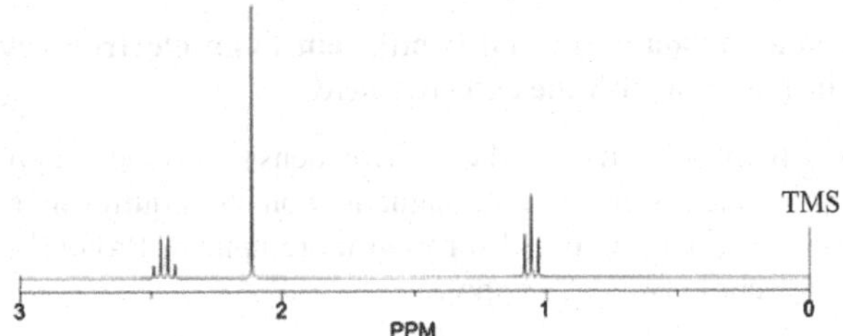

Where does the signal for TMS appear in a nmr spectrum at 100 MHz?

At all field strengths and all radio frequencies, TMS appears at 0 ppm. The instrument is adjusted to *make* the signal for TMS appear at 0 ppm.

If a nmr spectrum is recorded at 60 MHz and a signal appears at 345 Hz, what is the absorption in ppm?

This signal will appear at $(345 \text{ Hz}/60 \times 10^6 \text{ Hz}) = 5.45 \times 10^{-6} = 5.45$ ppm.

If a signal appears at 4.50 ppm at 60 MHz, where is the signal, in ppm, at 500 MHz?

The position of the signal in ppm will not change with field strength. This signal will, therefore, also appear at 4.50 ppm at both 500 MHz and at 60 MHz.

If a signal appears at 3.25 ppm at 60 Hz, where is the signal, in Hz, at 400 MHz?

A signal at 3.25 ppm (3.25×10^{-6}) appears at $(3.25 \times 10^{-6})(60 \times 10^{6}) = 195$ Hz. At 400 MHz, the 3.25 ppm signal appears at $(3.25 \times 10^{-6})(400 \times 10^{6}) = 1300$ Hz.

What is chemical shift?

The position of an absorption peak for a molecule in ppm, relative to TMS, is referred to as the chemical shift for that signal.

What is an upfield signal? A downfield signal?

An upfield signal appears at low ppm relative to TMS (close to TMS). A downfield signal appears at larger ppm relative to TMS, so a signal at 7.0 ppm is downfield of TMS. These terms can be used in a relative sense. A signal at 5.0 ppm is upfield of a signal at 7.0 ppm. A signal at 5.0 ppm is downfield of a signal at 2.45 ppm.

Is high field associated with signals closer to 8 ppm or closer to 1 ppm?

High field (upfield) is associated with signals closer to 1 ppm.

Why are ppm for a given group reported as a range of numbers?

For a given group, local variation in structure can lead to a range of absorption frequencies. If the hydrogen attached to the α carbon of a bromide (Br—C—<u>H</u>) appears at about 3.5 ppm, for example, the signal could vary between about 3.2–3.9 ppm, depending on how many other carbon atoms are attached to the carbon, and also what other groups or atoms are in proximity to this proton. Usually, the variation is about 0.5–1.0 ppm for a given functional group.

If a proton is attached to a carbon atom that is adjacent to an electron-releasing group, how does that influence the interaction with the external field?

An electron-releasing substituent will increase the electron density around the proton, increasing the net magnetic moment of the proton. This increase in magnetic moment requires more of an external field to bring the proton into resonance, making the absorption more upfield. Protons adjacent to an electron-releasing group generally appear between 2–3 ppm.

If a proton is attached to a carbon atom that is adjacent to an electron-withdrawing group, how does that influence the interaction with the external field?

The electron-withdrawing substituent will decrease the electron density around the proton, decreasing the net magnetic moment of the proton. This decrease in magnetic moment requires less of an external field to bring the proton into resonance, making the absorption more downfield relative to TMS. Protons adjacent to an electron-withdrawing group generally appear between 2–6 ppm, although the signal can be as far downfield as 15–18 ppm.

What is the ppm range for various common functional groups?

Typical chemical shifts for protons that are adjacent to various functional groups are shown in the table.

^{1}H NMR Chemical Shifts (in ppm)

Cyclopropane	0.2	Primary, RCH_3	0.9
Secondary, R_2CH_2	1.3	Tertiary, R_3CH	1.5
Vinylic, C=C—H	3.5–5.9	Alkynyl, CJC—H	2.0–3.0
Aromatic, Ar—H	6.0–8.5	Benzylic, Ar—C—H	2.2–3.0
Allylic, C=C—C—H	1.7	Fluorides, F—C—H	4.0–4.5
Chlorides, Cl—C—H	3.0–4.0	Bromides, Br—C—H	2.5–4.0
Iodides, I—C—H	2.0-4.0	Alcohols, HO—C—H α-H of alcohols	3.4–4.0
Ethers, C—O—C—H	3.3–4.0	Esters, RCOO—C—H H on carbon of alcohol unit	3.7–4.1
Carboxylic acids, HOOC—C—H α-H of acids	2.0–2.2	Esters, ROOC—C—H α-H of esters	2.0–2.7
Carbonyls, O=C—C—H α-H of aldehydes and ketones	2.0–2.7	Aldehydes, O=C—H Aldehyde proton	9.0–10.3
Hydroxyl, O—H	1.0–5.5	Phenols, ArO—H	4.0–12.0
Enols, C=C—O—H	15.0–17.0	Carboxylic acids, RCOO—H Acidic proton of the OH	10.5–15.0
Amino, R—N—H Proton on nitrogen	1.0–5.0	Amines, N—C—H α-H of amines	2.5

Methyl Signals for Common Fragments

To determine signals for funtional groups to a methylene, add 0.4 to these numbers
To determine signals for funtional groups to a methine, add 0.6 to these numbers

C_6H_5–CH_3	2.3	R–O–CH_3	3.3	R–C(=O)–CH_3	2.15
HO–C(=O)–CH_3	2.3	R_2N–CH_3	2.2	Ar–O–CH_3	3.85
RO–C(=O)–CH_3	2.6	R–C(=O)–O-CH_3	3.6		

What is a shielding effect?

A shielding effect is the label for an electron releasing group that causes the absorption to occur upfield. *A shielded proton will absorb upfield.*

What are common functional groups that cause shielding effects?

The silane (R_4Si) group of tetramethylsilane induces a large shielding effect. For this reason, TMS appears far upfield relative to most other organic molecules. Alkyl groups are shielding relative to C—O, C—N, C–halogen, C—C=O, etc.

What is a deshielding effect?

A deshielding effect is associated with an electron-withdrawing group, pushing the absorption downfield. A deshielded proton absorbs downfield.

What are common functional groups that cause deshielding effects?

Most electron-withdrawing groups induce downfield shifts via deshielding. These include C=O, C≡N, OR, NR_2, Ph, C=C, etc.

Which functional group will cause a greater downfield shift, C=O or Br?

The Br substituent is more deshielding and the proton signal will resonate further downfield. However, oxygen is more electronegative than bromine: 3.44 vs. 2.96. Remember that the signal of interest is a hydrogen atom attached to a carbon. With a bromine substituent, the H—C—Br unit has the electron withdrawing Br separated from H by two bonds. In the carbonyl unit, the H—C—C=O unit has the electron-withdrawing oxygen atom three bonds away from the hydrogen. Therefore, the bromine will have a greater effect. A proton adjacent to a bromine (H—C—Br) absorbs at about 2.70–4.10 ppm whereas the carbonyl leads to chemical shifts of 2.10–2.50 ppm for H—C—C=O.

Why is the signal for a proton attached to a C=C group further downfield than that attached to a Cl?

The π-electrons in the C=C double bond induce a secondary magnetic field that is opposed to the external field, as shown in the figure. The outer position of this secondary field enhances the field and a lower magnetic field is required for resonance and the signal will be more downfield. Conversely, if a proton is held in the center part of this secondary field, it will be shielded and moved upfield. Since the proton attached to the C=C is held in the deshielding portion of the secondary field, that hydrogen atom will absorb further downfield than is usual. This effect is in addition to the usual electron withdrawing effects and H—C=C absorbs between 4.5–6.5 ppm whereas H—C—Cl absorbs between 3.1–4.1 ppm since chlorine does not generate a secondary field.

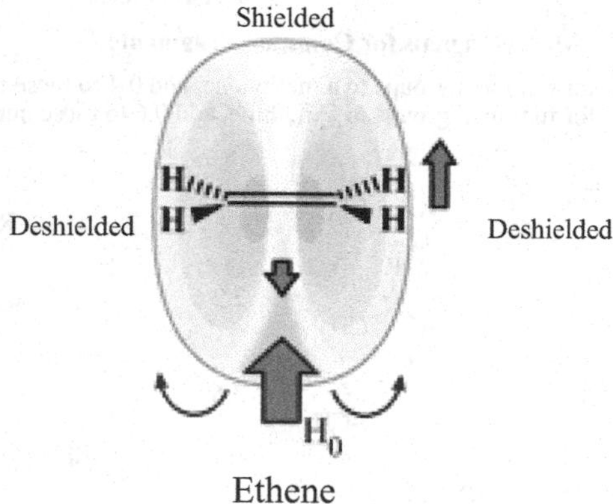

Ethene

What is the name of this secondary field effect?

Magnetic anisotropy.

Why does the hydrogen on a benzene ring appear at 6.8–7.2 ppm?

There are more π-electrons in benzene than in ethene (six vs. two) so the secondary magnetic field that is generated is expected to be larger. For this reason, the magnetic anisotropy effect is much greater. As shown in the figure, the protons on the benzene ring are in the deshielding portion of the secondary field, pushing the signal further downfield to 6.5–8.5 ppm.

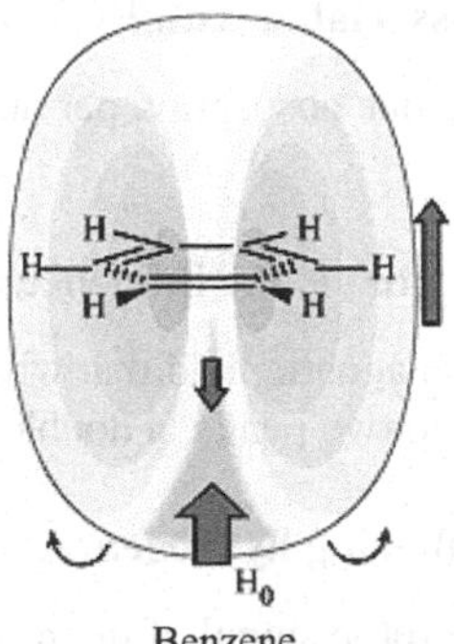

Benzene

Why does the proton attached to an alkyne appear upfield of the proton absorption for an alkene?

The presence of two π-bonds changes the orientation of the molecule with respect to the external field (H_o). A shown in the figure the secondary magnetic field is set up such that the proton attached to C≡C unit is held in the shielding portion of the secondary field and is shielded. For this reason, the signal is more upfield than the analogous H—C=C signal.

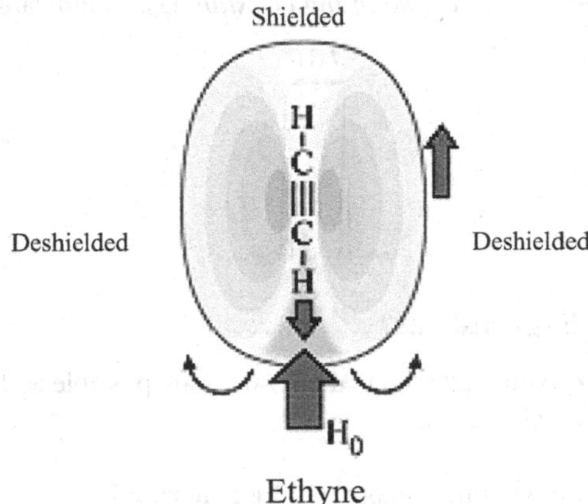

Ethyne

What is multiplicity?

Multiplicity is defined as the number of peaks that appears for each absorption (each signal). A signal that gives only one peak is called a singlet, two peaks is a doublet, three peaks is a triplet, four peaks is a quartet, five peaks is a pentet, etc.

Why does a proton give only one signal per absorption?

With a spin quantum number (I) of ½, there are only two orientations for the spin moment of the proton [Number of orientations = (2 × I)+1]. For two orientations (for and against the external field, A and B) there is only one possible signal (A to B). Each proton (^{1}H) therefore gives one signal (one absorption).

Explain why one deuterium gives rise to three signals.

Deuterium (^{2}H) has a spin of 1 and gives three orientations [(2 × 1)+1]. For three orientations (A, B, C) there are three signals (A to B, A to C, B to C). Each atom of ^{2}H therefore gives three signals per absorption.

How many signals per absorption are associated with ^{13}C? With ^{15}N? With ^{16}O?

Both ^{13}C and ^{15}N has a spin of ½ and give one absorption per nuclei. Since ^{16}O has a spin of zero (0), it does not exhibit a signal in the nmr.

If a proton has one hydrogen neighbor, what is the influence of that neighbor?

The neighboring proton exerts a separate magnetic field that will exhibit a small external field and will split the signal for the proton of interest into two peaks (a doublet).

How many peaks appear for each neighboring hydrogen?

Each neighboring hydrogen will split the proton signal of interest into two peaks (a doublet).

Why does a methyl group give only one peak?

All three of the protons of the methyl group are magnetically equivalent so they give only one signal. For this reason, the protons are not considered to be neighbors, but are identical and absorb as one peak.

What is the coupling constant?

When a signal is split into two peaks, the two peaks will be separated by some number of Hz. This distance (measured in Hz) is referred to as the *coupling constant* (*J*), as indicated in the figure.

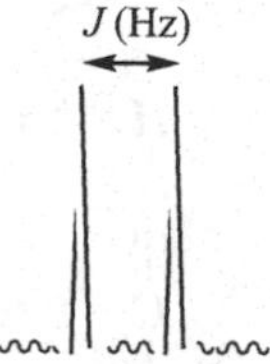

Of what magnitude are coupling constants?

Typical values of *J* are 0–15 Hz. Although much larger values are possible and are occasionally observed, *J* values are typically in the range indicated.

If a proton has one neighbor, how many peaks will be generated?

For *n* neighbors, a proton signal will be split into *n+1* peaks. A proton that appears as a single peak (a singlet) will have no neighbors. One neighbor gives two signals (a doublet).

What is the *n*+1 rule?

For a given proton signal with n neighbors, there will be *n*+1 peaks *if the neighboring hydrogens all have the same coupling constant* (J).

If there are more than one neighbor for a given proton signal, how many peaks will be generated for that proton?

If the hydrogen atoms are chemically and magnetically equivalent, the coupling constants will be the same. If the coupling constants are the same, then the *n*+1 rule applies. Using the *n*+1 rule, two neighbors lead to three peaks (a triplet) for a given signal. With three neighbors, the proton signal will appear as four signals (a quartet), and so on. In each case, the *J* value for the distance between each peak of doublet, triplet, or quartet is the same.

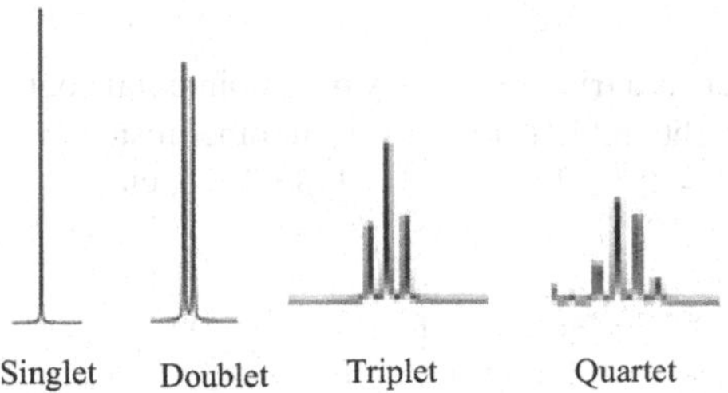

Why do three neighboring hydrogen atoms lead to four peaks for a given proton signal?

When each identical neighboring proton splits the signal of interest, the coupling constant will be identical, leading to overlap of the peaks for the signal. The overlap leads to a total of four peaks in an intensity ratio of 1:3:3:1 for a quartet. The ratio is 1:2:1 for a triplet and 1:1 for a doublet.

There is one signal in the nmr for $ClCH_3$. There are three hydrogen atoms, so why is there only one peak?

All three of the hydrogen atoms of the methyl group are chemically and magnetically identical. Therefore, all three of the hydrogen atoms give one signal and there are zero neighbors, so there is no spin–spin splitting and only one peak.

For the molecule $CH(CH_3)_3$, what is relationship of the hydrogen atoms on the methyl groups?

The three methyl groups are chemically and magnetically identical so all nine hydrogen atoms will appear as one signal.

For the molecule $CH(CH_3)_3$, there are two signals, a doublet and a heptet. Why are there only two signals and why does the CH signal appear as a multiplet?

The CH group has nine identical neighbors (three identical methyl groups), so the CH gives 9+1 = 10 peaks, which will likely show up as a multiplet. The nine identical hydrogen atoms of the three identical methyl groups are spit into a doublet by the one neighboring proton on CH.

For $ClCH(CH_3)_2$, there are two signals, a doublet and a heptet. Which signal is correlated with which hydrogen atom in the molecule?

The CH group has six identical neighbors (two identical methyl groups) so the CH gives 6+1 = 7 peaks, a heptet. The six identical hydrogen atoms of the two identical methyl groups are spit into a doublet by the one neighboring proton on CH.

Assuming the *n*+1 rule applies, how many neighboring hydrogens will there be for (a) a triplet, (b) a quartet, (c) a pentet, and (d) a singlet?

The neighbors will be 2 for (a), 3 for (b), 4 for (c), and 0 for (d).

Why are these multiple signals always symmetrical when the *n*+1 rule is applied?

Because the coupling constant is the same for all neighboring hydrogens. If J is not the same, the resulting signal will be asymmetric in that *the* n+*1 rule does not apply.*

What is Pascal's triangle?

In mathematics, Pascal's triangle is a triangular array of the binomial coefficients. It is a triangle of numbers bordered by ones on the right and left sides. Every number inside the triangle is the sum of the two numbers directly above it: 1 + 1 = 2; 1 + 2 = 3; 1 + 3 = 4, 3 + 3 = 6, etc.

1
1 1
1 2 1
1 3 3 1
1 4 6 4 1
1 5 10 10 5 1
1 6 15 20 15 6 1

How is Pascal's triangle related to spin–spin splitting in proton nmr?

The first-order patterns observed for the resonance of a nucleus that is coupled to *n* equivalent nuclei with spin = 1 may be described by the symmetrical Pascal-like triangle in the preceding question. In other words, two peaks will have a 1:1 relationship, three peaks will have a 1:2:1 relationship, four peaks will have 1:3:3:1 relationship, etc.

What is a multiplet?

A multiplet is a cluster of several peaks, but it is not possible to count them. This situation may be due to very low intensity for the outermost (satellite) signals or due to unsymmetrical overlap of peaks.

If a proton has two different kinds of hydrogen neighbors, what is the result?

The multiplet pattern will be asymmetric, reflecting one hydrogen splitting a proton into a doublet with one coupling constant. Each of those peaks will then be split into new doublets, but with a different coupling constant, leading to little or no overlap of peaks.

If the coupling constant for neighbor A is 2 Hz and the coupling constant for neighbor B is 5 Hz, what is the signal for a given proton if there are two neighboring H_A and one neighboring H_B?

The result of these asymmetric splitting patterns is the final six-peak multiplet shown in the figure, which is known as a double of triplets. Both the 2 Hz and 5 Hz coupling constants can be discerned in this multiplet. Working "backwards" from the multiplet, the number of neighbors and each coupling constant can be determined. Note that this double of triplets is the signal for one proton that has two different types of neighboring hydrogen atoms.

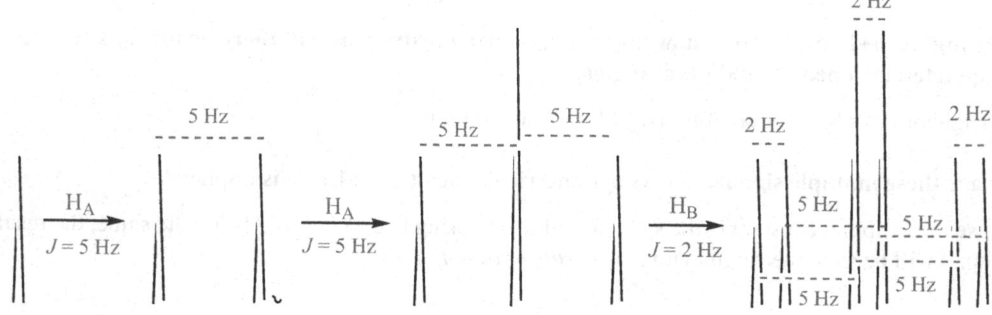

What is an AB quartet?

An AB quartet arises when two hydrogens have almost the same coupling constant, but those hydrogen atoms have slightly different magnetic environments. The asymmetric coupling leads to four peaks with the distinctive pattern shown in the figure.

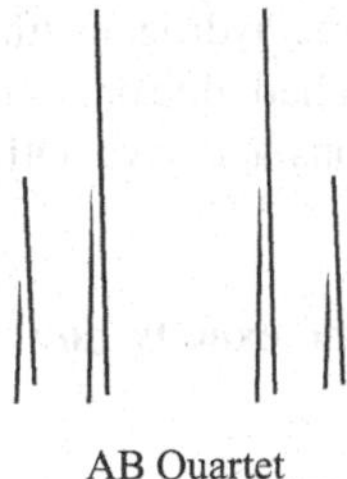

AB Quartet

What does integration of a signal in proton nmr mean?

Each absorption signal appears as a "peak" or a cluster of "peaks." The area under these peaks is measured (integrated) and is taken to be the integration for the signal. By comparing the peak area of one signal with another, the relative ratio of hydrogens for each signal can be determined (1:1, 1:2, 2:5, etc.). Integration does not give the actual number of hydrogens but only the relative ratio of hydrogens associated with each signal. Once this ratio is known, the empirical formula can be used to generate the actual ratio of hydrogen atoms for each signal.

Why is the integration always given as a ratio of signals?

The exact number of hydrogen atoms is unknown without the specific empirical formula and molecular weight. This information can be determined from the mass spectrum. Note that the integration is based on the ratio of the peak with the smallest area being divided into all other peaks.

How many different types of hydrogen atoms are there in (a), in (b), and in (c)?

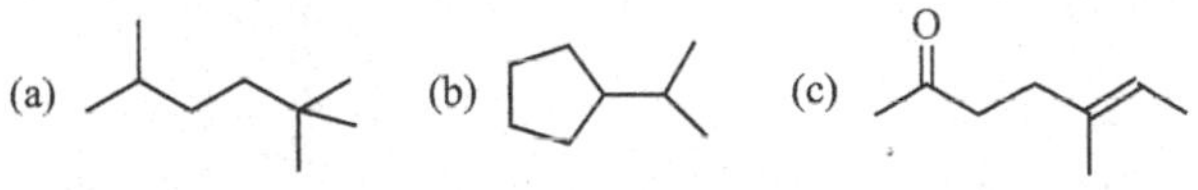

(a) (b) (c) O

Compound (a) has five different types of hydrogen atoms, each marked in a different color. Note that all six of the hydrogen atoms in the two methyl groups shown in light gray will give rise to one signal. Likewise, all nine hydrogen atoms in the three methyl groups of the tert-butyl group are identical and will give rise to one signal. Compound (b) has five different types of hydrogen atoms and will give rise to five different signals. Finally, compound (c) has six different types of hydrogen atoms and will give rise to six different signals. Note that each signal may be multiplet peaks depending on the number of neighbors.

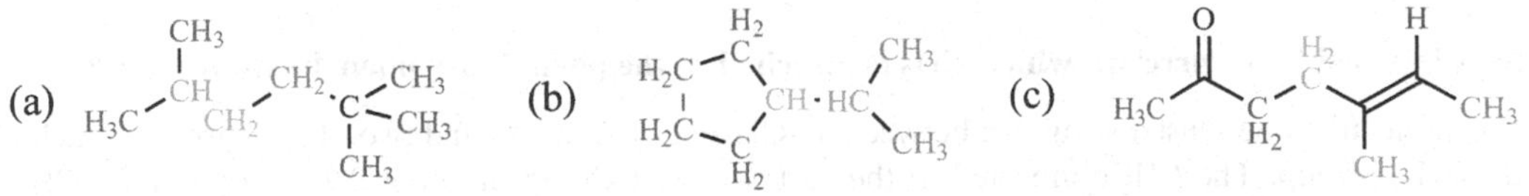

(a) CH_3 CH H_3C CH_2 CH_2 C CH_3 CH_3 CH_3 (b) H_2 H_2C C H_2C C H_2 CH·HC CH_3 CH_3 (c) O H H_3C C H_2 H_2 C CH_3 CH_3

If one signal (peak A) has a peak area of 120 and another (peak B) has a peak area of 40, what is the integration for the nmr?

The integration (ratio) of A:B = 120/40 : 40/40. Dividing both by the smaller number gives the ratio of hydrogen atoms to be 3:1. This ratio would be consistent with a molecule with 4 hydrogens, 8 hydrogens, 12 hydrogens, etc. that has two different types of hydrogen atoms.

Is the integration for the TMS signal counted for a sample?

No!

If there are three peaks with an integration of 1:2:6, what empirical formulas are possible?

This integration means there are a total of nine hydrogens (three different kinds of hydrogens in a ratio of 1:2:6). This ratio would fit any formula that had nine or a multiple of nine hydrogens in it (9, 18, 27, 36, 45, etc.). This integration refers only to protons and says nothing about the number of carbons or other atoms in the formula.

What information is required to determine exactly how many protons are associated with a given nmr spectrum?

The molecular weight and the empirical formula (usually determined from the mass spectrum) are required. In the example above, if given a choice between $C_9H_{18}O$ or $C_9H_{20}O$, the only possibility is $C_9H_{18}O$ for the example given above.

There are six protons in acetone, but acetone gives only one signal (a singlet) in the nmr. Why?

All six hydrogens in acetone are identical, magnetically and chemically (they have the same magnetic and chemical environments). All of the hydrogen atoms will therefore absorb the radio signal at exactly the same strength, leading to a single peak.

What is the nmr for 2,6-dimethylheptan-4-one?

This molecule has a formula of $C_9H_{18}O$. Since it is symmetrical, it will exhibit only three different signals: one for the two isopropyl groups and one for the two $-CH_2-$ groups attached to the carbonyl. The integration is 1:0.5:3 or 2:1:6. Since there are a total of 18 hydrogens, this represents four hydrogens for the doublet at 2.4 ppm, two hydrogens for the multiplet centered at about 2.0 ppm and 12 hydrogens for the doublet at about 0.9 ppm, as shown in the figure.

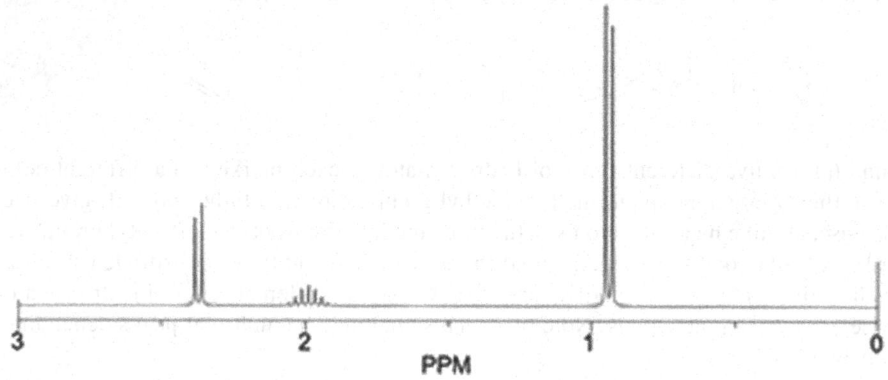

How is it possible to correlate which CH_2 is attached to the phenyl in 5-phenylpentan-1-one?

In this molecule, one must distinguish between a $-CH_2Ph$, $-CH_2-C{=}O$ and two $-CH_2-$ groups attached to a $-CH_2-$ group. The CH_2 connected to the carbonyl will absorb at about 2.2 ppm and the $-CH_2-$ groups connected to other $-CH_2-$ units will absorb below 2 ppm. The $-CH_2-$ group connected to Ph will have a chemical shift of 2.2–2.5 ppm and should set apart from the other signals and be easily identified. This $-CH_2-$ unit is marked light gray in the figure.

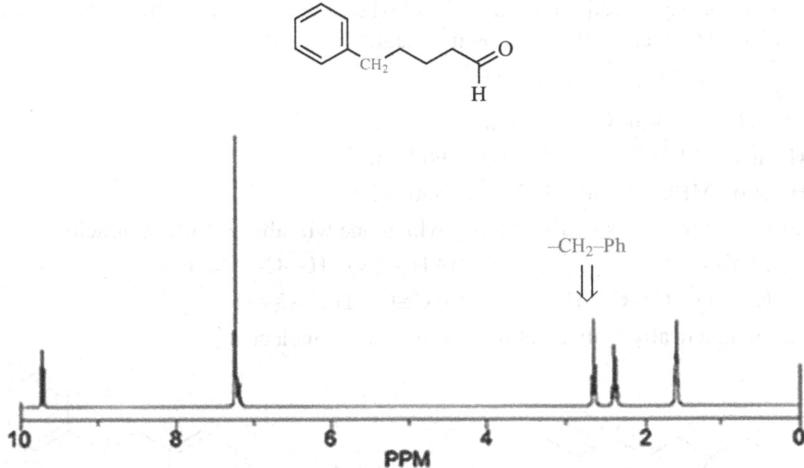

END OF CHAPTER PROBLEMS

1. Interchange each of the following:
   (a) 4.87×10^{-8} m = ___Hz (b) 2350 Å = ___cm (c) 6.91×10^{14} Hz = ___nm
   (d) 3800 nm = __ μ (e) 6.43 m = ___ Hz (f) 1641 cm^{-1} = ___ m
   (g) 875 cm^{-1} = ___ nm.
2. Interchange each of the following:
   (a) 70 eV = ___ kcal = ___ kJ (b) 30 eV = ___ kcal = ___ kJ
   (c) 1200 kcal = ___ eV (d) 2145 kcal = ___ eV
3. Draw the molecular ion for each of the following:
   (a) butan-2-one (b) *N,N*-dimethylbutanamine
   (c) prop-1-ene (d) ethanenitrile
4. Calculate the M, M+1, and M+2 ratios for each of the following:
   (a) $C_5H_{10}O$ (b) $C_8H_{17}N$ (c) $C_5H_{12}O_2$ (d) $C_{10}H_{21}NO$
5. Calculate the empirical formula for each of the following (molecular weight in brackets):
   (a) M (136) 100%, M+1 (137) 8.88%, M+2 (138) 0.794%.
   (b) M (113) 14.5 mm, M+1 (114) 1.18 mm, M+2 (115) 0.044 mm.
   (c) M (98) 79.8 mm, M+1 (99) 5.02 mm, M+2 (100) 0.123 mm.
   (d) M (100) 100%, M+1 (101) 6.66%, M+2 (102) 0.22%.
6. What can be gleaned from the following data?
   (a) M 100%, M+1 7.78%, M+2 100%. (b) M 100%, M+1 1 1.1%, M+2 4.7%.
   (c) M 100%, M+1 8.88%, M+2 34%.
7. Suggest possible fragments for each of the following:
   (a) M-15 (b) M-18 (c) M-28 (d) M-29 (e) M-43 (f) M-45
8. Why is it important *not* to take an infrared spectrum in an aqueous solution when using pressed KBr cells?
9. What is a "bending" vibration? A stretching vibration?
10. Does the C≡C or the C—O bond give the lowest energy infrared absorption?
11. Describe the important infrared absorption bands for (a) butan-2-one (b) 4-cyclohexylpentan-2-ol (c) 6-bromohexanoic acid.
12. Identify how many signals each of the following nuclei will generate in the nmr:
    (a) ^{2}H (b) ^{1}H (c) ^{13}C (d) ^{15}N (e) ^{6}Li (f) ^{12}C

13. If a 14,000-gauss magnet required a ΔE of 60 MHz for resonance, and this is taken as the standard, calculate ΔE for each of the following magnetic fields:

    (a) 28,574 (b) 125,672 (c) 297,113

14. Calculate each of the following in ppm:

    (a) 625 Hz at 120 MHz (b) 1475 Hz at 90 MHz
    (c) 432 Hz at 60 MHz (d) 2122 Hz at 500 MHz

15. For the following pairs of signals, identify which one will absorb further upfield.

    (a) HC—Br HC—NR_2 (b) H—C=O H—C—C=O
    (c) O=C—O—H C=C—C—H (d) C≡C—H C=C—H

16. Identify all magnetically equivalent hydrogens in each molecule.

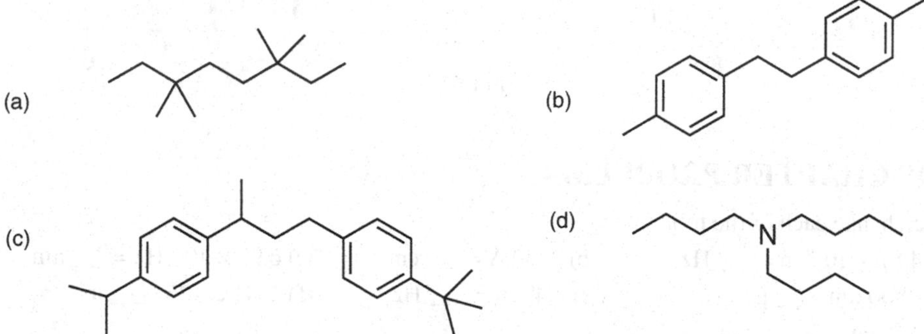

17. For each nmr signal indicate how many neighboring hydrogens it will have.

    (a) a pentet (b) a triplet (c) a septet (d) a singlet (e) a quartet

18. What is the actual signal for a hydrogen with three neighbors (J = 12.0 Hz) and also two neighbors (coupling constant 8.0 Hz)?

19. Give the chemical structure for each of the following based on the spectra provided.

    (a) $C_8H_{14}O_2$. Infrared stretching frequencies: 3350–2400 (bd, strong), 1675 (s), 1338–1220 (bd, strong), 996, 921, 683 cm^{-1}

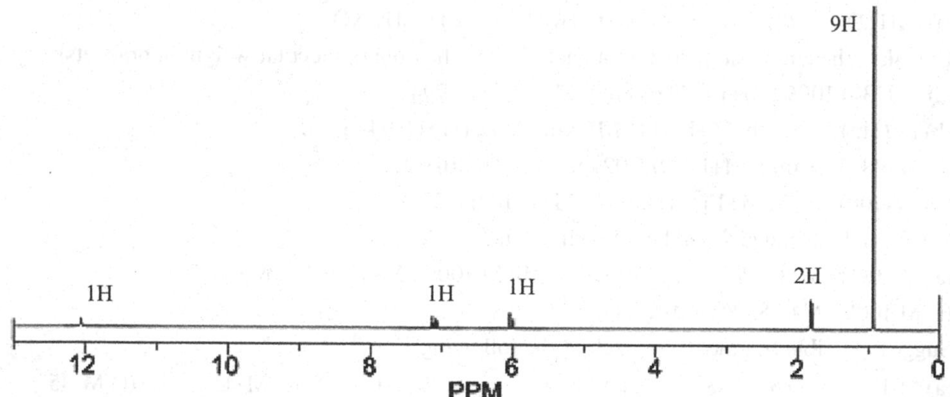

(b) $C_6H_{13}NO$. Infrared stretching frequencies: 2933, 2770, 1613, 813 cm^{-1}

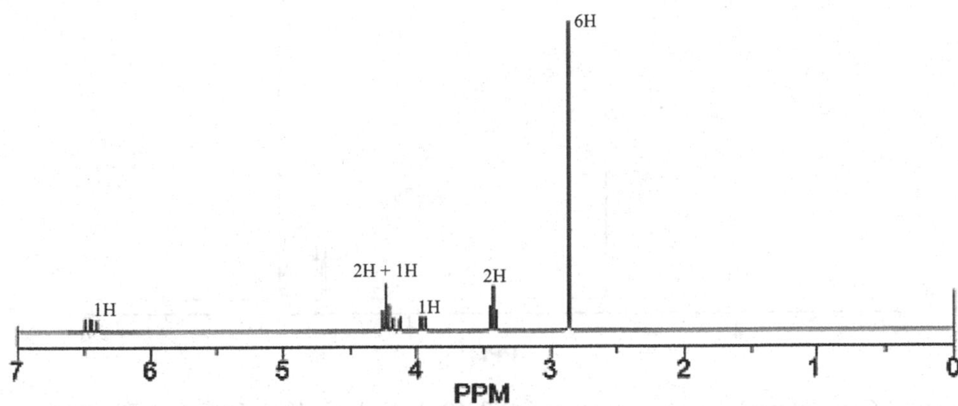

(c) $C_{10}H_{12}O$. Infrared stretching frequencies: 2950, 1721 (s), 1105, 735 695 cm^{-1}

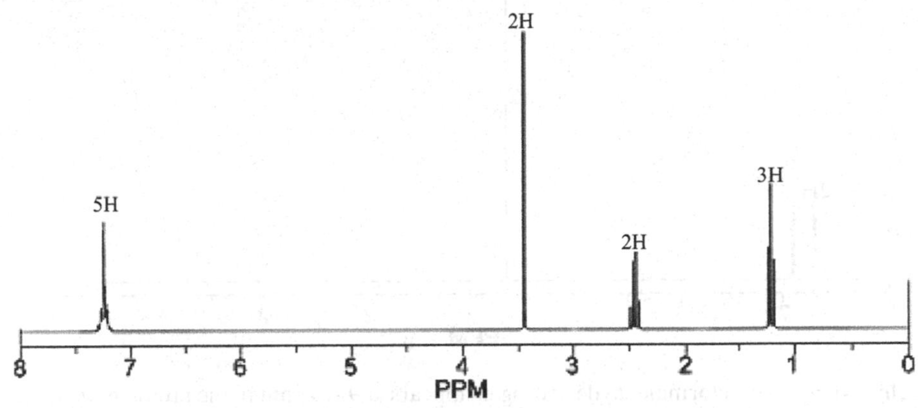

(d) $C_7H_{14}O_2$. Infrared stretching frequencies: 2941, 2833 (w), 1718 (s) 1366, 1220, 1079 cm^{-1}

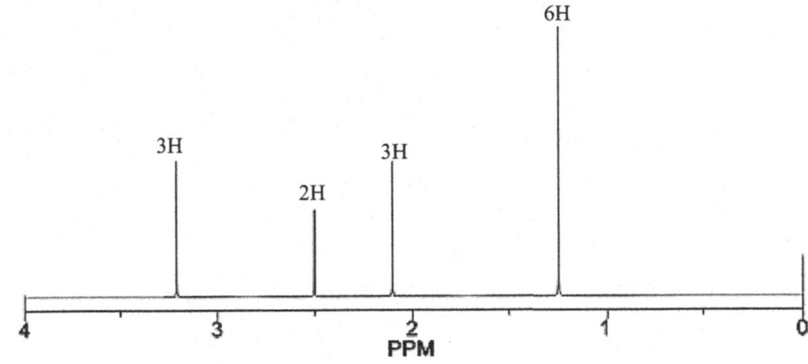

(e) $C_7H_{16}O_2$. Infrared stretching frequencies: 3448 (s), 2941, 1160, 1078, 833 cm^{-1}

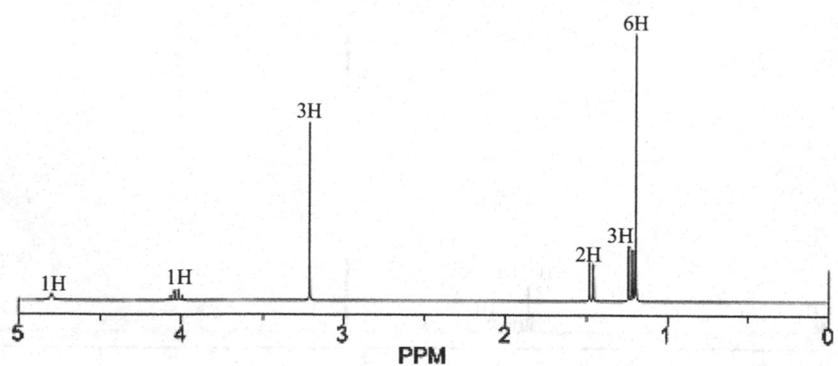

(f) C_8H_6ClN. Infrared stretching frequencies: 2262, 1493, 1412, 1071, 1015, 833, 794 cm^{-1}

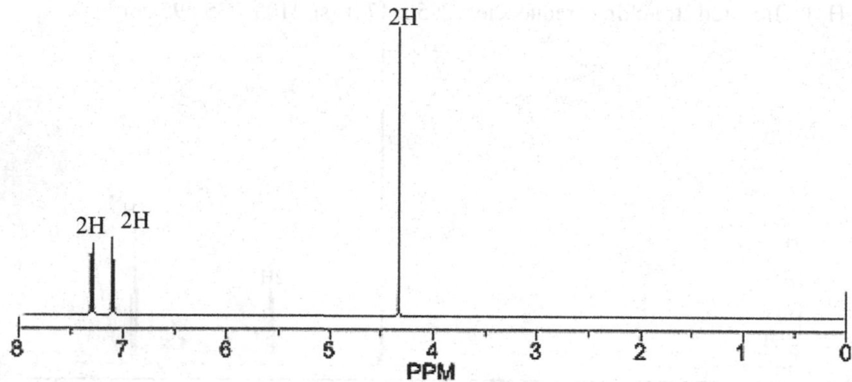

20. Briefly explain why a formaldehyde hydrogen appears at 9–10 ppm in the proton nmr while the hydrogen attached to carbon in an alcohol (the H—C—OH unit) appears at about 3.5 ppm. In other words, why is the aldehyde signal so far downfield?

12

Aldehydes and Ketones. Acyl Addition Reactions

Ketones and aldehydes, along with alkenes and alcohols, are among the most common and most used class of organic molecules. The carbonyl group (C=O) can be formed from alcohols by a variety of oxidative methods. The importance of ketones and aldehydes lies in the ability of nucleophilic reagents to add to the electrophilic carbon of the carbonyl, generating new carbon–carbon bonds. Many of the most important carbon–carbon bond forming reactions known in organic chemistry are based on reactions of aldehydes or ketones. The chemical and physical properties of carbonyl compounds will be discussed, along with methods for their preparation and their transformation into other molecules.

12.1 STRUCTURE AND NOMENCLATURE OF ALDEHYDES AND KETONES

What is a carbonyl?

The carbonyl group, C=O, is the main structural and reactive feature of aldehydes and ketones. A ketone has two carbon groups on either side of the carbonyl [R(C=O)R] whereas an aldehyde has at least one hydrogen attached to the carbonyl [R(C=O)H].

How can a carbon–carbon double bond be contrasted and compared with a carbon–oxygen double bond?

The double bond of an alkene is very similar to that of a carbonyl in that there is a weak π-bond and a strong σ-bond. The carbonyl is polarized, however, due to the presence of the oxygen ($C^{\delta+}$ and $O^{\delta-}$), and the C=C unit of an alkene is not polarized. This difference leads to significant differences in reactivity since nucleophiles will attack the electropositive carbon of the carbonyl. Such chemistry is not possible with an alkene.

What is the generic structure of an aldehyde? Of a ketone?

An aldehyde has at least one hydrogen attached to the carbonyl carbon, as shown in the figure. This structure is usually abbreviated as RCHO. A ketone has two carbon groups attached to the carbonyl carbon.

$$\mathrm{R^1(H)C{=}O} \qquad \mathrm{R^1(R^2)C{=}O}$$

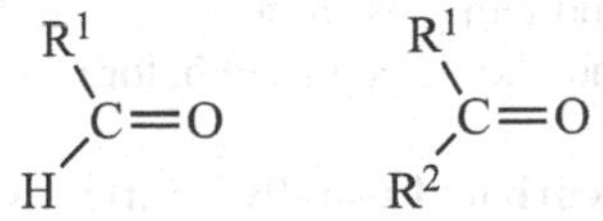

An Aldehyde   A Ketone

What is the name of the only aldehyde with two hydrogens attached to the carbonyl group?

The name is formaldehyde (HCHO). In the monomeric form, formaldehyde exists as a gas, but in the solid state or in solution it is can but also exists as a trimer [$(CH_2O)_3$] and as a solid polymer, paraformaldehyde [$(CH_2O)_n$].

What is a reasonable structure for $H_2C{=}O$?

As shown in the figure, a carbonyl consists of a C=O unit with one strong σ-bond and a weak π-bond. The geometry of the carbonyl is trigonal planar, and the bond angles are about 120°. The two attached hydrogen atoms are coplanar with the C and O. The lone electron pairs on oxygen are also in the same plane as the atoms but the electrons of the π-bond are perpendicular to the plane of the atoms.

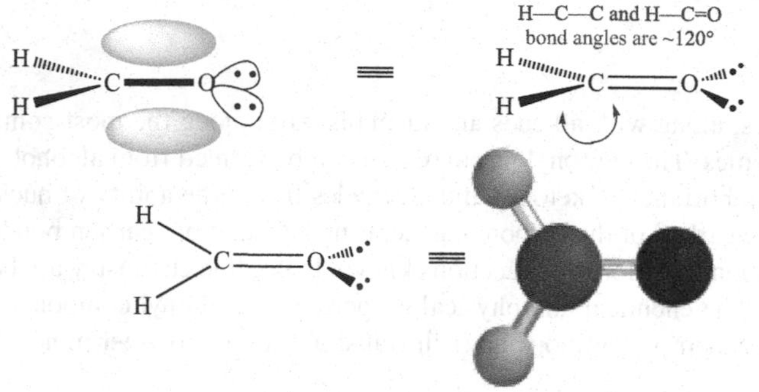

H—C—C and H—C=O
bond angles are ~120°

Which is more reactive, an aldehyde or a ketone? Explain!

An aldehyde is usually more reactive. There is less steric hindrance to approach of a reagent to the electropositive carbonyl since there is at least one hydrogen and only one carbon group (H is less sterically hindered than any alkyl or aryl group).

What are the generic IUPAC rules for naming aldehydes or ketones?

The longest continuous chain of carbons must contain the carbonyl carbon, so the carbonyl carbon is always C1 for an aldehyde. The carbonyl carbon of a ketone is assigned the lowest possible number. Substituents attached to the carbon chain of an aldehyde or ketone are numbered based on the carbonyl carbon and thereafter the normal rules of nomenclature apply. The suffix for an aldehyde is -al and the suffix for a ketone is -one.

What is the base name for an aldehyde?

The IUPAC name for an aldehyde uses the alkane, alkene, or alkyne prefix with the ending -al. Drop the (-e) ending and add -al, as in hexanal, hexenal, or hexynal.

What is the base name for a ketone?

The IUPAC name for a ketone uses the alkane, alkene, or alkyne prefix with the ending -one. The carbonyl carbon is assigned the lowest number possible and the number is placed before the -one suffix. Drop the (-e) ending and add -one, and name as in hexan-2-one, hex-3-en-2-one and hex-4-yn-2-one. Note that the number for the alkene and alkyne is placed before the -en- or the -yn-.

Why is the position number of the carbonyl usually omitted with an aldehyde but not with a ketone?

Since the carbonyl (C=O) is the functional group, the carbon of the carbonyl receives the lowest possible number as part of the longest continuous chain. Aldehydes always contain at least one hydrogen attached to the carbonyl carbon so it *must* be C1. For this reason, the number is usually omitted. The carbonyl carbon of a ketone can appear at many sites along the longest chain and, therefore, must be identified with a number.

What are the correct IUPAC names for (a), (b), (c), and (d)?

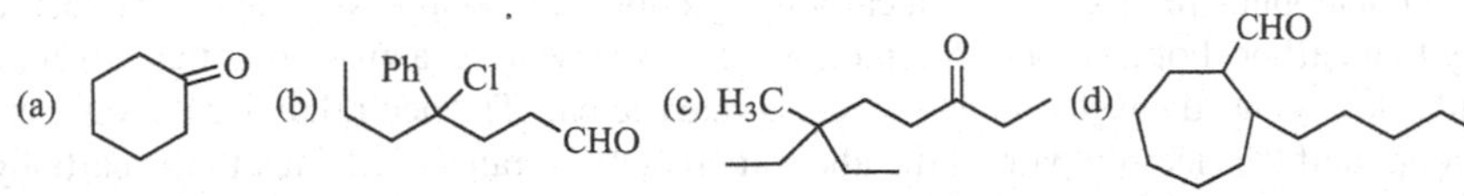

(a) (b) Ph Cl CHO (c) H_3C O (d) CHO

The name of (a) is cyclohexanone. For (b), this aldehyde is named 4-chloro-4-phenylheptanal. Ketone (c) is named 6-ethyl-6-methyloctan-3-one. *When an aldehyde is attached to a ring, the naming system is changed, and the aldehyde is named as a cycloalkyl carbaldehyde.* The parent aldehyde of (d) is cycloheptane carbaldehyde, but it has a hexyl substituent at C2. The name of (d) is, therefore, 2-hexyl-cylcoheptane carbaldehyde.

How are phenyl alkyl ketones named with the IUPAC system?

When the phenyl group is attached to C1, the ketone is named normally with the expectation that the carbonyl carbon is C1. An example is 1-phenylpropan-1-one (see the following problem). If the phenyl group is not attached to C1, the C_6H_5 unit is treated as a substituent and named as phenyl.

What is the IUPAC name of (a), (b) and (c)?

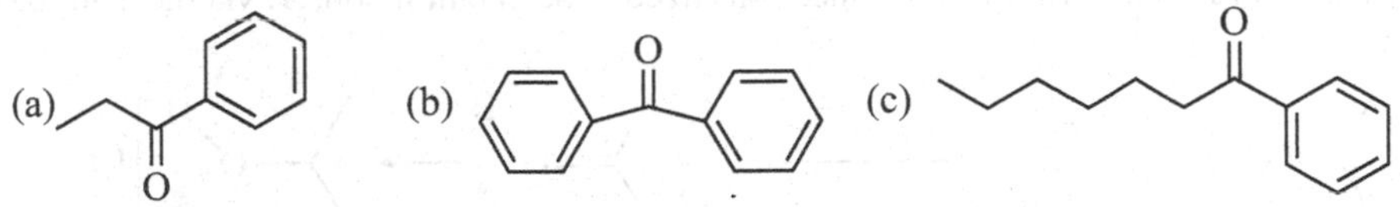

(a) O (b) O (c) O

1-phenylpropan-1-one (propiophenone) 1,1-diphenylmethanone (benzophenone) 1-phenylheptan-1-one

The IUPAC name of (a) is 1-phenylpropan-1-one, but the common name is propiophenone. In (b), both phenyl groups are attached to a single carbon, so it is a methanone, and the IUPAC name is 1,1-diphenyl-methanone. However, this compound is well-known by the common name, which is benzophenone. In (c), the long chain precludes a simple or common name. This example illustrates why the IUPAC name is necessary; the IUPAC name of (c) is 1-phenylheptan-1-one.

12.2 REACTION OF ALDEHYDES AND KETONES WITH WEAK NUCLEOPHILES

What is the major reaction of the carbonyl group in aldehydes and in ketones that involves carbon?

Nucleophilic acyl addition.

What is nucleophilic acyl addition?

Aldehydes and ketones react primarily by the polarized carbonyl group. This reaction involves the addition of a nucleophile to the carbon of a carbonyl, accompanied by cleavage of the π-bond to form an alkoxide. The most common reactions are nucleophilic acyl addition to the carbonyl and acid–base reactions involving protonation of the carbonyl oxygen to form an oxocarbenium ion.

What is a convenient classification of nucleophiles for reactions of aldehydes and ketones?

There are weak nucleophiles that tend to add reversibly to carbonyl groups and strong nucleophiles that tend to react irreversibly to give an alkoxide product.

Does water react with a ketone such as acetone?

Water is a weak nucleophile in reactions with carbonyl groups. This weakness is due to the fact that water adds reversibly to a carbonyl of a ketone. Addition would give rise to ***A***, a zwitterion that is very unstable, and the alkoxide "kicks out" the water moiety to regenerate acetone. The neutral molecule water is an excellent leaving group, and the electron pair on the alkoxide moiety is transferred back to the carbonyl carbon with concomitant expulsion of water. In other words, water does not react with acetone to give an isolable product but only acetone is observed in the reaction medium, so there is no reaction to give a product.

OH_2 H A

Apart from nucleophilic acyl addition, what is another major reaction of the carbonyl group?

The oxygen atom of a carbonyl is electron rich and can react as a base with a suitable acid: the carbonyl oxygen reacts as a Brønsted–Lowry base with a protonic acid such as HCl or H_2SO_4, and as a Lewis base with a suitable Lewis acid such as BF_3.

What initial product is formed with propane-2-one (acetone) reacts with H_2SO_4?

Acetone reacts with HCl to form the resonance stabilized oxocarbenium ion, ***A***, via the acid–base reaction shown.

O H—Cl H O+ + O H Cl^- A

What is an oxocarbenium ion?

An oxocarbenium ion, illustrated by ***A*** in the preceding question, is a carbocation attached to an oxygen atom that is resonance stabilized as shown. An oxocarbenium ion is very reactive since there is significant positive character on the carbon, reacting with even weak nucleophiles.

When a catalytic amount of a Brønsted–Lowry acid is added to aqueous acetone, a product can be detected but not isolated. What is the product?

In the presence of an acid catalyst, water adds to the carbonyl of acetone to form a *hydrate*, propane-2,2-diol. This hydrate is unstable and regenerates acetone, but it can be detected as a transient product. Indeed, the presumed product of this reaction is a hydrate, but it is very unstable and loses water to revert back to acetone. In general ketones and aldehydes are in equilibrium with a hydrate and the equilibrium favors the carbonyl form.

O cat. H^+, H_2O HO OH

propane-2,2-diol

What is a hydrate?

A hydrate is the product of the reaction of water with an aldehyde or ketone. Formally, it has the structure $R_2C(OH)_2$, with two OH units on the carbonyl carbon atom.

What is the mechanism of reaction between acetone and water with a catalytic amount of acid present? What is the product called?

The mechanism of reaction involves initial protonation of the carbonyl oxygen with a proton of the acid to give an oxocarbenium ion ***A***, which is resonance stabilized. The carbon of an oxocarbenium ion is electropositive and readily reacts with nucleophiles, even weak nucleophiles. The reactive oxocarbenium ion reacts with water to give oxonium ion ***B***. This intermediate loses a proton to give the hydrate. Hydrates are rather unstable and in the presence of an acidic medium, one of the oxygen atoms is protonated to give ***B***, and loss of water regenerates ***A*** and thereby the starting ketone, acetone.

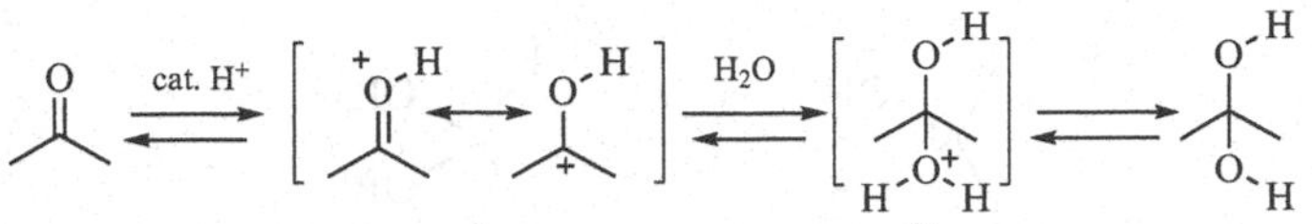

Why is it not possible to isolate most hydrates?

Hydrates are in equilibrium with the carbonyl precursor. The two OH groups withdraw a significant amount of electron density from the central carbon, destabilizing it. Hydrates are usually formed in acidic media, and the acid readily protonates an oxygen, which leads to loss of water and regeneration of the carbonyl precursor.

Why is chloral hydrate a stable product that can be isolated?

Choral hydrate (2,2,2-trichloroethane-1,1-diol) is the hydrate of choral (2,2,2-trichloroethanal). There are no β-hydrogens that allow loss of water. In addition, the chlorines withdraw electrons from the α-carbon which, in turn, pulls electrons from the carbonyl carbon. The carbonyl carbon withdraws electrons from both oxygens of the C—O bonds, strengthening those bonds and stabilizing the hydrate (the equilibrium is shifted in favor of the hydrate). In general, hydrates are stable enough to be isolated only when strongly electron-withdrawing groups are attached to the α-carbon of the ketone or aldehyde and there are no hydrogen atoms on the carbons attached to the carbonyl carbon.

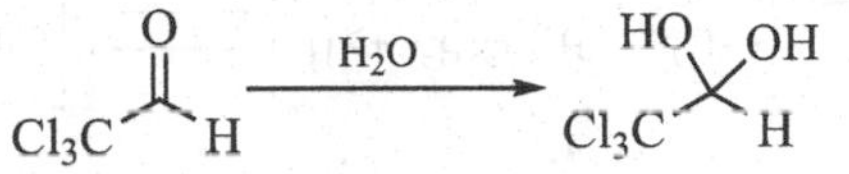

2,2,2-trichloroacetaldehyde 2,2,2-trichloroethane-1,1-diol

Alcohols are weak nucleophiles in reactions with carbonyls. Can the products be isolated?

Yes! Alcohols can add to a carbonyl to give a product known as an acetal, but the reaction usually requires an acid catalyst.

What is the product when butanal is reacted with an excess of ethanol in the presence of a catalytic amount of sulfuric acid?

This reaction is analogous to the hydrate-forming reaction, but due to a reactive intermediate the reaction takes a different course. Rather than water, the alcohol (ethanol) is the nucleophilic species, leading to a geminal diethoxy compound called an acetal, formed by the addition of two equivalents of ethanol to the aldehyde carbonyl. In this case, the acetal of butanal is 1,1-diethoxybutane.

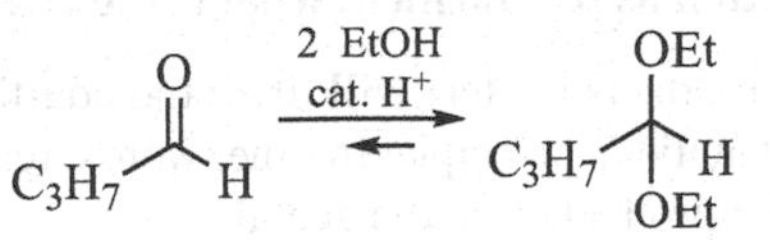

1,1-diethoxybutane

What is an acetal?

An acetal has the structure $R_2C(OR')_2$, and it the product of the reaction of two equivalents of an alcohol with an aldehyde or ketone, with acid catalysis.

What is a hemiacetal?

A hemiacetal has the structure $R_2COH(OR')$. A hemiacetal is formed by the reaction of one equivalent of an aldehyde or ketone with an alcohol. However, a hemiacetal is not stable to the acidic reaction conditions and loses a molecule of water that allows reaction with a second equivalent of an alcohol to give an acetal.

hemiacetal acetal

What is a ketal?

The nomenclature of these compounds originally classified an acetal as the product of an alcohol with an aldehyde $[RHC(OR')_2]$ and a ketal as the product of an alcohol with a ketone $[R_2C(OR')_2]$. Nowadays, the term acetal applies to the product of both an aldehyde or a ketone and the term ketal is considered to be a subclass of an acetal.

What is the complete mechanism for the reaction of butanal with ethanol to give an acetal?

Initial protonation of butanal gives oxocarbenium ion ***A***, which adds ethanol to give oxonium ion ***B***. Loss of a proton generates ***C***, which is called a *hemiacetal.* If ***C*** reacts with a proton, ***B*** can be formed again since the reaction is reversible and this reversible process will regenerate the aldehyde. However, if the OH group in ***C*** is protonated, the product is oxonium ion ***D***. Oxonium ion ***D*** can lose water (remember that neutral water is a good leaving group) to generate a new resonance-stabilized oxocarbenium ion ***E***. Addition of a second molecule of ethanol gives oxocarbenium ion ***E*** and loss of a proton from this intermediate completes the sequence to give the acetal, 1,1,-diethoxybutane. *This entire multi-step mechanism is reversible in every step.*

If water is removed from this reaction as it is formed, what is the effect on the reaction?

The removal of one of the reaction products (water) will drive the equilibrium toward the right, to the acetal product, consistent with Le Châtelier's principle. In other words, removal of the water product will shift the equilibrium toward the other product, here the acetal.

What is Le Châtelier's principle?

The principle is stated as: If a chemical equilibrium is disturbed by changing the conditions of concentration, temperature, volume, or pressure, the position of equilibrium moves to counteract the change.

What are some methods that can be used to remove water from a reaction?

Drying agents such as calcium chloride ($CaCl_2$) or magnesium sulfate ($MgSO_4$) can be added, although these are not very efficient. A zeolite (molecular sieve) can be added that has a pore size sufficiently large to accommodate water but not the larger organic molecules present in the mixture. The molecular sieves most commonly used are molecular sieves 3Å and 4Å. Another method for removing water is the use of a Dean-Stark trap. This glass apparatus relies on azeotropic distillation (ethanol-water mixtures form an *azeotrope*, which is a constant boiling mixture of the two liquids boiling lower than each individual liquid. The azeotropic distillate is a fixed ratio of the two liquids. The Dean–Stark trap relies on a mixture of a solvent (such as benzene) in which water is mostly insoluble, but with which it forms an azeotrope. The azeotropic mixture distills off and is collected, the water sinks to the bottom (it is denser than benzene), and the benzene eventually overflows back into the reaction vessel. The water collected in this manner is removed from the reaction.

What is a Dean–Stark trap?

A Dean–Stark trap is an apparatus for separating water from an azeotropic mixture. The boiling mixture condenses and is returned to a trap rather than the boiling flask. As the distillate collects in the trap, two layers separate and if water is one layer, it separates on the bottom of the trap and can be removed. The other liquid is insoluble in water and collects at the top of the trap. Once the trap is full, the water-insoluble liquid spills back into the boiling flask. In this way the apparatus allows azeotropic separation and removal of water.

What is an azeotrope?

An azeotrope is a constant boiling mixture of liquids because the vapor has the same composition as the liquid mixture. An example is water, ethanol, and benzene

What is the azeotrope of ethanol and water?

The mixture of ethanol (bp, 78.4°C) and water (bp, 100°C) forms a 95.6 ethanol:4.4 water azeotrope that boils at 78.1°C.

What is the ternary azeotrope of cyclohexane, ethanol, and water?

The mixture of cyclohexane (bp, 177.8°C), ethanol (bp, 78.4°C), and water (bp, 100°C) forms a 7(water):17 (ethanol): 76 (cyclohexane) ternary azeotrope mixture that boils at 61.1°C.

What solvents are commonly used in a Dean–Stark trap to remove water as an azeotropic mixture?

Common solvents are benzene, toluene, and cyclohexane.

What is the product when an acetal is reacted with aqueous acid where water is present in large excess?

The reaction described in a preceding question to form an acetal is completely reversible in every step. If water is removed from the reaction, the equilibrium is shifted toward the acetal. However, in the presence of a large excess of water, the equilibrium shifts back toward the carbonyl compound. The consequence of adding a large excess of water to an acetal is to remove the acetal group, shifting the equilibrium back to the carbonyl group. Using the mechanism shown in the preceding question, replace ethanol with water as the reagent and lose ethanol rather than water, and the equilibrium shifts toward the aldehyde.

What is the product when acetal 1,1-dimethoxyhexane is heated with aqueous acid?

The product is hexanal along with two equivalents of methanol via hydrolysis of the acetal.

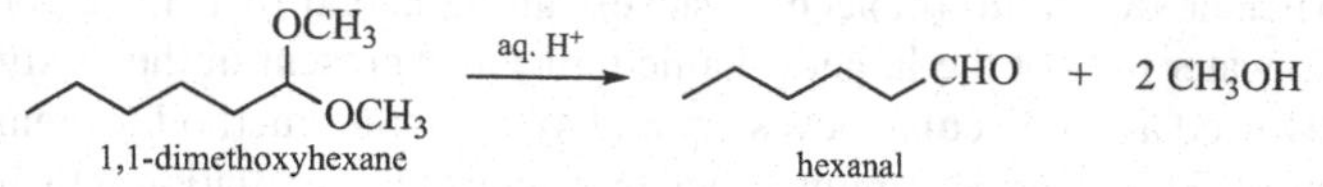

1,1-dimethoxyhexane —(aq. H^+)→ hexanal (CHO) + 2 CH_3OH

What is the product when butanal is treated with 1,2-ethanediol and a catalytic amount of acid?

In this case, the two alcohol units are part of the same molecule. In the mechanism given in a preceding question for acetal formation, one OH unit adds to the carbonyl carbon while the second OH is part of the same molecule. Intramolecular attack of the second OH unit on the electrophilic carbon leads to a cyclic acetal called a 1,3-dioxolane. In this reaction, the product is 2-propyl-1,3-dioxolane.

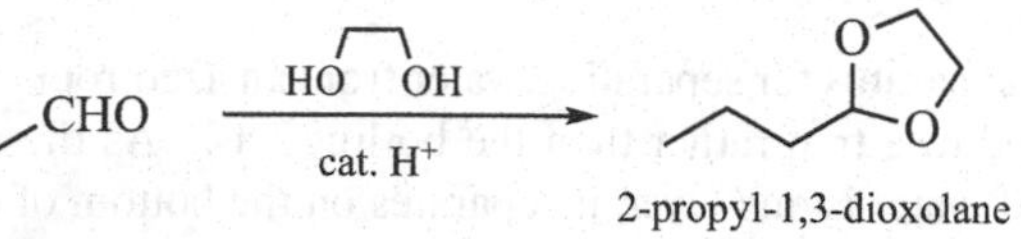

CHO —(HO OH, cat. H^+)→ 2-propyl-1,3-dioxolane

What is a dioxolane?

A dioxolane is a cyclic acetal: a five-membered ring with two oxygen atoms in a 1,3-relationship.

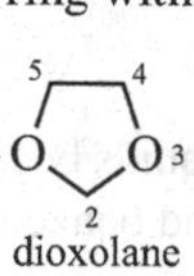

dioxolane

What is the mechanism and final product of the acid-catalyzed reaction of butanal with ethane-1,2-diol?

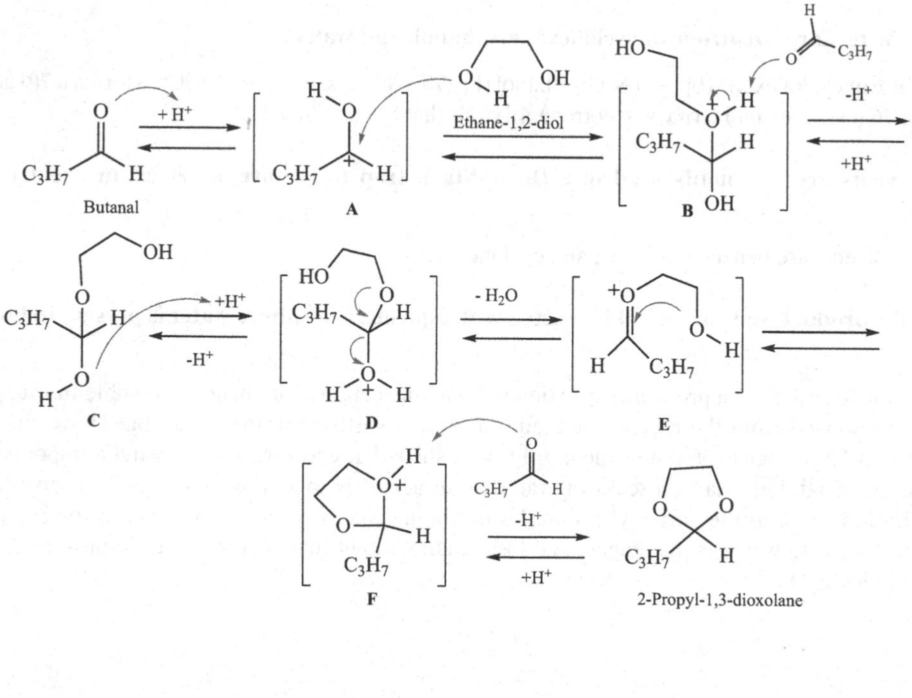

Butanal; A; Ethane-1,2-diol; B; C; D; E; F; 2-Propyl-1,3-dioxolane

The initial reaction of butanal with the acid catalyst leads to the oxocarbenium ion, ***A***, which reacts with ethanediol to give oxonium ion ***B***. Loss of a proton leads to the hemiacetal, ***C***. Protonation of the OH unit gives oxonium ion D and loss of water leads to oxocarbenium ion ***E***. The intramolecular reaction of the OH unit gives oxonium ion **F**, and loss of the proton gives the final product, the acetal: 2-propyl-1,3-dioxolane.

What is the product when pentan-2-one reacts with an excess of propanol in the presence of a catalytic amount of p-toluenesulfonic acid?

The product is 2,2-dipropoxypentane.

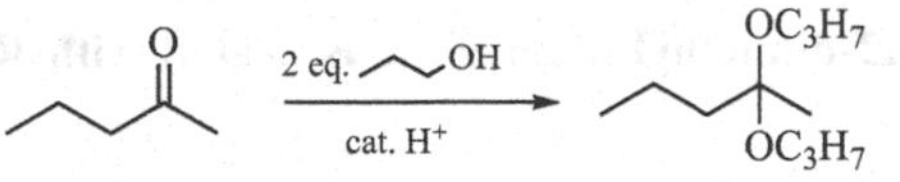

2 eq. OH, cat. H^+ → OC_3H_7 / OC_3H_7

2,2-dipropoxypentane

What is the product when cyclohexanone is treated with 1,2-ethanediol and a catalytic amount of acid?

As with dioxolane formation from the reaction of diols with aldehydes, ketones also form dioxolanes upon treatment with ethylene glycol (1,2-ethanediol). The acetal product is named 1,4-dioxaspiro[4,5] decane.

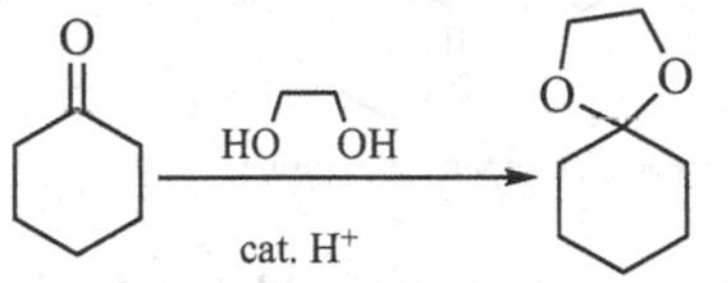

HO OH, cat. H^+ →

1,4-dioxaspiro[4.5]decane

What is the structure of a thiol?

A thiol (R–SH) is the sulfur analog of an alcohol with the functional group –SH. Thiols are named by taking the hydrocarbon name and adding the word thiol to it. The thiol $CH_3CH_2CH_2SH$ is, for example, propane-1-thiol and CH_3SH is methanethiol.

What is a common name for thiols?

The common name for these compounds is *mercaptan*. The thiol CH_3SH is named methyl mercaptan.

How should a thiol react?

Since sulfur is in Group 16, just under oxygen, a sulfur compound should behave similarly to an oxygen compound. A thiol should react, more or less, in a manner similar to an alcohol, at least in reactions with carbonyl derivatives.

What is the product when cyclopentanone is treated with an excess of ethanethiol and a catalytic amount of acid?

The product is a dithioketal, 1,1-diethylthiocycopentane, exactly analogous to formation of an acetal from treatment with an alcohol.

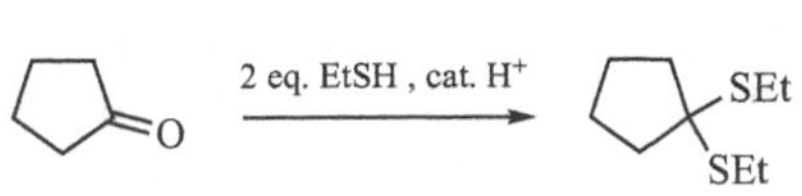

2 eq. EtSH , cat. H^+ → SEt / SEt

What is the product when pentanal is treated with 1,3-propanedithiol in the presence of a catalytic amount of acid?

The product of propane-1,3-dithiol and pentanal is a cyclic dithioacetal, 2-butyl-1,3-dithiane, exactly analogous to formation of an acetal from treatment with a cyclic diol. Six-membered rings with two sulfur atoms are called 1,3-dithianes.

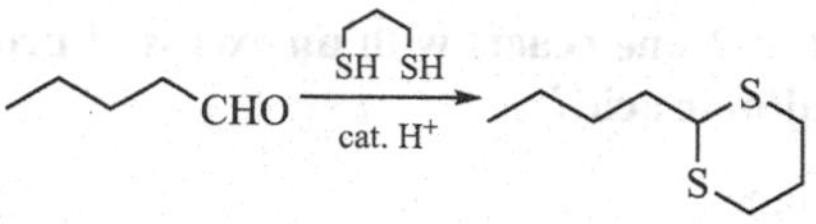

What is the product when 2,2-di(methylthio)hexane is heated with Raney nickel in acetone? Explain!

Raney nickel is specially prepared and has a considerable amount of hydrogen adsorbed on the surface of the finely divided nickel. Nickel has a strong affinity for sulfur. When a dithioketal is treated with this reagent, complete removal of the sulfur (desulfurization) occurs, with reduction (see Chapter 14) to a -CH_2- group. In this case, the final product is the alkane, hexane.

What is an imine?

An imine is an organic molecule that has a C=N unit, such as that in (*E*)-*N*-ethylpentane-2-imine.

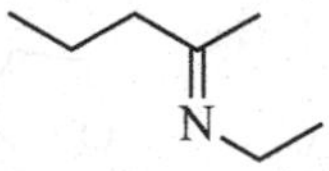

(*E*)-*N*-ethylpentan-2-imine

What is the product formed when pentan-2-one reacts with butylamine and an acid catalyst?

In general, when a ketone or aldehyde reacts with a *primary amine*, the product is an imine. In this case, butan-2-one reacts to give (*E*)-*N*-butylpentan-2-imine.

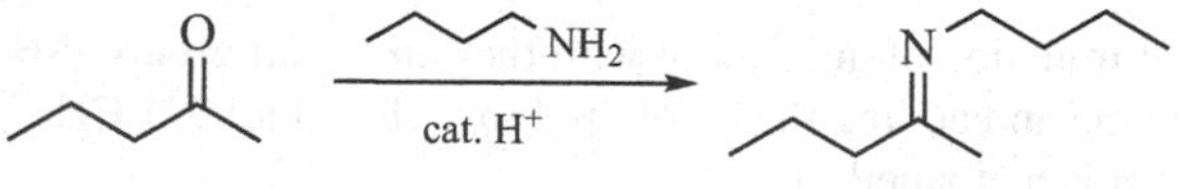

(*E*)-*N*-butylpentan-2-imine

What is the mechanism and final product of the acid-catalyzed reaction of acetone with methylamine?

The reaction of acetone with the acid catalyst gives oxocarbenium ion ***A***, which reacts with methylamine to give cation ***B***. Loss of a proton leads to the amino-alcohol, 2-methylamino)propan-2-ol. The reaction of the acidic catalyst with the OH unit leads to oxonium ion ***C***, which loses water to form iminium salt, ***D***. Loss of the proton from the nitrogen leads to the neutral product, the imine: N-(propan-2-ylidene) methanamine.

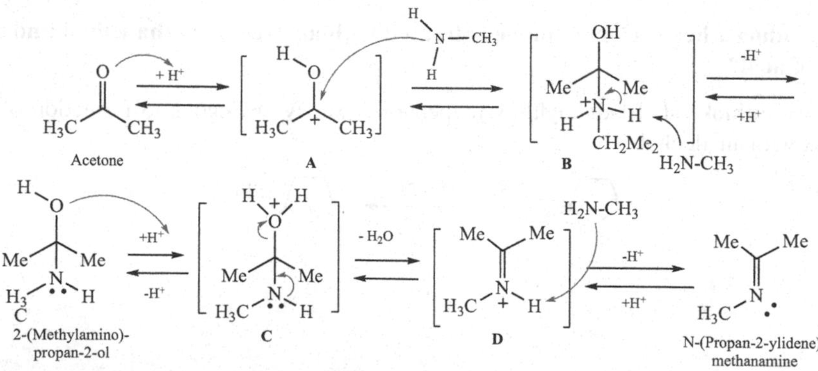

Is butylamine a primary or a secondary amine? What is the difference?

Butylamine is a primary amine. A primary amine has only one carbon group attached to nitrogen and two hydrogen atoms (RNH_2). A secondary amine has two carbon groups attached to nitrogen and only one hydrogen atom.

What is an enamine?

An enamine is a molecule that has an amino group (NR_2) attached directly to a carbon–carbon double bond. This particular example is the diethylamino enamine of pentan-2-one, named *N,N*-diethylpent-1-en-2-amine.

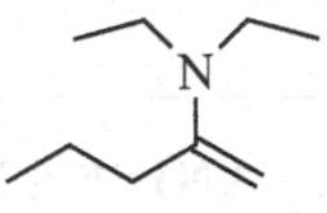

N,N-diethylpent-1-en-2-amine

How are enamines formed?

Enamines such as *N,N*-diethylpent-1-en-2-amine are formed by reaction of a ketone with a *secondary amine* (HNR_2), usually in the presence of an acid catalyst. In this case, pentan-2-one reacts with N,-diethylamine.

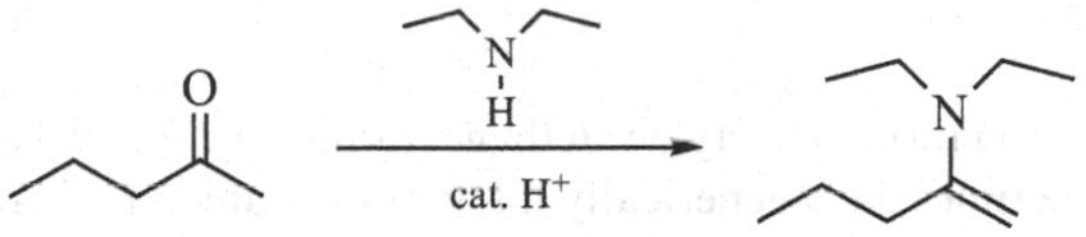

cat. H^+

N,N-diethylpent-1-en-2-amine

Give the mechanism for the reaction of pentane-3-one and diethylamine in the presence of a catalytic amount of acid.

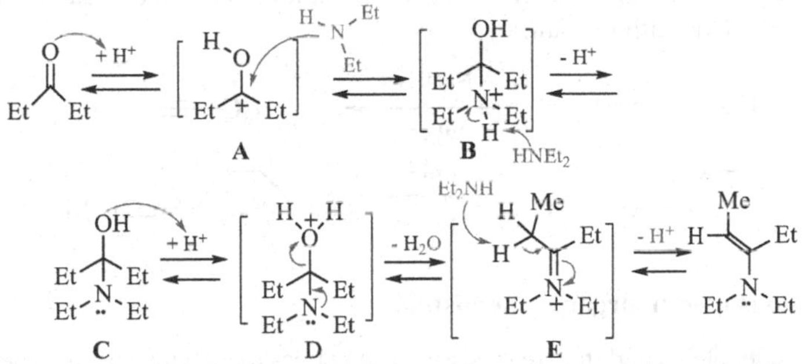

The reaction begins by formation of the oxocarbenium ion, ***A***, by reaction with the acid catalyst. Diethylamine adds to the electrophilic carbon to give ***B*** and loss of the proton gives the amino alcohol ***C***. Reprotonation of the amine leads back to the carbonyl in a reversible process, but protonation of the OH group to give oxonium ion ***D*** allows expulsion of water by the electron pair on the amine to give iminium salt ***E***. Excess amine or even water can remove the hydrogen as H^+ to give the final enamine product. This is a general mechanism for the reaction of secondary amines and ketones.

Why does a primary amine react with a ketone to give an imine and a secondary amine reacts to give an enamine?

Using the mechanism presented in the preceding question, a primary reacts to give an iminium salt, such as ***A***, that has a hydrogen atom attached to nitrogen. Conversely, a secondary amine reacts to give an iminium salt, such as ***B***, where there is no hydrogen atom attached to nitrogen. In the final step, a hydrogen atom is lost from the nitrogen atom of the iminium salt (the proton from ***A***) and the product is an imine. In ***B***, there is no hydrogen on the nitrogen of this iminium salt to remove, but there are hydrogen atoms on carbon and loss of a hydrogen leads to the enamine.

N-(1-Methylethyl)-propan-2-imine

(E)-N,N-Diethylpent-2-en-3-amine

12.3 REACTIONS OF ALDEHYDES AND KETONES. STRONG NUCLEOPHILES

What is a strong nucleophile?

A strong nucleophile reacts with a carbonyl via acyl addition to give a stable alkoxide product in an essentially non-reversible reaction. The most common strong nucleophiles in this book are carbon nucleophiles.

What is an acetylide?

Acetylide is formally the carbanion form of acetylene (ethyne) formed by removal of a hydrogen atom by base. The term acetylide is sometimes used generically for an alkyne anion R–C≡C:⁻.

How are alkyne anions formed?

The hydrogen atom of a terminal alkyne is acidic with a pK_a of about 25. When reacted with a strong base, such as $NaNH_2$ or butyllithium, a terminal alkyne reacts to form an alkyne anion. Examples are the reaction of prop-1-yne with $NaNH_2$ to give prop-1-yne sodium salt, and the reaction of hex-1-yne with butyllithium to give hex-1-yne lithium salt.

$$H_3C-C\equiv C-H \xrightarrow[\text{Ether}]{NaNH_2} H_3C-C\equiv C:^- Na^+$$

$$\text{hex-1-yne} \xrightarrow[\text{Ether}]{BuLi} \text{hex-1-ynyl}:^- Li^+$$

How are alkyne anions used in organic chemistry?

Alkyne anions are nucleophiles and they react with alkyl halides to give internal alkynes. Alkyne anions also react as a nucleophile with aldehydes or ketones to give an acyl addition product, the alkoxide.

What is acyl addition?

Acyl addition is the reaction of a nucleophile (Nuc) with the electrophilic carbon of a carbonyl (C=O) to give an alkoxide product, Nuc–C—O⁻.

What is the product when the sodium salt of ethyne (acetylene) reacts with pentan-2-one?

When the sodium salt of ethyne (Na⁺⁻C≡CH) reacts with pentan-2-one, the nucleophilic acetylide attacks the electropositive carbonyl carbon to produce an alkoxide, the sodium salt of 3-methylhex-1-yn-3-ol.

What is the product when the sodium salt of ethyne (acetylene) reacts with pentan-2-one followed by hydrolysis in a second step?

When the sodium salt of ethyne ($Na^+ \, ^-C{\equiv}CH$) reacts with pentan-2-one, the nucleophilic acetylide attacks the electropositive carbonyl carbon to produce an alkoxide. Hydrolysis liberates the alcohol product, 3-methylhex-1-yn-3-ol.

What is the product when pent-1-yne reacts first with butyllithium, then with benzaldehyde, and finally with dilute aqueous acid?

The terminal alkyne reacts with butyllithium to give the alkyne anion, which reacts with benzaldehyde to give the acyl addition product. Hydrolysis of the alkoxide product gives the final product, 1-phenylhex-2-yn-1-ol.

1. BuLi, THF
2. CHO
3. dil. aq. H^+

1-phenylhex-2-yn-1-ol

Why is this type of reaction important in organic chemistry?

It is important because it is one of the chemical reactions that forms a new carbon–carbon bond. In addition, the product contains other functionality that will allow further chemical transformations. In this case, two functional groups, an alcohol and an alkyne, are introduced into the same molecule.

What is a Grignard reagent?

A Grignard reagent is an organomagnesium compound, RMgX, formed by the reaction of magnesium metal with an alkyl halide (see Section 10.2).

What characteristics of a Grignard reagent are pertinent to reactions with aldehydes or ketones?

Grignard reagents have polarization $^{\delta-}C{-}Mg^{\delta+}$, so the carbon reacts as a carbon nucleophile with an aldehyde or a ketone.

What is the product when 1-bromobutane reacts with magnesium in diethyl ether? What is the name of this product?

The product is a Grignard reagent, butylmagnesium bromide, $CH_3CH_2CH_2CH_2MgBr$.

What is the role of the ether in this reaction?

The ether solvent acts as a Lewis base, donating electrons to the electron deficient magnesium, assisting formation of the Grignard reagent in the insertion reaction of the metal between C—Br, and also stabilizing the organomagnesium compound once it is formed.

What product results from the reaction of methylmagnesium bromide and acetone (propan-2-one)?

In the first step, the nucleophilic carbon of the Grignard reagent attacks the δ^+ carbon of the ketone (acetone). When the $C^{\delta-}$and $C^{\delta+}$ collide, the π-bond of the carbonyl is broken and those two electrons are transferred to the more electronegative oxygen, making the alkoxide ***A***, which is the product of the reaction. A second step is required in which aqueous acid is added to ***A*** to protonate the alkoxide and generate the alcohol product (*hydrolysis*). The final product is therefore 2-methylpropan-2-ol in a two-step reaction.

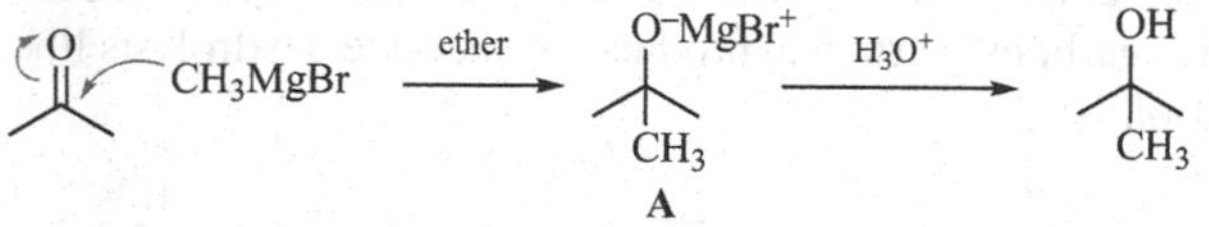

What is the name associated with the reaction of a Grignard reagent and an aldehyde or ketone?

This reaction is called a *Grignard reaction*. It is named after Victor Grignard.

What is the mechanism of reaction when methylmagnesium bromide reacts with acetone?

There is no intermediate when the Grignard reagent reacts with the carbonyl to form the alkoxide. The course of the reaction is therefore examined by inspecting the transition state. The nucleophilic carbon of the Grignard is attracted to the electropositive carbon of the carbonyl and the electropositive magnesium is attracted to the electronegative oxygen of the carbonyl, leading to a four-centered transition state as shown, allowing formation of a new carbon–carbon bond in the alkoxide product, ***A***. Hydrolysis of the alkoxide is required in a second step to give the alcohol product. Once again, this entire reaction sequence is known as a *Grignard reaction*.

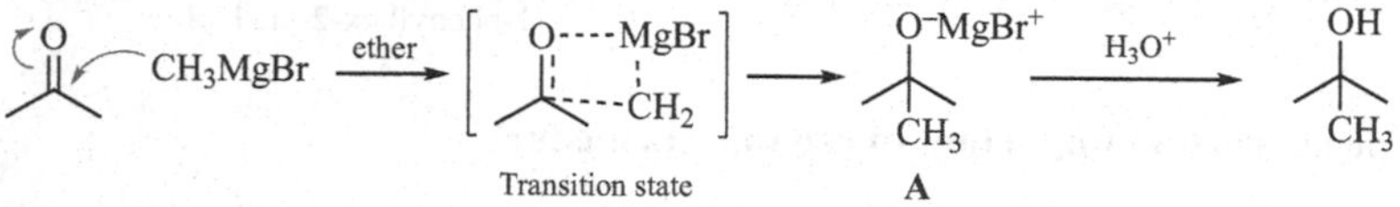

What is the Schlenk equilibrium?

The *Schlenk equilibrium* describes several organometallic species that comprise the actual structure of a "Grignard reagent" in solution. In its most simple form, the Schlenk equilibrium for a Grignard reagent (RMgX) is: $2RMgX \rightleftarrows R_2Mg + MgX_2$

What is the product of the Grignard reaction between ethylmagnesium bromide and cyclohexanone?

The product is 1-ethylcyclohexanol where the nucleophilic carbon of the Grignard reagent attacks the electropositive carbonyl carbon, forming a new carbon–carbon bond and producing an alkoxide. Hydrolysis gives the alcohol product.

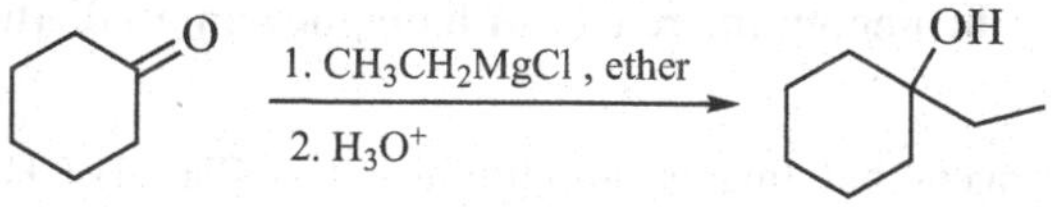

What is the product of the reaction between 1-chlorobutane and (1) Mg, ether, and in a second step (2) hexanal?

The reaction with magnesium generates the Grignard reagent, BuMgCl, which reacts with hexanal to give the alkoxide product shown. In order to form the alcohol, decan-5-ol, the alkoxide must be reacted with aqueous acid. This reaction sequence is just another way to present a Grignard reaction, but the starting material is the alkyl halide and the Grignard reagent must be formed first.

$$\text{CH}_3\text{CH}_2\text{CH}_2\text{CH}_2\text{Cl} \xrightarrow[\text{2. Hexanal, ether}]{\text{1. Mg, ether}} \text{O}^- \text{MgCl}^+$$

What aldehyde reacts with ethylmagnesium bromide to produce a primary alcohol?

Formaldehyde! When ethylmagnesium bromide reacts with formaldehyde (HCHO), hydrolysis gives the alcohol, propan-1-ol. Formaldehyde is the only aldehyde that generates a primary alcohol since all other aldehydes give a secondary alcohol in a Grignard reaction. Ketones react to give a tertiary alcohol.

Why is the reaction of a ketone or aldehyde and a Grignard reagent not reversible?

A strong carbon–carbon bond is formed when the nucleophilic Grignard reagents attacks the π-bond of the carbonyl. The strength of the carbon–carbon bond makes the reverse reaction (cleavage of the C—C bond) highly endothermic and it also has a high activation energy relative to the forward reaction. For this reason, the reaction of a Grignard reagent with an aldehyde or ketone tends to be irreversible.

12.4 THE WITTIG REACTION

What is an ylid?

An ylid is a neutral compound with a negatively charged carbon atom directly bonded to a positively charged atom of phosphorus, sulfur, and nitrogen, primarily. It is noted that ylid can also be spelled ylide.

What is a phosphine?

A phosphine has the structure R_3P, where R is a carbon group. Primary phosphines are RPH_2, secondary phosphines are R_2PH, and tertiary phosphines are R_3P. In this section, the primary focus will be on tertiary phosphines. Note that a phosphine is the phosphorus analog of an amine, since phosphorus appears right under nitrogen in Group 15 of the periodic table.

What is the structure of triphenylphosphine?

Triphenylphosphine is Ph_3P.

What is the product when triphenylphosphine reacts with iodomethane?

The phosphorus of triphenylphosphine behaves as a nucleophile, displacing iodide from iodomethane to form methyltriphenylphosphonium iodide [$Ph_3PMe^+ I^-$].

What is the product when methyltriphenylphosphonium bromide reacts with a strong base such as *n*-butyllithium (1-lithiobutane)?

The proton (on the methyl group) that is α- to the phosphorus in methyltriphenylphosphonium iodide is acidic (a weak acid, $pK_a \approx 25–32$) and requires a strong base such as *n*-butyllithium to remove it. When this proton is removed, the remaining carbanion is stabilized by the adjacent positively charged phosphorus in the ylid product, triphenylphosponium methylid. The ylid is resonance stabilized as shown.

$$Ph_3P \quad + \quad CH_3I \longrightarrow Ph_3\overset{+}{P}\text{-}CH_3 \; \overset{-}{I} \xrightarrow{\text{n-BuLi}} \left[Ph_3P\text{-}CH_2 \longleftrightarrow Ph_3P{=}CH_2 \right]$$

methyltriphenyl-phosphonium iodide

triphenylphosphonium methylid

What is the final product when an ylid reacts with cyclohexanone?

An ylid reacts with cyclohexanone to produce an alkene (in this case methylenecyclohexane) and triphenylphosphine oxide ($Ph_3P{=}O$) in what is known at the *Wittig reaction* or *Wittig olefination.*

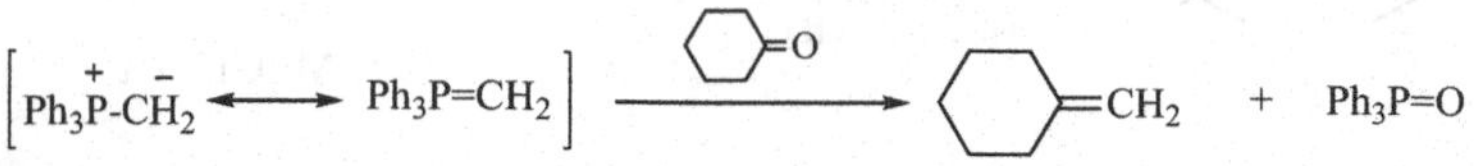

$$\left[Ph_3\overset{+}{P}\text{-}\overset{-}{C}H_2 \longleftrightarrow Ph_3P{=}CH_2 \right] \xrightarrow{\text{cyclohexanone}} \text{cyclohexane}{=}CH_2 \;+\; Ph_3P{=}O$$

What is the mechanism for the reaction of triphenylphosphonium methylid with cyclohexanone?

When triphenylphosphonium methylid reacts with cyclohexanone, the carbanion carbon of the ylid adds to the electrophilic carbon of the ketone to give a zwitterion known as a *betaine*. The alkoxide moiety quickly reacts with the positive phosphorus atom of the betaine to give a four-membered ring compound known as an *oxaphosphetane*. Formation of a P=O bond is exothermic, leading to cleavage to the C—P and C—O bond of the oxaphosphetane to give triphenylphosphine oxide along with the alkene product, methylenecyclohexane. Note that the reaction of the ylid and the carbonyl may go directly to an oxaphosphetane without the intermediacy of a betaine, but for this book, the betaine–oxaphosphetane mechanism shown is presumed to be correct for all phosphorus ylids unless otherwise stated.

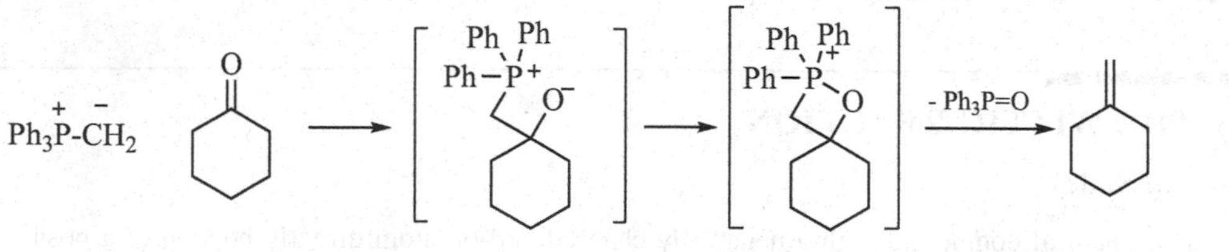

$$Ph_3\overset{+}{P}\text{-}\overset{-}{C}H_2 + \text{cyclohexanone} \longrightarrow [\text{betaine}] \longrightarrow [\text{oxaphosphatane}] \xrightarrow{-\,Ph_3P{=}O} \text{methylenecyclohexane}$$

betaine — oxaphosphatane — methylenecyclohexane

What is the distinction between an oxaphosphetane and a betaine?

The betaine is the dipolar ion, a zwitterion shown in the preceding question. An oxaphosphetane is a four-membered ring containing both a phosphorus and an oxygen, as shown in the preceding question.

What is the "driving force" for the Wittig olefination reaction, i.e., why does it react to give the alkene?

Formation of the very strong P–O bond, which is a strongly exothermic reaction. The energy released as a consequence of the exothermic reaction drives the cleavage of the oxaphosphetane to the alkene and triphenylphosphine oxide.

Give the major product of the reaction of (a), (b), and (c).

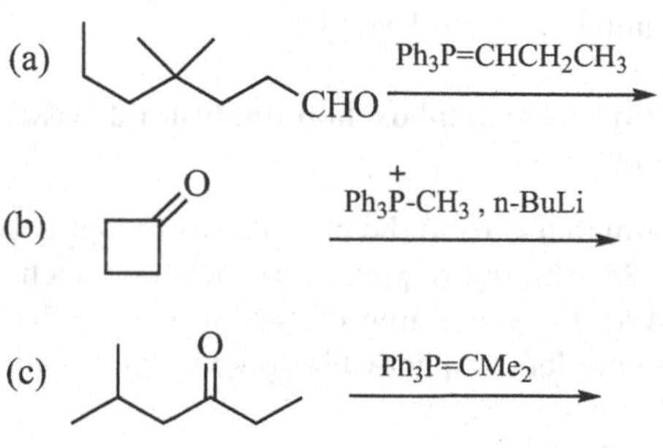

(a) aldehyde (CHO) $\xrightarrow{Ph_3P{=}CHCH_2CH_3}$

(b) cyclobutanone $\xrightarrow{Ph_3\overset{+}{P}\text{-}CH_3\text{ , n-BuLi}}$

(c) ketone $\xrightarrow{Ph_3P{=}CMe_2}$

In (a), the aldehyde 4,4-dimethylheptanal reacts with the ylid to produce the linear alkene, 7,7-dimethyl-dec-4-ene as a mixture of cis- and trans-stereoisomers. In (b), cyclobutanone reacts to form the exocyclic methylene compound, methylenecyclobutane. In (c), a methyl group is incorporated in the conversion of 5-methylhexan-3-one to the tetrasubstituted alkene, 3-ethyl-2,5-dimethylhex-2-ene.

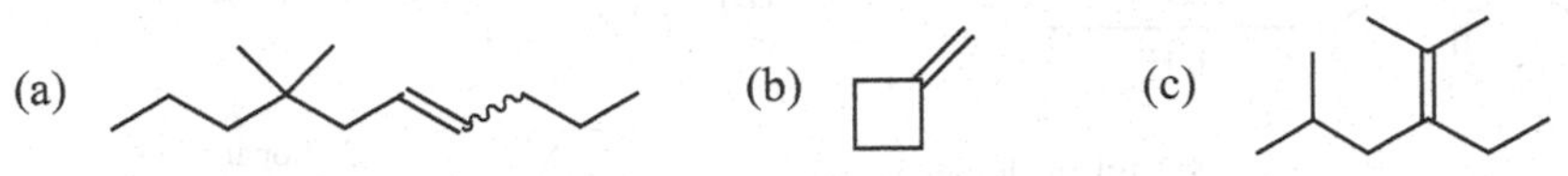

(a) 7,7-dimethyldec-4-ene (b) methylenecyclobutane (c) 3-ethyl-2,5-dimethylhex-2-ene

What does the term exocyclic mean?

The term literally means "outside the ring." In this case, the C=C unit is attached to the ring rather than within the ring.

END OF CHAPTER PROBLEMS

1. Give the IUPAC name for each of the following:

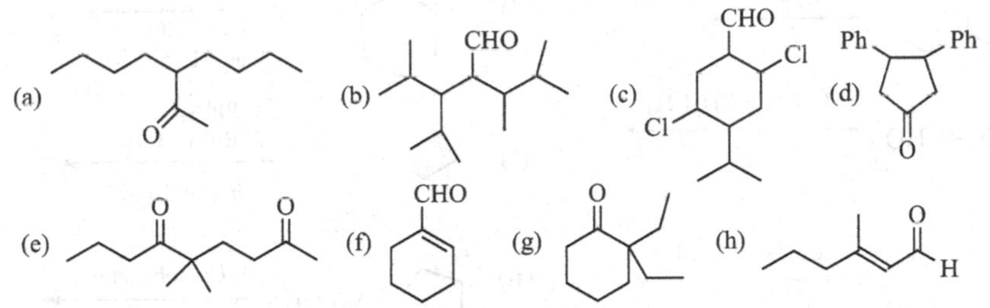

(a) (b) CHO (c) CHO, Cl, Cl (d) Ph, Ph, O

(e) O, O (f) CHO (g) O (h) O, H

2. Give the mechanism of the following reaction. Note that Me is methyl.

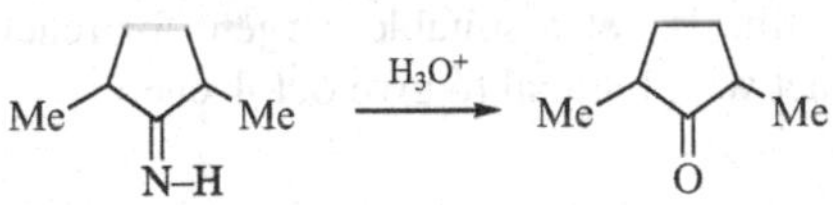

Me, Me, N–H $\xrightarrow{H_3O^+}$ Me, Me, O

3. Give a complete mechanism for the following reactions:

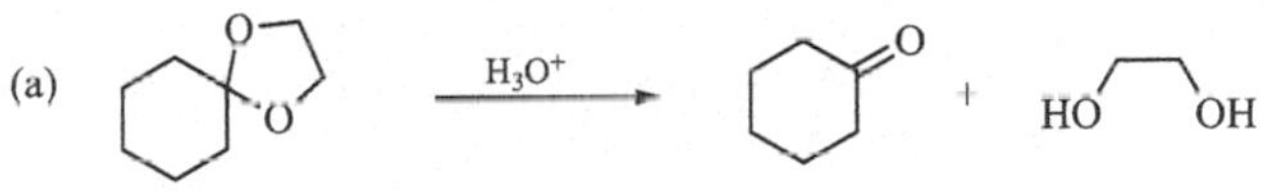

(a) O, O $\xrightarrow{H_3O^+}$ O + HO OH

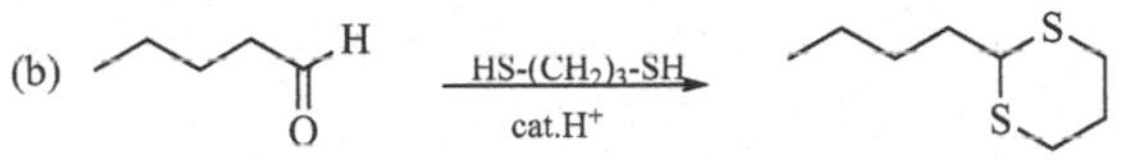

(b) H, O $\xrightarrow[\text{cat.}H^+]{HS\text{-}(CH_2)_3\text{-}SH}$ S, S

4. What is the initial product when the hydrate of butan-2-one loses water? How is this product converted back to butan-2-one?
5. Give the structures of 1,3-dioxane, of 1,3-dioxolane, of 1,3-dithiane, and of 1,3-dithiolane.

6. In each case, give the major product. Remember stereochemistry where appropriate and if there is no reaction, indicate by N.R.

(a) [pentan-3-one] $\xrightarrow[\text{cat. } H^+]{\text{EtOH}}$

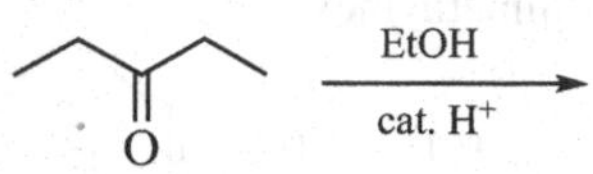

(b) Cl_3C–C(=O)–H $\xrightarrow{H_2O}$

(c) [pentanal] CHO $\xrightarrow[\text{cat. } H^+]{\text{1,2-Ethanedithiol}}$

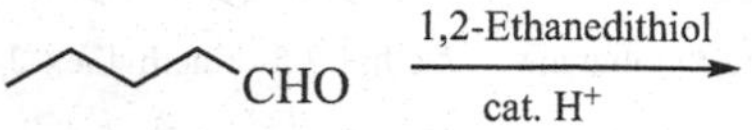

(d) [cyclohexanone] =O $\xrightarrow[\text{cat. } H^+]{\text{1,3-Propanediol}}$

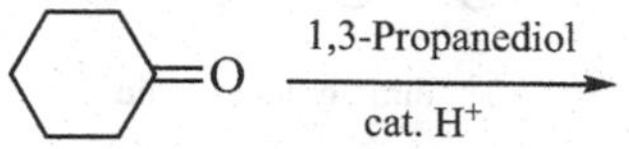

(e) [pentan-2-one] $\xrightarrow[\text{2. aq. } H^+]{\text{1. } \text{MgBr (butyl)}, \text{ THF}}$

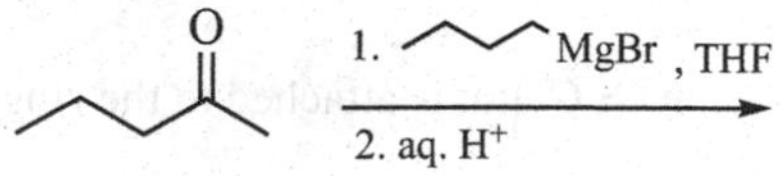

(f) [cyclopentanone] =O $\xrightarrow[\text{cat. } H^+]{\text{N,N-dipropylamine}}$

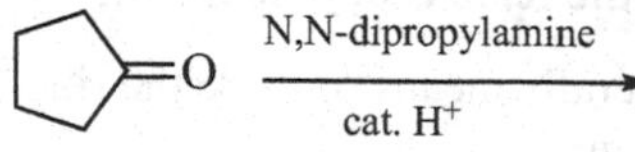

(g) [heptan-4-one] $\xrightarrow[\text{cat. } H^+]{\text{butane-1-amine}}$

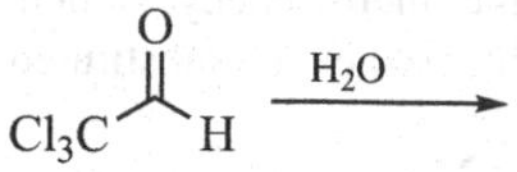

(h) [pent-1-yne] $\xrightarrow{\text{1. } NaNH_2\text{, THF; 2. cyclopentanone; 3. aq. } H^+}$

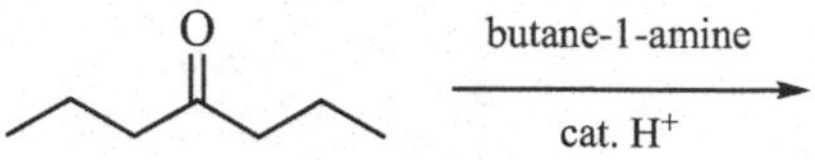

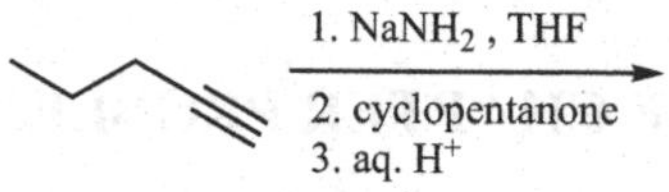

(i) [pentan-3-one] $\xrightarrow{H_2O}$

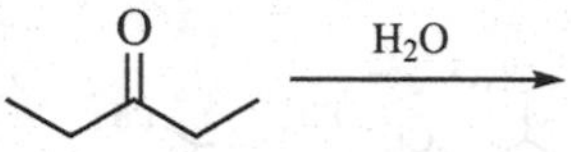

(j) [bromocyclohexane] Br $\xrightarrow{\text{1. Mg°, ether; 2. } CH_3CHO\text{; 3. aq. } H^+}$

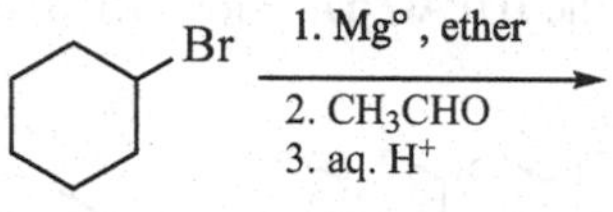

(k) [cyclopentane]–CHO $\xrightarrow{PH_3P{=}CHCH_2CH_3}$

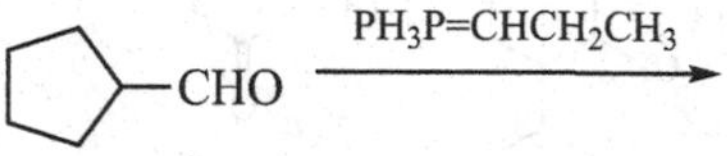

(l) [2-bromopentane] Br $\xrightarrow{\text{1. } PPh_3\text{; 2. BuLi, THF; 3. hexan-2-one}}$

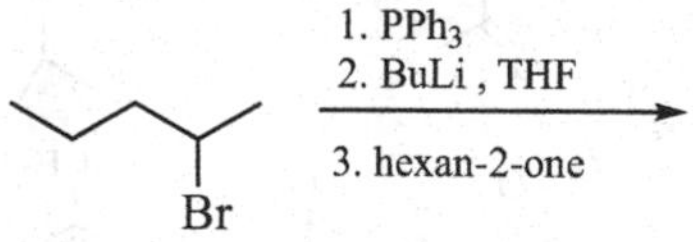

(m) [1,1-dimethoxycyclopentane] OCH_3, OCH_3 $\xrightarrow{\text{excess } H_2O\text{, } H^+}$

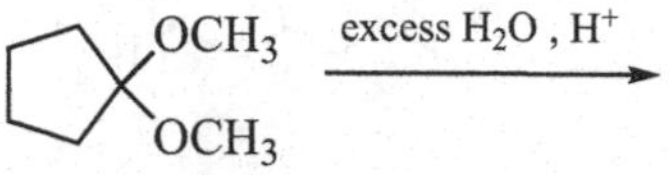

(n) [cyclopentyl]–MgCl $\xrightarrow[\text{2. aq. } H^+]{\text{1. Cyclohexanone}}$

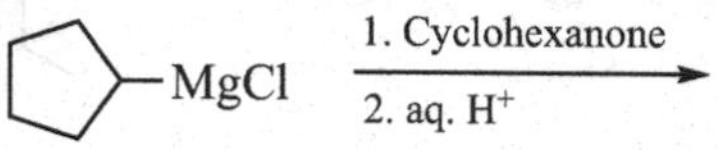

7. Explain why triethylphosphine is not a suitable reagent for reaction with 1-bromobutane to form an ylid that would react with butanal to give oct-4-ene.

Part B

A Q&A Approach to Organic Chemistry

13

Oxidation Reactions

Oxidation reactions are extremely important in organic chemistry. A molecule, such as an alcohol in a lower oxidation state, is converted to an aldehyde or ketone, for example, which is in a higher oxidation state. The conversion of an alkene to a diol is another example of an oxidation. It is also possible to prepare carboxylic acids by the oxidation of an aldehyde or even directly from an alcohol. This chapter will discuss oxidation reactions and their use in various organic chemical reactions.

What is the definition of an oxidation?

Oxidation is the loss of two electrons in the course of a chemical reaction. Oxidation can also be defined as the loss of hydrogen or the gain of heteroatoms such as oxygen. Loss of hydrogen atoms or the replacement of a hydrogen atom bonded to carbon with a more electronegative atom also correlates with oxidation. Note that oxidation is the reverse of reduction.

How can an oxidation reaction be identified?

Loss of hydrogen atoms or the replacement of a hydrogen atom bonded to carbon with a more electronegative atom, usually a heteroatom, constitutes an oxidation. Indeed, an easy way to identify an oxidation is incorporation of a heteroatom into a molecule. Common heteroatoms include oxygen, halogen, nitrogen, sulfur, and so on

Another way to measure an oxidation or reduction reaction is to monitor changes in the oxidation state of the starting materials and the products. Oxidation state is a number assigned to the carbon atoms involved in the transformation, and the formal rules for determining oxidation state are 1. The oxidation state of a carbon is taken to be zero. 2. Every hydrogen atom attached to a carbon is given a value of −1. 3. Every heteroatom attached to a carbon is assigned a value of +1.

What types of functional groups are involved in typical oxidation reactions or organic molecules?

Alkenes react with aqueous acid to give alcohols, which is a formal oxidation, and this reaction was discussed with the chemistry of alkenes in Section 7.3. Alkenes can also be oxidized to three-membered ethers known as oxiranes (epoxides; Section 7.4.2) or to vicinal diols (Section 7.4.3). Alkenes can also be oxidized to 1,2-diols or oxidatively cleaved to aldehydes, ketones, or carboxylic acids. Alcohols can be oxidized to aldehydes or ketones or to carboxylic acids. Aldehydes can be oxidized to carboxylic acids under some conditions.

13.1 OXIDATION REACTIONS OF ALKENES

What is dihydroxylation?

Dihydroxylation is the addition of two hydroxyl groups across an alkene, giving a vicinal diol as introduced in Section 7.4.3. There are two major reagents that give this product, $KMnO_4$ (potassium permanganate) and OsO_4 (osmium tetroxide).

What is the structure of potassium permanganate?

The structure is $KMnO_4$, with the structure shown.

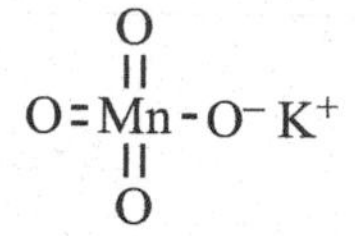

O=Mn(=O)(=O)-O⁻ K⁺

What is vicinal diol?

A vicinal diol is a dihydroxy compound with OH units on adjacent carbon atoms. An example is ethanediol, $HOCH_2CH_2OH$.

What is the major product when dilute $KMnO_4$ reacts with cyclopentene in aqueous KOH?

The major product of this reaction is one diastereomer, the *cis*-1,2-cyclopentanediol. In other words, the two OH units are on the same side of the molecule. This oxidation is a diastereospecific reaction since none of the diastereomer, the trans-diol, is formed. The cis- diol is racemic since reaction (both the 1*R*,2*S* and the 1*S*,2*R* stereoisomers are formed) can occur from the "top" face of the alkene and also from the "bottom" face equally well. Note that the cis- diol derived from cyclopentene is a meso compound since the 1*R*,2*S* and the 1*S*,2*R* stereoisomers are the same compound (they are superimposable).

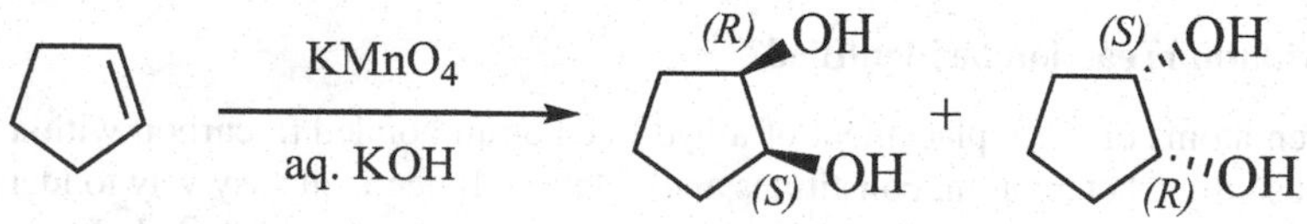

KMnO4, aq. KOH → (R) OH, (S) OH + (S) OH, (R) OH

Is there an intermediate in the reaction of dilute $KMnO_4$ with cyclopentene in aqueous KOH?

Yes! The reaction proceeds by initial formation of a cyclic manganese compound that reacts with hydroxide to decompose the manganate ester to give the diol.

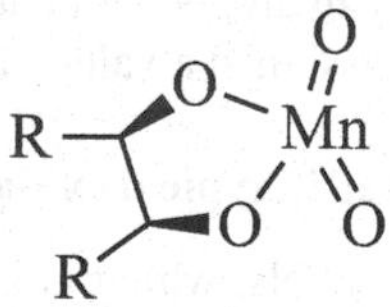

Manganate ester

What is the purpose of the aqueous KOH in this reaction?

Hydroxide attacks the manganese of the manganate ester, ***A***, to give intermediate ***B*** via cleavage of the O—Mn bond. In the presence of additional hydroxide, attack of the manganese in ***B*** leads to cleavage of the second O—Mn bond to remove manganese from the molecule. In the presence of water, the initially formed alkoxides protonated in both reactions, and the final product is the diol.

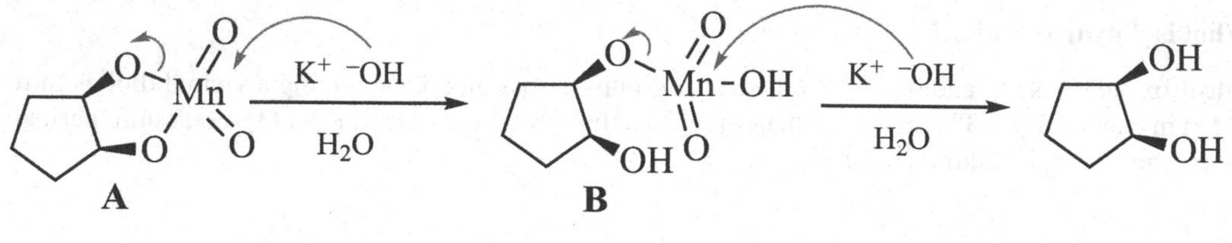

A —K⁺ ⁻OH, H_2O→ **B** —K⁺ ⁻OH, H_2O→ diol

Why does this reaction produce the cis- diol?

As seen in the figure, the alkene reacts with two of the oxygens on MnO_4^-. There is no intermediate in the reaction of cyclopentene to form ***A*** because the reaction is a synchronous [3+2]-cycloaddition (see Section 18.5). Therefore, the two bonds are formed close together in time (probably in a concerted manner), generating the cis- stereochemistry shown in manganate ester, ***A***. The cis- stereochemistry is therefore set by the synchronous reaction that forms ***A***. The trans- compound could form only if there were a bond rotation prior to formation of the second C—O bond. The bond-making process is too fast to allow this, and the cis- stereochemistry is characteristic of this reaction. Since hydroxide attacks Mn rather than carbon, the stereochemistry at the carbon atom is retained and the cis- diol is the final product.

K+ −OH, H2O → A; K+ −OH, H2O → B; → cis-diol

What sort of reaction is the synchronous reaction of an alkene with permanganate to form the cyclic product?

This reaction is called a *1,3-dipolar cycloaddition*, although the reaction is usually called a [3+2]-cycloaddition (Section 18.5). In this reaction, the p-orbitals of the alkene react with the orbitals of the manganese or osmium reagent to give the manganate ester or the osmate ester.

Is dihydroxylation of alkenes with $KMnO_4$ stereoselective?

Yes! For the reaction of potassium permanganate with a cyclic alkene such as cyclohexene, the product is the cis- diol, as described. There is none of the trans- diol. This result indicates that of two possible products, only the cis- diol is formed. The dihydroxylation reaction is a diastereospecific reaction since of the two diastereomers (cis- and trans-), only the cis- product is formed.

What does the term "diastereospecific" mean? "Diastereoselective?"

"Diastereospecific" means that of two or more possible products, one and only one is formed. "Diastereoselective" means that of two or more possible products, there is a major product and one or more minor products. Note that dihydroxylation occurs from either side of the C=C unit, so the reaction yields both enantiomers. Only one diastereomer is formed (diastereospecific), but that diastereomer is racemic.

Does an acyclic cis- alkene give the same product as an acyclic trans- alkene upon reaction with $KMnO_4$?

No! The reaction is diastereospecific. Therefore, an acyclic cis- alkene will react to give one diastereomer and an acyclic trans-alkene will give a different diastereomer. Note that the diastereomers are stereoisomers of each other.

What product is formed when pent-2*E*-ene reacts with $KMnO_4$/aq. KOH? What is the product when pent-2*Z*-ene reacts with $KMnO_4$/aq. KOH?

The reaction of pent-2*E*-ene gives pentan-2*S*,3*S*-diol, whereas pent-2*Z*-ene gives pentan-2*S*,3*R*-diol. These diols are different diastereomers, but each is racemic.

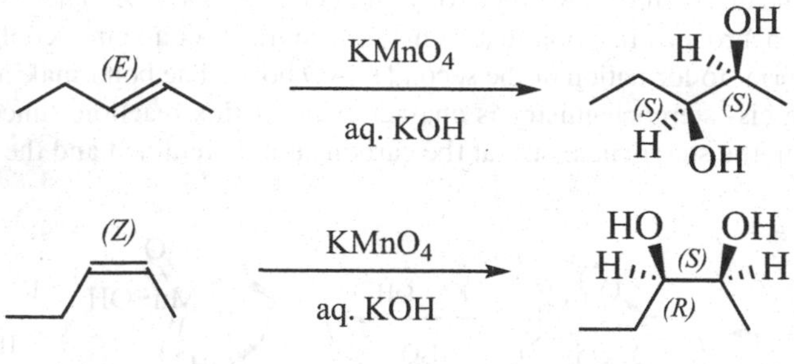

Will the diastereomer formed from a cis- or a trans- alkene be enantiopure?

No! The C=C unit of an alkene is planar, so the permanganate can approach from either the top or the bottom (different faces) of the molecule. Therefore, the diastereomer that is formed will be racemic. In other words, both enantiomers of the diastereomer will be formed in equal amounts.

What is the major product when trans-hex-3-ene reacts with $KMnO_4$ followed by aqueous KOH?

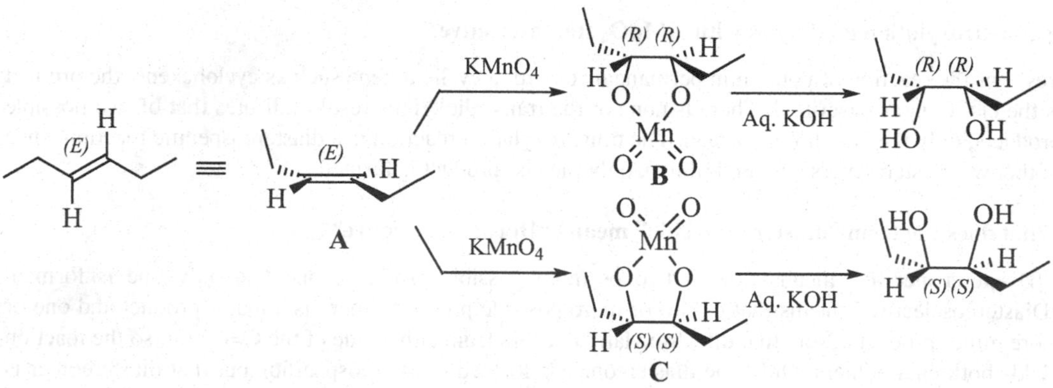

For an acyclic alkene, cis- addition of the hydroxyl groups applies, but the terms cis- and trans- do not apply to the diol product. To sort out the stereochemistry of the product, first rotate the alkene as shown in ***A***, such that one ethyl group is projected to the front of the page and one ethyl group is projected to the rear, reflecting the trans- geometry. If permanganate reacts from the bottom face of the alkene as it is drawn manganate ester ***B*** is formed, with the (3*R*,4*R*) stereochemistry. If permanganate reacts from the top face, manganate ester ***C*** is formed, with the (3*S*,4*S*) stereochemistry. Structures ***B*** and ***C*** are enantiomers of a single diastereomer. When these manganate esters react with hydroxide, the stereochemistry at carbon is retained since hydroxide attacks manganese rather than carbon. The final products are (3*R*,4*R*)-hexanediol and (3*S*,4*S*)-hexanediol, in equal amounts. The cis- addition has led to a single diastereomer, but it is racemic, reflecting the fact that the planar alkene can be attacked from two opposite faces.

Why does the conversion of an alkene to the corresponding 1,2-diol use relatively low temperatures and dilute solutions of permanganate?

Permanganate is a powerful oxidizing agent. It is important to understand that the reaction of potassium permanganate to yield a diol must be done in a relatively dilute solution (typically 0.1–0.5 M) and the temperature must be kept relatively "cold" (usually room temperature or lower). If the concentration is too high and the temperature too great, oxidative cleavage can occur and a variety of products can be formed, so there is much less diol and more unwanted byproducts.

What is the structure of osmium tetroxide?

The structure is OsO_4, with the structure shown in the figure.

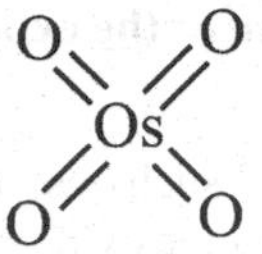

How does OsO_4 react with cyclohexene?

Osmium tetroxide (OsO_4) reacts very similarly to $KMnO_4$. The alkene reacts with the oxygens of OsO_4 to form an osmate ester via a [3+2]-cycloaddition, giving cis- addition of the two oxygen atoms to the alkene (see Section 18.5). A reagent other than KOH is required to decompose this osmate and generate the diol. The usual reagent is aqueous sodium thiosulfite ($NaHSO_3$), which is added in a second chemical step. The thiosulfate attacks the osmium, cleaving both O—Os bonds to liberate the diol. The combination of OsO_4 and aqueous $NaHSO_3$ converts alkenes to vicinal cis- diols.

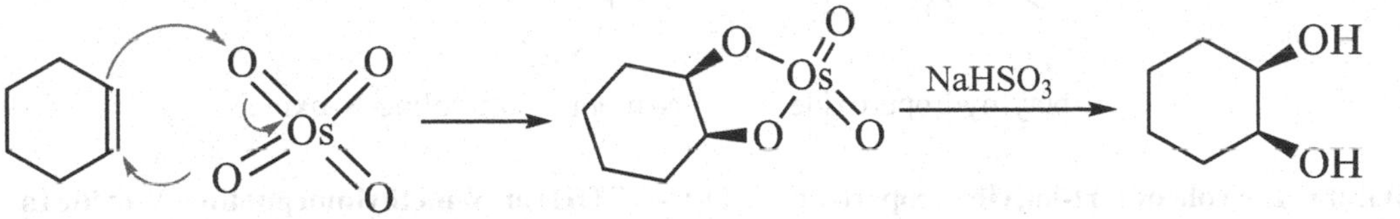

$NaHSO_3$

What is an osmate ester?

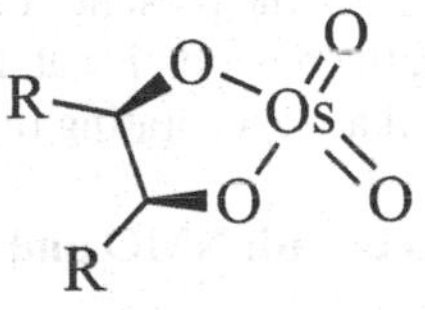

Osmate ester

An osmate ester (see the figure) is the product formed when OsO_4 reacts with an alkene via [3+2]-cycloaddition.

What is the major product of the reaction of pent-2*E*-ene and osmium tetroxide?

The 1,2-diol is formed, and dihydroxylation with OsO_4 is diastereospecific, as with the permanganate hydroxylation. In this case, pent-2*E*-ene is converted to the racemic diastereomer (3*R*,4*R*)/(3*S*,4*S*)-pentanediol via the cis- addition of osmium tetroxide.

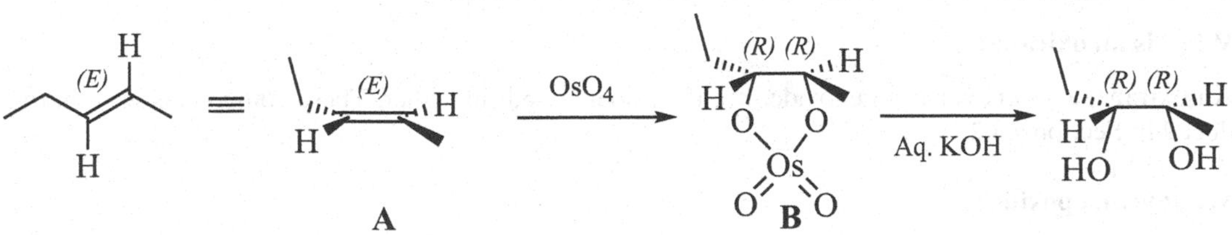

A OsO_4 B Aq. KOH

If $KMnO_4$ and OsO_4 lead to the same products, why use OsO_4?

The yields of cis- diol are generally higher with OsO_4 and there are fewer side reactions. If permanganate reactions become too hot or too concentrated, oxidative cleavage of the alkene can result. This is rarely a problem with OsO_4. However, OsO_4 is expensive and toxic. For these two reasons, OsO_4 is used for small scale applications in reactions with very expensive alkenes or when the $KMnO_4$ reaction cannot be controlled. Otherwise, potassium permanganate is commonly used. Note that reagents have been developed for use with OsO_4 dihydroxylation so that the oxidation is catalytic in osmium, making the reaction more practical.

Is it necessary to use a stoichiometric amount of the expensive OsO_4 in the conversion of alkenes to diols?

No! In the presence of catalytic agents such as *tert*-butylhydroperoxide (Me_3C—OOH) or *N*-methylmorpholine-*N*-oxide (NMO), osmium tetroxide reacts with an alkene to give an osmate ester. These two reagents not only covert the osmate ester to the diol but recycle the osmium tetroxide for reaction with additional alkene. Therefore, the reaction is catalytic in osmium tetroxide.

What are the structures of *tert*-butylhydroperoxide (Me_3C—OOH) or *N*-methylmorpholine-*N*-oxide (NMO)?

CH_3 OH O N^+ O^- O

tert-butylhydroperoxide N-methylmorpholine-N-oxide

What is the role of tert-butylhydroperoxide (Me_3C—OOH) or *N*-methylmorpholine-*N*-oxide in reactions of OsO_4 with alkenes?

Osmium tetroxide is a rather expensive reagent, and using a full molar equivalent is not always practical. If the reaction of an alkene with OsO_4 is done in the presence of *tert*-butylhydroperoxide (Me_3C—OOH) or *N*-methylmorpholine-*N*-oxide, however, the reaction is catalytic in osmium. Both reagents react with the osmate ester to generate the diol, as well as regenerating the OsO_4 reagent.

What is the product when pen-1-ene reacts with NMO and 5% aqueous OsO_4?

The product is pentane-1,2-diol, as shown.

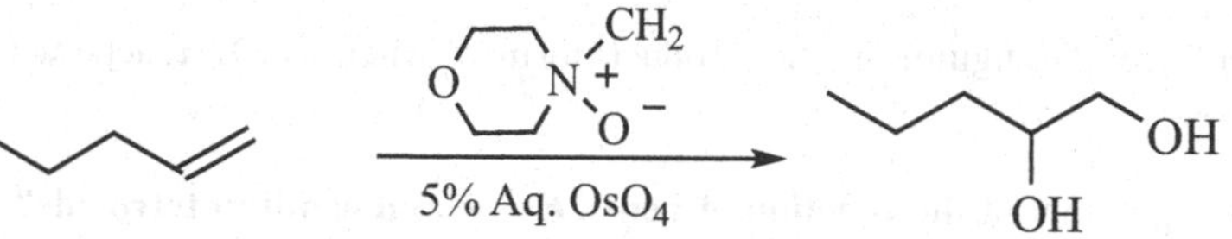

CH_2 O N + O −

5% Aq. OsO_4

OH OH

13.2 OXIDATION OF ALKENES: EPOXIDATION

What is an oxirane?

An oxirane, also known as an epoxide, is a three-membered ring ether. These compounds were introduced in Section 7.4.2.

What is an epoxide?

An epoxide is the common name for an oxirane.

What is a peroxycarboxylic acid?

A peroxycarboxylic acid or peroxyacid is class of chemical compound in which the —OH group of a carboxyl (–COOH) has been replaced by ——O——O——H.

What is the structure of peroxyacetic acid? Peroxyformic acid? meta-Chloroperoxybenzoic acid?

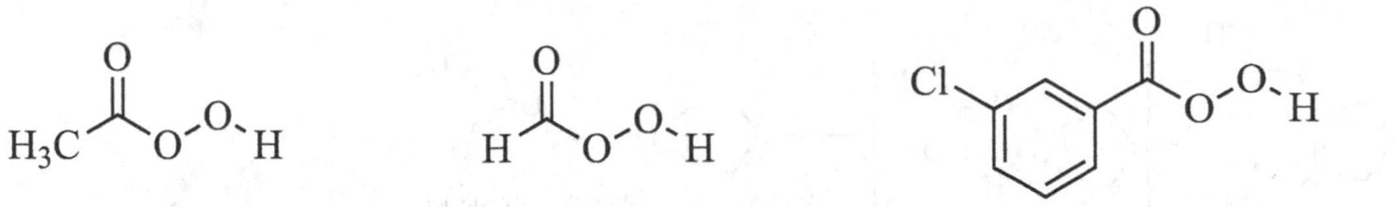

Peroxyacetic acid   Peroxyformic acid   *meta*-Chloroperoxybenzoic acid

What is the product when 2-methylhex-2-ene reacts with peroxyacetic acid?

The product is the epoxide (oxirane), 2,2-dimethyl-3-propyloxirane.

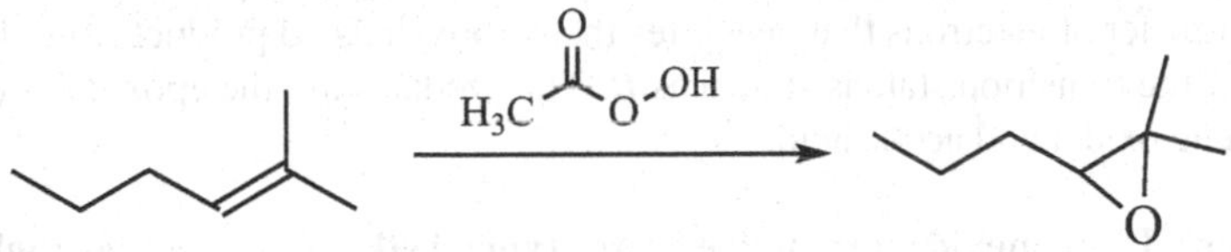

What structural feature of peroxycarboxylic acids is important for the oxidation of alkenes to oxiranes?

Peroxyacids shown have an electrophilic oxygen atom (δ^+) that will react with the electron-rich π-bond of an alkene. The electrophilic oxygen is a consequence of an induced dipole that originates with the carbonyl oxygen. The bond polarization that leads to an electrophilic oxygen is shown with peroxyformic acid.

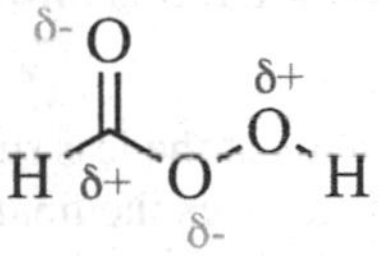

Apart from the oxirane, what is the other product formed when a peroxyacetic acid reacts with an alkene?

The reaction of 2-methylhex-2-ene with peroxyacetic acid gives 2,2-dimethyl-3-propyloxirane along with acetic acid, the carboxylic acid precursor to peroxyacetic acid, as shown in the figure. Therefore, there are two isolated products from the reaction of alkenes with peroxycarboxylic acids. Also see Section 7.4.2.

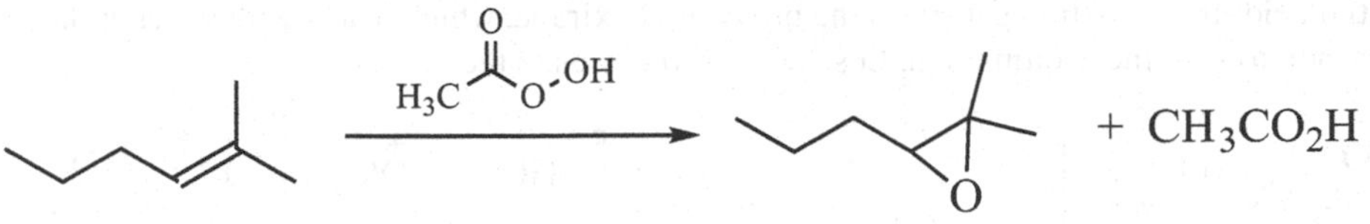

$+ CH_3CO_2H$

Does the reaction of a peroxycarboxylic acid and an alkene have an intermediate?

No! There is no intermediate for this reaction and the observed products are explained by a complex transition state.

What is the transition state for the epoxidation of alkenes?

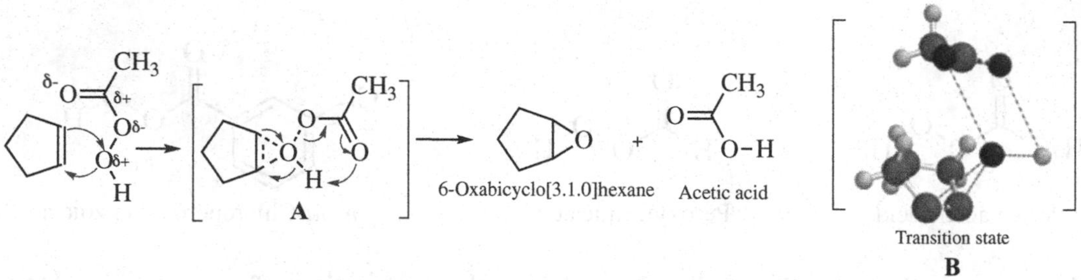

6-Oxabicyclo[3.1.0]hexane Acetic acid

Transition state

B

The reaction of cyclopentene and peroxyacetic acid is shown as an example. The transition state ***A*** must involve synchronous formation of both bonds between the alkene and the electrophilic O of the peroxyacid, as well as a transfer of electrons that generates the carboxylic acid product from the peroxyacid. A molecular model of the transition state is shown as ***B***. The products are the epoxide, 6-oxabicyclo[3.1.0] hexane (cyclopentene oxide) and acetic acid.

Epoxides are ethers. Is an epoxide unreactive as are typical ethers, or are they highly reactive?

Epoxides are strained three-membered rings with polarized C—O bonds. Epoxides are, therefore, very reactive. Epoxides undergo ring-opening reactions in the presence of acids, via an acid–base reaction. To circumvent this problem, buffers are added to react with the carboxylic acid byproduct and suppress secondary reactions. Common buffers include the salt of the carboxylic acid, such as sodium acetate $CH_3CO_2^-Na^+$. Epoxides also react with nucleophiles, as discussed in Sections 8.3 and 10.5.

What is the product formed when but-1-ene oxide (2-ethyloxirane) reacts with phenylmagnesium bromide? What is the product formed when this initial product reacts with dilute aqueous acid?

Initial reaction with the Grignard reagent occurs at the less substituted carbon of the oxirane to give the alkoxide ***A***. Aqueous hydrolysis of the alkoxide gives the final product, 1-phenylbutan-2-ol.

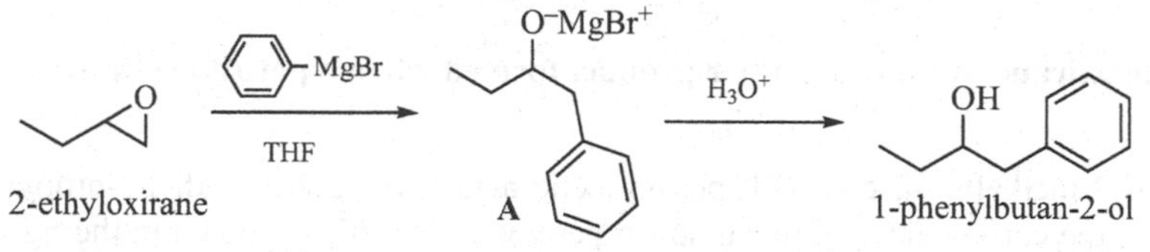

2-ethyloxirane **A** 1-phenylbutan-2-ol

What is the product formed when 2,3-ddimethyloxirane reacts with aqueous acid?

The initial acid–base reaction generates the protonated oxirane, which reacts with water at the less hindered carbon to give the oxonium ion. Loss of a proton leads to the 1,2-diol.

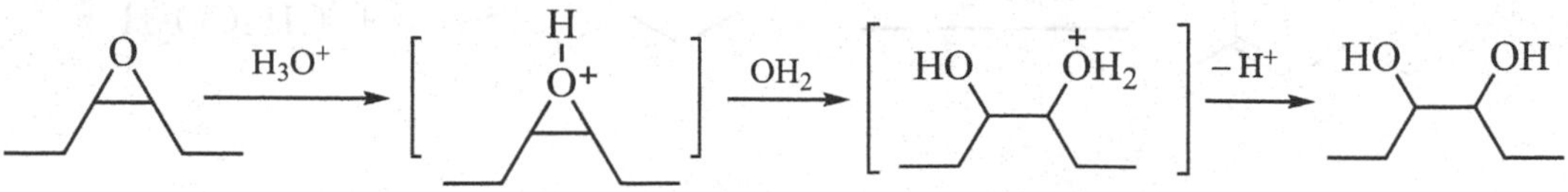

13.3 OXIDATIVE CLEAVAGE: OZONOLYSIS

What is ozonolysis?

Ozone (O_3) adds to alkenes, but the initially formed product rearranges to a more stable product called an ozonide, even at low temperatures. Subsequent treatment with an oxidizing or reducing agent leads to net cleavage of the carbon–carbon double bond and formation of aldehydes, ketones, or carboxylic acids. The process of cleavage of alkenes by reaction with ozone into carbonyl derivatives is called ozonolysis.

How many resonance forms can be drawn for ozone?

There are four resonance forms that bear positive and negative charges.

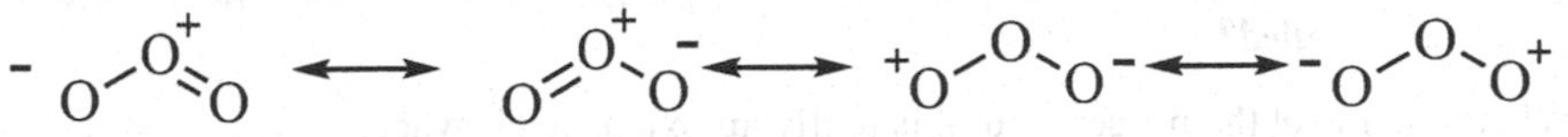

What product is formed initially when cyclohexene reacts with ozone?

In a process that is similar to the one observed with OsO_4 and MnO_4^-, ozone reacts with alkenes, such as cyclohexene, and the π-bond of an alkene attacks one terminal oxygen, and the other terminal oxygen of ozone in turn attacks the developing positive charge on the carbon to form a cyclic species, a 1,2,3-trioxolane. This reaction is a [3+2]-cycloaddition as described in Section 18.5.

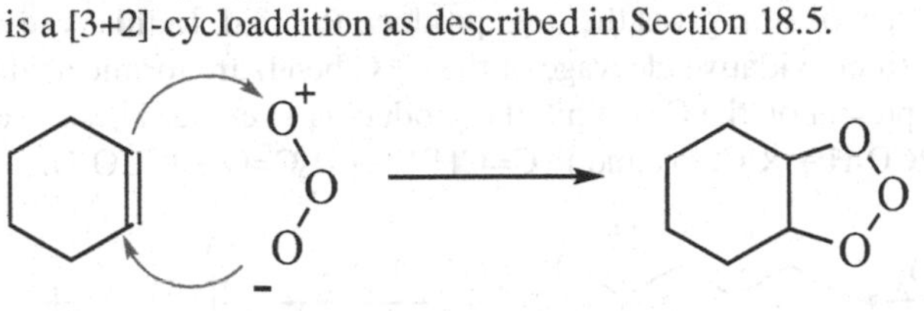

What is a trioxolane?

The term trioxolane refers to a five-membered ring with three oxygen atoms in the ring.

When ozone reacts with-but-2-ene, why is the observed product not the initial 1,2,3-trioxolane?

The initially formed 1,2,3-trioxolane is unstable and rearranges to a more stable 1,2,4-trioxolane. This final product is more commonly called an *ozonide.*

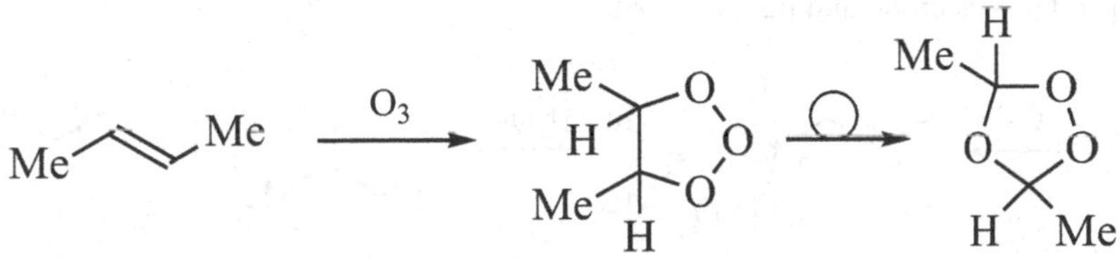

a 1,2,3-Trioxolane

a 1,2,4-Trioxolane (an ozonide)

What is the mechanism for transformation of 1,2,3-trioxolane to 1,2,4-trioxolane, an ozonide?

In this mechanism, the ozonide cleaves at the weak O—O bond to give a zwitterion (a dipolar ion), ***A***. The alkoxide moiety transfers electrons to form a carbonyl (ethanal) and zwitterion ***B***. The alkoxide of ***B*** attacks the carbonyl of ethanal and the oxygen of ethanal attacks the C=O moiety of ***B*** to give the ozonide. This latter reaction occurs before the two molecules (ethanal + ***B***) can "drift apart." The experimentally determined mechanism for this transformation is called the *Criegee mechanism* after Rudolf Criegee (1902–1975; Germany) who proposed it.

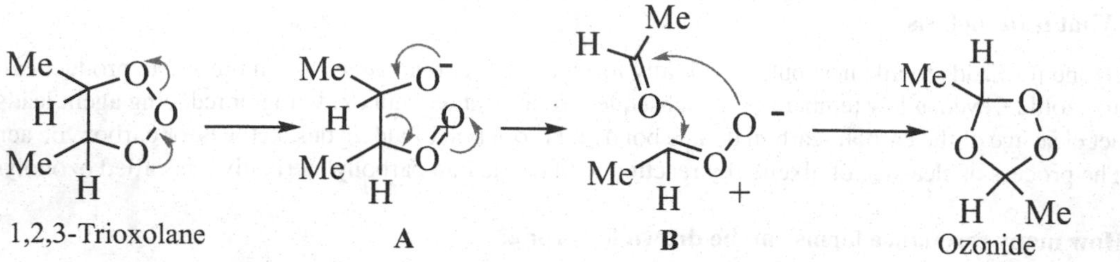

1,2,3-Trioxolane → A → B → Ozonide

When an alkene is converted to an ozonide and the ozonide is decomposed to give two products, what is this process called?

Ozonolysis is the name of the process, but it is really an oxidative cleavage.

When the ozonide derived from hex-1-ene is treated with hydrogen peroxide, what are the products?

Both C1 and C2 in *A* (the ozonide of hex-1-ene) have at least one hydrogen attached to the C=C unit. With an oxidizing agent such as hydrogen peroxide, both C1 and C2 are initially oxidized to an aldehyde but subsequent rapid oxidation, *in situ*, gives the final product, the acid. In this case, the two acid products (two carbonyl products from oxidative cleavage of the C=C bond) are formic acid and pentanoic acid. If a hydrogen atom is not present on the C=C unit, the product is a ketone. These reactions can be generalized: $RCH{=}CHR^1 \rightarrow RCO_2H + R^1CO_2H$ and $R_2C{=}CHR^1 \rightarrow R_2C{=}O + R^1CO_2H$.

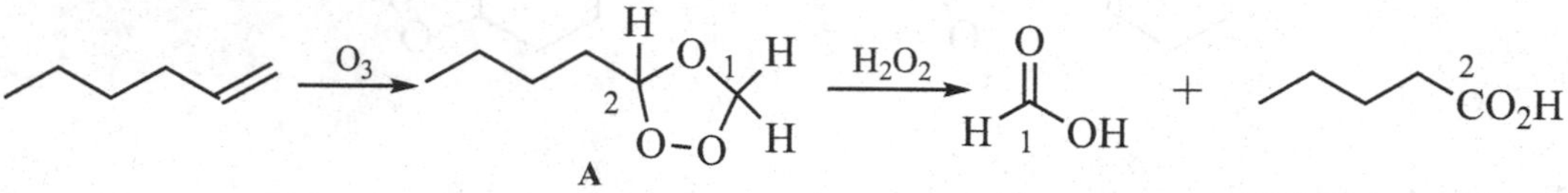

O_3 → A → H_2O_2 → H(C=O)OH + CO_2H

When the ozonide derived from 2,3-dimethylpent-2-ene is treated with hydrogen peroxide, what are the products?

Cleavage of the C=C bond in 2,3-dimethylpent-2-ene leads to the ozonide *A*. In this case, both C1 and C2 have two alkyl groups attached and no hydrogens, which is clear since no hydrogen atoms are attached to the C=C unit in the alkene. Oxidation of *A* with hydrogen peroxide therefore leads to the two oxidative cleavage ketone products, acetone and pentan-2-one.

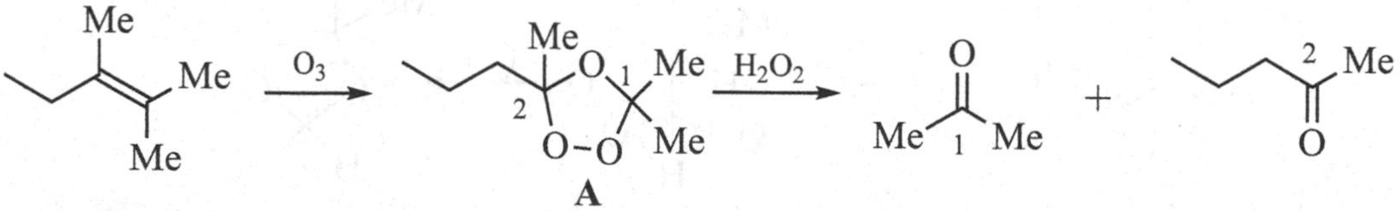

O_3 → A → H_2O_2 → Me(C=O)Me + pentan-2-one

When the ozonide derived from hex-1-ene is treated with zinc and acetic acid, what are the products?

The ozonide derived from-hex-1-ene is *A*, which can be reduced rather than oxidized. When *A* is treated with zinc metal in acetic acid, reduction of the ozonide leads to formaldehyde and pentanal. Note that the hydrogen atoms on the C=C unit of the alkene remain unchanged. In other words, the initially formed aldehyde products are *not* oxidized to an acid.

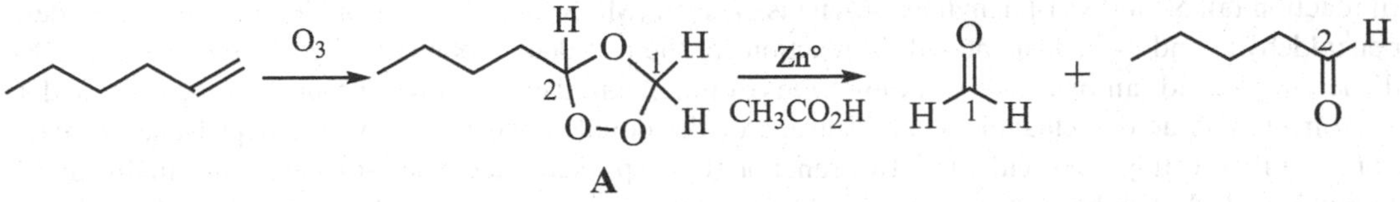

When the ozonide derived from 2,3-dimethylpent-2-ene is treated with zinc and acetic acid, what are the products?

The ozonide derived from 2,3-dimethylpent-2-ene is *A*, and reduction with zinc metal in acetic acid gives acetone and pentan-2-one. Note that these are the same products obtained when the ozonide was oxidized with hydrogen peroxide (see earlier). This experiment shows that oxidation or reduction of an ozonide derived from an alkene with no hydrogen atoms on the C=C unit will give the same products.

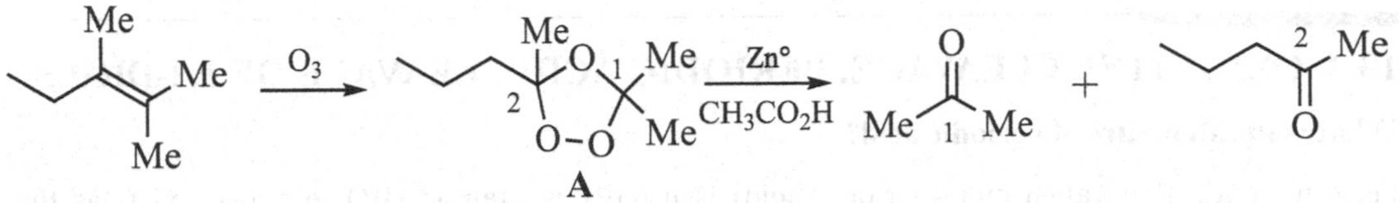

What is another common reagent used to reduce ozonides?

Dimethyl sulfide, CH_3—S—CH_3 (Me_2S). In the preceding questions, if the ozonide is treated with dimethyl sulfide, the oxidative cleavage products are the same as those shown above.

Ozonolysis of a cyclic alkene gives how many products?

One! Cleavage of the cyclic alkene gives a product with two aldehyde units, two ketone units, and aldehyde and a ketone, a ketone or aldehyde and an acid, or two acid groups at distal ends of the molecule.

What is the product when cycloheptene is reacted with (1) ozone and (2) zinc and acetic acid?

Ozonolysis of cycloheptene gives the ozonide *A*, and reduction with dimethyl sulfide gives one product, the α,ω-dialdehyde, heptanedial. Note that if the ozonide formed from cycloheptene is reduced with zinc and acetic acid, heptanedial is also formed.

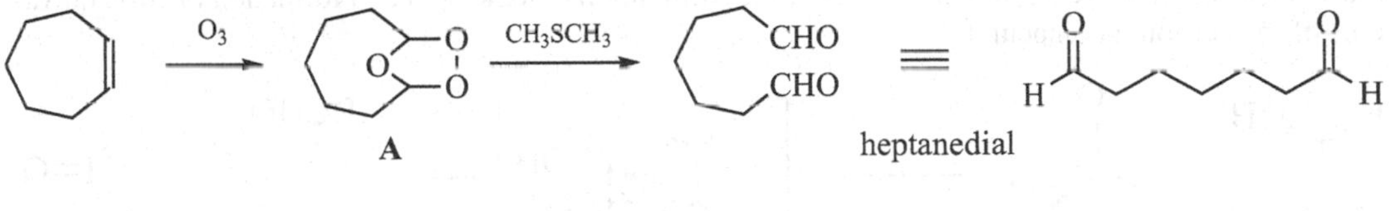

heptanedial

What is (are) the product(s) of the reactions of (a), (b), (c), and (d)?

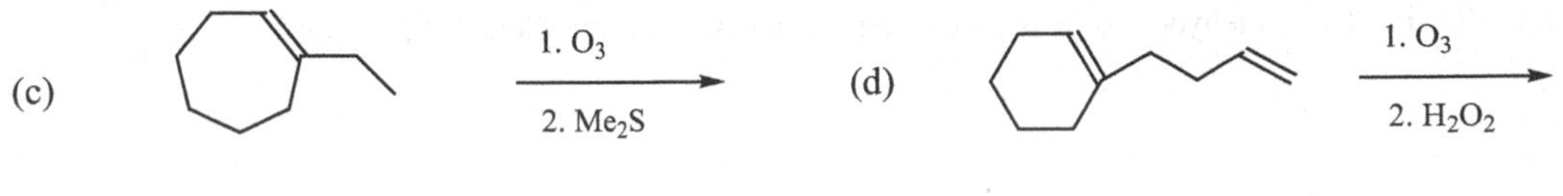

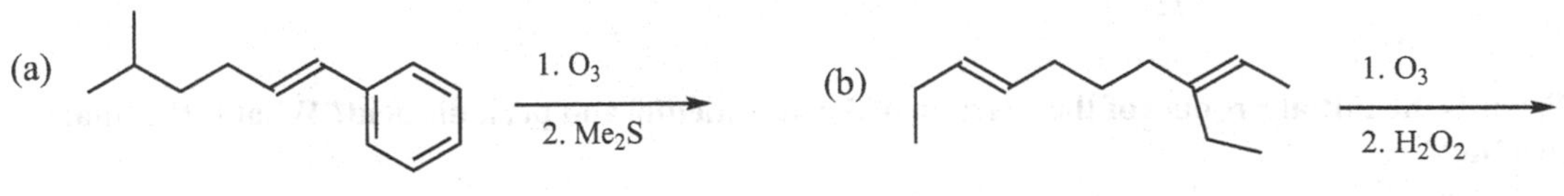

(a) 1. O_3 2. Me_2S

(b) 1. O_3 2. H_2O_2

(c) 1. O_3 2. Me_2S

(d) 1. O_3 2. H_2O_2

In reaction (a), 5-methyl-1-phenylhex-1*E*-ene is cleaved (Me_2S reduces the ozonide) into two aldehydes: benzaldehyde and 4-methylpentanal. In reaction (b) the two double bonds in diene 3-ethyldeca-2*E*,7*E*-diene are cleaved (an oxidative workup of the ozonide), and there are three products: propionic acid + 5-oxoheptanoic acid + ethanoic acid. Cleavage of the double bond in 1-ethylcyclohept-1-ene, in reaction (c), gives a single molecule with two functional groups, keto-aldehyde 7-oxononanal. Finally, diene 1-(but-3-en-1-yl)cyclohex-1-ene in reaction (d) is cleaved to two products, ethanoic acid and keto-diacid 4-oxononanedioic acid.

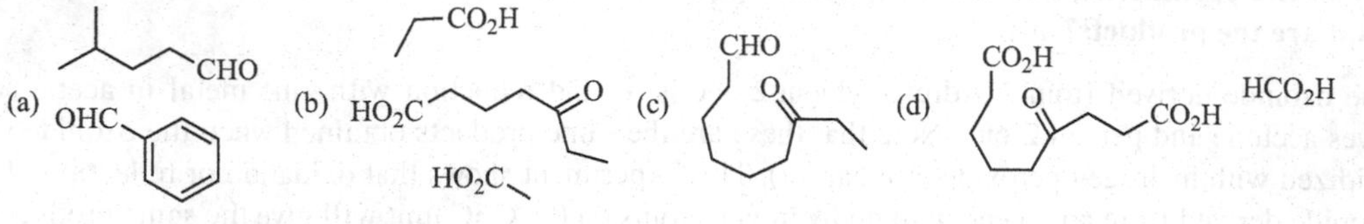

13.4 OXIDATIVE CLEAVAGE. PERIODIC ACID CLEAVAGE OF 1,2-DIOLS

What is the structure of periodic acid?

Periodic acid (also called meta-periodic acid) is usually written as HIO_4 but also exists as the dihydrate, orthoperiodic acid, written as H_5IO_6. The structure of both compounds is shown in the figure. The two structures are used interchangeably for the reaction discussed in the following questions.

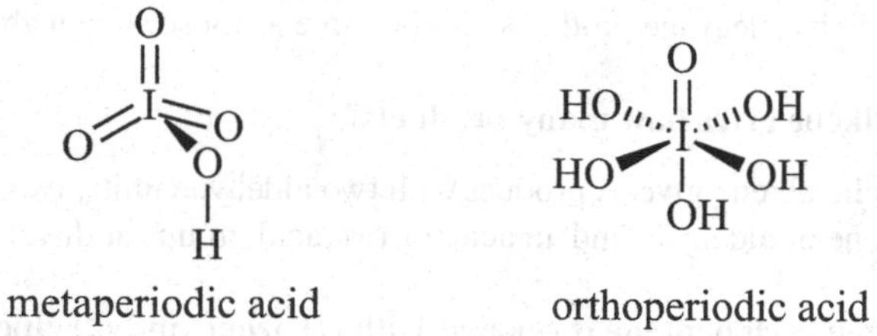

metaperiodic acid orthoperiodic acid

What is the general mechanism of the reaction of periodic acid with a 1,2-diol?

Periodic acid reacts with the 1,2-diol to form a cyclic periodate ester, ***A***. A concerted rearrangement allows cleavage of the carbon–carbon bond with elimination of iodic acid and formation of two equivalents of the carbonyl compound.

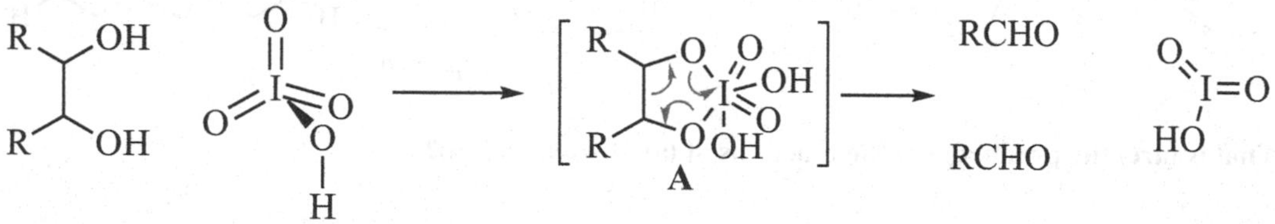

What is the initial product of the reaction of 3,4-hexanediol and periodic acid? What is the final product?

The initial reaction with periodic acid generates complex ***A***, which decomposes and leads to cleavage of the 1,2-diol into two aldehydes. In this case, the product is two equivalents of propanal.

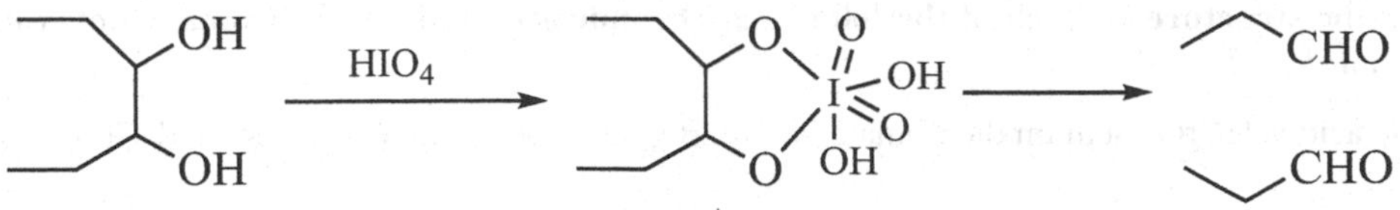

What is the initial product of the reaction of 1,2-cyclohexanediol and periodic acid? The final product?

Periodic acid cleaves 1,2-diols into aldehydes via the initially formed complex *A*. In this case, the product is a dialdehyde, hexane-1,6-dial [OHC-$(CH_2)_4$-CHO].

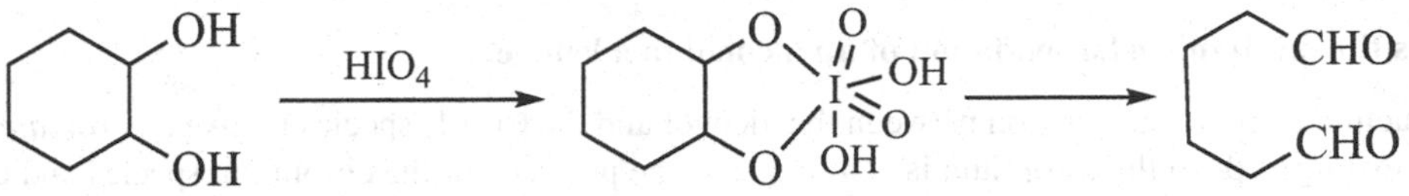

How are 1,2-diols usually formed?

As discussed in Sections 7.4.3 and 13.1, 1,2-diols are usually formed by treatment of an alkene with dilute $KMnO_4$ and hydroxide or with OsO_4 and sodium thiosulfite.

What is the product when hept-2-ene is treated with a mixture of osmium tetroxide and HIO_4?

In this case the OsO_4 converts hept-2-ene to heptane-2,3-diol, in the presence of HIO_4. The HIO_4 then cleaves the diol into carbonyl compounds, in this case ethanal and pentanal.

13.5 OXIDATION OF ALCOHOLS TO ALDEHYDES OR KETONES

What is the most common preparation of aldehydes or ketones?

The most common method for the preparation of a ketone or aldehyde is the oxidation of a primary or secondary alcohol. In general, oxidation of a secondary alcohol is expected to give a ketone, and oxidation of a primary alcohol gives either an aldehyde or a carboxylic acid, depending on the oxidizing agent.

What is the structure of chromium trioxide?

The basic structure of chromium trioxide is CrO_3, but this reagent is generally considered to be a polymer, $(CrO_3)_n$ where *n* is a large number. Chromium trioxide is a Cr (VI) reagent.

What species are present in solution when chromium trioxide is dissolved in water?

There are several Cr(VI) species, including CrO_3, $HCrO_4$ (chromic acid) and dichromate (CrO_7^{-2}). In a large excess of water, dichromate is usually the major species, but this depends on what is added to the solution. In very dilute solutions, more CrO_3 and chromic acid are present.

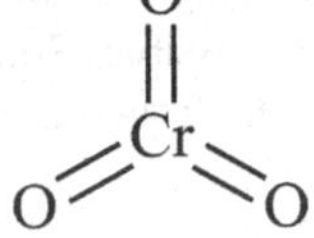

What is the structure for each of the following: chromic acid, sodium dichromate, potassium dichromate?

Chromic acid is $HCrO_4$, sodium dichromate is Na_2CrO_7, and potassium dichromate is K_2CrO_7.

What is the Jones reagent?

Mixing an acid, such as HCl or aqueous sulfuric acid with CrO_3 or dichromate, in an organic solvent, such as acetone, generates the oxidizing agent shown as Jones reagent. It is a powerful oxidizing medium.

What is the product when cyclohexanol is treated with Jones reagent?

The Cr(VI) in Jones reagent converts cyclohexanol into cyclohexanone.

What is the mechanism for oxidation of an alcohol to a ketone?

This reaction begins with reaction between the alcohol and the Cr(VI) species to give a *chromate ester*, *A*. The hydrogen β- to the chromium is acidic due to the presence of the chromium species and can be removed by the water that is in the system (water behaves as a base in this reaction). The reaction expels the CrO_3H leaving group concomitantly with formation of the carbonyl of an aldehyde or a ketone.

$$R_1R_2CH{-}O{-}H \xrightarrow[CrO_3]{H_2O} \left[R_1R_2CH{-}O{-}CrO_3H \right]_{\mathbf{A}} \xrightarrow{-HCrO_3} R_1R_2C{=}O$$

What is the importance of formation of a chromate ester in this oxidation reaction?

The presence of the chromium species makes hydrogen of the H—C—O—Cr moiety (the α-hydrogen) acidic. This hydrogen can react as an acid with a base, in this case water, and CrO_nH moiety is a good leaving group. This sequence facilitates the oxidation of the H—C—O—H unit to C=O.

How is a chromate ester converted to the ketone?

The hydrogen β- to the chromium atom is acidic and is removed by a base (usually water) to form a carbonyl π-bond and expel the chromium (III) species, which disproportionates. In this reaction, the chromium is a good leaving group. Since acid (H_3O^+) is formed, the reaction proceeds best in acid media.

Does the reaction of a tertiary alcohols a chromium trioxide form a chromate ester?

Yes!

Why is it not possible to oxidize a tertiary alcohol to a ketone?

There is no hydrogen β- to the chromate ester of this alcohol and formation of a carbonyl would require breaking a C—C bond.

Why is there a difference in reaction rate for chromate esters *A* and *B*?

The chromate ester in *A* has a hydrogen that is "underneath" the ring and is very difficult to approach due to steric hindrance imposed by shape of the ring system. In chromate ester *B* that hydrogen is on the outer face of the molecule and it is relatively accessible. Since the hydrogen in *A* in hard to remove, the rate of oxidation is slower since removal of the hydrogen atom is the rate determining step.

H₃C OCrO₃H / **A** H   H₃C H / **B** OCrO₃H

What is the major product for the reactions of (a), (b), and (c)?

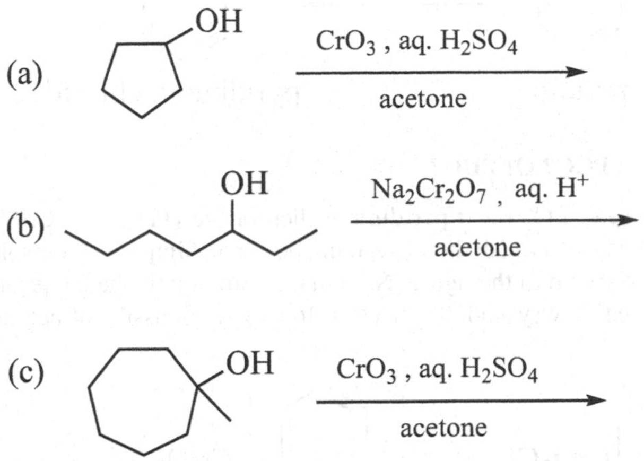

(a) OH — CrO_3, aq. H_2SO_4 / acetone →

(b) OH — $Na_2Cr_2O_7$, aq. H^+ / acetone →

(c) OH — CrO_3, aq. H_2SO_4 / acetone →

In the first reaction, cyclopentanol is converted into cyclopentanone by the Jones reagent. In the second reaction octan-3-ol is converted into octan-3-one, and in the final example, 1-methylcycloheptanol is treated with Jones reagent. Since this is a tertiary alcohol, no oxidation takes place and the correct answer is no reaction.

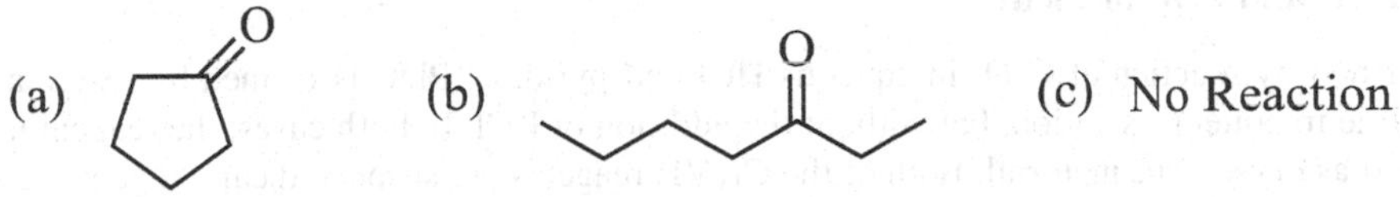

(a) O (b) O (c) No Reaction

What is the expected product when a primary alcohol is oxidized with Cr(VI)?

A primary alcohol is expected to be oxidized into an aldehyde ($RCH_2OH \rightarrow RCHO$), but the aldehyde is often *not* the observed product unless special precautions are taken. The actual product isolated when a primary alcohol is oxidized with Jones reagent is often a carboxylic acid ($RCH_2OH \rightarrow RCO_2H$) via initial oxidation to the aldehyde and *in situ* oxidation of the aldehyde to the carboxylic acid. Chromium (VI) in acidic media is a powerful oxidizing medium and aldehydes are very susceptible to oxidation to acids. Indeed, many low molecular weight aldehydes are oxidized to acids by exposure to oxygen in the air. In the presence of Cr(VI), therefore, the initially formed aldehyde from the oxidation will be further oxidized to a carboxylic acid. This unwanted oxidation can be avoided if the contact time for the reaction is short, the reaction temperature is kept low, or if the aldehyde product is removed from the reaction medium.

What is the structure of pyridine?

The structure of pyridine is shown in the figure and it is essentially the compound formed by replacing on of the carbon atoms of benzene with nitrogen. Pyridine is an aromatic amine (see Section 16.6) and the nitrogen is basic.

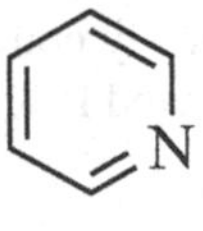

N

What is the product when the amine, pyridine, reacts as a base with HCl?

The acid–base reaction of pyridine with HCl is shown in the figure. The product is the ammonium salt, pyridinium chloride.

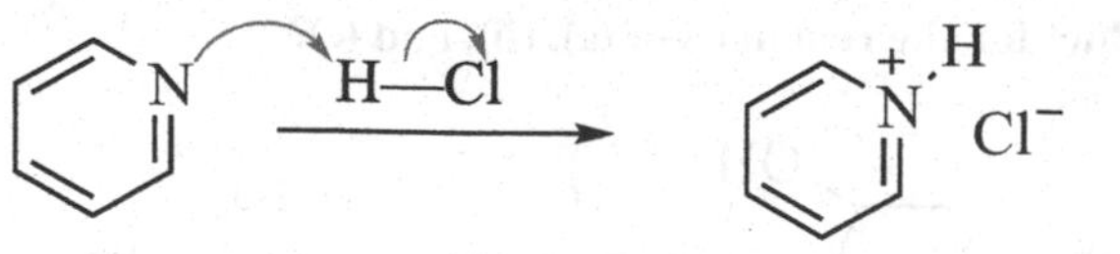

pyridine → pyridinium chloride (H—Cl; Cl⁻)

What is the structure of PCC? Of PDC?

Pyridinium chlorochromate (PCC) and pyridinium dichromate (PDC) are Cr(VI) reagents that have been structurally modified to diminish their oxidizing power and improve their solubility in organic solvents. The structures are shown in the figure. Note that pyridinium is the conjugate acid of the reaction of pyridine and a Brønsted–Lowry acid. See Section 16.6 for a discussion of heteroaromatic compounds such as pyridine.

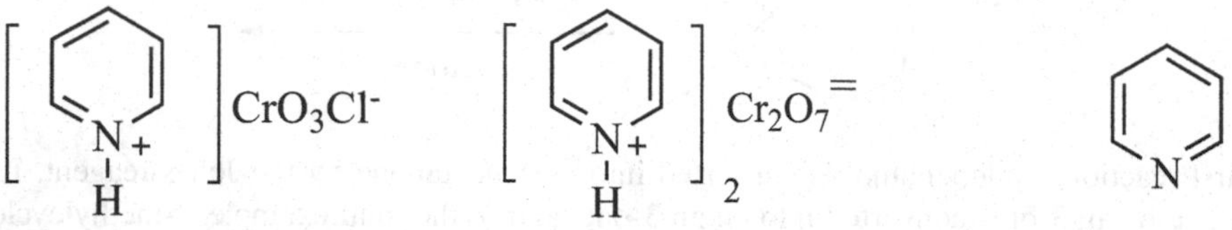

CrO_3Cl^- $Cr_2O_7^{=}$

Pyridinium chorochromate Pyrdium dichromate Pyridine

How are PCC and PDC formed?

PCC is formed by reaction of CrO_3 in aqueous HCl and pyridine. PDC is formed by reaction of CrO_3 with pyridine in aqueous solution, but without the addition of HCl. In both cases, the reagent is isolated and purified as crystalline material. Both of the Cr(VI) reagents are suspected carcinogens, however.

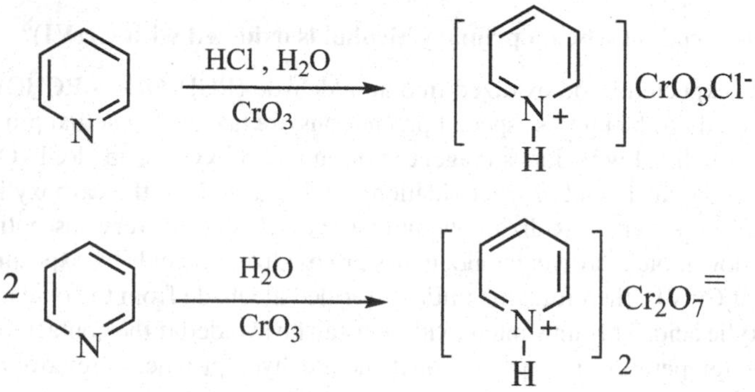

HCl, H_2O / CrO_3 → CrO_3Cl^-

2 (pyridine) H_2O / CrO_3 → $Cr_2O_7^{=}$

Why are PCC and PDC used for the oxidant of primary alcohols, especially allylic primary alcohols rather than a Jones reagent?

Both PCC and PDC are significantly milder oxidizing agents and will convert a primary alcohol to an aldehyde without further oxidation to the carboxylic acid using dichloromethane as a solvent. It is known that allylic alcohols (C=C—C—OH) are more reactive and more susceptible to over-oxidation than simple primary alcohols. Both PCC and PDC easily convert allylic primary alcohols to the conjugated aldehyde in dichloromethane solvent. Both PCC and PDC will convert a secondary alcohol to a ketone.

What is the product of the reactions of (a), (b), (c), and (d)?

(a) 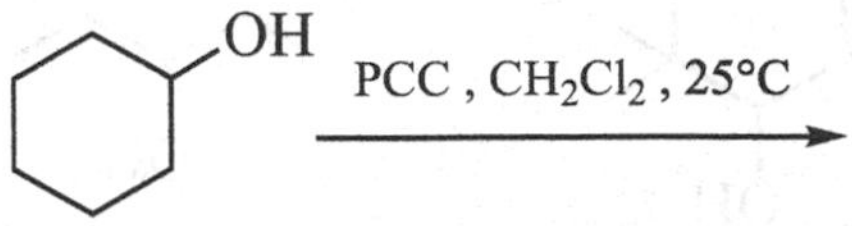 OH — PCC , CH_2Cl_2 , 25°C →

(b) 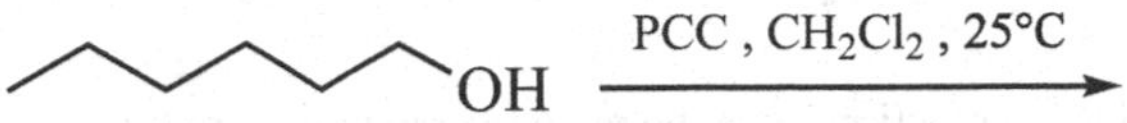 OH — PCC , CH_2Cl_2 , 25°C →

(c) CH_2OH — PDC , CH_2Cl_2 , 25°C 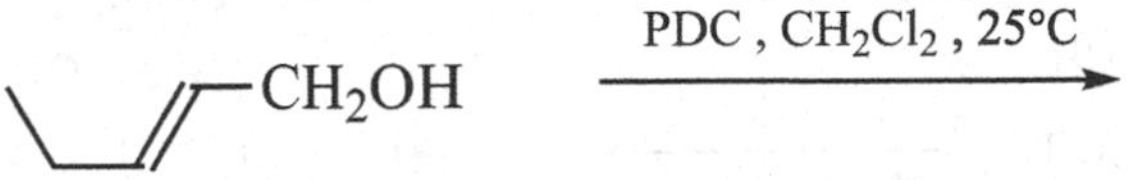 →

(d) 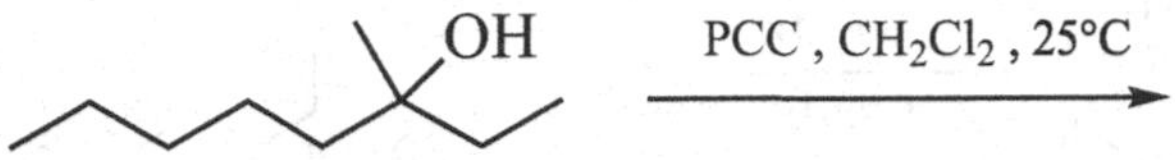 OH — PCC , CH_2Cl_2 , 25°C →

Cyclohexanol is oxidized to cyclohexanone with PCC. Hexan-1-ol is oxidized to the aldehyde (hexanal) with PCC. PDC will oxide pent-2*E*-en-1-ol to pent-2*E*-al. 3-Methyloctan-3-ol is a tertiary alcohol and neither PCC nor PDC will oxidize this alcohol. The answer here is no reaction. In all cases, the reactions are performed at 25°C using dichloromethane as a solvent. These are typical reaction conditions.

(a) 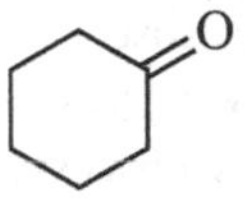 O (b) 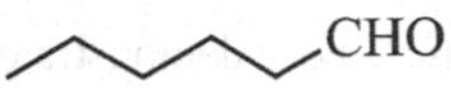 CHO (c) 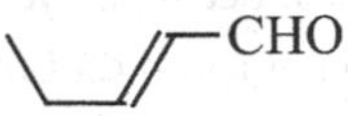 CHO (d) No Reaction

END OF CHAPTER PROBLEMS

1. In each of the following reactions, give the major product. Remember stereochemistry and if there is no reaction, indicate by N.R.

(a) 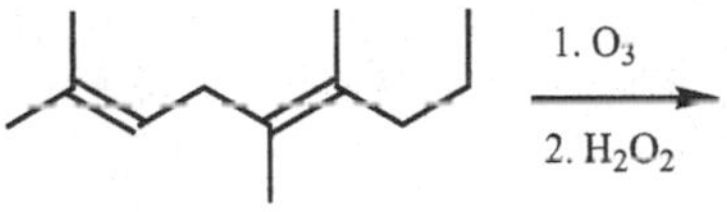 1. O_3 2. H_2O_2 →

(b) 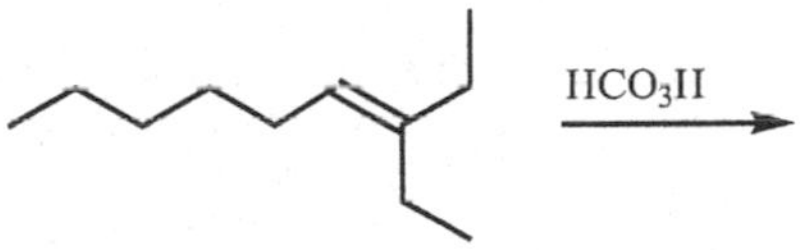 $IICO_3II$ →

(c) 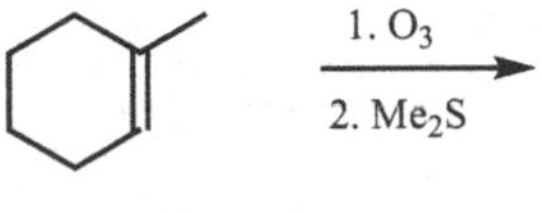 1. O_3 2. Me_2S →

(d) 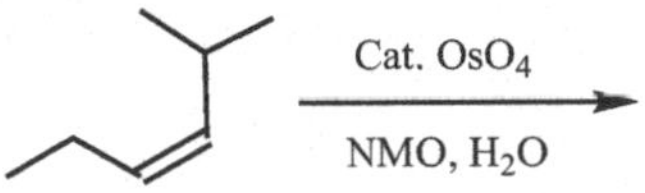 Cat. OsO_4 NMO, H_2O →

(e) 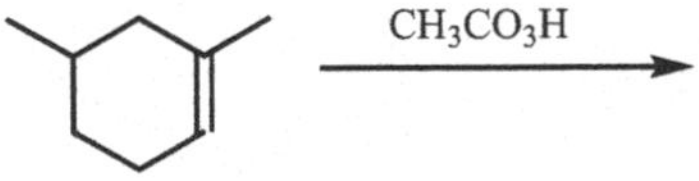 CH_3CO_3H →

(f) 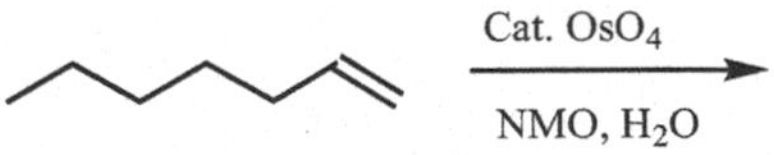 Cat. OsO_4 NMO, H_2O →

(g) 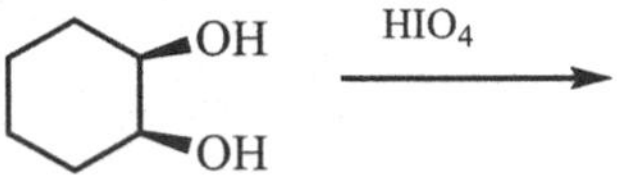 OH OH — HIO_4 →

(h) OH OH — HIO_4 →

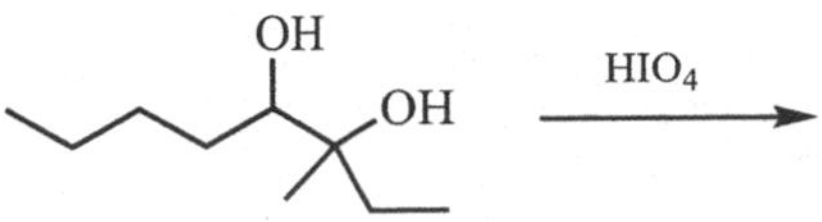

2. Explain why alcohol ***A*** is oxidized much slower than alcohol ***B***.

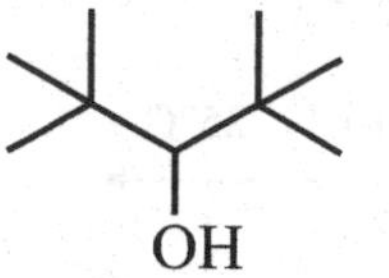

OH
A

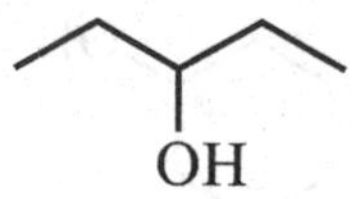

OH
B

3. For each of the following reactions give the major product. If there is no reaction, indicate by N.R.

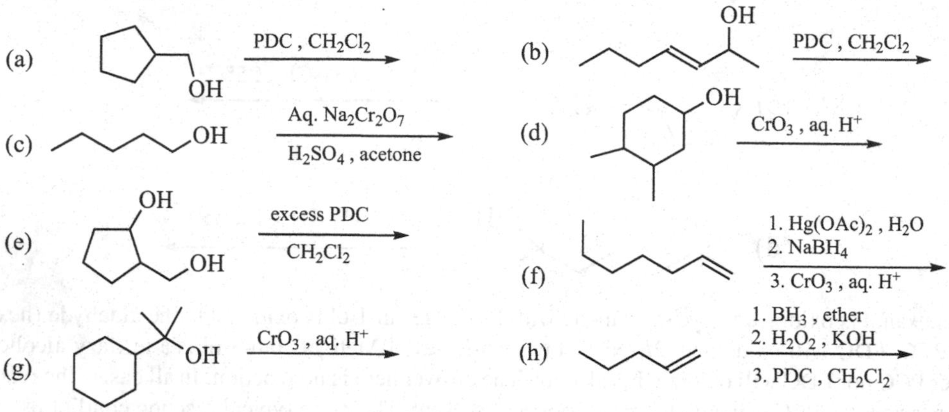

(a) OH — PDC , CH_2Cl_2 →

(b) OH — PDC , CH_2Cl_2 →

(c) OH — Aq. $Na_2Cr_2O_7$ / H_2SO_4 , acetone →

(d) OH — CrO_3 , aq. H^+ →

(e) OH, OH — excess PDC / CH_2Cl_2 →

(f) 1. $Hg(OAc)_2$, H_2O 2. $NaBH_4$ 3. CrO_3 , aq. H^+ →

(g) OH — CrO_3 , aq. H^+ →

(h) 1. BH_3 , ether 2. H_2O_2 , KOH 3. PDC , CH_2Cl_2 →

4. How can one distinguish between cyclohexanone and cyclohexen-2-one using spectroscopy?
5. How does the isolation of a cis- diol from a cyclic alkene demonstrate that hydroxide does not attack carbon when the manganate ester is decomposed in the reaction of $KMnO_4$ with a cyclic alkene?
6. Why is sodium acetate often added to the epoxidation of alkenes with peroxycarboxylic acids?
7. Which reacts faster with peroxyacetic acid, pent-1-ene or pent-2-ene?

14

Reduction Reactions

Reduction reactions are extremely important in organic chemistry. A molecule, such as an aldehyde or ketone, in a higher oxidation state is converted to an alcohol, which is in a lower oxidation state. It is also possible to prepare alcohols by reduction of carboxylic acids. The conversion of an alkene to an alkane is a reduction, as is the conversion of an alkyne to an alkene or to an alkane. This chapter will discuss reduction reactions and their use in various organic chemical reactions.

What is the definition of a reduction?

Reduction is defined as a reaction in which two electrons are gained in the final product. A more practical definition is a reaction that adds hydrogen to the molecule or loses an electronegative element (such as oxygen) from the molecule.

What is an oxidation state?

Oxidation state is a number associated with gain or loss of electron density. The usual formalism involves assigning a −1 to each attached element that is less electronegative than carbon (such as H); +1 to each attached element that is more electronegative than carbon (such as O, N, Br, etc.). Another attached carbon is assigned a value of 0. These numbers are added together to give the oxidation state for each carbon.

What is the change in oxidation state when acetone is converted to propan-2-ol?

In acetone, the two C—C bonds attached to the carbonyl carbon are assigned a value of 0 and the two bonds to oxygen (C=O) give a value of +2. The oxidation level for the carbonyl carbon is, therefore, +2. Examination of propan-2-ol (isopropanol) shows the C—O bond is valued at +1, the C—H bond at −1 and each C—C bond, 0. The central carbon of isopropanol has an oxidation level of 0. The conversion from +2 to 0 is a net *gain* of electrons (electrons are negatively charged and increasing electron density leads to a more negative number) and is, therefore, a reduction.

O +2
H3C 0, CH3 0 ⟶ +1 OH; H3C 0, H −1, CH3 0

In general, if the change in oxidation number is positive, it is an oxidation (see Chapter 13) and if it is negative it is a reduction.

If the alcohol is oxidized, what happens to the reagent that causes the oxidation to occur?

Oxidation and reduction are linked. If the alcohol is oxidized, the reagent that caused that transformation must be reduced. Conversely, if a ketone is reduced, the reagent that caused that transformation must be oxidized.

What is this reagent called?

A reducing agent is a molecule that causes another molecule to be reduced. An oxidation agent is a molecule that causes another molecule to be oxidized.

14.1 CATALYTIC HYDROGENATION

Does but-1-ene or but-2-yne react with hydrogen gas in ethanol with no other additives?

No! Alkenes and alkynes do not react with hydrogen gas if no other additives are present.

Does but-1-ene or but-2-yne react with hydrogen gas in ethanol in the presence of a transition metal?

Yes! Hydrogen does not react directly with the π-bond of an alkene or alkyne but it does react with many transition metals. In the presence of a transition metal catalyst, the π-bond of an alkene or alkyne reacts to form a metal complex and the metal also reacts with diatomic hydrogen, breaking the H—H bond to give hydrogen atoms bound to the metal. Once this complex is formed, hydrogen is transferred to the π-bond of the metal-bound complex leading to the transfer of two hydrogen atoms to the π-bond. This reaction is known as *catalytic hydrogenation.*

Explain why hex-1-ene does not react with hydrogen gas when no other reagents are present.

Diatomic hydrogen gas (H—H) is not polarized and is not polarizable. Because H_2 is not polarized, when the alkene comes into close proximity to H_2, there is no "$H^{\delta+}$—$H^{\delta-}$" for the alkene to react with. The only way H_2 can react with an alkene is when another reagent is present than can react with H_2 to break the H—H bond.

Can diatomic hydrogen react with an alkene if the H—H unit is cleaved by some other molecule added to the reaction?

Yes! Transition metals such as nickel, palladium, platinum, or metal salts such as platinum oxide react with hydrogen gas, breaking the H—H bond and forming metal–H bonds. Once the hydrogen bond is broken by the metal, the alkene can react with the hydrogen atoms on the surface of the metal.

In the reaction with hydrogen gas with a transition metal, is a catalytic or a stoichiometric amount of the metal required?

The reaction with the metal and hydrogen gas leads to a complex, and after the transfer of hydrogen atoms to the carbon atom of a π-bond from the complex, the metal is free to react with more hydrogen gas and the alkene or alkyne is further reduced. Therefore, only a catalytic amount of the metal is required.

What is the major product when 3-methyloct-3*E*-ene reacts with hydrogen gas in the presence of a catalytic amount of palladium metal adsorbed on carbon black?

The platinum oxide is a *catalyst* for the addition reaction of hydrogen gas to the alkene, converting (*E*)-3-methyloct-3-ene to the alkane (3-methyloctane). Only a catalytic amount of palladium metal is required to promote this reaction, which is known as *catalytic hydrogenation.*

H_2, Pd-C

3*E*-Methyloct-3-ene → 3-Methyloctane

What is adsorption?

Adsorption is the adhesion of a chemical species onto the surface of a particle or particles. Adsorption creates a thin film of the adsorbate (the species that is adsorbed) on the surface of the adsorbent (the surface that adsorbs the species). This process differs from absorption, in which a fluid is dissolved by or permeates a liquid or solid, respectively.

What is heterogeneous catalysis?

In heterogeneous catalysis, the phase of the catalyst is different from the phase of the reactants or products. In practical terms, particles of the catalyst are insoluble in the reaction medium.

What are some common catalysts used for heterogeneous catalytic hydrogenation?

The most common catalysts are the transition metals platinum (Pt), palladium (Pd), and nickel (Ni).

Why are fine powders rather than larger lumps of catalyst used?

The expensive metals used as catalysts are finely divided since catalytic hydrogenation occurs in heterogeneous systems as a surface reaction. In other words, the hydrogen and the alkene or alkyne are adsorbed on the surface of the metal catalyst. Therefore, the higher the surface area of the catalyst, the greater the adsorption of the reactants and the faster the rate of hydrogenation. The metals are often converted to metal compounds such as platinum oxide (PtO_2) or palladium chloride ($PdCl_2$), which can also serve as catalysts.

What is the purpose of the carbon in the catalyst palladium on carbon (Pd/C)?

Since palladium and platinum are expensive, the finely divided metal is often mixed with inert materials that have a high surface area, such as carbon black. The carbon is called a *solid support*, and mixing a small amount of the catalyst with the carbon "dilutes" the catalyst as well as increases the relative surface area. Metals can also be adsorbed or mixed with calcium carbonate ($CaCO_3$), barium carbonate ($BaCO_3$), alumina (Al_2O_3), or Kieselguhr (a form of diatomaceous earth).

What solvents are commonly used in heterogeneous catalysts?

Typical solvents are methanol or ethanol. Other solvents are possible of course but these simple alcohol solvents are common.

What is a mechanistic rationale for the catalytic hydrogenation of but-2-ene with palladium on carbon?

If the catalyst is treated as a surface hydrogen approaches the metal. The metal transfers electrons to hydrogen and a homolytic cleavage leads to hydrogen atoms, which bind to the metal as hydrogen atoms. When the alkene approaches the metal, the π-bond binds to the surface of the metal and a hydrogen atom is transferred to the alkene, generating a carbon radical, which is also bound to the metal as a complex. Transfer of a second hydrogen liberates the alkane product (here, butane) and regenerates the catalyst, which can react with more hydrogen.

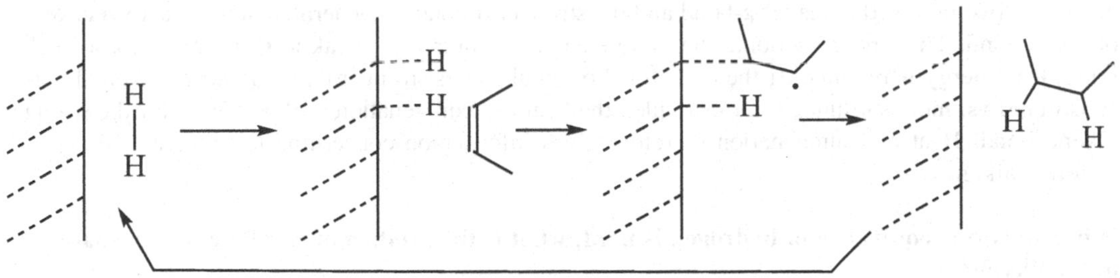

What is the major product of the reactions of (a), (b), (c), and (d), shown?

(a) cyclopentene $\xrightarrow[\text{EtOH}]{H_2\text{, Pd/C}}$

(b) $\xrightarrow[\text{BaSO}_4\text{, EtOH}]{H_2\text{, Pt}}$

(c) $\xrightarrow[\text{MeOH}]{2\ H_2\text{, Pd/BaSO}_4}$

(d) cyclohexene $\xrightarrow[\text{MeOH}]{H_2\text{, Carbon black}}$

Reaction (a) generates cyclopentane. Reaction (b) gives 2,5-dimethylhexane. Diene (c) has two double bonds, and with two equivalents of hydrogen, both are hydrogenated to give 2-methylheptane. In the reaction of (d), there is no metal catalyst, so there is no reaction and the cyclohexene starting material is isolated.

(a) Cyclopentane (b) 2,5-Dimethylhexane (c) 2-Methylheptane (d) No Reaction

What is heat of hydrogenation?

Each covalent bond requires that a certain amount of energy be added to break it. That same amount of energy is inherent to the bond and is called the *bond dissociation energy*. When a carbon–carbon double bond is broken during catalytic hydrogenation, the bond dissociation energy for that bond is released and is called *heat of hydrogenation* (alternatively, the amount of heat that must be added to disrupt the C=C bond).

What information does heat of hydrogenation provide about alkenes?

There are two bonds, the weaker π-bond and the stronger σ-bond. In general, alkenes react via cleavage of the π-bond. The stronger a bond, the more energy is required to break it. Conversely, for a weaker bond, less energy is required. If the C=C bond of an alkene is stronger than another C=C bond (tetra-substituted vs. monosubstituted, for example), the heat of hydrogenation will be higher for the stronger alkene bond. Heat of hydrogenation therefore gives information concerning the inherent strength of different alkenes.

When only one equivalent of hydrogen is used, what is the product of catalytic hydrogenation of an alkyne?

A single equivalent of hydrogen, with an appropriate catalyst, will give an alkene as the final product; also, some alkane may be formed since the alkene is also subject to reaction with hydrogen and the catalyst. If the stoichiometry is maintained and the reaction conditions are controlled, the alkene is usually the major product. The reaction is: R-C≡C-R + H_2 + Pd/C → RCH=CHR.

How many equivalents of hydrogen are required to convert an alkyne to an alkane?

The conversion of an alkyne to an alkane is R-C≡C-R → RCH_2CH_2R and requires a minimum of two equivalents of hydrogen gas, along with an appropriate catalyst.

What catalysts can be used for hydrogenation of an alkyne?

In general, the same catalysts used for hydrogenation of an alkene: nickel, platinum, and palladium.

What is the major product in the reactions of (a), (b), and (c)?

(a) H_2, EtOH

(b) 2 H_2 Pd/C, EtOH

(c) H_2, Pd/C, EtOH

In the reaction hex-1-yne in (a), there is no catalyst so there is no reaction with hydrogen, and hex-1-yne is recovered. The answer is, therefore, no reaction. In the reaction of the alkyne in (b), reaction with two equivalents of hydrogen, in the presence of a palladium catalyst, leads to the alkane (2-cyclopentylethyl) cyclohexane. When 3-hex-3-yne in (c) reacts with one equivalent of hydrogen in the presence of the palladium catalyst, the product is an alkene, hex-3-ene. However, there is little selectivity, and hex-3-ene is a mixture of cis- and trans- isomers.

(a) No Reaction (b) (2-Cyclopentylethyl)cyclohexane (c) Major: Hex-3*Z*-ene; Minor: Hex-3*E*-ene

How many products are possible when hex-3-yne is treated with one equivalent of hydrogen in the presence of a platinum catalyst?

There are three possible products, two major and one minor. The two major products are cis- and trans-hex-3-ene and the minor product is hexane. In this case, reduction of the alkyne group in hex-3-yne to the alkene gives either a cis- alkene or a trans- alkene. In this case, there is no way to control the reaction and *both* stereoisomers are formed. Depending on the metal catalyst, the thermodynamically more stable trans- isomer is formed in greater amount than the cis-, but both are formed.

Why is it important to carefully control the number of equivalents of hydrogen added to an alkyne when the alkene is the desired product?

If too much hydrogen gas is used, the alkene product of the reduction can be further reduced to give the alkane, as seen earlier. Another problem is that the alkene product may be more reactive to the catalyst (or to hydrogen after being bound to the catalyst) and react faster than unreacted alkyne. For this reason, the alkane often accompanies the alkene as a minor product.

If one equivalent of hydrogen gas is used but the reaction conditions are vigorous (heat, pressure), what types of products are possible?

Since the alkene product may be more reactive than the alkyne starting material, vigorous conditions (heat and pressure) may cause over-reaction to give the alkane product. To minimize this problem, both the temperature and the pressure of the reaction are controlled, along with the number of equivalents of hydrogen gas. Another important factor in this reaction is the nature of the catalyst. In general, palladium catalysts are used to reduce alkynes to alkenes and although a platinum catalyst works, it is less selective. Note that rhodium and ruthenium catalysts are also very useful.

What is the Lindlar catalyst?

The original *Lindlar catalyst* was a mixture of palladium chloride ($PdCl_2$), which was precipitated on calcium carbonate ($CaCO_3$) in acidic media and deactivated with lead tetraacetate [$Pb(OAc)_4$] to give the named Pd-$CaCO_3$-PbO catalyst. Later, the so-called *Rosenmund catalyst* was developed with palladium on barium carbonate ($BaCO_3$) or calcium carbonate ($CaCO_3$) was deactivated with quinoline and found to give similar reactivity. This latter catalyst is often referred to as the *Lindlar catalyst*. The structure of quinoline is shown, and similar aromatic compounds are discussed in Section 16.6.

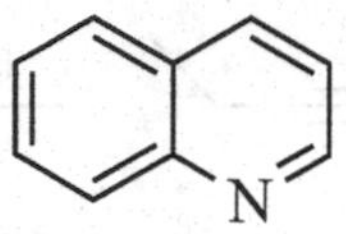

N

Quinoline

Why are the Lindlar catalyst and the Rosenmund catalyst important?

The importance of these catalysts is shown by the conversion of 1,2-dicyclohexylethyne to (*Z*)-1,2-dicyclohexylethene. Both catalysts give almost exclusively the cis- alkene from the alkyne, with little or no contamination by the trans- alkene or from the over-reduction product (in this case (*Z*)-1,2-dicyclohexylethene). The preferred use of the Lindlar catalyst or the Rosenmund catalyst is, therefore, formation of Z-alkenes from alkynes.

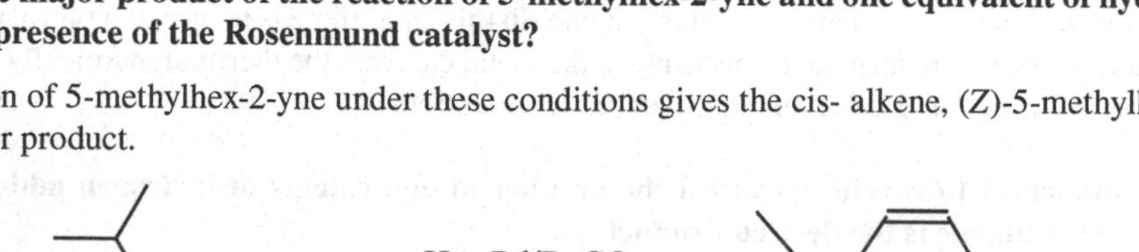

H_2 , Pd/$BaCO_3$

EtOH

N

What is the major product of the reaction of 5-methylhex-2-yne and one equivalent of hydrogen gas in the presence of the Rosenmund catalyst?

The reaction of 5-methylhex-2-yne under these conditions gives the cis- alkene, (*Z*)-5-methylhex-2-ene, as the major product.

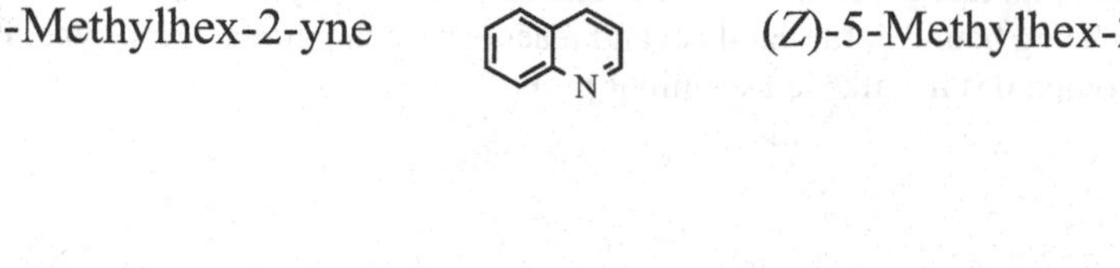

H_2 , Pd/$BaCO_3$

EtOH

N

5-Methylhex-2-yne

(*Z*)-5-Methylhex-2-ene

What is homogeneous catalysis?

Homogeneous catalysis has the catalyst, reactants, and products in the same phase. Typically, the catalyst is soluble in the reaction medium and reactions occur by discrete and detectable steps. In other words, the mechanism of homogeneous catalytic hydrogenation can be determined.

What is Wilkinson's catalyst? What is Vaska's catalyst?

Wilkinson's catalyst is a rhodium catalyst with one chlorine and three triphenylphosphine units: chloridotris(triphenylphosphino)rhodium (I). Vaska's catalyst is an iridium catalyst with two triphenylphosphine units, one chlorine and one carbon monoxide unit: carbonylchlorobis(triphenylphosphine) iridium (I). Both of these molecules are examples of homogenous catalysts.

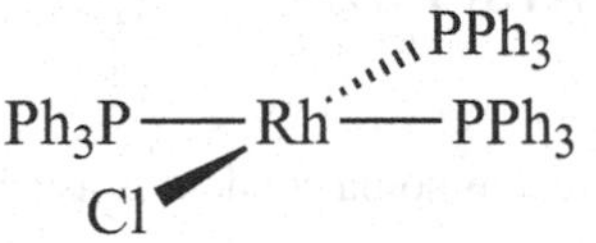

PPh_3
Ph_3P—Rh—PPh_3
Cl

Wilkinson's catlyst

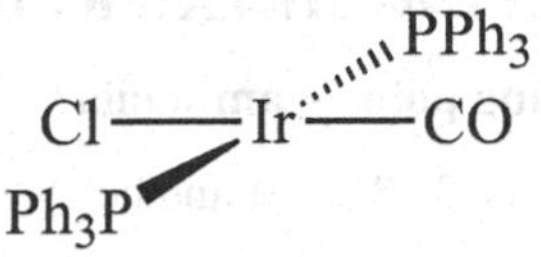

PPh_3
Cl—Ir—CO
Ph_3P

Vaska's catlyst

Why are homogeneous catalysts attractive?

As seen in the preceding question, homogenous catalysts are typically discrete molecules and they are soluble in the reaction medium. Homogenous catalysts react by predictable reactions called organometallic reactions, which will not be discussed further in this book, but their predictable reactions allow a discrete mechanism to be determined for the catalytic hydrogenation.

What are the major product(s) of the following reactions?

(a) 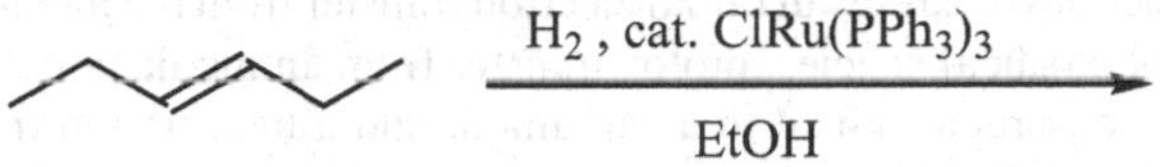 $\xrightarrow[\text{EtOH}]{H_2\text{, cat. ClRu(PPh}_3)_3}$

(b) 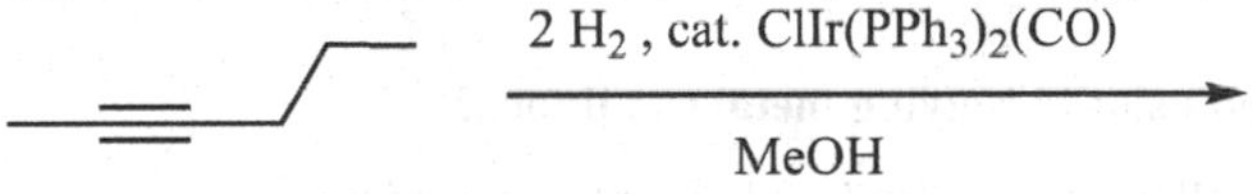 $\xrightarrow[\text{MeOH}]{2\,H_2\text{, cat. ClIr(PPh}_3)_2\text{(CO)}}$

(c) 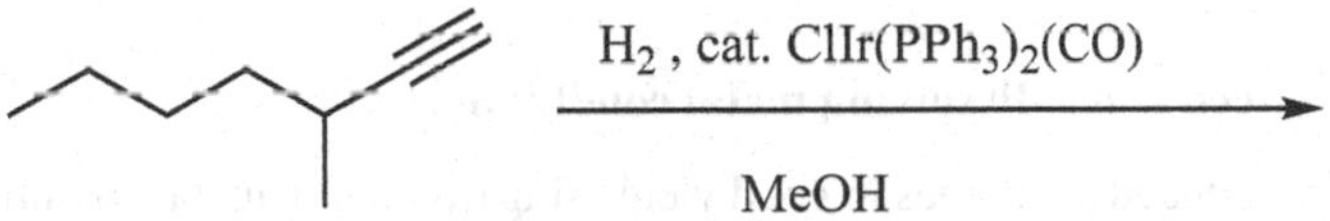 $\xrightarrow[\text{MeOH}]{H_2\text{, cat. ClIr(PPh}_3)_2\text{(CO)}}$

(d) 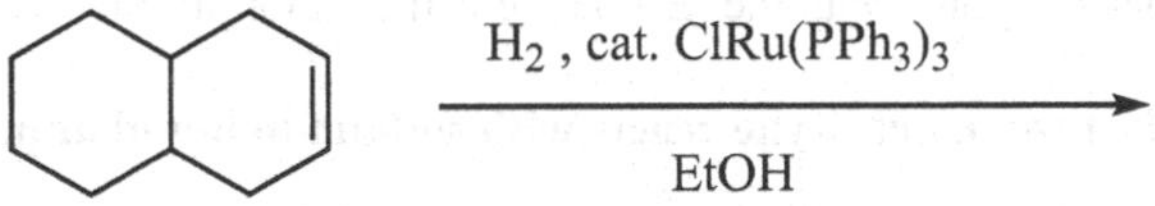 $\xrightarrow[\text{EtOH}]{H_2\text{, cat. ClRu(PPh}_3)_3}$

(e) 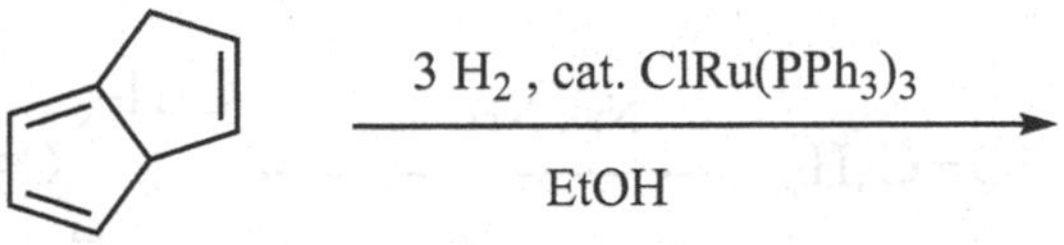 $\xrightarrow[\text{EtOH}]{3\,H_2\text{, cat. ClRu(PPh}_3)_3}$

Hydrogenation of the alkene in (a) with one equivalent of hydrogen gas and hydrogenation of alkyne with excess hydrogen gas in (b) both lead to hexane. Hydrogenation of the alkyne in (c) with only one equivalent of hydrogen leads to the alkene 3-methylhept-1-ene. Hydrogenation of (d) reduces the single C=C unit to give the bicyclic compound decahydronaphthalene, and hydrogenation of (e) with an excess of hydrogen gas leads to the bicyclic compound octahydropentalene.

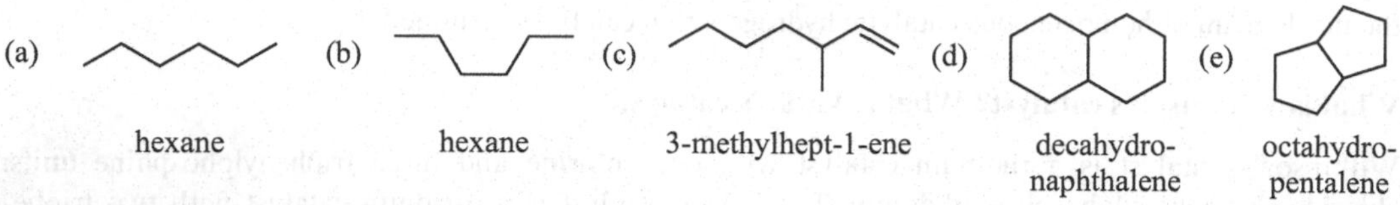

(a) hexane (b) hexane (c) 3-methylhept-1-ene (d) decahydro-naphthalene (e) octahydro-pentalene

14.2 DISSOLVING METAL REDUCTION: ALKYNES

What is the boiling point of ammonia?

The boiling point is -33.3°C. At and below this temperature, ammonia condenses as a blue liquid.

What is the most common reaction of sodium metal?

Sodium is in Group 1 and is characterized by the transfer of a single electron.

What is a dissolving metal reduction?

Dissolving metal reduction is the reduction of organic molecules (alkynes, aldehydes or ketones, and aromatic compounds are typical substrates) primarily with sodium, potassium, or other Group 1 or 2 metals (e.g., Na, Li, or K) in a liquid ammonia solvent. The technique can be done with or without added ethanol.

How does a dissolving metal reduction work?

Dissolving metal reductions occur by an initial electron transfer from the metal. The mechanism involves the initial formation of a radical species, proton transfer from ammonia or ethanol, a subsequent second electron transfer that converts a radical to a carbanion, and a final proton transfer giving the product. The proton source is the protic solvent in an acid–base reaction with the carbanion to give the product.

Are alkenes reduced using dissolving metal conditions?

In general, no! Most alkenes are not reduced under these conditions.

Are alkynes reduced using dissolving metal conditions?

Yes! Alkynes are reduced to alkenes in good yield using dissolving metal conditions, and the experimental evidence shows that where appropriate the (*E*)-alkene is the major product.

What is the major product when oct-4-yne reacts with sodium in liquid ammonia?

The product is oct-4*E*-ene.

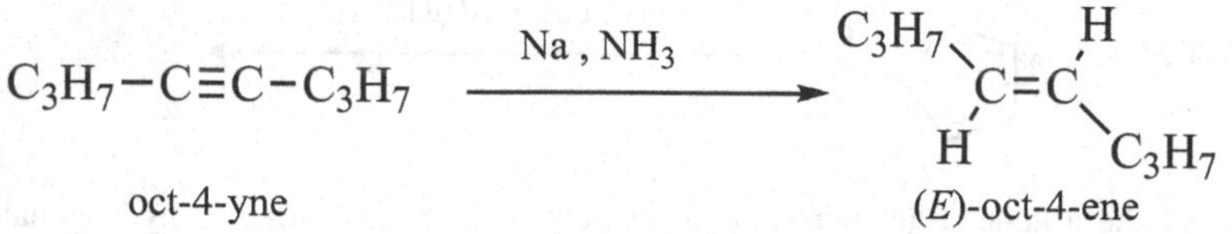

$$C_3H_7{-}C{\equiv}C{-}C_3H_7 \xrightarrow{Na\ ,\ NH_3} (C_3H_7)HC{=}CH(C_3H_7)$$

oct-4-yne (*E*)-oct-4-ene

What is the mechanism for the dissolving metal reduction to oct-4-yne with sodium in ammonia?

Electron transfer from the sodium to one π-bond of oct-4-yne leads to a radical anion *A* by transfer of a single electron. The radical anion is resonance stabilized as shown in the figure. The radical anion has one orbital that contains a single electron (a radical) and a second orbital that contains two electrons (an anion). The two orbitals can be either on the same side or on opposite sides. Formation of the observed (*E*)-product is most easily explained by minimizing the electronic repulsion between the two orbitals, making the anti- or trans- relationship of the orbitals the lowest energy and most prevalent species. Reaction with ethanol via an acid–base reaction with the carbanion leads to radical intermediate ***B***. A second electron transfer to radical ***B*** from a second Na atom leads to carbanion ***C***, and protonation gives the final product, oct-(4*E*)-ene.

$C_3H_7-C{\equiv}C-C_3H_7 \xrightarrow{\bullet Na} [\text{A}] \xrightarrow{EtOH} [\text{B}] \xrightarrow{\bullet Na} [\text{C}] \xrightarrow{EtOH} (C_3H_7)HC{=}CH(C_3H_7)$

What is the significance of this reaction with alkynes?

This method is an interesting counterpoint to the Lindlar reduction discussed in Section 14.1. The Lindlar reduction of an alkyne gives a (*Z*)-alkene, but dissolving metal reduction of an alkyne yields an (*E*)-alkene. The reduction process can therefore be controlled, and either a (*Z*)- or an (*E*)-alkene can be prepared.

What is the product when benzene reacts with sodium metal in liquid ammonia and ethanol?

The product is cyclohexa-1,4-diene in what is known as the Birch reduction. The Birch reaction is discussed in Section 16.5.

14.3 HYDRIDE REDUCTION OF ALDEHYDES AND KETONES

Why is the conversion of a ketone to an alcohol considered to be a reduction?

The C=O → H—C—O—H conversion involves the gain of two electrons, which is a reduction. The structural change is the formation of two bonds, C—H and O—H, with concomitant cleavage of the π-bond. Clearly, the reaction adds two hydrogen atoms to the carbonyl and therefore fits that definition.

What is a hydride reagent?

A hydride reagent is an "ate" complex that is usually derived from BH_3 (borane) or alane (AlH_3), with structures such as BH_4^- or AlH_4^-. The feature of such reagents that is most useful for this chapter is the bond polarization of B—H or Al—H, which gives the hydrogen a δ^- dipole. Such reagents react as nucleophiles with electrophilic atoms such as the carbonyl carbon of aldehydes or ketones.

What is the structure of lithium aluminum hydride?

The structure is $LiAlH_4$, where the active species is tetrahydridoaluminate, AlH_4^-.

$$[AlH_4]^- \; Li^+$$

What is the bond polarization for the Al—H bond of lithium aluminum hydride?

Aluminum is less electronegative than hydrogen and the hydrogen takes the negative pole ($H^{\delta-}$). The polarization is $^{\delta+}Al—H^{\delta-}$.

What is the structure of sodium borohydride?

Sodium borohydride is $NaBH_4$ and the active agent is tetrahydridoborate, BH_4^-.

H
| –
H-Na-H Na^+
|
H

What solvents are used for $LiAlH_4$? For $NaBH_4$?

Ether solvents such as diethyl ether or THF are used with $LiAlH_4$ whereas protic solvents such as ethanol, methanol, or sometimes water are used with $NaBH_4$.

Can water or methanol be used as a solvent with $LiAlH_4$?

No! Lithium aluminum hydride reacts violently with water or methanol to produce hydrogen gas. Since $LiAlH_4$ is much more reactive than $NaBH_4$, water cannot be used as a solvent, although water is commonly used in $NaBH_4$ reactions.

Is sodium borohydride a stronger or a weaker reducing agent when compared to lithium aluminum hydride? Explain.

Sodium borohydride is a much weaker reducing agent than lithium aluminum hydride. It is capable of reducing only a few functional groups (aldehydes, ketones, acid chlorides). Esters can sometimes be reduced, but with difficulty, but the yields of alcohol product are often poor. In general, the B—H bond is less polarized than the Al—H bond, and the hydrogen of the B—H bond is a weaker hydride species.

What is the product when cyclohexanone is treated with (1) $LiAlH_4$ in THF (2) water?

The product is cyclohexanol.

What is the product when cyclopentanone is treated with (1) $NaBH_4$ in THF (2) aqueous NH_4Cl?

The product is cyclopentanol.

Why is aqueous NH_4Cl used for hydrolysis with $NaBH_4$ but water is used with $LiAlH_4$?

Sodium borohydride is much less reactive than lithium aluminum hydride, and the complex obtained by the reaction of $NaBH_4$ with a ketone or aldehyde is also much less reactive than the complex formed by the reaction of $LiAlH_4$ with an aldehyde or ketone. For this reaction, the stronger acid aqueous NH_4Cl solution is required to decompose the $NaBH_4$ complex with the less reactive B—H units.

Is there an intermediate in the reaction when lithium aluminum hydride reacts with butan-2-one?

The initial product is not the alcohol but rather an alkoxyaluminate, ***B***, that requires a second chemical reaction with water to give the alcohol. The alkoxyaluminate ***B*** is a formal product of the reaction and not a formal intermediate to the product. The reaction proceeds by a four-centered transition state such as ***A*** to form the alkoxyaluminate ***B***, which is the initial product formed by this reaction. Note that for this reaction to occur, the electropositive aluminum is attracted to the electronegative oxygen. Likewise, the electronegative hydrogen (a hydride) is attracted to the electropositive carbon.

AlH_4^-

A

B

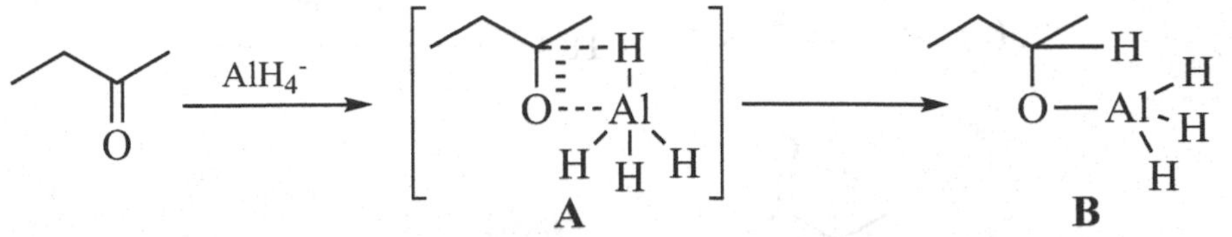

What is the product of the initial reaction between lithium aluminum hydride and butan-2-one after hydrolysis with water?

Butan-2-one is reduced to butan-2-ol after hydrolysis.

Why is ethanol used as a solvent with $NaBH_4$ reductions rather than ether or THF?

Sodium borohydride is more soluble in ethanol. It is less reactive than $LiAlH_4$ and although $NaBH_4$ can react with ethanol to give an alkoxyborate, it is sufficiently reactive for reduction of aldehydes or ketones. The fact that a protic (acidic) solvent such as ethanol is used with $NaBH_4$ is a clear indication that $NaBH_4$ is less reactive since $LiAlH_4$ will react violently with ethanol.

What is the mechanism of the reaction between sodium borohydride and cyclohexanone? What is the product after hydrolysis?

The initial product is the alkoxyborate ***B*** that requires a second chemical reaction with water to give the alcohol. The reaction proceeds by a four-centered transition state such as ***A*** to form the alkoxyborate ***B***, which is the initial product formed by this reaction. Note that for this reaction to occur, the electropositive boron is attracted to the electronegative oxygen. Likewise, the electronegative hydrogen (a hydride) is attracted to the electropositive carbon.

BH_4^-

A

B

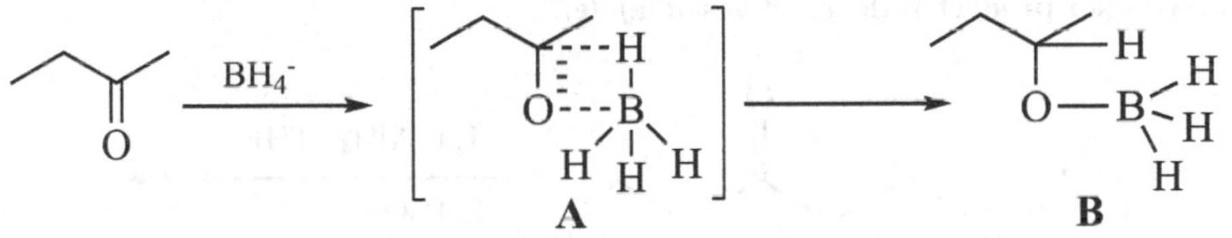

What is the product when an aldehyde is reduced? A ketone?

When an aldehyde reacts with a reducing agent such as lithium aluminum hydride or sodium borohydride, the product after hydrolysis is a primary alcohol. A similar reaction with a ketone will give a secondary alcohol.

What is the major product when cycloheptanone is reacted with $LiAlH_4$ and then water?

The product is an alcohol resulting from "nucleophilic" attack of the hydride on the electropositive carbonyl carbon. In this case, cycloheptanone is reduced to cycloheptanol.

What is the major product when 3-methylhexanal is reacted with $NaBH_4$ and then aqueous ammonium chloride?

The product is 3-methylhexan-1-ol.

What is the major product from the reactions of (a) and (b)?

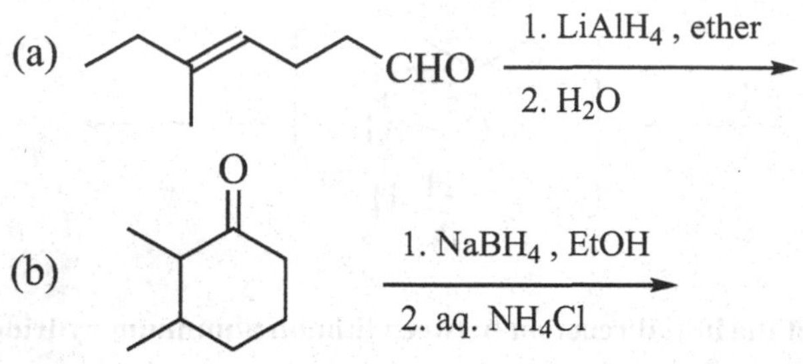

(a) CHO; 1. $LiAlH_4$, ether; 2. H_2O

(b) O; 1. $NaBH_4$, EtOH; 2. aq. NH_4Cl

(a) 5-Methylhept-4*E*-enal is reduced with $LiAlH_4$ to give the corresponding alcohol, 5-methyl-hept-4*E*-en-1-ol. (b) 2,3-Dimethylcyclohexanone is reduced with $NaBH_4$ to the alcohol, 2,3-dimethylcyclohexan-1-ol.

(a) OH (b) OH

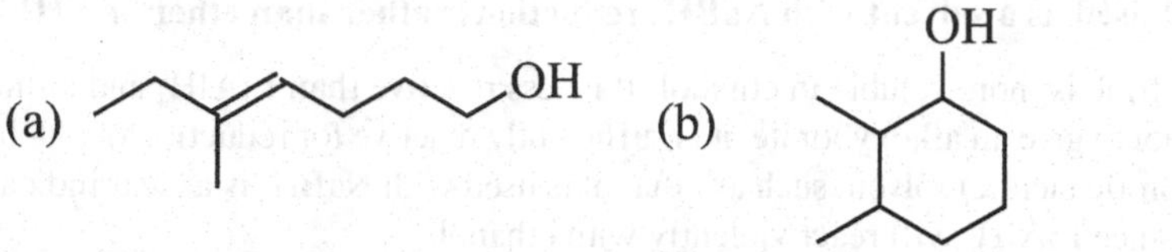

(*E*)-5-methylhept-4-en-1-ol 2,3-dimethylcyclohexan-1-ol

What is the reaction product when sodium borohydride reacts with ethyl butanoate?

The best answer is no reaction since $NaBH_4$ generally does not reduce esters very well. In fact, some esters are reduced to the primary alcohol with $NaBH_4$, although the reaction is often slow. However, no reaction is usually the first assumption. Alternatively, $LiAlH_4$ easily reduces esters to an alcohol, as will be presented in Section 15.6.

What is the major product of the reactions of (a)–(e)?

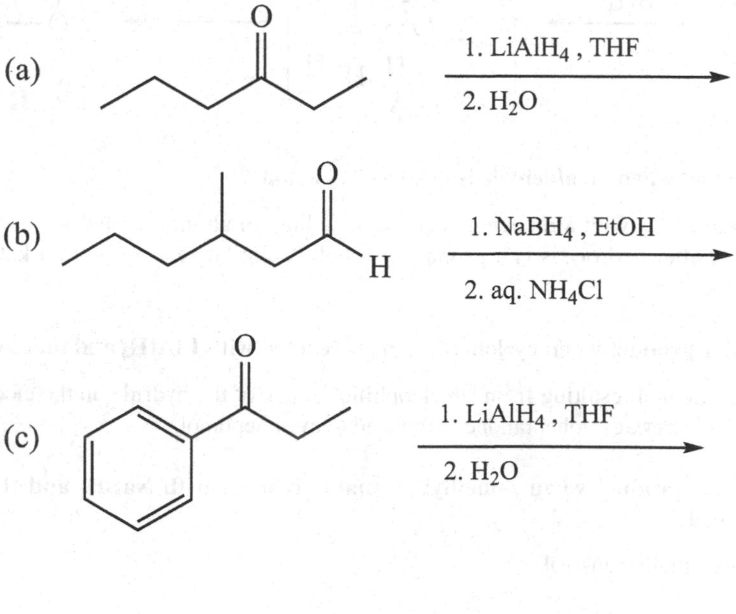

(a) O; 1. $LiAlH_4$, THF; 2. H_2O

(b) O, H; 1. $NaBH_4$, EtOH; 2. aq. NH_4Cl

(c) O; 1. $LiAlH_4$, THF; 2. H_2O

(d) 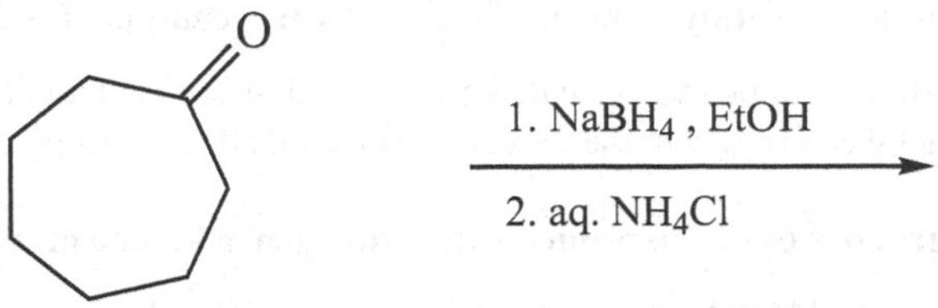 cycloheptanone $\xrightarrow[\text{2. aq. } NH_4Cl]{\text{1. } NaBH_4\text{ , EtOH}}$

(e) 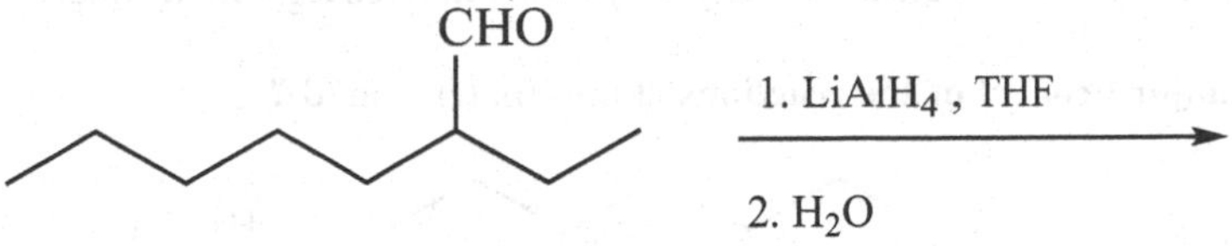 CHO $\xrightarrow[\text{2. } H_2O]{\text{1. } LiAlH_4\text{ , THF}}$

In (a), the product of the reduction of hexan-3-one is hexan-3-ol. In (b), reduction of 3-methylhexanal is 3-methylhexan-1-ol. In (c), reduction of 1-phenylpropan-1-one leads to phenyl-1-propan-1-ol as the product. In (d), the $NaBH_4$ reduction of cycloheptanone leads to cycloheptanol and in (e) reduction of 2-ethylheptanal gives 2-ethylheptan-1-ol.

(a) 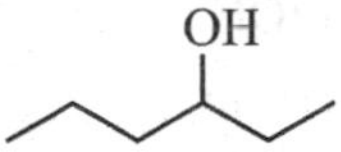 OH (b) 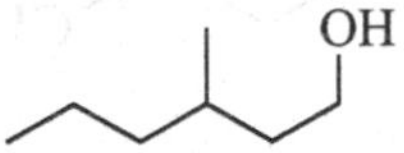 OH (c) 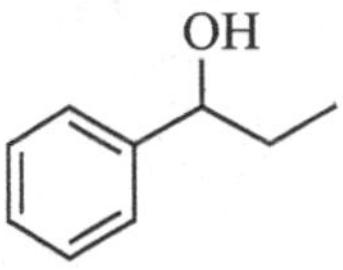 OH

(d) 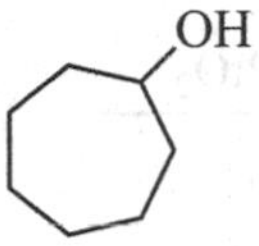 OH (e) 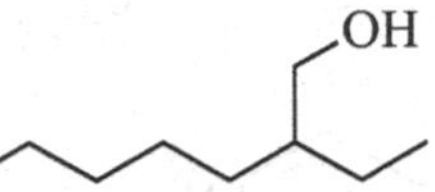 OH

Are aldehydes and ketones reduced to the corresponding alcohol by catalytic hydrogenation?

Yes! See Sections 14.1 and 14.4. As with alkenes, hydrogen in the presence of a suitable transition metal catalyst (usually platinum) reduces carbonyls of aldehydes and ketones to the corresponding alcohol.

14.4 CATALYTIC HYDROGENATION AND DISSOLVING METAL REDUCTIONS. ALDEHYDES AND KETONES

Can catalytic hydrogenation be used for the reduction of aldehydes and ketones?

Yes! Catalytic hydrogenation can be used for the reduction of ketones and aldehydes, and the reaction also requires a catalyst. The most efficient catalyst for the reduction of carbonyl compounds is usually platinum. The reduction gives the corresponding alcohol, and the mechanism with heterogeneous catalysts is very similar to that shown for alkenes in Section 14.1.

What is the product when pentan-2-one is treated with hydrogen gas and no other additive?

There is no reaction! As with the hydrogenation of alkenes, hydrogen gas does not react with ketones or aldehydes unless a catalyst is present. As described, this attempted hydrogenation gives no reaction.

What is the product when pentan-2-one is reacted with platinum oxide and hydrogen gas?

In the presence of the platinum derivative catalyst, pentan-2-one is reduced to pentan-2-ol. Note that platinum oxide is commonly known as Adam's catalyst.

Can other transition metal catalysts be used for the hydrogenation of aldehydes or ketones?

Yes! Aldehydes or ketones can be hydrogenated using the catalysts used for alkenes, including Pd, Pt, Ni, or other transition metal catalysts, but the reduction is usually done with platinum derivatives.

Which functional group is easier to reduce with hydrogen, a ketone or an ester?

The carbonyl group of an aldehyde or a ketone is much easier to reduce by catalytic hydrogenation than is the carbonyl of an ester. Esters are usually very difficult to reduce with hydrogen (see Section 15.6).

What is the major product of the reactions of (a), (b), (c), and (d)?

(a) O — H_2 , Ni / CH_3OH →

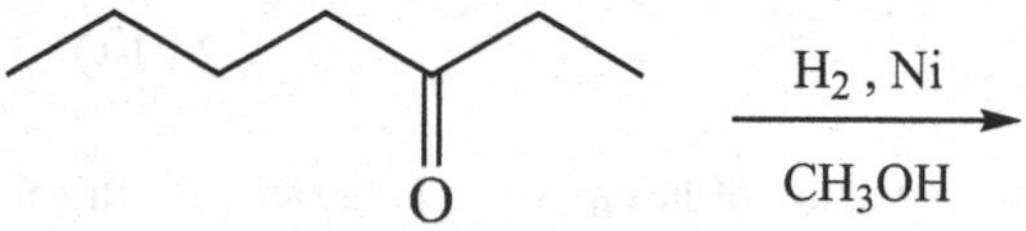

(b) CHO — H_2 , PtO_2 / EtOH →

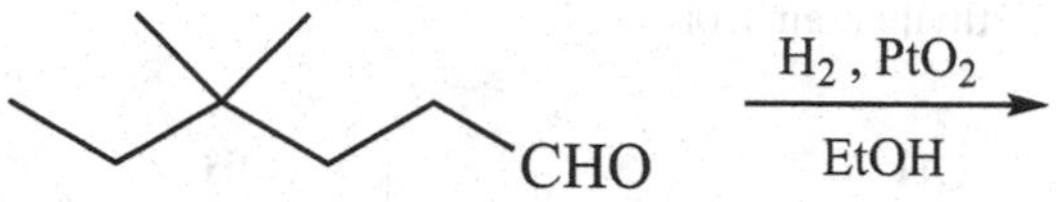

(c) O — H_2 , PtO_2 / EtOH →

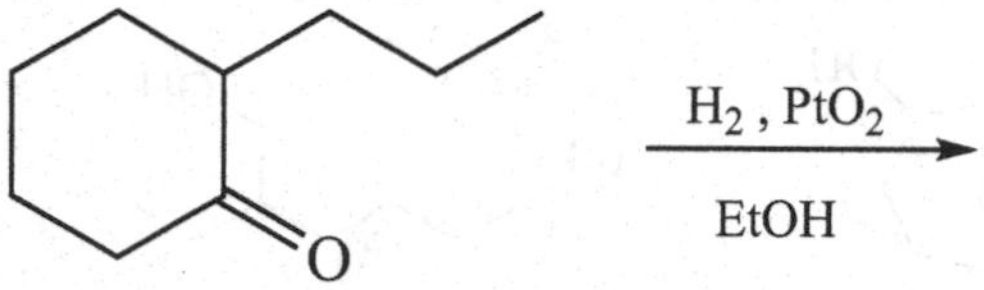

(d) O — H_2 / EtOH →

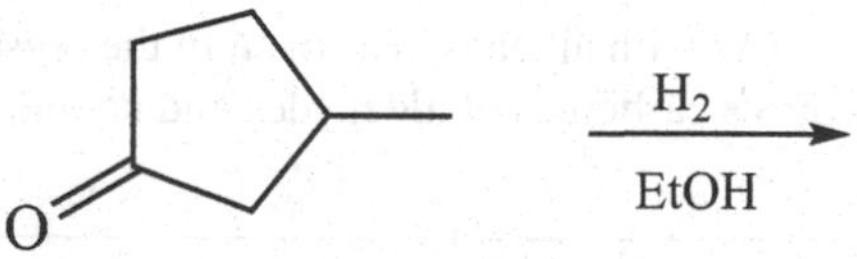

In (a), catalytic hydrogenation of octan-3-one gives octan-3-ol. In (b), reduction of 4,4-dimethylhexanal gives 4,4-dimethyl-hexan-1-ol. In (c), reduction of 2-propylcyclohexanone leads to 2-propylcyclohexanol. In (d), there is no metal catalyst so there is no reaction.

(a) OH

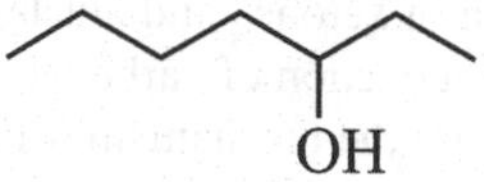

(b) OH

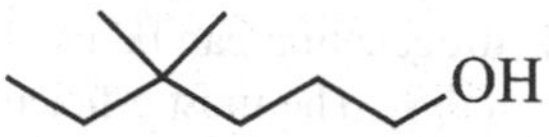

(c) OH

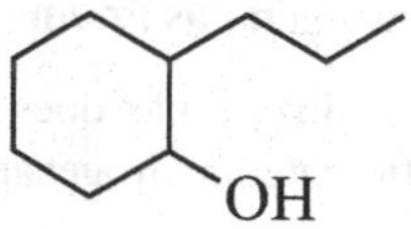

(d) No Reaction

What is the major product from the hydrogenation of (a) and (b)?

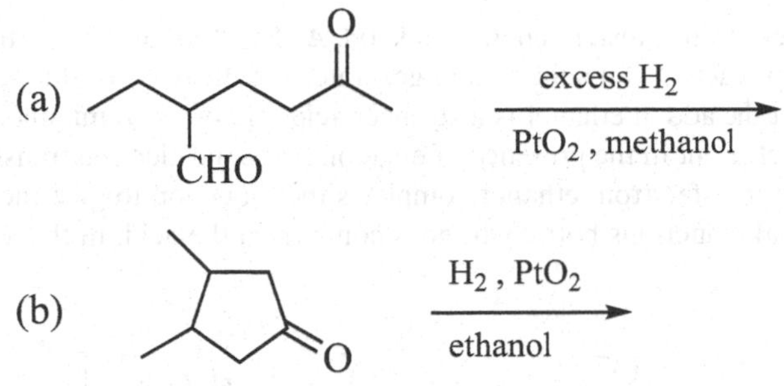

(a) CHO, O — excess H_2 / PtO_2, methanol →

(b) O — H_2, PtO_2 / ethanol →

In (a), keto-aldehyde 2-ethyl-5-oxohexanal contains two carbonyl groups, an aldehyde and a ketone. When reduced with excess hydrogen with platinum oxide, a diol (2-ethylhexane1,5-diol) is formed. In (b), reduction of 3,4-dimethylcyclopentanone gives 3,4-dimethylcyclopentan-1-ol.

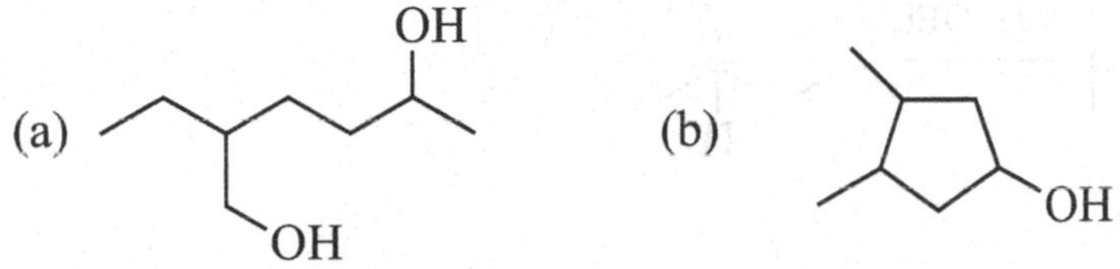

(a) OH, OH — 2-ethylhexane-1,5-diol

(b) OH — 3,4-dimethylcyclopentan-1-ol

When sodium metal is mixed with acetone, what is the initial product?

Sodium transfers one electron to the carbonyl, forming a *ketyl* (*A*). This resonance stabilized intermediate is highly reactive and has characteristics of both a radical and a carbanion (it is an example of a radical anion).

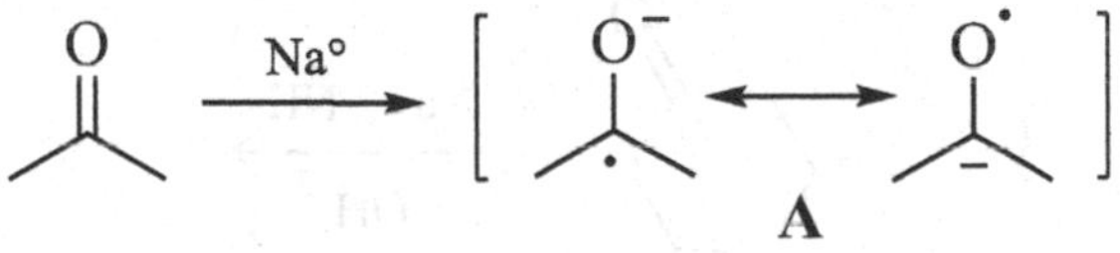

O — Na° → [O^- ↔ O•] **A**

What is a radical anion?

A radical anion is a negatively charged species that is a radical; this is, it is a radical that carries a negative charge.

What is the final product of the reaction of acetone with sodium metal when the reaction is done in liquid ammonia and ethanol?

The reaction leads to reduction of the ketone to the alcohol; in this case the product is propan-2-ol (isopropanol).

Why does sodium metal transfer an electron to the carbonyl π-bond?

Sodium metal lies in Group 1 of the periodic table. Energetically, it is easier to lose one electron (ionization potential) than to gain seven electrons (electron affinity) to achieve a full octet in the outer shell. Indeed, Group 1 metals such as Li, Na, or K are well known electron transfer reagents.

What is the complete mechanism for the reduction of butan-2-one to butan-2-ol with sodium metal in liquid ammonia and ethanol?

In this process, initial electron transfer generates a ketyl, ***A***. The "carbanion" portion of this ketyl reacts with the ethanol, which reacts as an acid, which generates a radical, ***B***. In this reaction, ammonia can function as an acid, but the added ethanol is a stronger acid relative to ammonia and the overall reduction is faster and more efficient in the presence of ethanol. A second electron transfer from sodium gives alkoxide ***C***, and proton transfer from ethanol completes the reduction to give the final product, butan-2-ol. In dissolving metal reductions both hydrogens come from the acid, in this case ethanol. Also see Section 16.5.

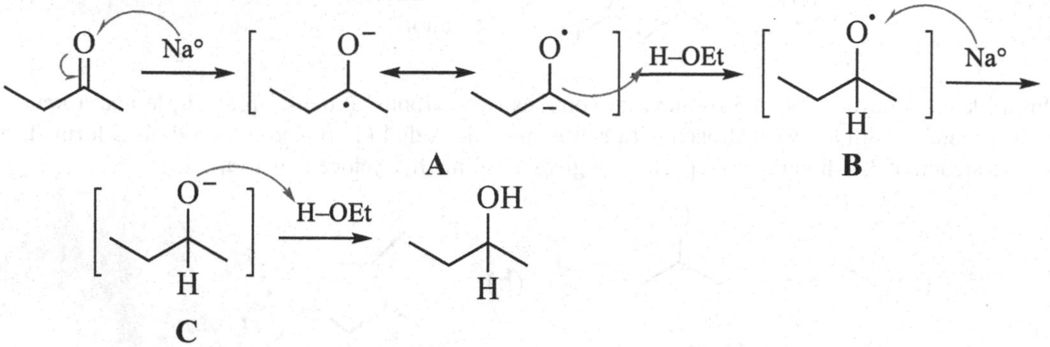

Na° → A → H–OEt → B → Na° → C → H–OEt

Why is ethanol added to this reaction?

In this reaction, ammonia can function as an acid, but the added ethanol is a stronger acid relative to ammonia and the overall reduction is faster and more efficient in the presence of ethanol.

What are the major products of the reactions of (a) and (b)?

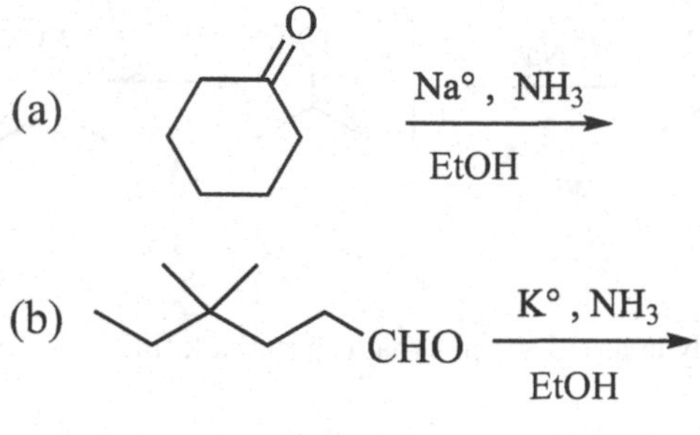

(a) Na° , NH_3 / EtOH

(b) CHO K° , NH_3 / EtOH

In (a), the dissolving metal reduction of cyclohexanone with sodium in ammonia/ethanol leads to cyclohexanol. In (b), reduction of 4,4-dimethylhexanal with potassium in ammonia/ethanol leads to 4,4-dimethylhexan-1-ol.

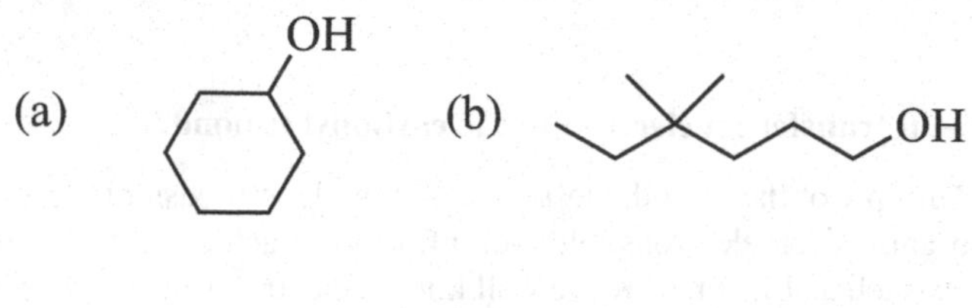

(a) OH (b) OH

END OF CHAPTER PROBLEMS

1. In each case give the major product of the reaction. Remember stereochemistry and if there is no reaction, indicate by N.R.

(a) 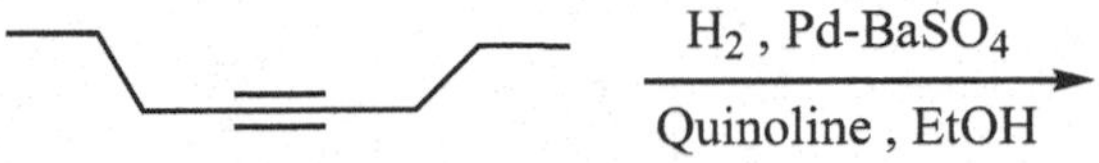 $\xrightarrow[\text{Quinoline , EtOH}]{H_2\text{ , Pd-BaSO}_4}$

(b) 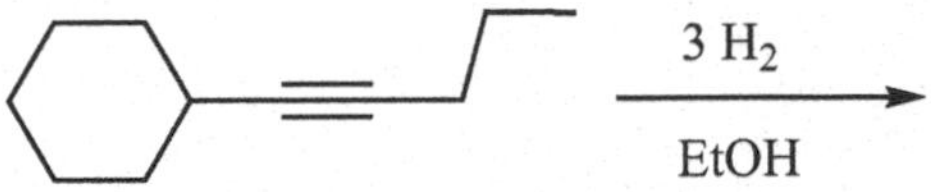 $\xrightarrow[\text{EtOH}]{3\ H_2}$

(c) 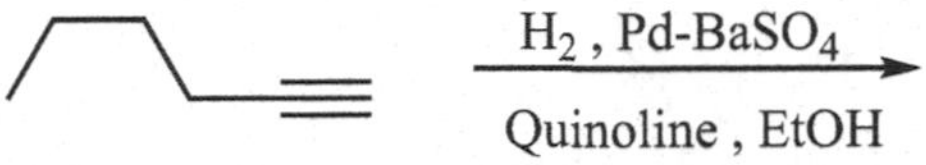 $\xrightarrow[\text{Quinoline , EtOH}]{H_2\text{ , Pd-BaSO}_4}$

2. In each case give the major product of the reaction. Remember stereochemistry and if there is no reaction, indicate by N.R.

(a) 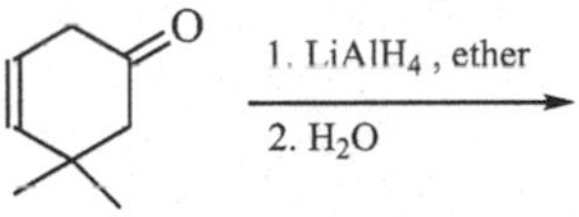 O $\xrightarrow[\text{2. } H_2O]{\text{1. LiAlH}_4\text{ , ether}}$

(b) CHO $\xrightarrow[\text{EtOH}]{H_2\text{ , PtO}_2}$

(c) CHO $\xrightarrow[\text{2. Aq, NH}_4\text{Cl}]{\text{1. NaBH}_4\text{ , EtOH}}$

(d) O $\xrightarrow[\text{EtOH}]{\text{Na}^\circ\text{ , NH}_3}$

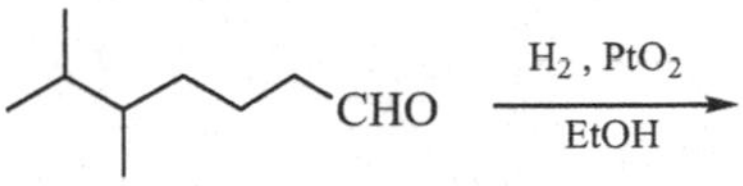

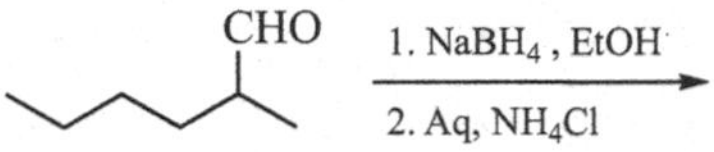

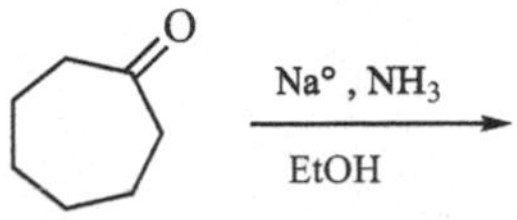

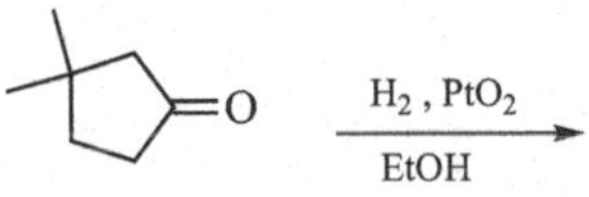

(e) =O $\xrightarrow[\text{EtOH}]{H_2\text{ , PtO}_2}$

(f) 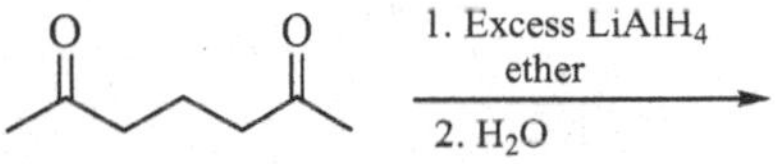 O O $\xrightarrow[\text{2. } H_2O]{\text{1. Excess LiAlH}_4\text{ ether}}$

(g) CHO $\xrightarrow[\text{EtOH}]{\text{Na}^\circ\text{ , NH}_3}$

(h) O $\xrightarrow[\text{2. Aq, NH}_4\text{Cl}]{\text{1. NaBH}_4\text{ , EtOH}}$

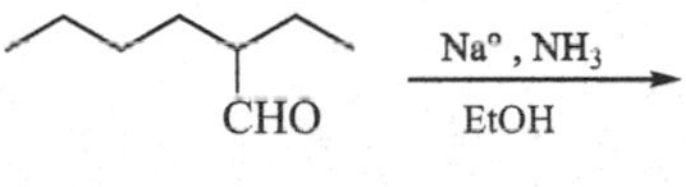

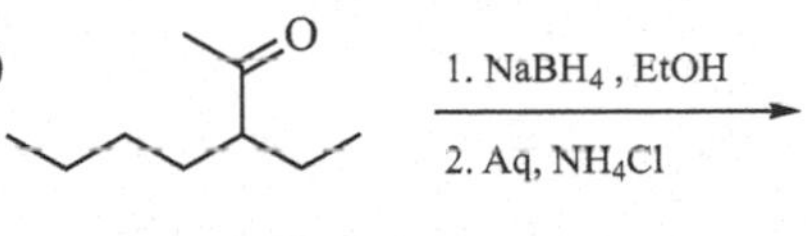

3. Reduction of 5-chloropentanal with sodium borohydride may produce a by-product other than the expected 5-chloropentan-1-ol. What is this product and how is it formed?

4. Give the mechanism for the following reaction.

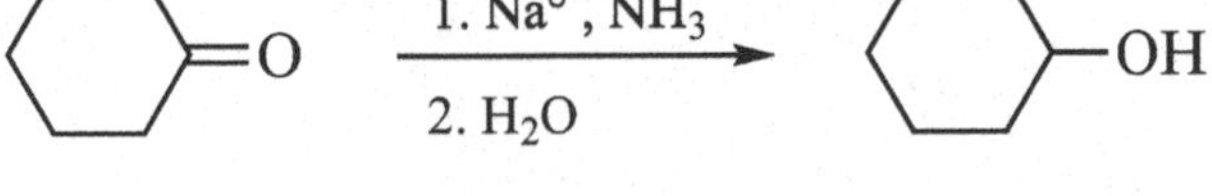

=O $\xrightarrow[\text{2. } H_2O]{\text{1. Na}^\circ\text{ , NH}_3}$ OH

15

Carboxylic Acids, Carboxylic Acid Derivatives, and Acyl Substitution Reactions

Carboxylic acids are the prototype organic acid. They are the parent compounds of an entire family of molecules called acid derivatives. The name "acid" describes much of their chemistry. These organic acids are important building blocks for the formation of other functional groups. Their acid properties are important in such diverse applications as giving important physical and chemical properties to amino acids (see Chapter 18) to their use as acid catalysts in cationic reactions of alcohols and alkenes. This chapter will focus on the acid properties of carboxylic acids and the factors which influence acidity. This chapter will also show how carboxylic acids can be transformed into other acid derivatives, such as acid chlorides, esters, anhydrides, and amides and the reactions of those derivatives.

15.1 STRUCTURE OF CARBOXYLIC ACIDS

What is the fundamental unit referred to as a carboxyl group?

A carbonyl with an OH attached to it, HO-C=O.

What is the distinguishing feature of a carboxyl group?

A carboxyl group is characterized by the presence of a very acidic hydrogen on an O—H unit, along with an electropositive carbonyl carbon of the C=O.

What is the characteristic chemical reaction of a carboxylic acid?

Carboxylic acids are Brønsted–Lowry acids.

Describe the bond polarity in a carboxyl group.

The O—H group in the figure is polarized as shown such that the H is acidic, and the carbonyl carbon is electrophilic.

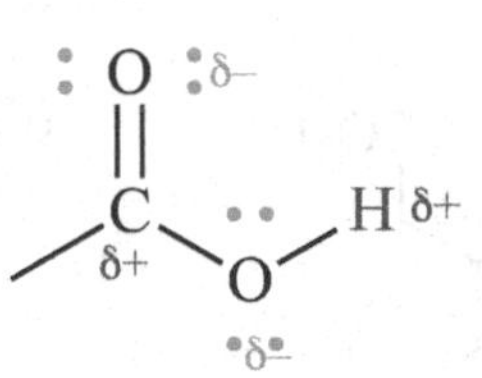

:O: δ–
C δ+
O δ–
H δ+

How extensive is the hydrogen bonding capability of a carboxyl group?

The acidic hydrogen of the OH group is strongly hydrogen bonded to the carbonyl oxygen of a second carboxyl, and hydrogen bonding is possible in protic solvents such as water or an alcohol.

When compared to an alcohol of similar molecular weight, a carboxylic acid generally has a much higher boiling point. Why?

A carboxyl group is capable of extensive hydrogen bonding, much more extensive and stronger than observed with alcohols. This strong hydrogen bonding must be disrupted to bring the carboxylic acid into equilibrium with both gas and liquid (boiling point), requiring higher temperatures than with an alcohol. For example, the boiling point of CH_3COOH (molecular weight 60) is 118.1°C whereas the boiling point of ethyl methyl ether ($CH_3OCH_2CH_3$, methoxy ethane, molecular weight 60) is 7.6°C. The molecular weight of these two compounds is identical and the greater boiling point of CH_3COOH is due to the extensive hydrogen bonding that must be overcome to volatize this compound.

What is the IUPAC ending that is correlated with a carboxylic acid?

The IUPAC ending for a carboxylic acid is -oic acid. The alkane, alkene, or alkyne carbon chain is used, and the terminal -e is dropped and replaced with -oic acid. Using a five-carbon chain, the generic names are pentanoic acid, pentenoic acid, or pentynoic acid.

Why is a linear C6 acid called hexanoic acid rather than hexoic acid?

As with any acid, there could be an alkane, alkene, or alkyne backbone. The -an, -en, or -yn must be included to properly identify the carboxylic acid. For the linear C6 acid, this requirement will lead to the names hexanoic acid, hexenoic acid, and hexynoic acid for the three cases mentioned. For this specific question, hexanoic acid refers to a carboxylic acid with an alkane backbone: $CH_3CH_2CH_2CH_2CH_2COOH$.

Why is the numerical position of the carboxyl group usually omitted from the name of a carboxylic acid?

Since the carbonyl carbon of the carbonyl *must* have the lowest number (it is the functional group) and that carbon contains the OH, it *must* be C1. For this reason (as with aldehydes), the number is usually omitted.

What is the correct IUPAC name for (a), (b), (c), and (d)?

(a) Ph CO_2H

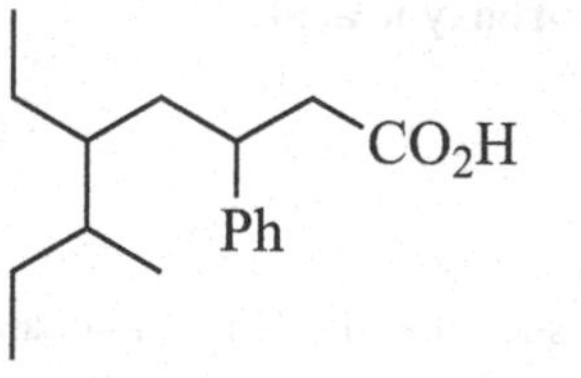

(b) Cl Cl CO_2H

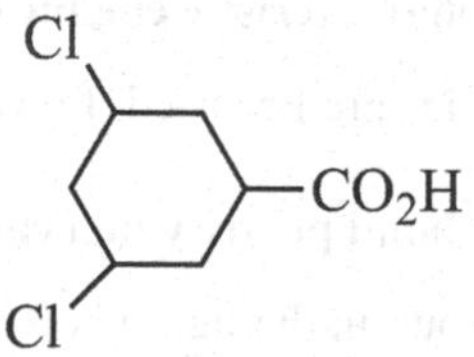

(c) CO_2H

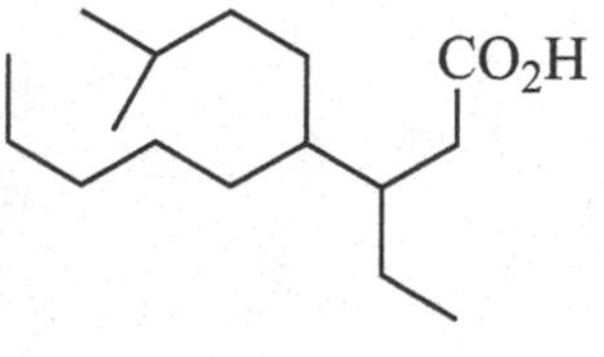

(d) CO_2H

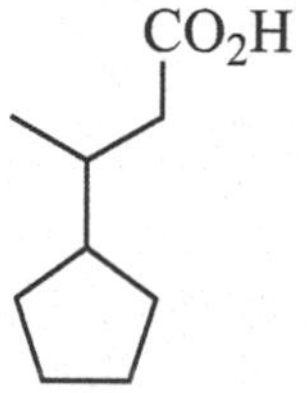

(a) 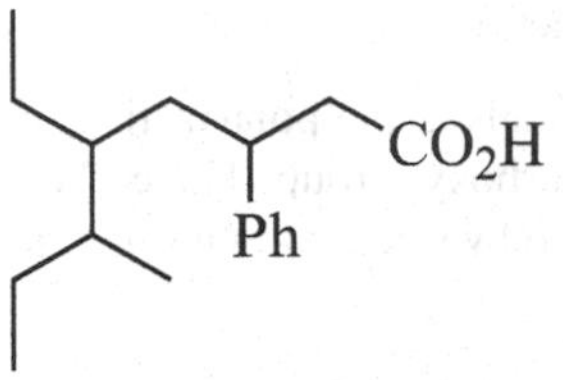 CO_2H, Ph

5-ethyl-6-methyl-3-phenyloctanoic acid

(b) 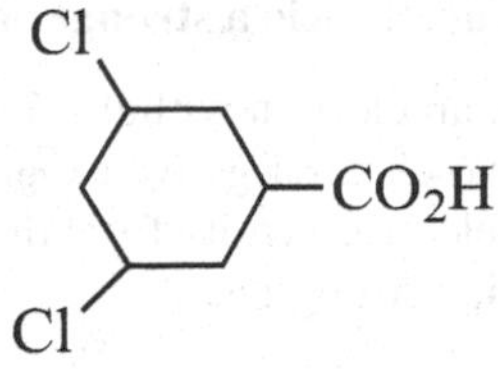 Cl, CO_2H, Cl

3,5-dichlorocyclohexane-1-carboxylic acid

(c) 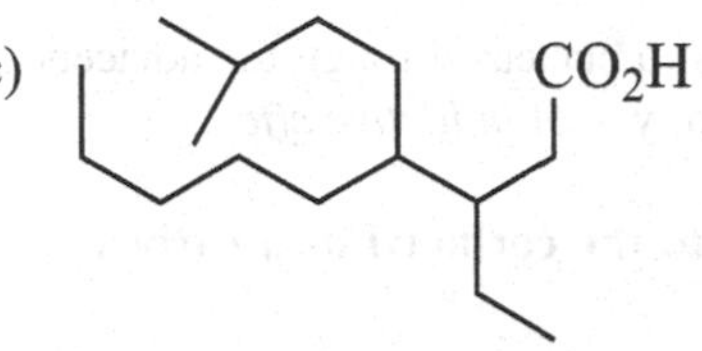 CO_2H

3-ethyl-4-(3-methylbutyl)-nonanoic acid

(d) 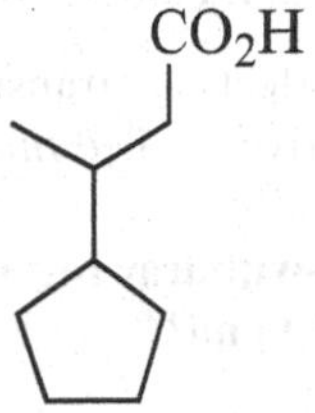 CO_2H

3-cyclopentyl-butanoic acid

What is the common name of HCO_2H and of CH_3CO_2H?

These two acids have been known since the nineteenth century and are so ubiquitous that common names are well known and often used rather than the IUPAC names of methanoic acid and ethanoic acid. The common name of (a) is acetic acid and (b) is called formic acid. Formic acid is an ant venom and acetic acid is found in vinegar.

What is the most distinguishing chemical feature of carboxylic acids?

Perhaps the most distinguishing feature of carboxylic acids is that they are Brønsted–Lowry (protonic) acids and react with a variety of suitable Brønsted–Lowry bases.

What is the pK_a of acetic acid (ethanoic acid)?

The pK_a of acetic acid (ethanoic acid) is 4.76.

What are the pK_a values of the following carboxylic acids: (a) propanoic acid, (b) butanoic acid, and (c) formic acid?

(a) propanoic = 4.89; (b) butanoic acid = 4.82; (c) formic acid = 3.75.

Why is acetic acid a weaker acid than formic acid?

Acetic acid has a methyl group attached to the electropositive carbonyl. Relative to hydrogen (in formic acid), methyl is an electron-releasing group relative to the carbonyl carbon. This inductive effect "pushes" electrons toward the O—H bond, strengthening it, and making that hydrogen less acidic (less positive = less like H^+).

What is the pK_a of 2-chloroethanoic acid (chloroacetic acid)?

The pK_a of chloroacetic acid is 2.85.

Why is 2-chloroacetic acid a stronger acid than acetic acid?

The chlorine has an electron-withdrawing effect. The Cl adds to the polarization of the α-hydrogen δ^+, along with the two electronegative oxygen atoms of the carboxyl group. The carbonyl carbon therefore withdraws more electron density from the O—H bond, thereby weakening it (more positive H, more like H^+) and making it a stronger acid.

What are inductive effects?

Bond polarization of σ-bonds leads to a so-called *inductive effect*, an electronic effect that is typically due to a difference in electronegativity between the atoms of that bond.

What are through-bond inductive effects?

Certain electronic effects are transmitted from nucleus to nucleus through the adjacent covalent bonds and these are collectively called *through-bond effects*, a type of *inductive effect*.

When an electron-withdrawing group is attached to the carbonyl of a carboxyl, what is the effect on the O—H bond?

The electron-withdrawing group induces a δ^+ charge on the α-carbon, accentuating the effect of the two electron-withdrawing oxygen atoms of the carboxyl group. This greater δ^+ charge is adjacent to the δ^+ charge on the carbonyl carbon, which is destabilizing. To compensate, electron density is drawn from neighboring atoms to diminish the electron-withdrawing effects of the α-carbon, which makes the O—H bond more polarized, the H more positive and more acidic.

Will an electron-withdrawing substituent increase or decrease acidity?

In general, electron-withdrawing groups make the carboxylic acid a stronger acid (larger K_a, smaller pK_a).

Why is 3-chloropropanoic acid a weaker acid than 2-chloropropanoic acid?

The electron-withdrawing chlorine atom is further away from the carbonyl carbon in 3-chloropropanoic acid than in 2-chloropropanoic acid. The electron-withdrawing ability of an atom or group diminishes as the distance from the O—H group and the carbonyl increases, so the inductive effect for 3-chloropropanoic acid is less than in 2-schloropropanoic acid, which makes it a weaker acid. The pK_a is 2.83 for 2-chloropropanoic acid and 3.98 for 3-chloropropanoic acid.

Why is 2,2,2-trichloroethanoic acid a stronger acid than 2-chloroethanoic acid?

If one chlorine atom withdraws electrons from the α-carbon and this makes the O—H bond weaker, the presence of three electron-withdrawing chlorines will withdraw even more electron density. This structural difference will make the α-carbon more positive and the O—H bond weaker, and therefore more acidic. The pK_a of 2-chloroethanoic acid (see the preceding question) is 2.89 and the pK_a of 2,2,2-trichloroethanoic acid is 0.64, making the latter a significantly stronger acid.

Will an electron-releasing substituent on the α-carbon of a carboxylic acid increase or decrease acidity?

An electron-releasing substituent "feeds" electrons toward the electropositive carbonyl so that carbonyl carbon will withdraw *less* electron density from the O—H bond. The O—H bond is stronger, and the acid is a weaker acid (more difficult to remove the H from O—H).

In each of the following series, what is the strongest acid? (a) 3-chloropropanoic acid or 3-chloropentanoic acid (b) 2-methoxyethanoic acid or propanoic acid.

In (a), both acids have an electron-withdrawing chlorine at C3 but 3-chloropentanoic acid also has an ethyl group attached to C3. The presence of the electron releasing alkyl group, which is missing in 3-chloropropanoic acid, will make 3-chloropentanoic acid a weaker acid. Therefore, 3-chloropropanoic acid is the stronger acid. In (b), methoxy is electron-withdrawing, primarily by through-space effects (see the next question), whereas the methyl (attached to the α-carbon of acetic acid) is electron releasing. In (c), since the oxygen of the methoxy group is more electronegative than the adjacent carbon, it is electron-withdrawing in this system. Therefore, 2-methoxyethanoic acid is expected to be the stronger acid (pK_a of methoxyacetic acid = 3.6; pK_a of propionic acid = 4.9).

What is a "through-space" field effect?

When an atom or group with a δ^- dipole is sufficiently close in space to the acidic hydrogen of the carboxyl, there is a significant attractive force "through-space" between the atoms This effect is a strong electronic effect, often called a field effect. Such field effects will enhance the acidity of the acid. These through-space effects are usually a stronger influence on the acidity than the through-bond effects.

How can the relative acidity of ethanoic acid and 2-chloroethanoic acid be compared in terms of a through-space effect?

Examination of the figure shows that in one conformation of this molecule the chlorine and the H of the OH can hydrogen bond (through space) in what is effectively a five-membered ring. This interaction is conformationally accessible and the electron-withdrawing effect of this through-space hydrogen bonding is very strong, making 2-chloroacetic acid a stronger acid relative to acetic acid, which has no chlorine atom.

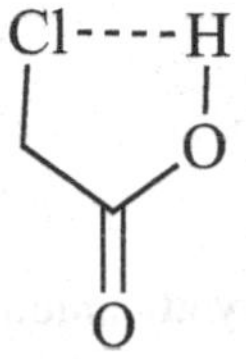

Cl----H
O
O

Why is the through-space effect in 4-chlorobutanoic acid weaker than in 2-chlorobutanoic acid?

In 2-chlorobutanoic acid, a pseudo five-membered ring is possible, as shown in *A*, which indicates that the through space effect between Cl and H—O is strong due to the proximity of the two groups in space. However, the chlorine is further apart in 4-chlorobutanoc acid and a pseudo seven-membered ring is required (see ***B***) to bring the two atoms close in space. The greater distance between the carboxyl group and the electron-withdrawing group mitigates the interaction, and the further the group is away from the carboxyl group, the weaker the acid.

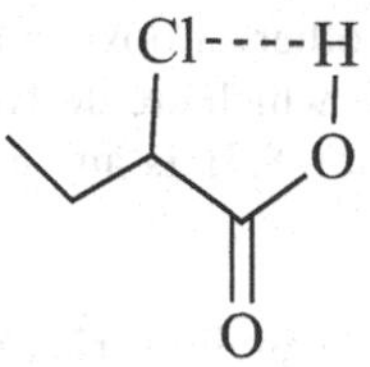

Cl----H
O
O
A

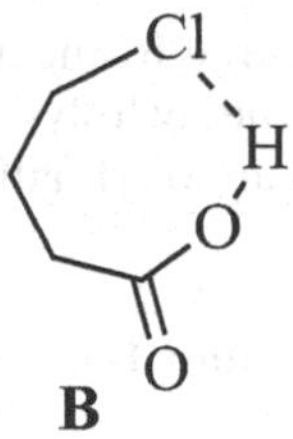

Cl
H
O
O
B

What is the structure of the carboxylate anion, formed by removal of the acidic hydrogen from the acid?

Treatment of a carboxylic acid with a base ($NaHCO_3$ is a sufficiently strong base for this reaction) generates a carboxylate anion. This ion is resonance stabilized, with the charge dispersed to both oxygens. Since the charge is dispersed and electrons are difficult to donate, the carboxylate anion is a weak nucleophile and a relatively weak base.

$$RC(=O)O{-}H \xrightarrow{NaHCO_3} \left[RC(=O)O^- \longleftrightarrow RC(O^-)=O \right] + H_2CO_3$$

Carboxylate anion

Why is the carboxylate anion considered to be very stable?

As shown in the figure for the carboxylate anion of formic acid (the formate anion), the carboxylate anion is resonance stabilized. The negative charge is delocalized over three atoms (O—C—O), which diminishes the net charge on each oxygen atom. Therefore, the electron-donating ability of the formate anion is diminished. Since it is a weaker electron donor, it is a weaker base.

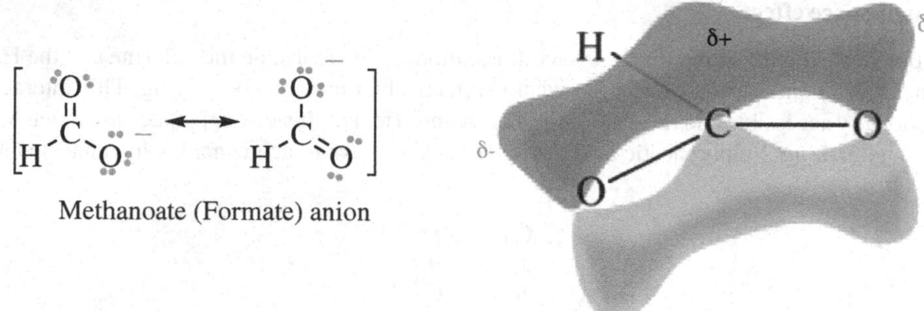

Methanoate (Formate) anion

How does the special stability of the carboxylate anion influence acidity?

The product (the carboxylate anion) is resonance stabilized and an equilibrium reaction will be influenced by the relative stability of the species that make up that equilibrium. A more stable product tends to shift the equilibrium toward that product. In this case, if the equilibrium is shifted toward the carboxylate, K_a is larger. A large K_a means a smaller pK_a, indicative of a stronger acid.

15.2 PREPARATION OF CARBOXYLIC ACIDS

How are carboxylic acids generally prepared?

Carboxylic acids can be prepared by the hydrolysis of other carboxylic acid derivatives or by oxidation of alcohols or alkenes. The hydrolysis of cyanides, which are derived from alkyl halides by the reaction of cyanide ion with an alkyl halide (see Section 8.3), is another very common preparative method.

What is the product when pentan-1-ol is heated with chromium trioxide in aqueous acid?

Chromium trioxide (in aqueous acid, it is usually called *Jones reagent*) is a powerful oxidizing agent. In this powerful oxidizing medium, the initially formed aldehyde (from the primary alcohol) is further oxidized to a carboxylic acid. The product of heating pentan-1-ol using Jones oxidation conditions is usually, but not always, pentanoic acid. Short contact times and lower temperatures can mitigate formation of the acid in this reaction. This chemistry was mentioned in Section 13.5.

Is the oxidation of primary alcohols a useful method for the preparation of carboxylic acids or does it usually give mixtures of products?

When Jones reagent is used for the oxidation of primary alcohols, the carboxylic acid is usually the major product, often the exclusive product, but not always as mentioned in the preceding question. The vigorous reaction conditions and the strongly acidic medium make this method less attractive as a general method. However, this oxidation is useful for relatively simple primary alcohols. In addition, the acidic carboxylic acid but the aldehyde product and alcohol starting material are both neutral, so the acid is easily separated, making this a useful preparative method for simple carboxylic acids.

Can ozonolysis of alkenes be used to generate carboxylic acids?

Yes, if the alkene has a hydrogen atom attached to the C=C unit, and the ozonide is treated with an oxidizing agent such as hydrogen peroxide in a second step. Ozonolysis is described in Section 13.3.

What is the major product or products when oct-2-ene is reacted with ozone and then with hydrogen peroxide?

Cleavage of oct-2-ene with ozone with an oxidative workup leads to a mixture of ethanoic acid and hexanoic acid. Ozonolysis is described in Section 13.3.

What are the major products from the ozonolysis of (a) and (b)?

(a) 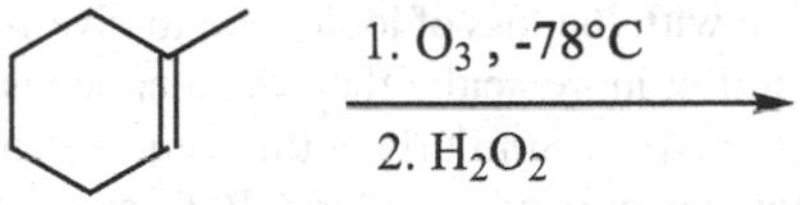 1. O_3, -78°C; 2. H_2O_2

(b) 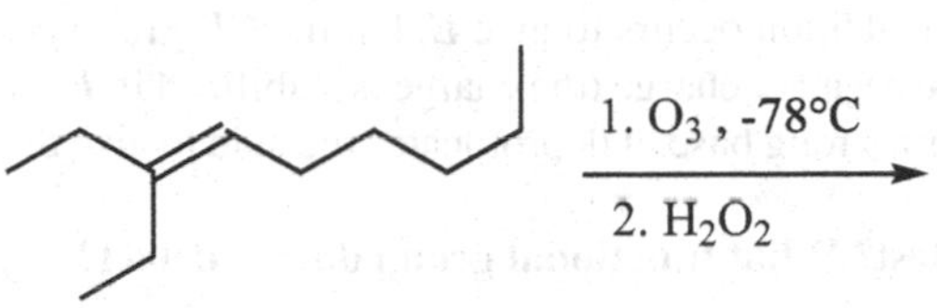 1. O_3, -78°C; 2. H_2O_2

In (a), oxidative cleavage of methylcyclohexene leads to a ketoacid (6-oxoheptanoic acid). In (b), oxidative cleavage of 3-ethylnon-3-ene leads to a mixture of two products, pentan-3-one and hexanoic acid.

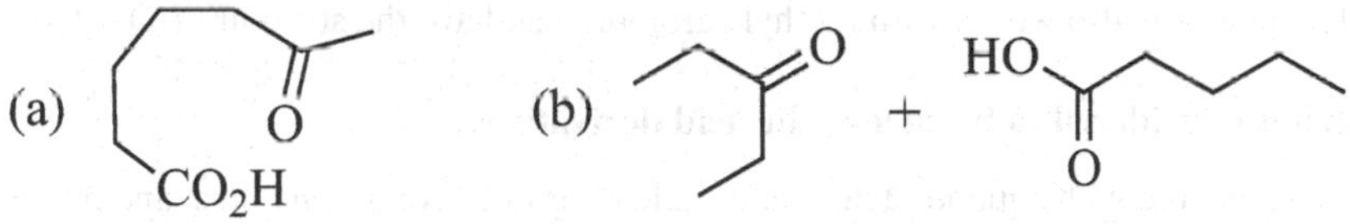

(a) O, CO_2H (b) O + HO, O

What is a haloform?

A haloform has the structure HCX_3 where X = F, Cl, Br, I.

What is the structure of iodoform? Of bromoform?

The structure of iodoform is HCI_3 and the structure of bromoform is $HCBr_3$.

What is the product when butan-2-one is treated with iodine and aqueous sodium hydroxide?

This reaction leads to oxidative cleavage of the C—C bond in methyl ketones. In this case there are two products, iodoform (HCI_3) and propanoic acid.

What is the product when acetone is treated with iodine and aqueous sodium hydroxide?

Iodine and base leads to oxidative cleavage to iodoform (HCI_3) and ethanoic acid.

What is the mechanism of this reaction with acetone?

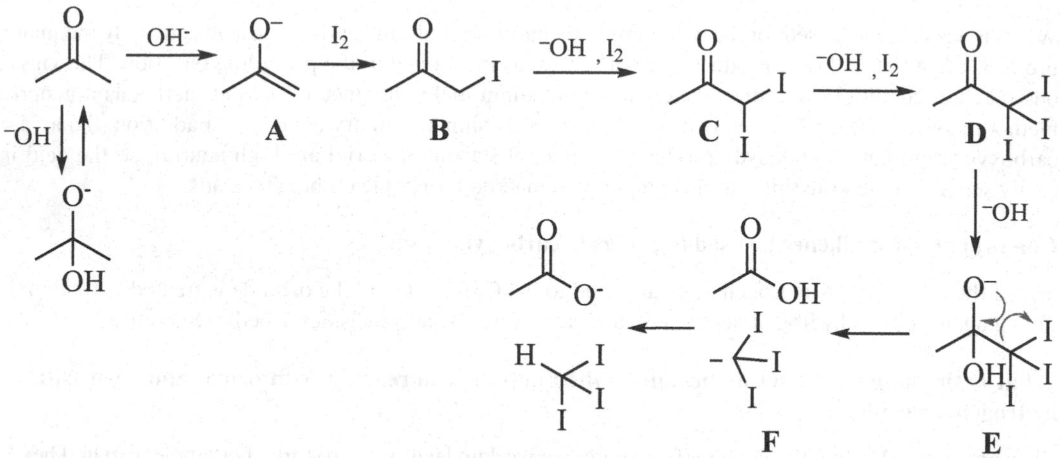

Acetone quickly reacts with hydroxide via nucleophilic acyl addition, but this reaction is reversible and favors the carbonyl starting material. Therefore, other reactions can occur. The iodoform reaction begins with formation of enolate *A* by deprotonation of acetone with hydroxide (see Section 17.1). The diatomic iodine reacts with the enolate anion with the loss of iodide ion to give 1-iodopropan-2-one (*B*). The presence of the iodine makes the α-proton more acidic than the analogous proton in acetone and a second iodine can add (via the enolate) to give *C*. Similarly, a third equivalent of iodine adds to give *D*. Acyl addition of hydroxide to the carbonyl occurs with acetone, *B*, *C*, and *D* throughout the process. When *D* is formed, however, acyl addition occurs to give *E*, but the CI_3 group is a good leaving group since it is able to accommodate the negative charge (the charge is stabilized in *F*). This fact allows cleavage to acetic acid and *F*. Since *F* is a strong base, it deprotonates the acid to give the carboxylate salt and iodoform.

What is the iodoform test? What functional group does it detect?

The iodoform test mixes a suspected methyl ketone with iodine and aqueous hydroxide. The functional group is a methyl group attached to a carbonyl (O=C—CH_3). If the methyl ketone functional group is present, a yellow precipitate of iodoform is observed when the ketone is mixed with iodine in aqueous hydroxide. The reaction also works with methyl carbinols that have the structure HO—C—CH_3.

How are nitriles considered to be carboxylic acid derivatives?

When a nitrile is reacted with aqueous acid, under rather vigorous conditions (heat and relatively concentrated acid), a carboxylic acid is formed. Often, the nitrile can be converted to an amide and then further hydrolyzed to the acid. See Section 15.5.

What is the product when 1-bromobutane is reacted with sodium cyanide in DMF?

Cyanide behaves as a carbon nucleophile, and the reaction product is pentanenitrile ($CH_3CH_2CH_2CH_2C{\equiv}N$) via a S_N2 reaction (see Sections 8.2 and 8.3).

What is the product when hexanenitrile is treated with cold and dilute aqueous HCl?

Nitriles can be hydrolyzed to carboxylic acids or amides, but this hydrolysis usually requires strong acid and vigorous reaction conditions. If any reaction occurs at all under the relatively mild conditions given in the question, the product will be the amide, hexanamide. It is more likely that the nitrile will be recovered unchanged from this reaction medium. Amides will be discussed later in this chapter, in Section 15.4.

What is the product when a 6N solution of HCl is added to pentanenitrile and heated to 100°C for several hours?

Under these vigorous reaction conditions, pentanenitrile is converted first to the amide and under the vigorous hydrolysis conditions the amide is converted to the carboxylic acid, pentanoic acid. Therefore, the isolated product of the reaction is pentanoic acid.

What is the product when methylmagnesium bromide reacts first with formaldehyde followed by reaction with aqueous acid?

The product is ethanol via acyl addition of the Grignard reagent to the carbonyl of formaldehyde (see Section 12.3).

In what way is carbon dioxide related to formaldehyde?

Carbon dioxide is a carbonyl compound (O=C=O), just as formaldehyde ($H_2C=O$) contains a carbonyl. Both compounds can react with nucleophilic reagents such as Grignard reagents.

When ethylmagnesium bromide reacts with carbon dioxide, what is the initial product? What is the product after hydrolysis?

The nucleophilic Grignard reagent will attack the carbonyl of CO_2 to produce a carboxylate salt. Hydrolysis will convert the salt to the acid, propanoic acid in this case.

BrMg
O=C=O — Ether → (propanoate) O⁻ — H_3O^+ → (propanoic acid) OH

What are the major products from the reaction of heptan-3-ol with the sequence of reagents shown?

OH (heptan-3-ol) — 1. PBr_3 2. Mg°, ether 3. CO_2 4. H_3O^+ →

When heptan-3-ol reacts with PBr_3, 3-bromoheptane is produced (see Section 8.3). Subsequent reaction with Mg leads to the Grignard reagent (see Section 10.2) and condensation with CO_2 followed by hydrolysis leads to 2-ethylhexanoic acid.

Br — 1. PBr_3 2. Mg°, Ether 3. CO_2 4. H_3O^+ → CO_2H

15.3 CARBOXYLIC ACID DERIVATIVES

What are acid derivatives?

Carboxylic acid derivatives are compounds where the OH of the acid has been replaced by another atom or group, including Cl, OCOR, OR, and NR_2. Replacement of the OH leads to the common acid derivatives: acid chlorides, acid anhydrides, esters, or amides.

What is an acid halide?

An acid halide has a halogen, usually chlorine or bromine, attached directly to a carbonyl (X—C=O).

What is an acid chloride?

An acid chloride has a chlorine attached directly to a carbonyl (Cl—C=O).

What is the IUPAC nomenclature system for an acid chloride?

The -oic acid ending of the parent carboxylic acid is dropped and replaced with -oyl chloride. The acid chloride of hexanoic acid is therefore hexanoyl chloride. Using the common name acetic acid, the acid chloride is acetyl chloride.

What is the structure of each of the following compounds? (a) 5-phenyl-3,3-dimethyloctanoyl chloride (b) malonyl chloride (c) oxalyl chloride (d) phenylacetyl chloride.

(a) Ph O Cl (b) O O Cl Cl

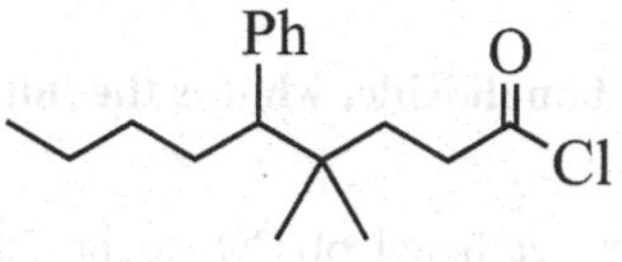

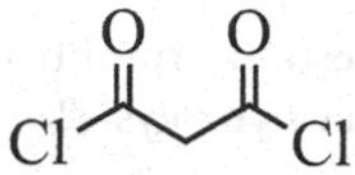

(c) O Cl Cl O (d) O Cl

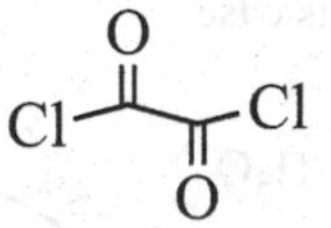

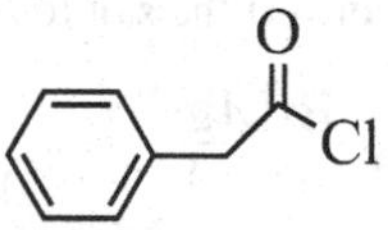

What is the basic structure of an acid anhydride?

An acid anhydride is characterized by the O=C—O—C=O structure. A generic example is shown, where R is alkyl or aryl.

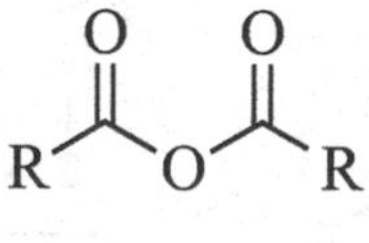

O O R O R

What is the IUPAC nomenclature system for a symmetrical acid anhydride?

Acid anhydrides are essentially composed of two acid functionalities that are joined together. There are, therefore, two acyl groups (RC=O). If both of the acyl groups are the same, the acid ending of the acid is dropped and replaced with the word anhydride. The first example is ethanoic anhydride (the common name is acetic anhydride) and the second example is butanoic anhydride (the common name is butyric anhydride).

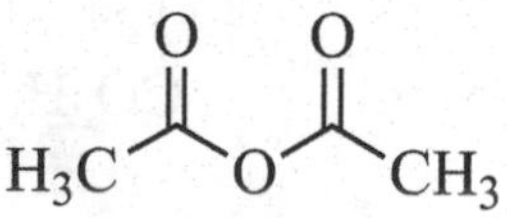

O O H_3C O CH_3 O O $H_3CH_2CH_2C$ O $CH_2CH_2CH_3$

ethanoic anhydride
(acetic anhydride)

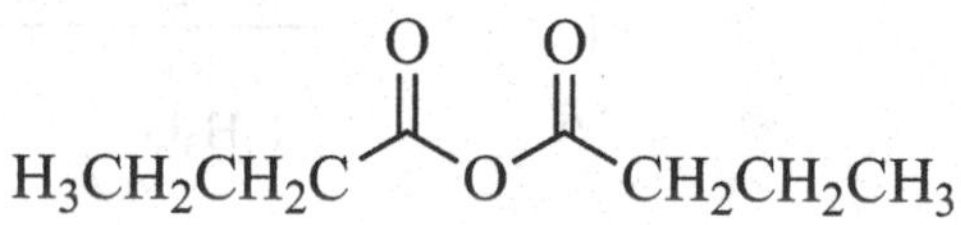

butanoic anhydride
(butyric anhydride)

What is a "mixed" anhydride?

A mixed anhydride has two different acyl groups as part of the anhydride, as in heptanoic pentanoic anhydride

How are mixed anhydrides named?

The two acyl groups are arranged in alphabetical order followed by the word anhydride. The example shown is named heptanoic pentanoic anhydride.

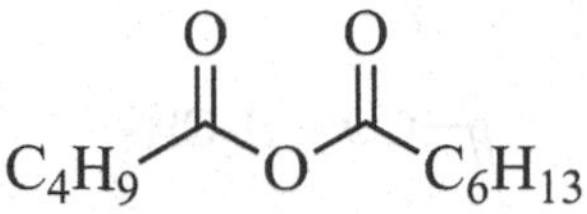

$C_4H_9C(=O)OC(=O)C_6H_{13}$

heptanoic pentanoic anhydride

What are the common cyclic anhydrides derived from succinic acid, maleic acid, and glutaric acid? Give their name.

Succinic acid gives succinic anhydride (a), maleic acid gives maleic anhydride (b), and glutaric acid gives glutaric anhydride (c). The IUPAC names are shown in parentheses under each common name. In general, dicarboxylic acids of 4–6 carbons give cyclic anhydrides. Diacids of less than four carbons would lead to highly strained three- or four-membered rings which are difficult to form. Larger chain diacids must form eight and larger membered rings, which is very difficult for C8–C13 compounds.

(a) 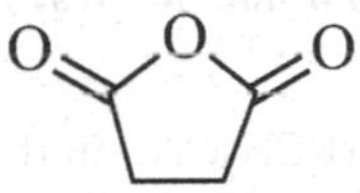 succinic anhydride (dihydrofuran-2,5-dione)

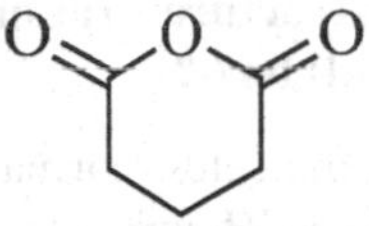

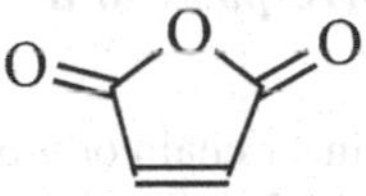

(b) maleic anhydride (furan-2,5-dione)

(c) glutaric anhydride (dihydro-2*H*-pyran-2,6(3*H*)-dione)

What is the basic structure of an ester?

An ester has an alcohol group (OR') attached to a carbonyl [R'O-C=O]. Therefore, a carboxylic ester has a carboxylic acid component and an alcohol component.

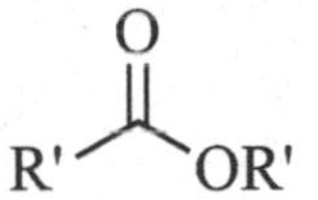

$R'C(=O)OR'$

What is the IUPAC nomenclature system for an ester?

The -oic acid ending of the parent acid is dropped and replaced with -oate. The "alcohol" portion of the ester is put in front of the "acid portion." $CH_3CO_2CH_3$ is an example where the "acid part" is ethanoic acid (acetic acid) and the "alcohol part" is methanol. The IUPAC name is methyl ethanoate whereas the common name is methyl acetate, based on the common name for the acid.

What is the name of the following ester?

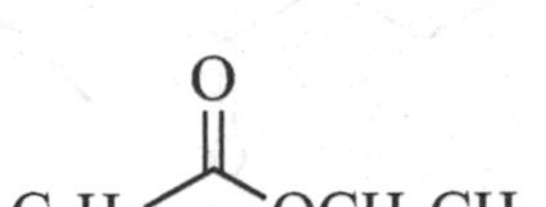

$C_4H_9C(=O)OCH_2CH_3$

The ester is derived from ethanol as the alcohol portion and pentanoic acid as the carboxylic acid portion. The name is ethyl pentanoate.

What is the IUPAC name of (a), (b), and (c)?

(a) 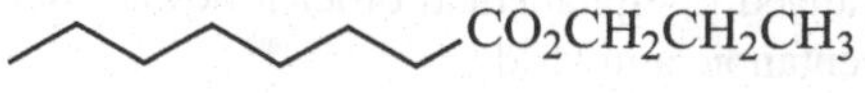 $CO_2CH_2CH_2CH_3$

(b) 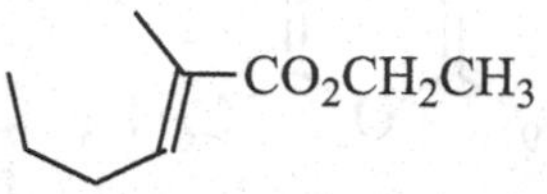 $CO_2CH_2CH_3$

(c) 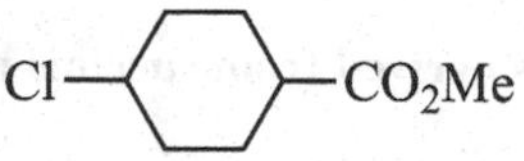 Cl CO_2Me

The name of (a) is propyl octanoate. The name of (b) is ethyl 2-methylhex-2*E*-enoate. The name of (c) is methyl 4-chlorocyclohexane-1-carboxylate. Note that an ester group attached to a ring is named as a carboxylate, just as a COOH unit attached to a ring, say cyclopentane, is named cyclopentane carboxylic acid.

What are the structural fragments that correspond to the following common names: (a) n- (b) iso- (c) sec- (d) tert-?

For (a), the "n-" indicates "normal," as in the linear chain of n-butane, $CH_3CH_2CH_2CH_3$. In (b), the iso indicates the $(CH_3)_2CH$- unit; (c) indicates the $CH_3CH_2(CH_3)CH$- unit; and, (d) indicates the $(CH_3)_3C$- unit.

What is the structure of the following: (a) tert-butyl benzoate (b) isopropyl butanoate (c) sec-butyl 3,3-dimethylhexanoate?

(a) 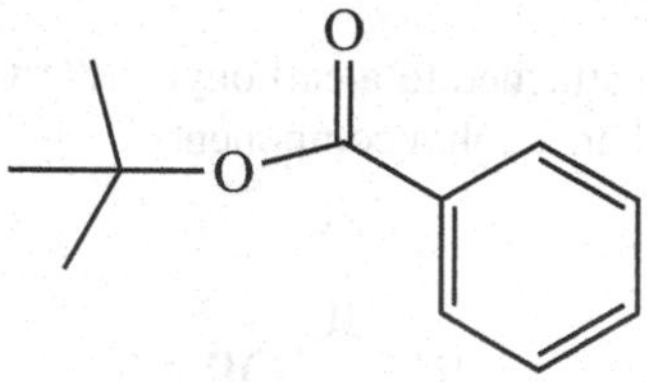 O O

(b) 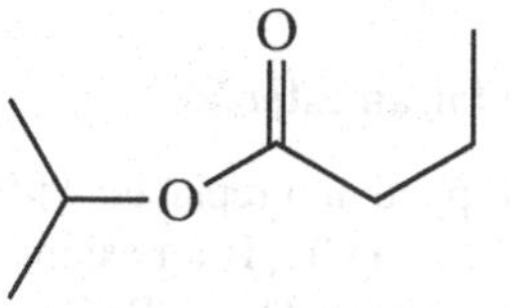 O O

(c) 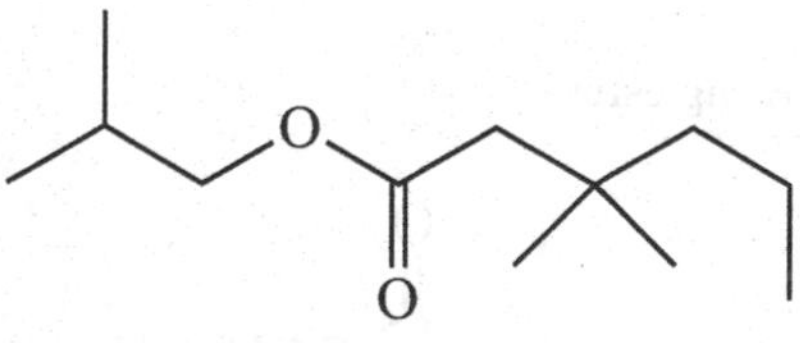 O O

What is the definition of a lactone?

A lactone is a cyclic ester.

How are lactones named?

Lactones are named by dropping the -oic acid ending and replacing it with -olide.

What is the name of (a), (b), and (c)?

(a) 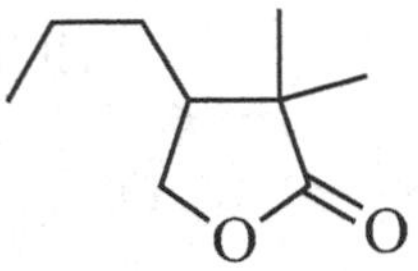 (b) 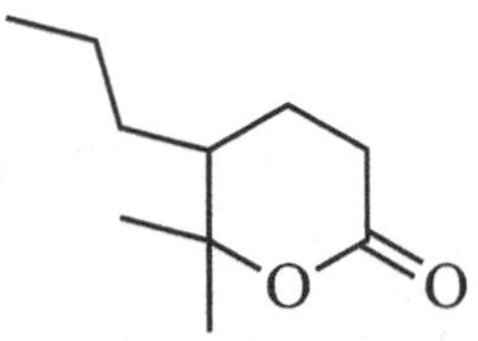 (c) 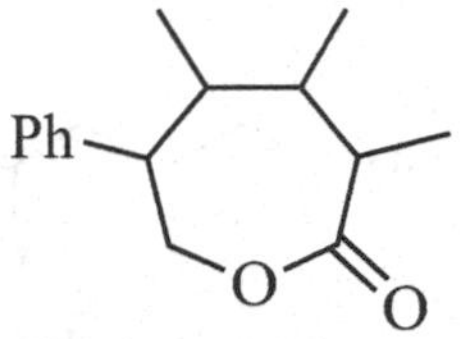 Ph

The name of (a) is 2,2-dimethyl-3-propylbutan-4-olide. The name of (b) is 6.6-dimethyl-5-propylpentan-5-olide. The name of (c) is 3,4,5-trimethyl-6-phenylhexan-6-olide.

What is the structure of each of the following: (a) 4-butanolide (b) 6-hexanolide (c) 4-ethyl-3-methyl-6-hexanolide (d) but-2-en-4-olide?

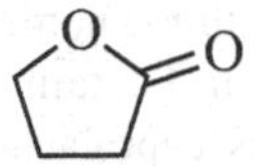

4-butanolide 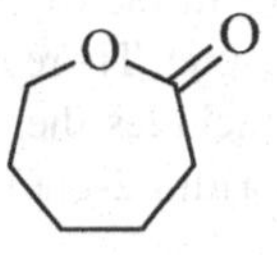 6-hexanolide 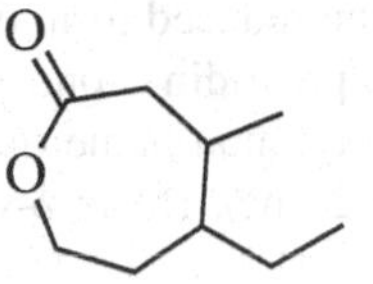 4-ethyl-3-methyl-6-hexanolide 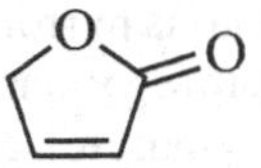 but-2-en-4-olide

What is the basic structure of an amide?

The fundamental structure of an amide has an amino group attached directly to a carbonyl, as shown (O=C—NR_2). There are primary amides (-NH_2), secondary amides (-NHR) and tertiary amides (NR_2).

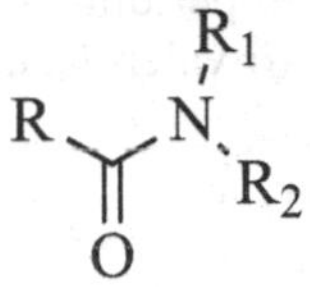

What is the IUPAC nomenclature system used to name an amide?

The -oic acid of the parent carboxylic acid is dropped and replaced with amide. The amide of propanoic acid is, therefore, propanamide (CH_2CH_2CONH). The structure of pentanamide, a primary amide, is shown.

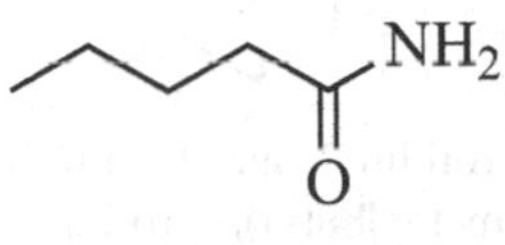

How are acyclic amides named?

The nomenclature system described in the preceding question is for acyclic amides (the -CON unit is not part of a ring). If pentanoic acid is the parent, replacing the -OH with NR_2 leads to dropping the -oic acid and replacing it with amide. If the common name of the acid is used (such as acetic acid), the -ic acid is dropped and replaced with amide. The NH_2 amide of acetic acid is, therefore, ethanamide or acetamide (CH_3CONH_2).

What is the nomenclature protocol when substituents appear on the nitrogen of an amide?

When substituents appear on the nitrogen the position of the substituent is given by using *N*- in front of the substituent. Amide (a) is *N*-ethyl-*N*-methylhexanamide and (b) is *N*,4-dimethylcyclohexane-1-carboxamide.

Note that the *N*- is used to position substituents on the nitrogen just as the traditional number and that an amide unit attached to a ring is named as carboxamide.

(a) 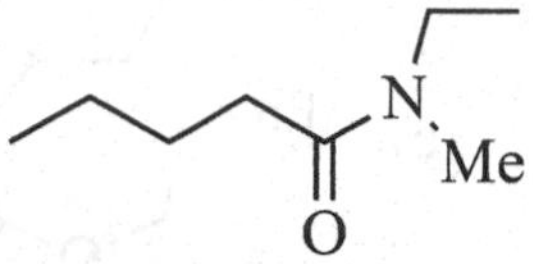 *N*-ethyl-*N*-methylpentanamide (b) *N*,4-dimethylcyclohexane-1-carboxamide

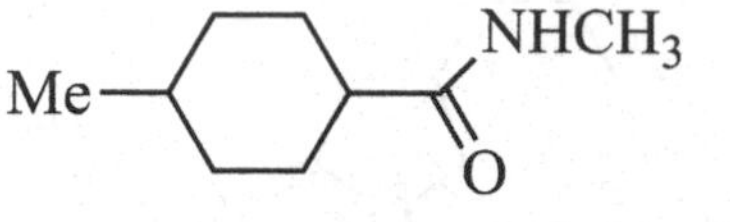

What is the definition of a lactam?

A lactam is a cyclic amide where the carbonyl carbon and the nitrogen are both part of a ring.

How are lactams named?

The names are derived from the reduced form of a heteroaromatic amine (see Section 16.6). The name of (a) is pyrrolidin-2-one, (b) is piperidin-2-one, and (c) is azepan-2-one. There is also a common nomenclature system, based on the common name of the acid, which includes the word lactam. Lactam (a) is γ-butyrolactam (pyrrolidin-2-one), (b) is δ-valerolactam (piperidin-2-one), and (c) is caprolactam (azepan-2-one).

(a) 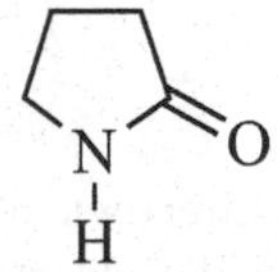 pyrrolidin-2-one (γ-butyrolactam) (b) 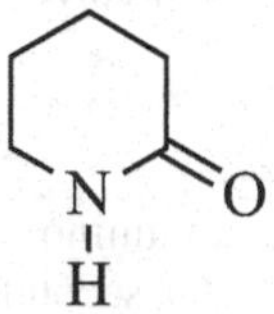 piperidin-2-one (δ-valerolactam) (c) 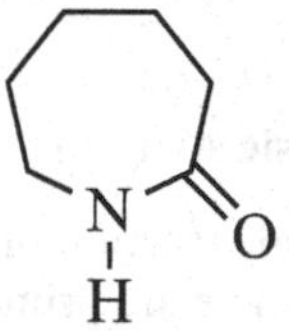 azepan-2-one (caprolactam)

What are the names of lactams (a), (b), and (c)?

(a) 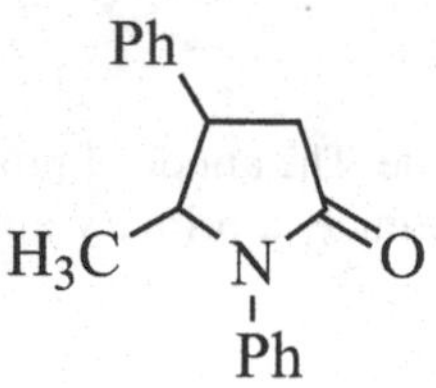 (b) 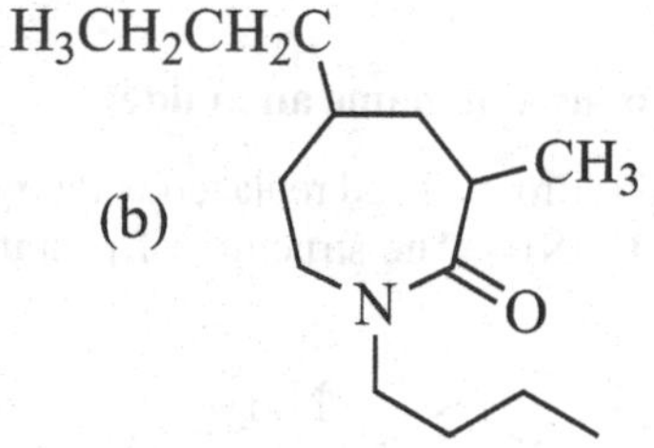 (c)

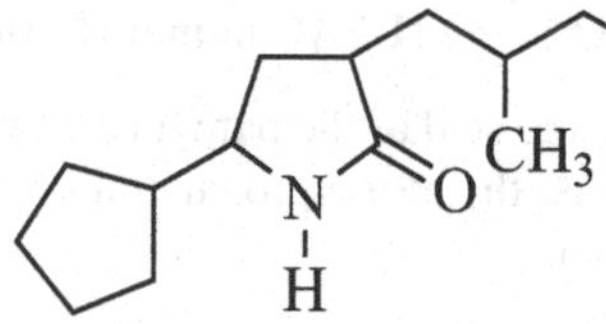

Lactam (a) is 5-methyl-1,4-diphenylpyrrolidin-2-one. Lactam (b) is 1-butyl-3-methyl-5-propylazepan-2-one. Lactam (c) is 5-cyclopentyl-3-(2-methylbutyl)pyrrolidin-2-one.

What is the definition of an imide?

An imide is the nitrogen equivalent of an anhydride and is characterized by the O=C—N—C=O moiety.

How are imides named?

The fundamental name of an imide uses the word imide. The name of EtCONHCOEt is diethylimide. Cyclic imides such the generic structure shown are also known, derived from α,ω-dicarboxylic acids.

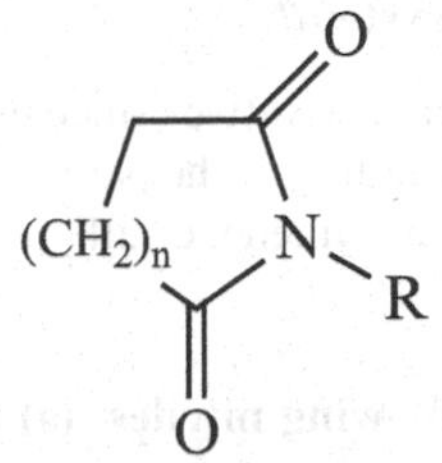

(CH2)n N R O O

What are the structures and names of the cyclic imides derived from the diacids succinic acid, glutaric acid, and adipic acid?

The imide derived from succinic acid is succinimide (pyrrolidine-2,5-dione), glutaric acid gives glutarimide (piperidine-2,6-dione), and adipic acid leads to adipamide (azepane-2,7-dione).

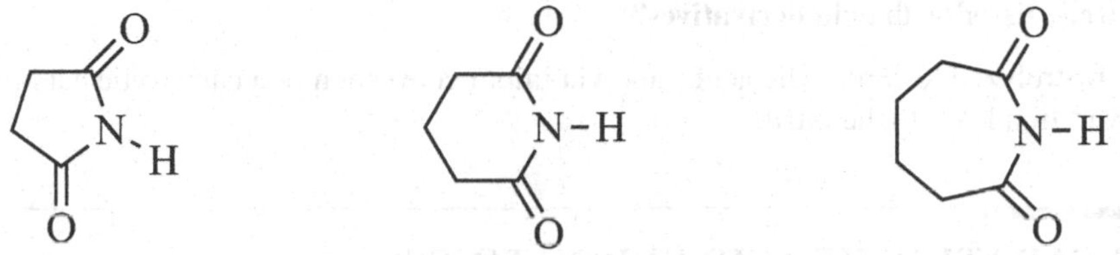

What is the structure of *N*-chlorosuccinimide (abbreviated NCS) and *N*-bromosuccinimide (abbreviated NBS)?

Both NCS and NBS are cyclic derivatives of succinic acid (see Section 8.6).

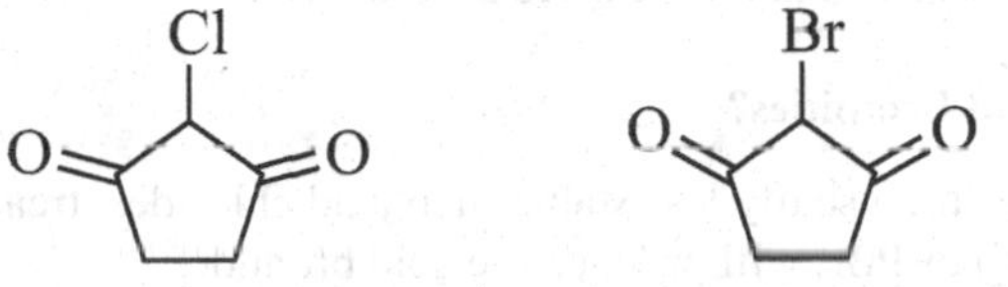

N-Chlorosuccinimide (NCS) N-Bromosuccinimide (NBS)

What is the structure of (a) 2-methylglutarimide, (b) *N*,3-diethyladipimide, and (c) *N*-phenylsuccinimide?

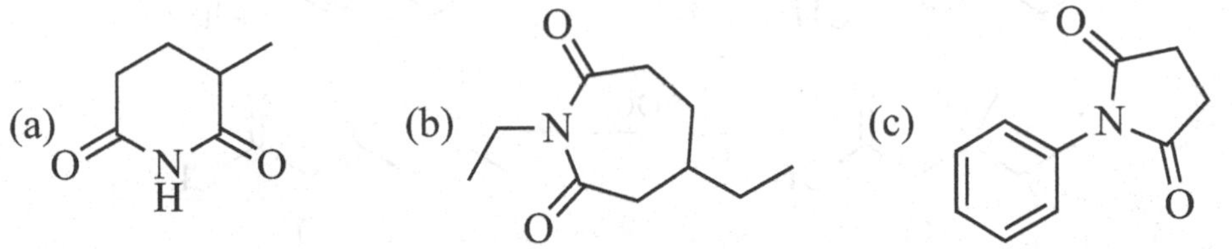

(a) 2-methylglutarimide (b) *N*,3-diethyladipimide (c) *N*-phenylsuccinimide

What is the basic structure of a nitrile?

A nitrile is characterized by the presence of a cyano group, -C≡N. An example of a nitrile is $CH_3CH_2CH_2CH_2C{\equiv}N$ (pentanenitrile).

How are nitriles named by the IUPAC system?

Nitriles are considered to be carboxylic acid derivatives since they can be hydrolyzed to carboxylic acids. They are named by dropping the -oic acid ending of the parent acid and replacing it with the word nitrile. The C5 nitrile is named by using the alkane, alkene, or alkyne base and adding the word nitrile. In this system, the C5 nitrile is pentanenitrile.

What is the structure of each of the following nitriles: (a) nonanonitrile (b) 3,5,diphenylhexanonitrile (c) 3,3-dimethylpentanenitrile?

(a) 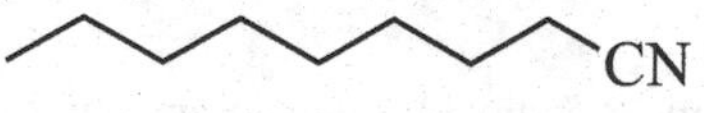 CN (b) 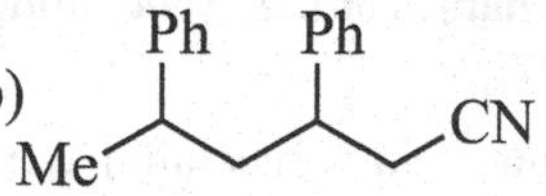 Ph Ph Me CN (c) 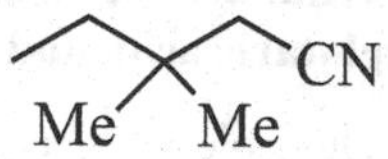 CN Me Me

Why is a nitrile listed with acid derivatives?

Nitriles are hydrolyzed to carboxylic acids, and via initial conversion of a carboxylic acid to a primary amide, dehydration leads to the nitrile.

15.4 PREPARATION OF ACID DERIVATIVES

What are at least three different reagents that transform a carboxylic acid into an acid chloride?

The same reagents used for conversion of alcohols to chlorides (see Section 8.3) are effective with acids: thionyl chloride, ($SOCl_2$), PCl_3, PCl_5, and $POCl_3$ are all effective.

Is it possible to prepare acid bromides?

Yes! Although acid bromides are usually less stable than acid chlorides, treatment of a carboxylic acid with thionyl bromide ($SOBr_2$) or PBr_3 will produce the acid bromide.

What reactions are used for the preparation of the acid chloride of pentanoic acid, 3,3-dimethylhexanoic acid, and cyclohexanecarboxylic acid? Give the structures of each acid chloride.

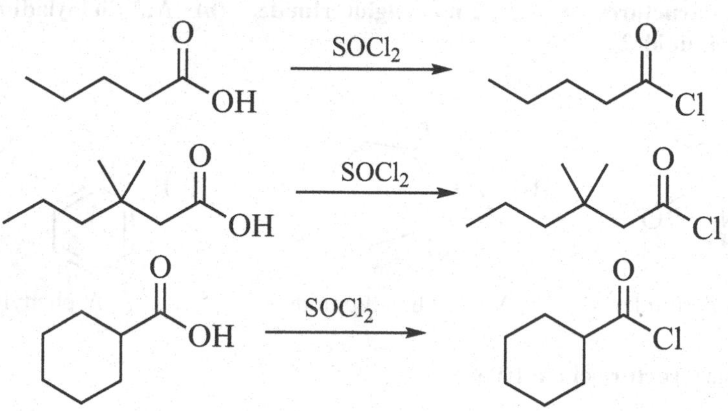

O OH $\xrightarrow{SOCl_2}$ O Cl

O OH $\xrightarrow{SOCl_2}$ O Cl

O OH $\xrightarrow{SOCl_2}$ O Cl

What are the names for the acid chlorides in the preceding question?

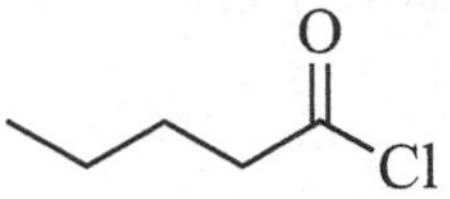

pentanoyl chloride 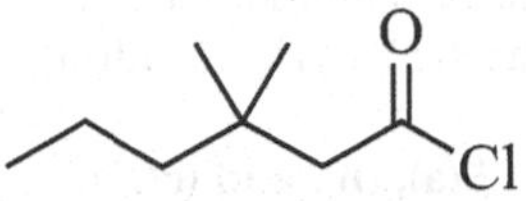   3,3-dimethylhexanoyl chloride 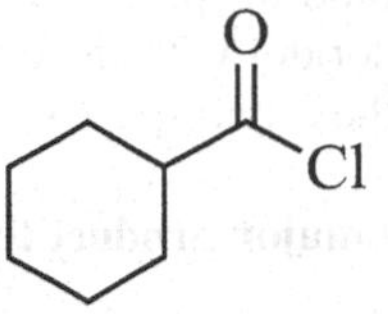   cyclohexanecarbonyl chloride

Why are acid fluorides and acid iodides almost never observed?

Both tend to be unstable and difficult to isolate. It is also true that thionyl fluoride or iodide are not usable reagents and phosphorus iodides are relatively unstable. The latter reagents are usually formed *in situ* by reaction of phosphorous with iodide. Although POF_3 is known, acid fluorides are typically too unstable to isolate.

What components are required for the preparation of an anhydride?

In a generic reaction two carboxylic acids combine, with loss of a molecule of water, to form the anhydride. The anhydride therefore consists of two acid fragments.

How are symmetrical anhydrides prepared?

A carboxylic acid can be heated with a dehydrating agent such as phosphorus pentoxide (P_2O_5) to produce the anhydride. Alternatively, the carboxylate salt of an acid can be reacted with the acid chloride of that same acid.

How can butanoic anhydride be prepared from butanoyl chloride?

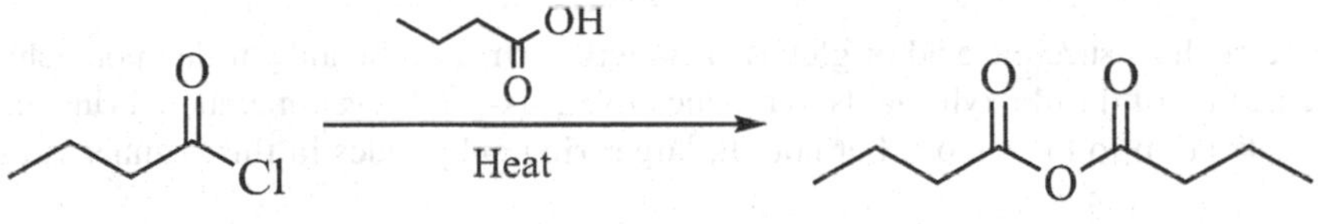

Heat

When butanoic acid is heated with an excess of butanoyl chloride, butanoic anhydride can be isolated.

Why is the preparation of mixed anhydrides often accompanied by low yields and significant amounts of symmetrical anhydrides?

If two different acids such as ethanoic acid and butanoic acid are heated with a dehydrating agent, ethanoic acid can condense with itself or with butanoic acid. Likewise, butanoic acid can condense with itself or with ethanoic acid. This reaction, therefore, produces three anhydrides in a 1:2:1 ratio: acetic anhydride, acetic butyric anhydride, and butyric anhydride, respectively. In other words, the targeted unsymmetrical anhydride is produced in diminished yield as a mixture of three compounds, requiring a difficult separation.

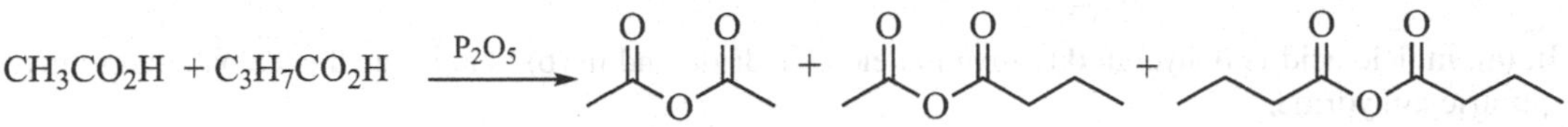

$CH_3CO_2H + C_3H_7CO_2H \xrightarrow{P_2O_5}$ + +

acetic anhydride   acetic butyric anhydride   butyric anhydride

How can the problems described in the preceding question be overcome?

A good method for producing mixed anhydrides is to condense the acid chloride of one acid (such as butanoyl chloride) with the carboxylate salt of the other (such as sodium ethanoate). In this example, reaction of these two species will produce acetic butyric anhydride exclusively.

What is the major product the reactions of (a), (b), and (c)?

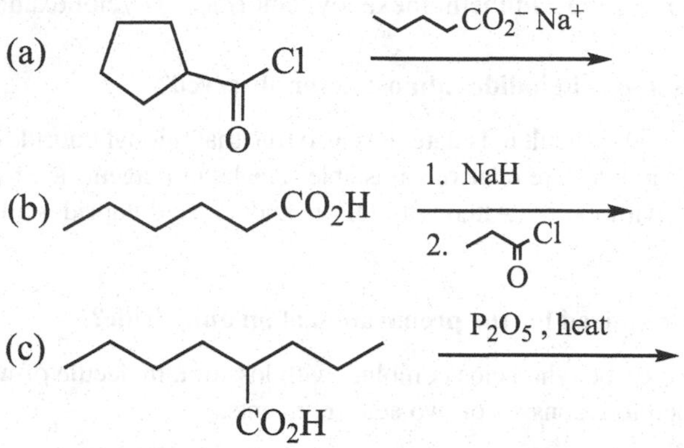

(a) cyclopentyl–C(=O)Cl, $CO_2^-\ Na^+$ →

(b) CO_2H, 1. NaH, 2. Cl, O →

(c) CO_2H, P_2O_5, heat →

In (a), cyclopentanecarboxylic acid chloride reacts with the sodium salt of pentanoic acid unsymmetrical anhydride, cyclopentanecarboxylic pentanoic anhydride. In (b), the mixed anhydride hexanoic propionic anhydride is formed by reaction of the carboxylic salt of hexanoic acid formed by reaction with sodium hydride (NaH), with propanoyl chloride. Example (c) produces a mixed anhydride 2-propylhexanoic 2-propylpentanoic anhydride by heating 2-propylhexanoic acid with phosphorus pentoxide.

What type of acid derivative leads to a cyclic anhydride?

A dibasic acid such as succinic acid or glutaric acid will form a cyclic anhydride upon dehydration. In general, cyclization of dicarboxylic acids to produce five-, six-, and seven-membered ring anhydrides is favorable. Cyclization to form most, but not all, larger ring anhydrides in this manner is usually very difficult.

What is the major product from the reactions of (a) and (b)?

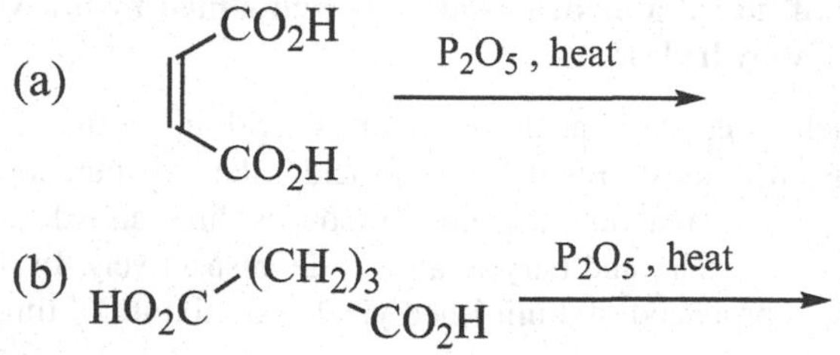

(a) CO_2H, CO_2H, P_2O_5, heat →

(b) HO_2C–$(CH_2)_3$–CO_2H, P_2O_5, heat →

In (a), maleic acid is dehydrated to give maleic anhydride and in (b) glutaric acid is dehydrated to give glutaric anhydride.

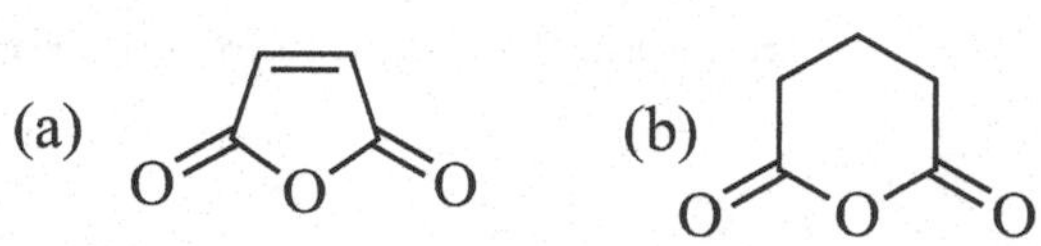

(a) O, O, O (b) O, O, O

Why does fumaric acid (*trans*-but-2-enedioic acid) *not* give a cyclic anhydride upon treatment with P_2O_5?

Unlike maleic acid, which has the carboxyl groups on the same side and close enough for those groups to interact to lose water, fumaric acid has the carbonyl groups on opposite sides of the double bond. The reactive units cannot get close enough to interact.

What are the structural components of an ester that are relevant to their preparation?

Esters are composed of a carboxylic acid part and an alcohol part.

What is an efficient method for the preparation of a carboxylic ester?

The reaction of an acid chloride and an alcohol typically in the presence of an amine, usually a tertiary amine, which reacts as a base with the HCl byproduct, is an efficient method for the preparation of an ester. Relatively simple esters can be prepared by heating a carboxylic acid in an alcohol solvent, with an acid catalyst, and the water byproduct is usually removed by addition of a dehydrating agent or with a Dean–Stark trap (see Section 12.2).

What is the product when pentanoyl chloride reacts with propanol in the presence of triethylamine?

The product is propyl pentanoate [$CH_3CH_2CH_2O_2C(CH_2)_4CH_3$]. The triethylamine reacts with the HCl by-product to produce triethylammonium chloride.

What is the product when butanoyl anhydride reacts with ethanol in the presence of triethylamine?

The anhydride reacts with ethanol, in the presence of an amine, to produce butanoic acid (from the anhydride) and ethyl butanoate ($CH_3CH_2O_2CCH_2CH_2CH_3$). The triethylamine will react with butanoic acid to produce triethylammonium butanoate (the acid salt), driving the reaction toward the ester.

Which is more reactive, an acid chloride or an ester? Explain.

An acid chloride is somewhat more reactive than an acid anhydride, but they are close in reactivity, and significantly more reactive than an ester. The reason for the enhanced reactivity of the acid chloride in acyl addition reactions is because chlorine is a better leaving group than an acyl group of the anhydride and much better than the OR group of an ester.

What is the major product of the reactions of (a) and (b)?

(a) OH —(acetic anhydride; NEt_3)→

(b) cyclohexanecarboxylic acid (OH) —(1. $SOCl_2$; 2. cyclohexanol (OH), NEt_3)→

Butan-1-ol reacts with acetic anhydride to form the ester, methyl butanoate (butyl acetate). Initial reaction of cyclohexanecarboxylic acid with $SOCl_2$ generates the acid chloride, which reacts with cycloheptanol to form cycloheptyl cyclohexanecarboxylate.

(a) butyl acetate

(b) cycloheptyl cyclohexanecarboxylate

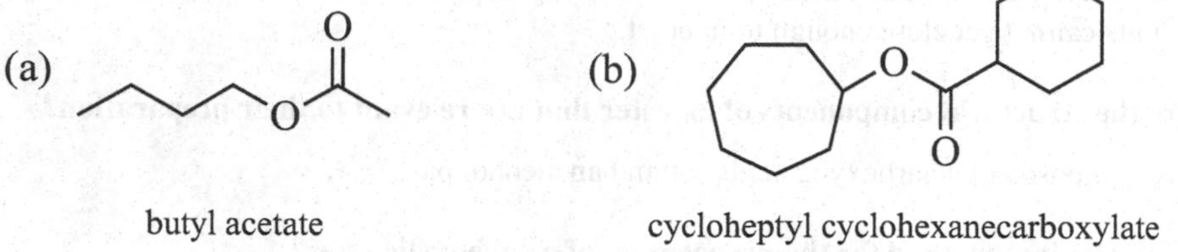

When butanoic acid is dissolved in ethanol and heated, in the presence of an acid catalyst, what is the major product?

The product is ethyl butanoate.

What is acyl substitution?

When an acid derivative reacts with a nucleophile, the nucleophile replaces the leaving group to give a new acyl derivative. The leaving group is Cl for an acid chloride, O(C=O)R for an anhydride, OR for an ester, and NR_2 for an amide.

What is a tetrahedral intermediate?

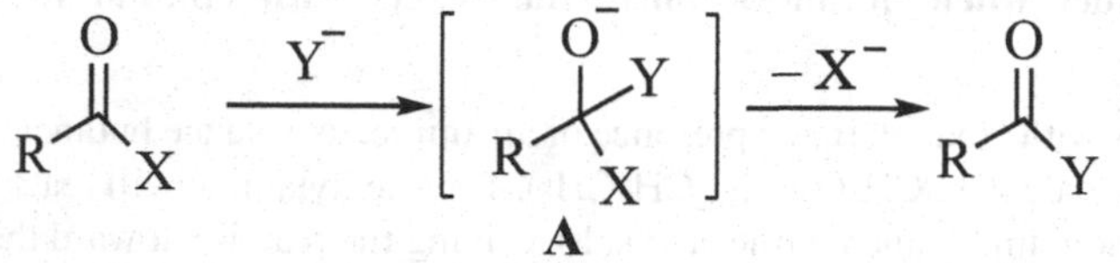

When a nucleophile (Y–) reacts with an acid derivative, acyl addition leads to an alkoxide intermediate (A) known as a *tetrahedral intermediate.* The key feature of ***A*** is the presence of a leaving group X in the tetrahedral intermediate. The alkoxide unit "kicks out" the leaving group (X) to give a new acyl derivative. Since X has been replaced with Y in the final product, this reaction is an acyl substitution reaction.

What is the mechanism for the acid catalyzed esterification of butanoic acid with ethanol?

Initial protonation of the acid gives oxocarbenium in ***A***, which reacts with ethanol to give oxonium ion ***B***. Loss of a proton gives the tetrahedral intermediate ***C***. Protonation of the OH moiety gives ***D***, which allows the loss of the product water to form oxocarbenium ion ***E***. Loss of a proton gives the product, ethyl butanoate.

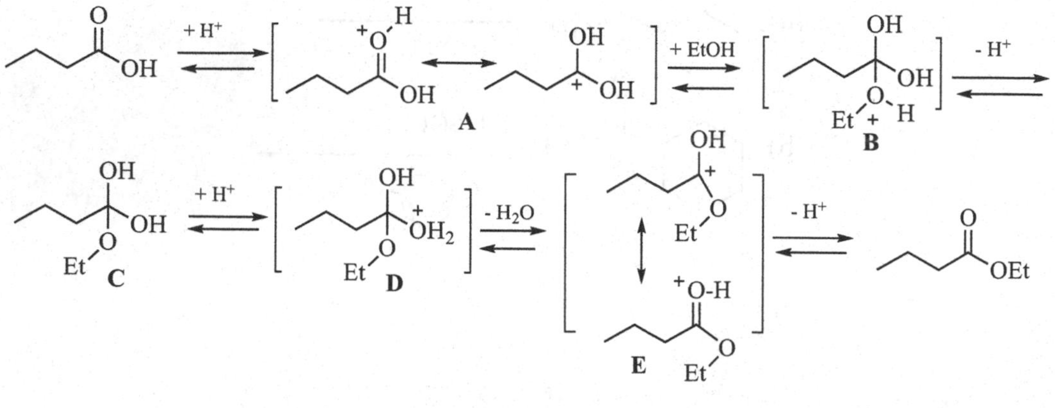

What is the major product of the reactions of (a) and (b)?

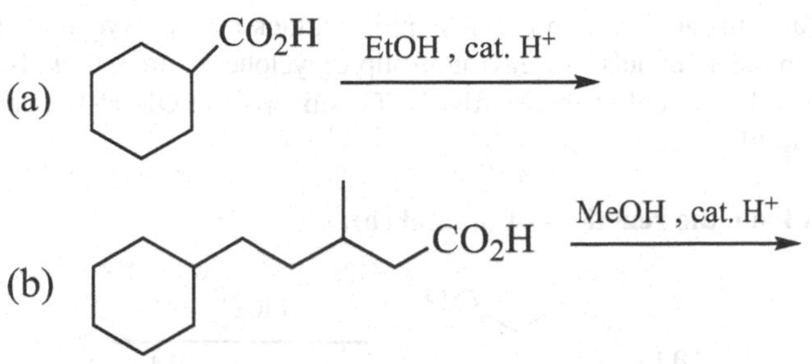

(a) CO_2H EtOH , cat. H^+

(b) CO_2H MeOH , cat. H^+

In (a), cyclohexanecarboxylic acid reacts with ethanol to form ethyl cyclohexanecarboxylate. In (b), 5-cyclohexyl-3-methylpentanoic acid reacts with methanol to form methyl 5-cyclohexyl-3-methylpentanoate.

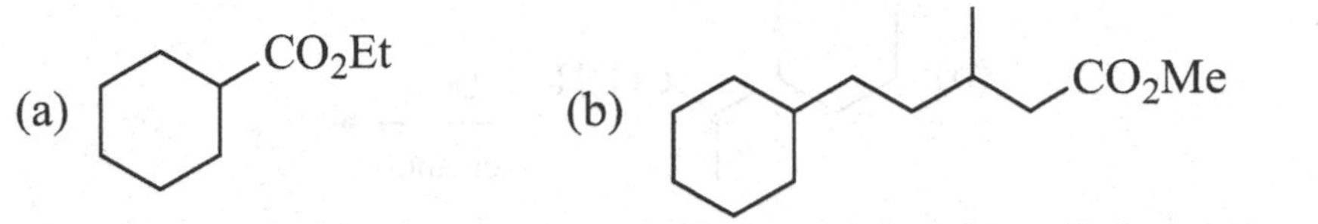

(a) CO_2Et (b) CO_2Me

ethyl cyclohexanecarboxylate methyl 5-cyclohexyl-3-methylpentanoate

What is the structure of dicyclohexyl carbodiimide (DCC)?

The structure of DCC is shown.

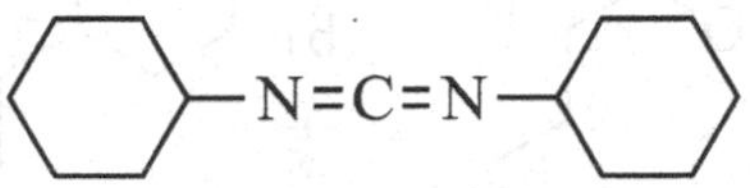

N=C=N

What is the product of the reaction between propanoic acid and ethanol in the presence of DCC?

The products are the ester, ethyl propanoate, and dicyclohexyl urea.

What is the mechanism of the reaction of propanoic acid and ethanol with DCC?

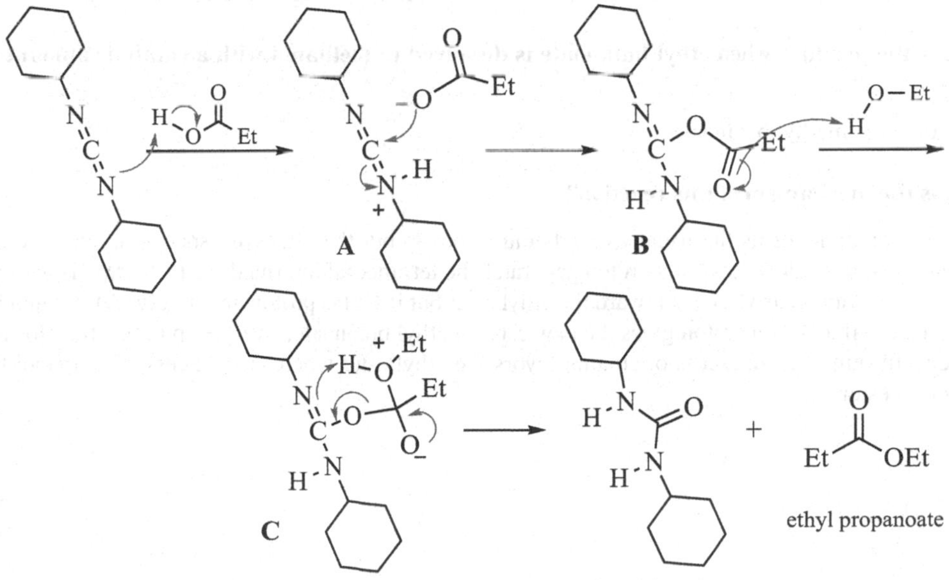

A B C

ethyl propanoate

dicyclohexyl urea

The initial reaction between DCC and the acid generates the protonated iminium ion ***A***. The central carbon of the protonated DCC is electrophilic, and reaction with the carboxylic acid generates ***B***. Intermediate A activates the acyl carbon to nucleophilic attack by the oxygen of the alcohol, giving ***C***. This tetrahedral intermediate expels the leaving group dicyclohexyl urea, and also generates the ester, ethyl propanoate. For all practical purposes, the DCC converts the OH of the carboxylic acid into an excellent leaving group (the urea).

What is the product from the reactions of (a) and (b)?

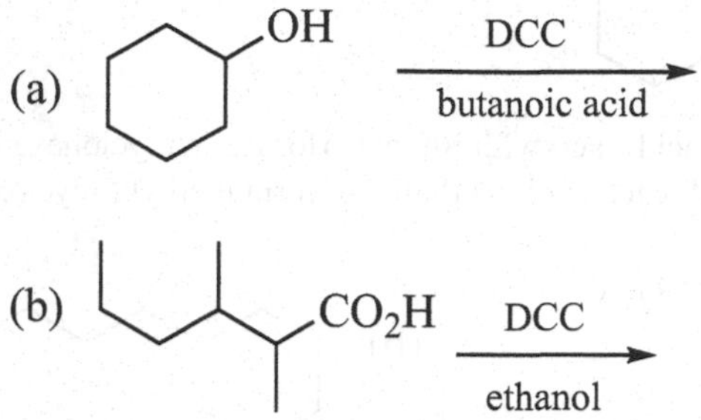

(a) OH — DCC, butanoic acid →

(b) CO_2H — DCC, ethanol →

In (a), cyclohexanol reacts with butanoic acid to form cyclohexyl butyrate. In (b), 2,3-dimethylhexanoic acid reacts with ethanol to give ethyl 2,3-dimethylhexanoate.

(a) O O (b) O O

cyclohexyl butyrate ethyl 2,3-dimethylhexanoate

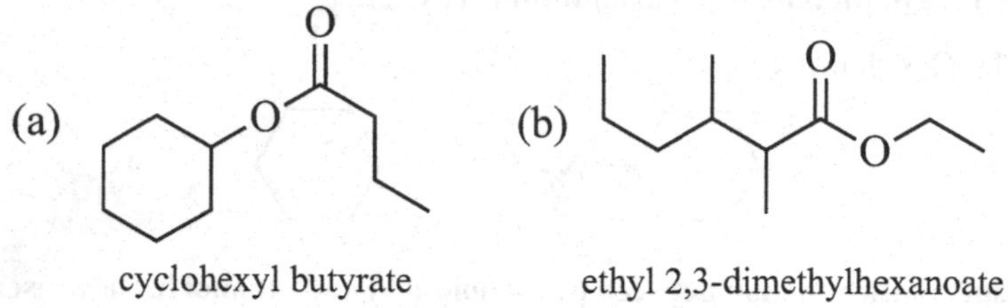

What does the term transesterification mean?

Transesterification refers to exchanging the OR group of an ester with a new alcohol group (OR^1). Conversion of a methyl ester to an ethyl ester is an example of transesterification.

What is the product when ethyl butanoate is dissolved in methanol with a catalytic amount of acid?

The product is methyl butanoate.

What is the mechanism of this reaction?

Initial protonation forms the usual oxocarbenium ion ***A***, but the attacking species is now methanol, forming oxonium salt ***B***. Loss of a proton generates the tetrahedral intermediate ***C***. If OMe is protonated again, the reaction is driven back toward the ethyl ester but if OEt is protonated (to give ***D***), ethanol is lost to give ***E***. Final loss of a proton gives the new ester, methyl butanoate. Every step in this transformation is an equilibrium and an excess of ethanol favors the ethyl ester whereas an excess of methanol favors the methyl ester.

What is the product when succinic acid is dissolved in ethanol with a catalytic amount of acid?

The product is the diester, diethyl succinate.

$$HO_2C\text{-}CH_2CH_2\text{-}CO_2H \xrightarrow{\text{EtOH , cat. } H^+} EtO_2C\text{-}CH_2CH_2\text{-}CO_2Et$$

Is it possible to form the "half-ester" of a dibasic acid?

Yes! It is usually difficult to stop an equilibrium reaction (catalytic H^+ and an alcohol, for example), but if the half-acid chloride can be made, the half ester can be prepared by standard techniques.

What is the product of the reactions of butanoic acid and dimethylamine at 25°C?

The acid–base reaction is the fastest reaction possible, giving the ammonium salt of the acid, dimethylammonium butanoate.

$$CH_3CH_2CH_2CO_2H \xrightarrow{HNMe_2} CH_3CH_2CH_2CO_2^- \; H_2\overset{+}{N}Me_2$$

How can dimethylammonium butanoate be converted to an amide?

Heating to about 200–250°C usually leads to dehydration of the salt and formation of the amide, *N,N*-dimethylbutanoic amide. In some cases, somewhat lower or higher temperatures are required.

$$CH_3CH_2CH_2CO_2H \xrightarrow{HNMe_2} CH_3CH_2CH_2CO_2^- \; H_2\overset{+}{N}Me_2 \xrightarrow[-H_2O]{250\ °C} CH_3CH_2CH_2C(=O)NMe_2$$

N,N-dimethylbutanoic amide

What is the product of the reactions of (a) and (b)?

(a) $CH_2=CHCH_2CH(CH_3)CH_2CH_2CO_2H \xrightarrow{Me_2NH\text{ , }250°C}$

(b) cyclooctyl-NHMe $\xrightarrow[225°C]{CH_3CH_2CH_2CO_2H}$

In (a), reaction of 4-methylhept-6-enoic acid and dimethylamine generates the dimethylammonium carboxylate salt. Thermolysis dehydrates the salt to produce *N*,*N*,4-trimethylhept-6-enamide. Similarly, in (b), reaction of *N*-methylcyclooctanamine with butanoic acid gives a salt, and thermolysis gives *N*-cyclooctyl-*N*-methylbutyramide.

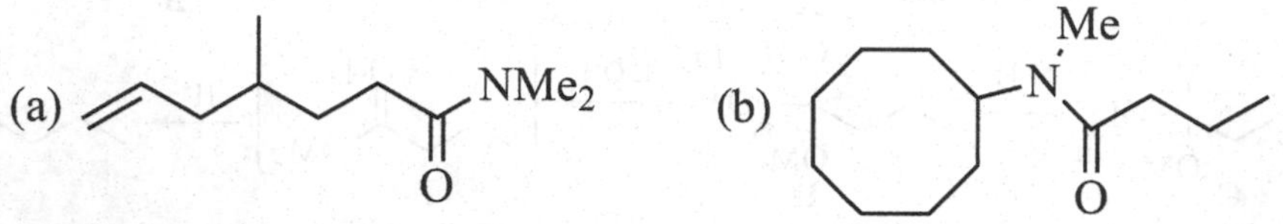

(a) NMe$_2$ O (b) Me N O

N,*N*,4-trimethylhept-6-enamide *N*-cyclooctyl-*N*-methylbutyramide

What is the major product when butanoyl chloride reacts with butylamine in the presence of triethylamine?

The product is the amide, *N*-butylbutanamide.

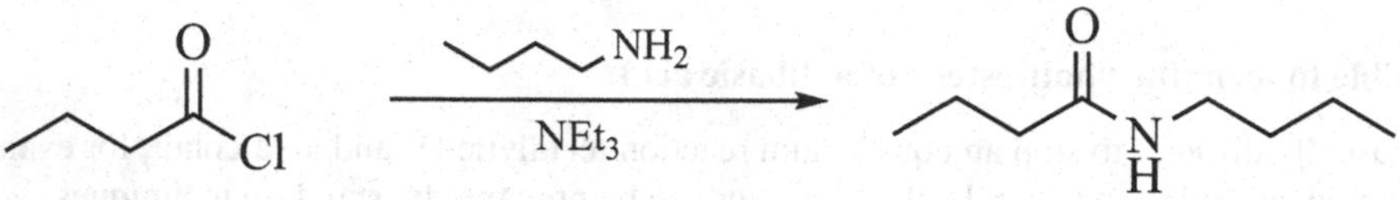

O Cl NH$_2$ NEt$_3$ O N H

What is the product when pentan-1-amine reacts with acetic anhydride?

Acetic anhydride reacts similarly to an acid chloride and the reaction with an amine provides the acyl portion of an amide. Therefore, reaction of acetic anhydride and pentan-1-amine gives *N*-pentylethanamide (*N*-acetylpentan-1-amine; *N*-pentanylacetamide).

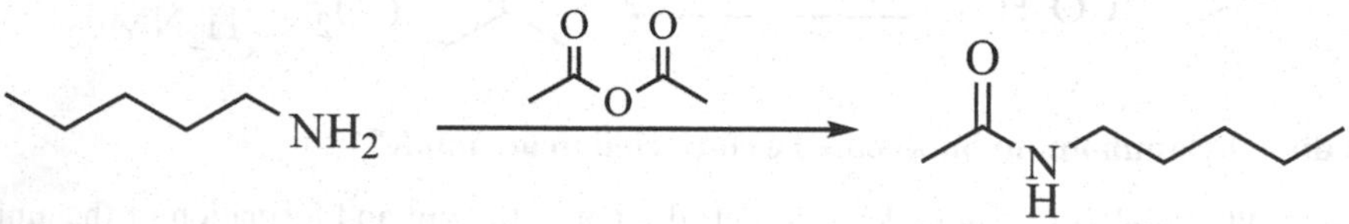

NH$_2$ O O O O N H

What is the product when ethyl pentanoate reacts with ammonia under conditions of high heat and pressure?

Under these conditions, an amide is formed (pentanamide) where the ammonia displaces ethanol via acyl addition and substitution.

What is the product when CH_3NH_2 reacts with γ-butyrolactone?

The nitrogen replaces the ester unit to form the cyclic amide, a lactam, (*N*-methyl-2-pyrrolidinone).

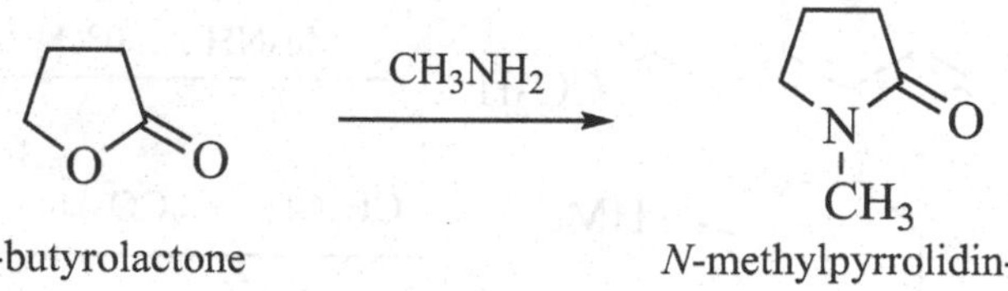

O O CH_3NH_2 N O CH_3

γ-butyrolactone *N*-methylpyrrolidin-2-one

What is the major product of the reactions of (a) and (b)?

(a) $CH_3(CH_2)_6CO_2Et$ —(Et_2NH, heat)→

(b) MeO–(cyclohexane)–CO_2H —(1. $SOCl_2$; 2. EtOH, NEt_3; 3. pyridine, $CH_3(CH_2)_4NH_2$)→

In (a), ethyl octanoate reacts with diethylamine to form the *N,N*-diethyl amide, *N,N*-diethyloctanamide. In (b), the reaction of 4-methoxycyclohexane-1-carboxylic acid to the acid chloride allows esterification to the ethyl ester. Subsequent reaction with pentylamine leads to the amide, 4-methoxy-*N*-pentylcyclohexane-1-carboxamide.

(a) $CH_3(CH_2)_6C(=O)NEt_2$ — *N,N*-diethyloctanamide

(b) MeO–(cyclohexane)–$C(=O)NHC_5H_{11}$ — 4-methoxy-*N*-pentylcyclohexane-1-carboxamide

By analogy with the DCC reaction of alcohols and acids, what is the product in the DCC reaction of cyclopentane-1-amine with propanoic acid?

Analogous to the coupling of acids and alcohols, when DCC reacts with the carboxylic acid and an amine, the products are *N*-cyclopentylpropionamide and dicyclohexylurea. In such reactions, the intermediate formed from DCC and the acid is attacked by the amine, giving a tetrahedral intermediate that leads to the products.

$CH_3CH_2C(=O)OH$ + cyclopentyl–NH_2 —(DCC)→ $CH_3CH_2C(=O)NH$–cyclopentyl

N-cyclopentylpropionamide

What is the product when δ-valerolactone is heated with ammonia? With methylamine?

A lactone is a cyclic ester. Reaction of an ester with an amine leads to formation of a cyclic amide, a lactam. When δ-valerolactone is heated with ammonia, the product is δ-valerolactam (piperidin-2-one). Similarly, when δ-valerolactam is heated with methylamine, *N*-methyl-2-piperidone is the product. Depending on the size of the ring, lactones of greater than eight members give an open chain amino acid.

piperidin-2-one ←(NH_3, heat)— δ-valerolactone (tetrahydro-2*H*-pyran-2-one) —(CH_3NH_2, heat)→ *N*-methylpiperidin-2-one

Why does heating a nine-membered ring lactone with ammonia lead to an open chain hydroxy amide rather than a lactam?

Nine-membered rings are high in energy due to *transannular* steric effects (the result of crowding hydrogen atoms inside the cavity of the ring). If a nine-membered ring is being formed, the molecule assumes a conformation analogous to a nine-membered ring in the transition state. The high transannular strain destabilizes the transition state that leads to that ring, which inhibits formation of the ring. Since cyclization to the nine-membered ring lactam is very difficult, the molecule simply opens to an amino acid (9-aminononanoic acid in this case).

What is transannular?

The term literally means across the ring. The term is used for cyclic compounds to identify interactions of groups or atoms that are not on adjacent atoms but rather across a ring.

When succinic anhydride is heated with ammonia, what is the product?

Just as lactones are converted to lactams, cyclic anhydrides are converted to cyclic imides upon heating with ammonia or an amine. In this case, succinic anhydride is converted to succinimide.

NH_3, heat

Why is it difficult to convert diethyl malonate into a lactam?

If diethyl malonate were to form a lactam, it would be a four-membered ring lactam (a so-called β-lactam). In general, the strain inherent to four-membered rings makes their formation by this route difficult, but not impossible.

How is a nitrile considered to be an acid derivative?

Strong hydrolysis of nitrile gives a carboxylic acid. A carboxylic acid is converted to a nitrile by initial conversion to a primary amide followed by dehydration.

What is a common method for the preparation of alkyl nitriles?

A S_N2 reaction of a cyanide ion with a primary or secondary alkyl halide.

What is the major product when 1-iodopentane is heated with KCN in THF?

The product is pentanenitrile, $CH_3CH_2CH_2CH_2C{\equiv}N$ via a S_N2 reaction (see Sections 8.2 and 8.3).

What is the product when (3*S*)-bromoheptane reacts with NaCN in THF?

Since the reaction is S_N2, it proceeds with 100% inversion of configuration. The product is (2*R*)-ethylpentanenitrile.

KCN , THF

Br

CN

3*S*-bromoheptane

2*R*-ethylhexanenitrile

What is a dehydration agent?

A dehydrating agent is a reagent that reacts with water and removes it from the reaction medium or reacts with a molecule to remove the elements of water.

What are common dehydrating agents?

The most common dehydrating agent is probably phosphorus pentoxide (P_2O_5). NOTE: the actual formula of this reagent is P_4O_{10} – the other formula was thought to be correct and accounts for the name. Sulfuric acid is sometimes used as a dehydrating agent in relatively simple molecules.

What is the reaction product when butanamide is heated with phosphorus pentoxide?

Under these conditions, butanamide is converted to butanenitrile, $CH_3CH_2CH_2C{\equiv}N$.

What is the product when pentanoic acid is treated with: 1. $SOCl_2$ 2. NH_3, heat 3. P_2O_5, heat?

The product is pentanenitrile, $CH_3CH_2CH_2CH_2C{\equiv}N$

What is the major product of the reactions (a) and (b)?

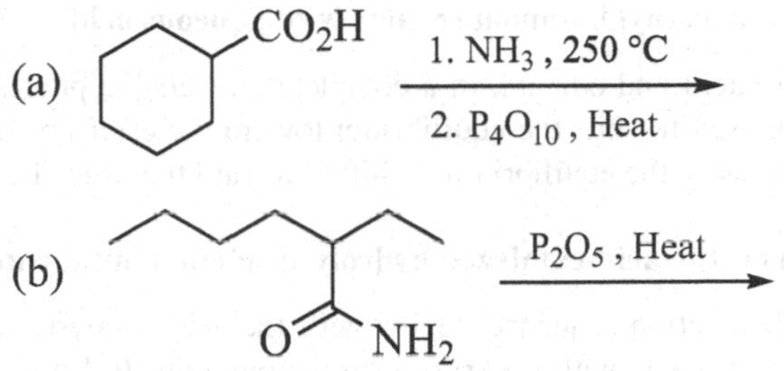

(a) CO_2H 1. NH_3, 250 °C 2. P_4O_{10}, Heat

(b) O NH_2 P_2O_5, Heat

In (a), the reaction of cyclohexanecarboxylic acid and ammonia leads to the amide when heated. Subsequent dehydration gives the corresponding nitrile, cyclohexanecarbonitrile. In (b), 2-ethylhexanamide is dehydrated to give 2-ethylhexanenitrile.

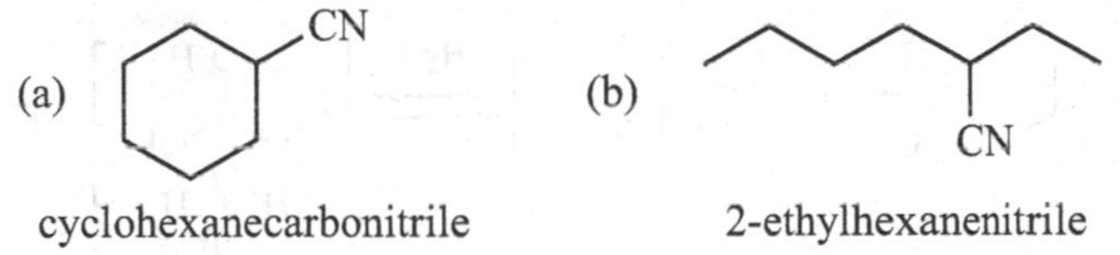

(a) CN

cyclohexanecarbonitrile

(b) CN

2-ethylhexanenitrile

15.5 HYDROLYSIS OF CARBOXYLIC ACID DERIVATIVES

When acid derivatives are heated with aqueous acid, what are the products?

Hydrolysis reactions of acid derivatives generally give the carboxylic acid parent of the derivative, along with HCl from acid chlorides, the acid from an anhydride, the alcohol from an ester, and the amine from an amide.

What is the product formed when pentanoyl chloride is heated with dilute aqueous acid?

The product is the parent acid of the acid chloride, in this case pentanoic acid.

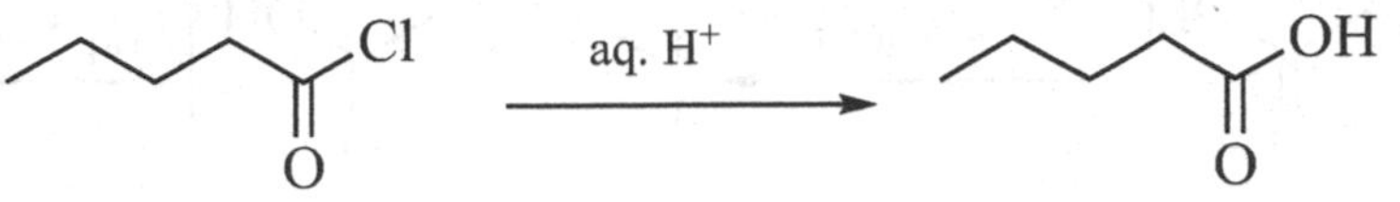

Cl O aq. H^+ OH O

What product is formed when pentanoyl chloride reacts first with aqueous NaOH and then dilute aqueous acid?

The initial product is pentanoic acid, but in an aqueous NaOH medium, the acid is quickly converted to the sodium salt of the acid, sodium pentanoate. Due to this conversion to the salt, a second chemical step is required to convert the salt to the acid, pentanoic acid.

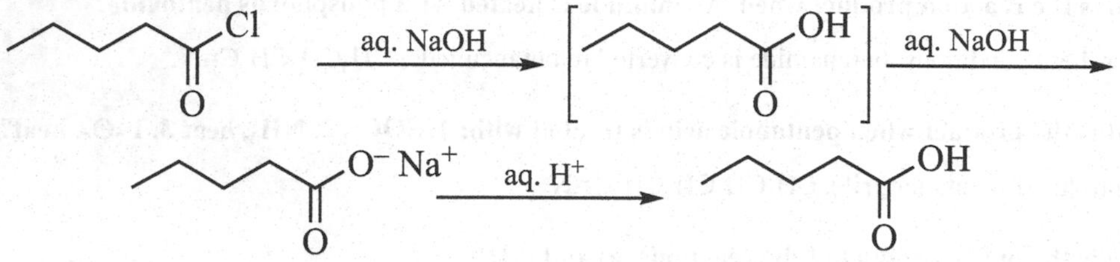

What are the products when ethyl butanoate reacts with aqueous acid?

The products are butanoic acid and ethanol, in a completely reversible process. A large excess of the alcohol (ethanol) must be used to shift the equilibrium toward the ester product, or the water product must be removed. In both cases, the equilibrium is shifted toward the ester (Le Châtelier's principle).

What is the mechanism for the acid-catalyzed hydrolysis of ethyl butanoate?

The completely reversible reaction sequence begins with the acid catalyst, and the reaction gives an oxocarbenium ion, ***A***, which reacts with water to form oxonium ion ***B***. Loss of a proton generates the *tetrahedral intermediate* ***C***. In order to lose the OEt group, protonation of that unit with acid generates oxonium ion ***D***. Loss of the leaving group ethanol, which is one product of the reaction, generates oxocarbenium ion ***E***, which loses a proton to give the acid product, butanoic acid. Note that this mechanism is the exact opposite of the acid-catalyzed esterification of an acid.

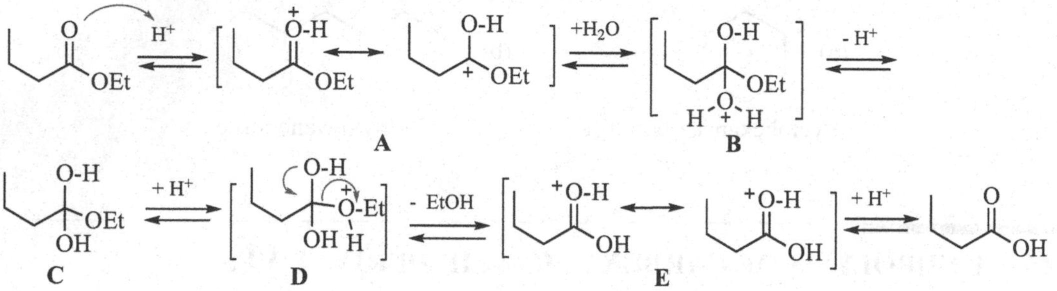

What is the product when ethyl butanoate is treated first with aqueous NaOH and then with aqueous acid?

The initial reaction of the ester with aqueous NaOH generates the carboxylic acid (butanoic acid) along with ethanol. However, in the presence of aqueous NaOH, butanoic acid reacts to give sodium butanoate via an acid–base reaction. Therefore, a second step is required to generate the acid product, butanoic acid.

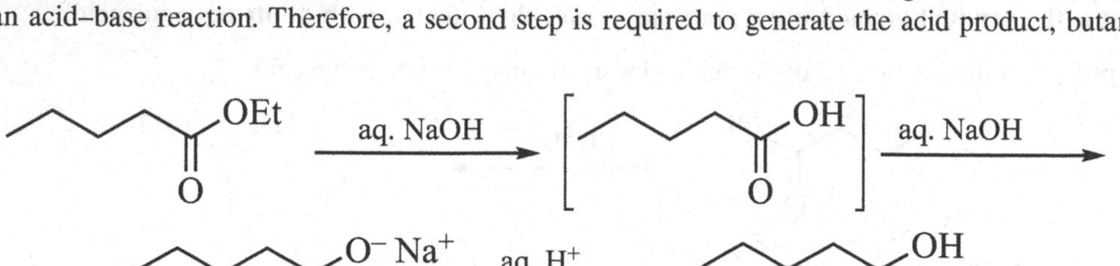

As a practical matter, it is more efficient to use the base hydrolysis of an ester rather than the acid-catalyzed reaction. Explain!

The acid catalyzed hydrolysis reaction is completely reversible and requires the use of a large excess of water, and more importantly for this question, the alcohol should be removed. Although there are methods for removing lower molecular weight alcohols, the process is not efficient with a wide range of alcohols or esters. The base hydrolysis process is essentially irreversible, and although two steps are required, the yield of the acid product is usually higher and requires less purification.

The two-step, base hydrolysis of esters has a special name. What is it?

The base hydrolysis of esters is called *saponification.*

What is saponification?

Saponification is a chemical reaction sequence that generates glycerol and a fatty acid salt, called a "soap," by the reaction of triglycerides, sodium, or potassium hydroxide (lye). Saponification is also used for the alkaline hydrolysis of the fatty acid esters.

What is a lipid?

A class of organic compounds including fatty acids or their derivatives that are insoluble in water but soluble in organic solvents. They include many natural oils, waxes, and steroids.

What is a fatty acid?

A long chain carboxylic acid that has a hydrocarbon chain composed of 4–28 carbon atoms and forms esters in fats and oils.

What is glycerol?

Glycerol is the common name of propane-1,2,3-triol. Glycerol is found in many lipids that are known as glycerides, diglycerides, and triglycerides.

What is a triglyceride?

A triglyceride is an ester derived from glycerol and three fatty acids. Triglycerides are the main constituents of body fat in humans and other animals, as well as vegetable fat.

What is an example of a triglyceride?

A generalized triglyceride is shown, along with glycerol. The specific triglyceride, cocoa butter, is shown. Cocoa butter is composed of three fatty acid esters of glycerol, oleic acid, palmitic acid, and stearic acid.

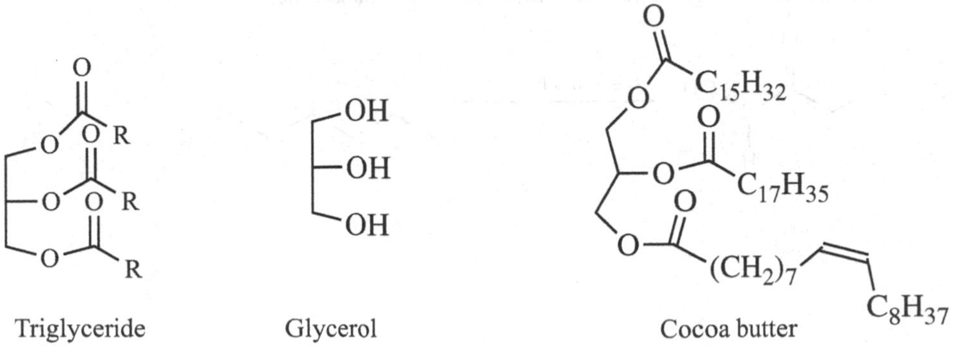

O O O R R R

Triglyceride

OH OH OH

Glycerol

O $C_{15}H_{32}$ O O $C_{17}H_{35}$ O O O $(CH_2)_7$ C_8H_{37}

Cocoa butter

What are the IUPAC names of oleic acid, palmitic acid, and stearic acid?

Oleic acid is cis-9-octadecenoic acid. Palmitic acid is hexadecanoic acid. Stearic acid is octadecanoic acid.

What is the product of the "partial hydrolysis" of hexanenitrile?

The complete hydrolysis of a nitrile gives a carboxylic acid. "Partial hydrolysis" refers to limiting the hydrolysis conditions to isolate the amide, which is an intermediate product on the path to the carboxylic acid. In this case, partial hydrolysis leads to hexanamide. In general, relatively dilute acid and relatively mild conditions give the amide.

What conditions are required for the conversion of a nitrile to a carboxylic acid?

If concentrated aqueous acid and vigorous reaction conditions (refluxing conditions for a long period of time) are used, the nitrile is converted directly to the carboxylic acid.

What is the pK_a of a typical amide N—H?

The pK_a of the hydrogen attached to an amide nitrogen is in the range of 15–17, very similar to the acidity of the O—H group of an alcohol.

Is the amide N—H more or less acidic than an amine?

An amide is significantly more acidic than the N—H of an amine (a typical amine N—H shows a pK_a of about 25–30). The carbonyl group on the nitrogen of the amide serves as an electron-withdrawing group to stabilize the amide base (after removal of the hydrogen) and to make the N—H more polarized (more acidic).

What type of base is required to deprotonate the N—H unit of an amide?

A relatively strong base is required, such as $NaNH_2$, $NaNR_2$, $LiNR_2$, an organolithium reagent such as *n*-butyllithium, or a base such as sodium hydride.

What conditions are required for the conversion of an amide to a carboxylic acid?

If concentrated aqueous acid and vigorous reaction conditions (refluxing conditions for a long period of time) are used, the amide is converted directly to the carboxylic acid.

What is the product formed when *N*-methylhexanamide is heated with aqueous acid?

Heating *N*-methylhexanamide with aqueous acid leads to hydrolysis and formation of the ammonium salt of methanamine and hexanoic acid. Note that generation of methanamine in an aqueous medium leads to an acid–base reaction that gives the ammonium salt of methanamine.

O
CH_3
N
H
aqueous H^+
O
OH
+
H + CH_3
N
H
H

15.6 REACTIONS OF CARBOXYLIC ACIDS AND ACID DERIVATIVES

What is the product when methylmagnesium bromide reacts with propanoic acid?

A Grignard reagent is a strong base, and the reaction with the carboxylic acid is fast, giving the conjugate base, $CH_3CH_2CO_2^-$ $MgBr^+$ and the conjugate acid CH_3—H. The acid–base reaction is faster and preferred to any other reaction of a carboxylic acid. The reaction with an excess of the Grignard reagent does not lead to further reaction since the Grignard reagent is not reactive with the carboxylate anion.

What is the product when methylmagnesium bromide reacts with propanoyl chloride? With ethyl propanoate?

The initial acyl addition of methylmagnesium bromide with the acid chloride gives a ketone, butan-2-one. However, ketones are as reactive or sometimes more reactive than the acid chloride. After one half-life (see Section 8.2), half of the unreacted Grignard reagent is available, and the ketone reacts to give the alkoxide product. After hydrolysis, 2-methylpropan-2-ol is isolated as the major product, along with some butan-2-one.

The identical reaction occurs with the ester, except that the ketone product is more reactive than the ester. Therefore, the major product is the alcohol, 2-methylpropan-2-ol.

Cl, O — CH_3MgBr / Ether → [CH_3, O] — CH_3MgBr → CH_3, CH_3, O^-MgBr^+ — H_3O^+ → CH_3, CH_3, OH

OEt, O — CH_3MgBr / Ether → [CH_3, O] — CH_3MgBr → CH_3, CH_3, O^-MgBr^+ — H_3O^+ → CH_3, CH_3, OH

What is the product when ethyl propanoate reacts with an excess of methylmagnesium bromide?

In the presence of an excess of Grignard reagent, the ester is converted exclusively to the alcohol, 2-methylpropan-2-ol.

What product is formed when lithium dimethylcuprate reacts with butanoyl chloride?

Lithium dialkyl cuprates react with acid chlorides to give the ketone. Organocuprates do not react with the ketone product, so the reaction is an excellent method for the preparation of ketones. In this example, butanoyl chloride reacts with lithium dimethylcuprate to give pentan-2-one.

Cl, O — $(CH_3)_2CuLi$ / Ether, –10 °C → CH_3, O

Do carboxylic acids and/or acid derivatives react with lithium aluminum hydride?

Yes!

What is the product of the reaction of pentanoic acid and $LiAlH_4$?

The powerful reducing agent $LiAlH_4$ reduces acids to the corresponding primary alcohol, in this case pentan-1-ol.

What is the product of the reaction between butanoic acid and $NaBH_4$?

Experiments have shown that $NaBH_4$ is not powerful enough to reduce the acid to the alcohol. However, $NaBH_4$ reacts with butanoic acid in an acid–base reaction to form the carboxylate salt of butanoic acid.

What is the product of the reaction of pentanoyl chloride and $LiAlH_4$? With ethyl butanoate?

This reagent reduces acid chloride to the corresponding alcohol and also reduces esters to alcohols. Reduction of pentanoyl chloride gives pentan-1-ol as the major product. Reduction of ethyl butanoate gives butan-1-ol as the major product, and the OEt unit is also converted to ethanol, so there are two products.

What is the product of the reaction of butanamide and $LiAlH_4$?

The reduction of amides takes a different course than carboxylic acids, acid chlorides, or esters. The reagent $LiAlH_4$ is strong enough to reduce amides, but the product is an amine, where the oxygen has been removed from the molecule. In this case, butanamide is reduced to butan-1-amine.

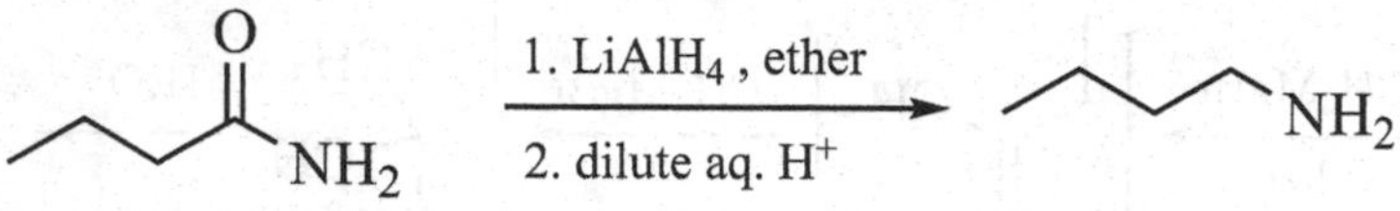

O NH$_2$ 1. $LiAlH_4$, ether 2. dilute aq. H^+ NH$_2$

What is the product of the following reaction?

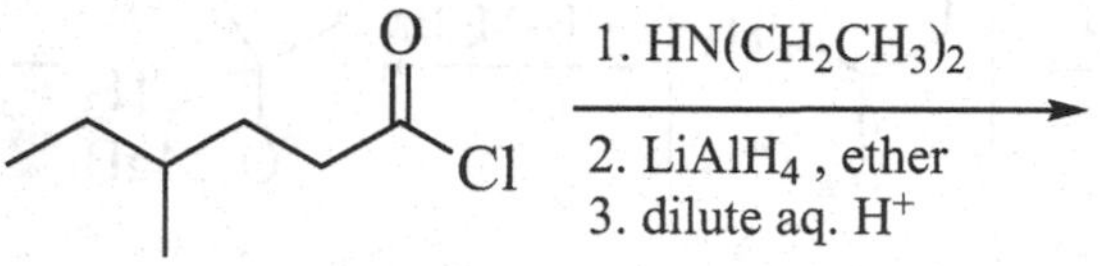

O Cl 1. $HN(CH_2CH_3)_2$ 2. $LiAlH_4$, ether 3. dilute aq. H^+

The final product is *N,N*-diethyl-4-methylhexan-1-amine. Initial reaction of the acid chloride and the secondary amine gives the tertiary amide. Subsequent reduction with $LiAlH_4$ gives the amine, *N,N*-diethyl-4-methylhexan-1-amine.

What is the product of the reaction of pentanolide and $LiAlH_4$?

Reduction of the lactone generates a diol. In this case, pentanolide is converted to pentane-1,5-diol.

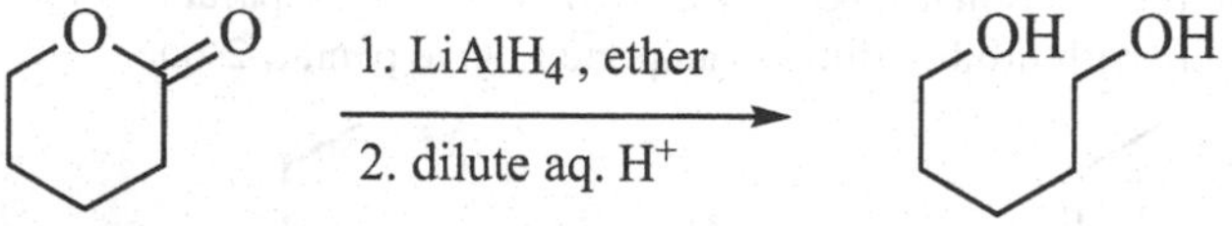

O O 1. $LiAlH_4$, ether 2. dilute aq. H^+ OH OH

pentanolide pentane-1,5-diol

What is the product of the reaction between butanoyl chloride and $NaBH_4$?

Sodium borohydride is a strong enough reducing agent to reduce acid chlorides to the primary alcohol, in this case butan-1-ol. At low temperatures, reduction may give good yields of the aldehyde, butanal, however. For problems in this book, assume that the product is the alcohol.

What is the product of the reaction between ethyl pentanoate and $NaBH_4$?

In general, $NaBH_4$ is not strong enough to reduce esters or amides, so *assume* the answer is no reaction. However, some highly reactive esters are reduced completely or in part upon treatment with $NaBH_4$.

Are there other reducing agents that can reduce carboxylic acids?

Yes!

What is the product when propanoic acid is treated with borane (BH_3) and then hydrolyzed with dilute acid?

Borane has a great affinity for the oxygen atoms of a carboxyl and readily reduces carboxylic acids. The product after hydrolysis is the corresponding alcohol. Borane will reduce propanoic acid to propan-1-ol.

Why is borane often called "the reagent of choice" for the reduction of carboxylic acids?

Borane will reduce an acid faster than an ester, a nitro compound, a nitrile, or many other functional groups. If both an ester and a carboxylic acid are present in the same molecule, a reaction with borane will give selective reduction of the acid. The reaction of 5-ethoxy-5-oxopentanoic acid with borane, followed by hydrolysis, leads to clean reduction of the carboxyl group, leaving the ester group untouched. The product will be ethyl 5-hydroxypentanoate.

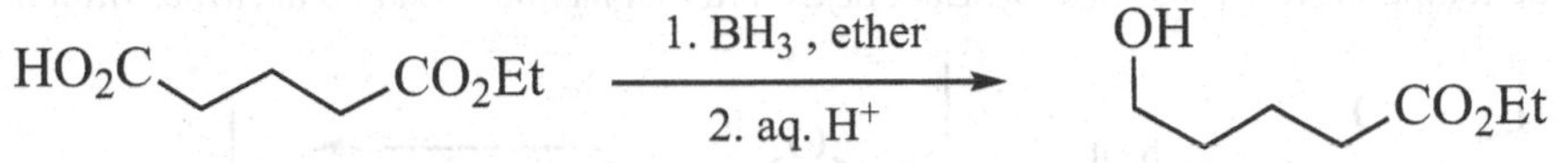

HO_2C–(CH₂)₃–CO_2Et → (1. BH_3, ether; 2. aq. H^+) → OH–(CH₂)₄–CO_2Et

5-ethoxy-5-oxopentanoic acid ethyl 5-hydroxypentanoate

What is decarboxylation?

When the carbonyl of a carboxyl group has a 1,3-relationship with another carbonyl, or if it is conjugated to a π-bond, heating often induces the loss of carbon dioxide in a reaction called *decarboxylation*.

Can 1,3-dicarboxylic acids be decarboxylated?

Yes! Heating dicarboxylic acids with a 1,3-relatinship of the carbonyl carbons leads to decarboxylation via a six-centered transition state to give an enol that tautomerizes to a monocarboxylic acid.

What is the structure of malonic acid?

Malonic acid is 1,3-propanedioic acid, $HO_2C\text{-}CH_2\text{-}CO_2H$. Note that since the carboxyl groups must be at each terminus, the numbers are not necessary, and this compound is simply propanedioc acid. The common name is malonic acid.

Is there an intermediate for the thermal decarboxylation described in the preceding question?

No! The reaction must be probed by examination of a six-centered transition state.

Draw the decarboxylation transition state and the final product for the thermal decarboxylation of 2-ethylpropanedioc acid.

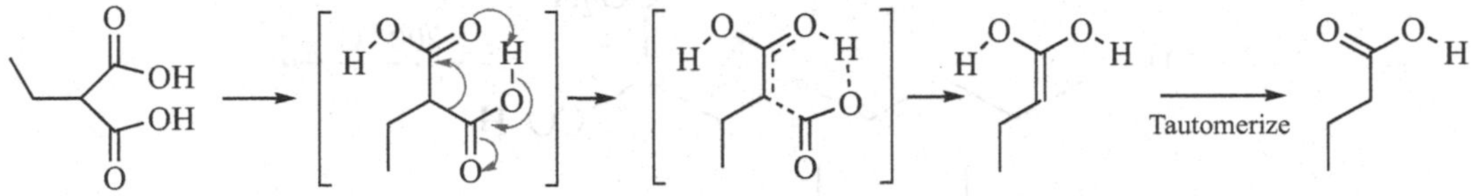

Conformational Change Transition State Enol Tautomerize butanoic acid

The final products are CO_2 and the enol of butanoic acid, which tautomerizes to butanoic acid.

What is the tautomerization step?

The initially formed product of decarboxylation is an enol, which is unstable. The enol tautomerizes via "keto-enol" tautomerism to the "keto" form, the carboxylic acid (butanoic acid).

What is the final product when 2-hexylmalonic acid is heated to 250°C?

The decarboxylation reaction of 2-hexylmalonic acid is facile since 1,3-diacids are capable of losing CO_2 thermally. The final isolated product is heptanoic acid.

How can CO_2 be lost from 3-ketopentanoic acid?

The carbonyl oxygen can attack the acidic hydrogen of the acid via a six-centered transition state (illustrated by the arrows in *A*). The electron flow will break the C—C bond, generate CO_2 (O=C=O) and the *enol*, ***B***. Since the enol is quickly transformed to the ketone via *keto-enol tautomerism*, the final product is butan-2-one. The acid *must* have a basic atom on a group that can form a six-membered or a five-membered transition state to facilitate the loss of CO_2. The more basic that atom is (O > C for example), the lower the temperature for loss of CO_2. Loss of CO_2 in this manner is called *decarboxylation*.

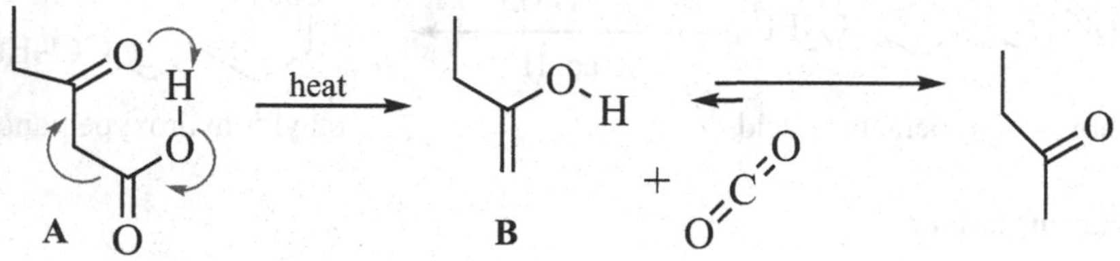

A heat B + O=C=O

Why is the final product of this reaction a ketone?

Since the initial product is an enol, tautomerism favors the carbonyl form (it is thermodynamically more stable), as introduced in Section 7.6; also see Section 12.2.

What are the requirements for thermal loss of carbon dioxide from β-ketoacids?

The acid must have a carbonyl, an alkene, or an aromatic ring in the β-position relative to the carbonyl. That group must have a basic atom that can form a six-membered or a five-membered transition state with the acidic hydrogen.

Is decarboxylation of malonic acid derivatives more or less facile than β-ketoacids? Explain.

In general, the carbonyl of an acid is somewhat less basic than the carbonyl of a ketone. For this reason, removal of the hydrogen via decarboxylation is slower with the carbonyl of a keto acid than with a dicarboxylic acid. It therefore requires somewhat higher reaction temperatures and is slightly less facile.

What is the major product from the reactions of (a) and (b)?

(a) CO_2H CO_2H 200 °C

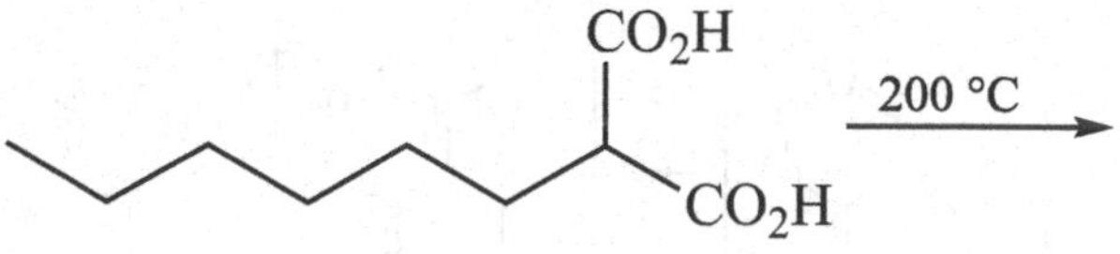

(b) CO_2H O 200 °C

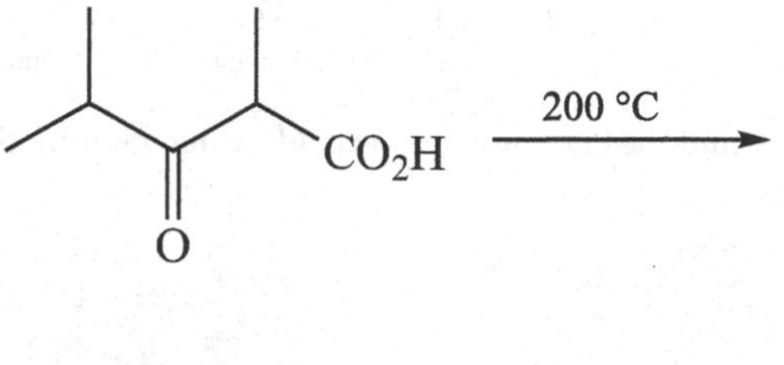

In the first case the carboxyl carbonyl at the β-position can remove the hydrogen from the OH group. Such 1,3-diacids decarboxylate thermally to give the mono-acid. Heating 2-hexylpropandoic leads to octanoic acid. The carbonyl that is β- to the acid group in 2,4-dimethyl-3-oxopentanoic acid is a ketone and decarboxylation by heating leads to 2-methylpentan-3-one.

(a) 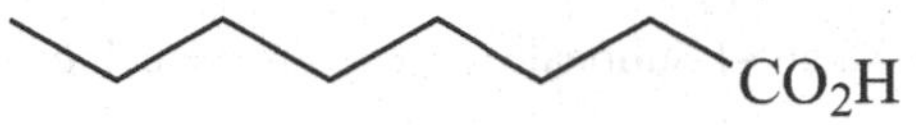 CO_2H (b) 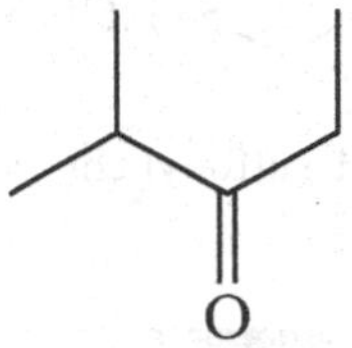 O

What is the structure of a sulfonic acid?

The structure is RSO_2OH. Sulfonic acids have many characteristics of carboxylic acids in that they are Brønsted–Lowry acids, and they form acid chlorides, esters, and amides.

What is the structure of methanesulfonic acid, ethanesulfonic acid, and 4-methylpentanesulfonic acid?

Methanesulfonic acid is CH_3SO_3H; ethanesulfonic acid is $CH_3CH_2SO_3H$; 4-methylpentanesulfonic acid is: SO_3H .

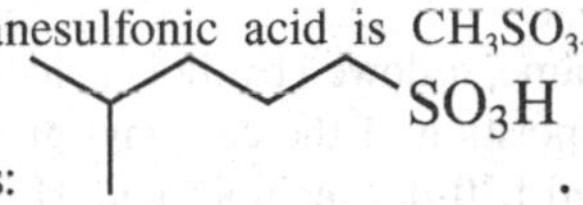

What is a sulfonyl halide?

A sulfonyl halide is the acid halide of a sulfonic acid. The generic structure is RSO_2Cl (or Br). The name of CH_3SO_2Cl is methanesulfonyl chloride. The name of $CH_3CH_2CH_2CH_2SO_3Cl$ is butanesulfonyl chloride. These two sulfonyl chlorides are derived from the corresponding sulfonic acids, methanesulfonic acid (CH_3SO_2H), and butanesulfonic acid ($CH_3CH_2CH_2CH_2SO_3H$).

What is a sulfonate ester?

A sulfonate ester is the alcohol derivative (an ester) of a sulfonic acid and is named sulfonate. The generic structure is RSO_2OR'. The name of $CH_3SO_2OCH_3$ is methanesulfonate. The name of $CH_3CH_2CH_2CH_2SO_2OCH_2CH_3$ is ethyl butanesulfonate.

What is the product when ethylsulfonyl chloride reacts with butan-1-ol in the presence of triethylamine?

Just as an acid chloride derived from a carboxylic acid reacts with an alcohol to produce an ester, a sulfonyl chloride reacts with an alcohol to produce a sulfonate ester, RSO_2OR'. In this case the product is butyl ethylsulfonate, $CH_3CH_2SO_2OCH_2CH_2CH_2CH_3$.

What is a sulfonamide?

A sulfonamide is the amine derivative (an amide) of a sulfonic acid. The generic structure is $RSO_2NR'_2$. The name of $CH_3SO_2NH_2$ is methanesulfonamide. The name of $CH_3CH_2CH_2CH_2SO_2NMe_2$ is *N,N*-dimethyllbutanesulfonamide.

What is the product when ethylsulfonyl chloride reacts with propan-1-amine?

Just as an acid chloride derived from a carboxylic acid reacts with an amine to produce an amide, a sulfonyl chloride reacts with an amine to produce a sulfonamide, $RSO_2NHCH_2CH_2CH_3$. In this case the product is butyl ethylsulfonamide, $CH_3CH_2SO_2NHCH_2CH_2CH_2CH_3$.

What is the structure of propanesulfonyl chloride, ethyl butanesulfonate, and *N*-methylbutanesulfonamide?

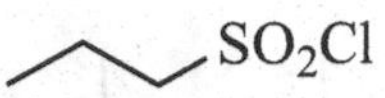

propane-1-sulfonyl chloride 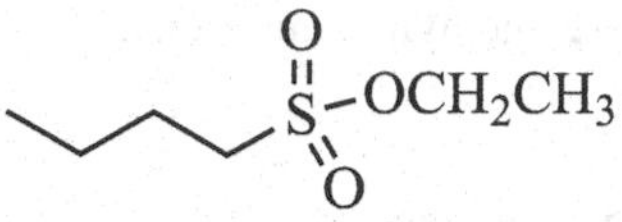 ethyl butane-1-sulfonate 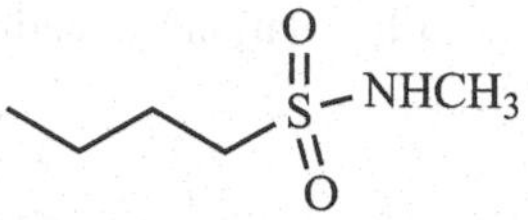 *N*-methylbutane-1-sulfonamide

15.7 DIBASIC CARBOXYLIC ACIDS

What is a dibasic acid?

When a molecule contains two carboxyl groups it is referred to as a *dibasic acid*, where the two carboxyl groups are at opposite ends of a chain of carbon atoms. The IUPAC nomenclature system uses the ending dioic acid.

What is the IUPAC nomenclature system for dibasic acids?

The carbon chain is indicted by the usual alkane, alkene, or alkyne name, followed by dioic acid, where di- indicates the presence of two carboxyl groups. Technically, the position of the carbonyl groups is given by numbers. An example is $HO_2C\text{-}(CH_2)_8\text{-}CO_2H$, which is named 1,10-decanedioic acid. However, the carboxyl groups must be at the end(s) of a carbon chain, so the numbers are not necessary and dodecanoic acid is an acceptable name.

What is the IUPAC name for compounds (a), (b), and (c)?

(a)

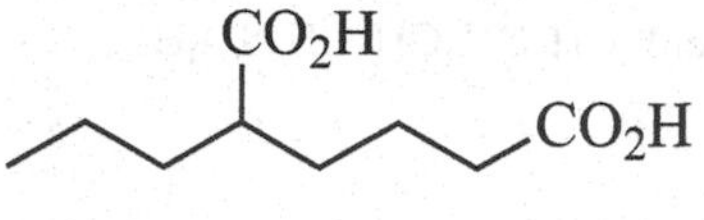

(b)

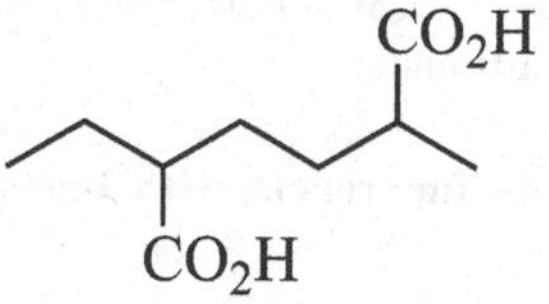

(c)

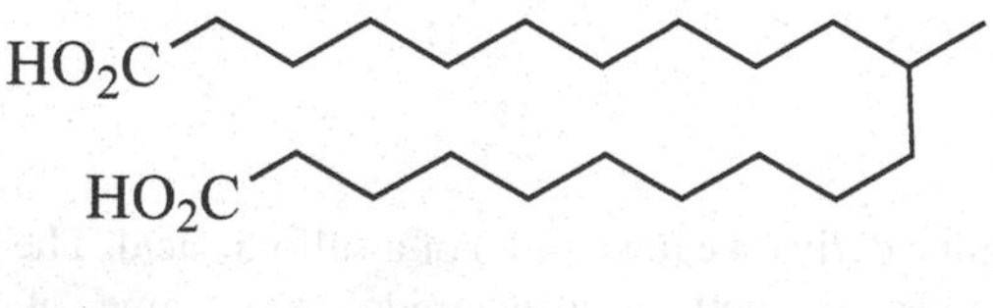

The name of (a) is 2-propylhexanedioic acid. Diacid (b) is named 2-ethyl-5-methylhexanedioic acid. Diacid (c) is named 11-methylhenicosanedioic acid.

What is the structure of oxalic acid?

Oxalic acid is the common name of ethanedioic acid, $HO_2C\text{-}CO_2H$.

What are the common names for the C3-C10 dibasic acids?

The common names are: propanedioic acid is malonic acid; butanedioic acid is succinic acid; pentanedioic acid is glutaric acid; hexanedioic acid is adipic acid; heptanedioic acid is pimelic acid; octanedioic acid is suberic acid; nonanedioic acid is azelaic acid; decanedioic acid is sebacic acid.

There are two different pK_a values for oxalic acid. Why?

There are two carboxyl groups and two acidic hydrogens. One of the hydrogens has a pK_a of 1.27 but the second pK_a is 4.27. Examination of oxalic acid shows that internal hydrogen bonding via a five-centered interaction is expected to greatly enhance the acidity of one of the carboxyl hydrogen atoms in the diacid. In addition, the carboxyl group is electron-withdrawing, strengthening the first pK_a by an inductive effect. The carboxylate formed after removal of the first hydrogen (***A***) is less electron-withdrawing and the internal hydrogen bonding is less extensive, weakening the acid. Removal of both acidic hydrogens generates the dicarboxylate salt, ***B***.

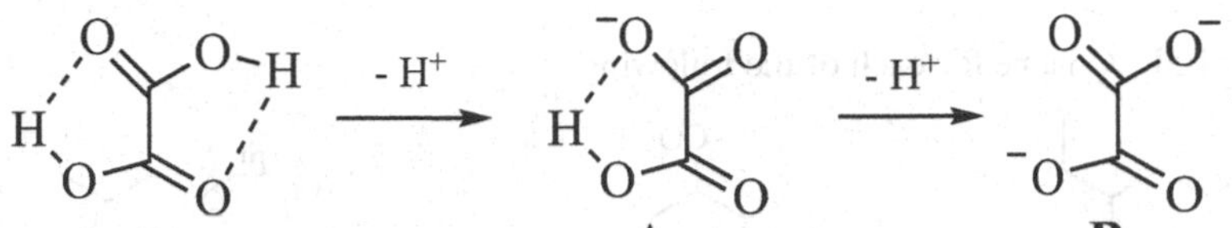

- H+ → **A** - H+ → **B**

Can the first pK_a of oxalic acid be compared with that of acetic acid (ethanoic acid)?

The pK_a of acetic acid is 4.76. By comparison, the first pK_a of oxalic acid is 1.27 and the second is 4.27. The low pK_a value is clear evidence of the strong electron-withdrawing effect of a second carboxyl. Even the second pK_a of oxalic acid indicates that the second carboxyl is more acidic than acetic acid, again the result of the electron-withdrawing carboxyl group.

What is the first and second pK_a of malonic acid?

The first pK_a is 2.86 and the second pK_a is 5.70.

Can the first and second pK_a value of malonic acid be compared with those of oxalic acid?

The first pK_a of malonic acid shows it to be a significantly weaker acid than oxalic. Likewise, the second pK_a is much higher, again reflecting a much weaker acid, weaker even than acetic acid. The reason for these changes is the presence of the -CH_2- group between the carboxyl groups. The increased distance between the acidic hydrogens and the carboxyl groups diminishes the inductive effects, and hydrogen bonding is weaker due to the increased distance between the carbonyl group and the acidic hydrogen.

Why is glutaric acid a significantly weaker acid than malonic acid?

The first pK_a of glutaric acid is 4.34 and the second pK_a is 5.27. This decrease in acidity reflects the increased distance between the carboxyl groups and the diminished inductive effects.

What is the structure of maleic acid? Give the IUPAC name. What is the structure of fumaric acid? Give the IUPAC name.

Maleic acid is the common name of cis-but-2-en-1,4-dioic acid. Fumaric acid is the common name of trans-but-2-en-1,4-dioic acid.

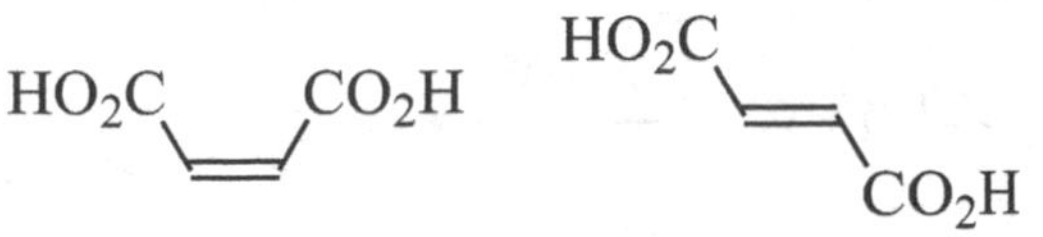

HO_2C CO_2H HO_2C CO_2H

maleic acid fumaric acid

Why does maleic acid have a lower pK_a than fumaric acid (compare first pK_as)?

In maleic acid, the carboxyl groups are on the same side of the molecule, and intramolecular hydrogen bonding (a through-space inductive effect) will make the acid much stronger (see the figure). When the carboxyl groups are on opposite sides of the molecule as in fumaric acid, this intramolecular interaction is not possible, and the result is a weaker acid. The first pK_a of maleic acid is 2.0 and the second pK_a is 6.3. The first pK_a of fumaric acid is 3.0 and the second pK_a is 4.4.

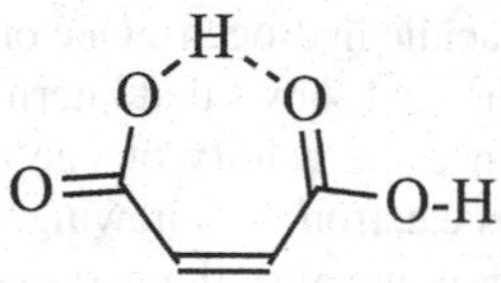

END OF CHAPTER PROBLEMS

1. Give the IUPAC name for each of the following:

(a) 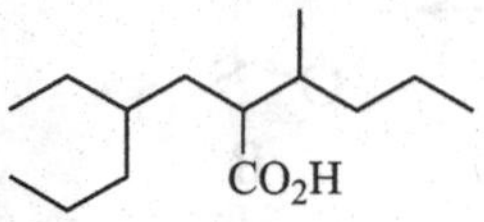 (b) 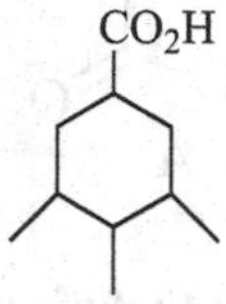 (c) 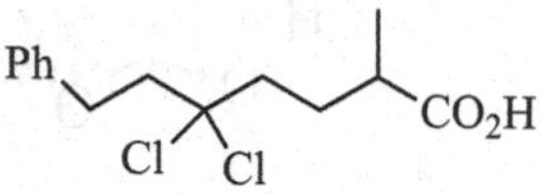 (d) 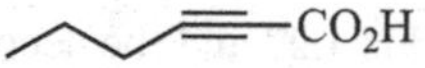 (e) 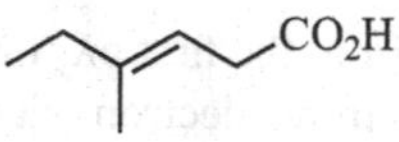 (f) 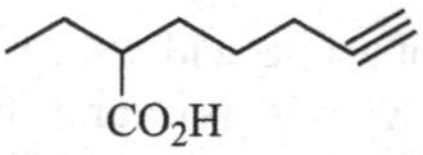 (g)

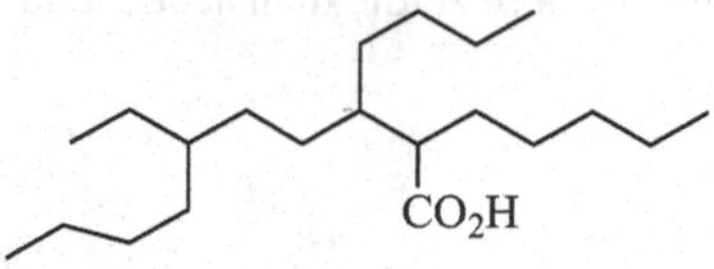

2. Which of the following is the strongest acid? Explain.

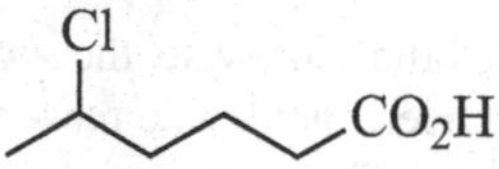

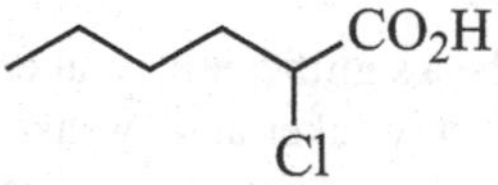

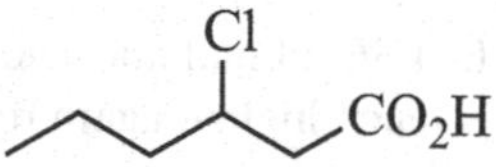

3. Draw a diagram to illustrate through-space inductive effects in 4-chloropropanoic acid.
4. Why is acetic acid a stronger acid in water than in ethanol?
5. When 4-hydroxybutanoic acid was prepared and heated, the final product was not acidic as expected. Explain this observation.
6. Give the complete mechanism for the following reaction:

$$\xrightarrow{H_3O^+}$$

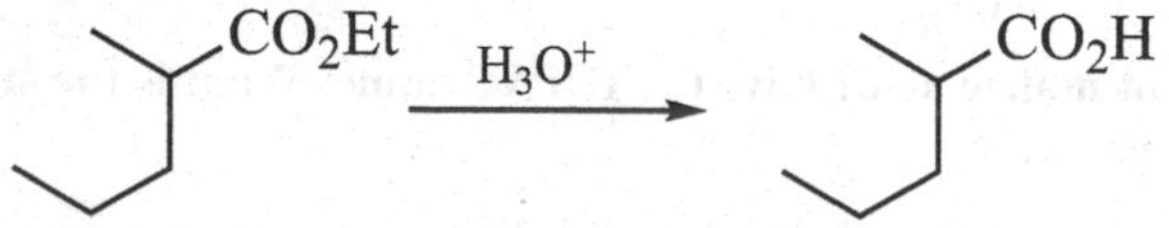

7. Give the complete mechanism for the following reaction:

$$\xrightarrow{NH_2Me}$$

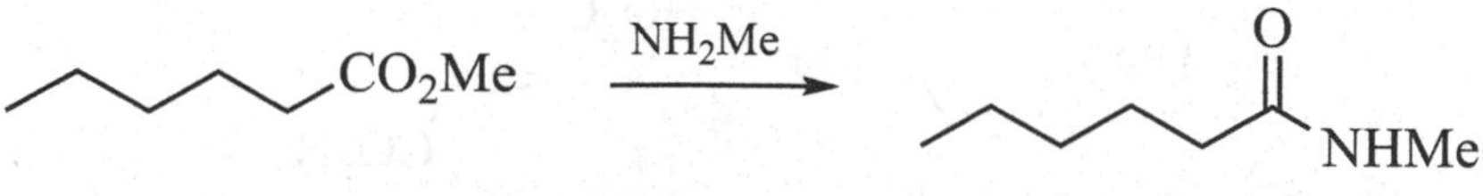

8. Give the correct IUPAC name for each of the following. Also give the common name.

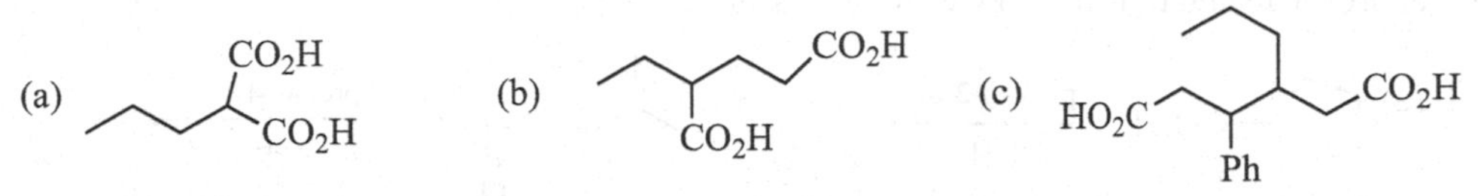

(a) (b) (c)

CO_2H CO_2H CO_2H CO_2H HO_2C CO_2H Ph

9. Why is the first pK_a of malonic acid lower than the first pK_a of glutaric acid?
10. In each case give the major product. If there is no reaction, indicate by N.R.

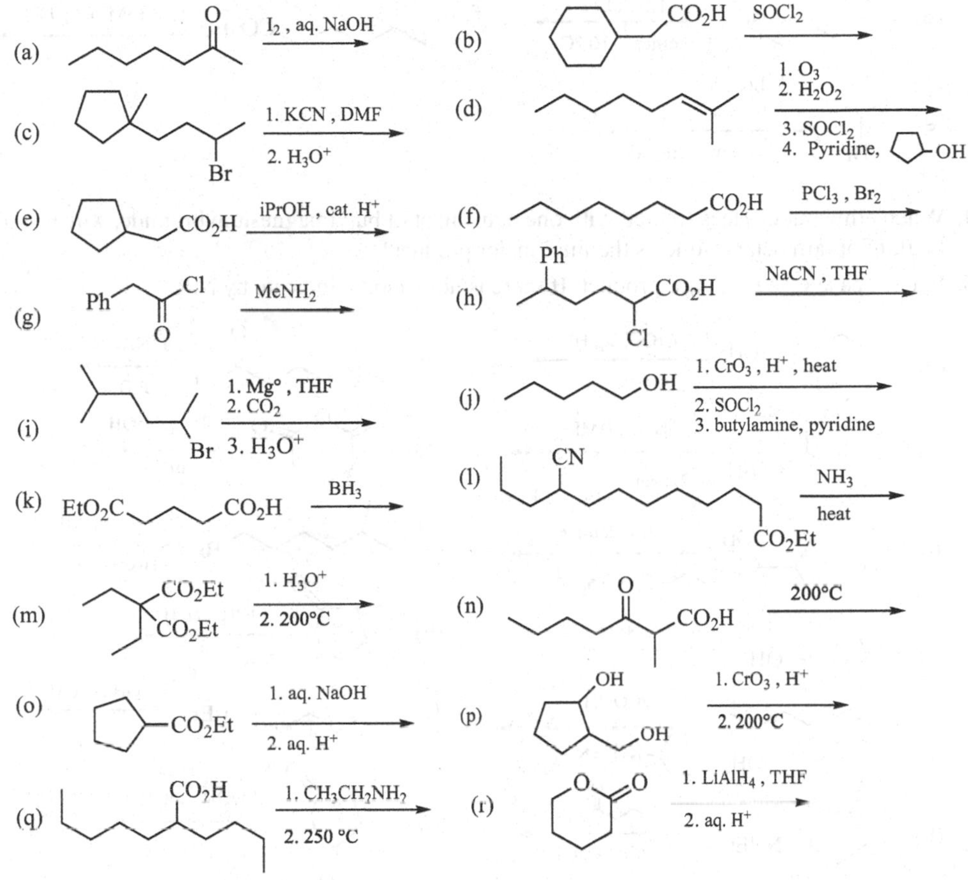

(a) O; I_2, aq. NaOH

(b) CO_2H; $SOCl_2$

(c) Br; 1. KCN, DMF; 2. H_3O^+

(d) 1. O_3; 2. H_2O_2; 3. $SOCl_2$; 4. Pyridine, OH

(e) CO_2H; iPrOH, cat. H^+

(f) CO_2H; PCl_3, Br_2

(g) Ph, Cl, O; $MeNH_2$

(h) Ph, CO_2H, Cl; NaCN, THF

(i) Br; 1. Mg°, THF; 2. CO_2; 3. H_3O^+

(j) OH; 1. CrO_3, H^+, heat; 2. $SOCl_2$; 3. butylamine, pyridine

(k) EtO_2C, CO_2H; BH_3

(l) CN, CO_2Et; NH_3, heat

(m) CO_2Et, CO_2Et; 1. H_3O^+; 2. 200°C

(n) O, CO_2H; 200°C

(o) CO_2Et; 1. aq. NaOH; 2. aq. H^+

(p) OH, OH; 1. CrO_3, H^+; 2. 200°C

(q) CO_2H; 1. $CH_3CH_2NH_2$; 2. 250 °C

(r) O, O; 1. $LiAlH_4$, THF; 2. aq. H^+

11. Give the complete mechanism for the following reaction:

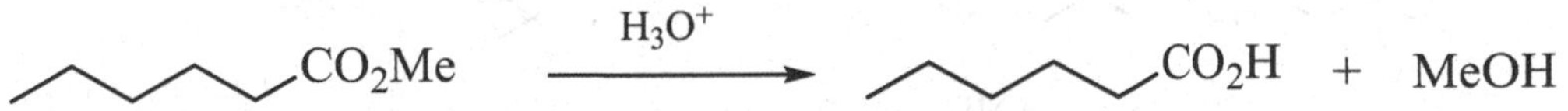

$$\text{CO}_2\text{Me} \xrightarrow{H_3O^+} \text{CO}_2\text{H} + \text{MeOH}$$

12. Why are esters more reactive than amides to base hydrolysis?

13. For each of the following reactions give the major product. Remember stereochemistry where appropriate and if there is no reaction, indicate by N.R.

(a) cyclopentyl–CO_2H → propan-2-ol, cat. H^+

(b) acid chloride (–Cl, =O) → propan-1-amine, NEt_3

(c) SO_3H → 1. $SOCl_2$ 2. propan-1-ol

(d) alcohol (OH) → butanesulfonyl chloride, NEt_3

(e) acid chloride (O, Cl) → Et_2CuLi, ether, -10 °C

(f) CO_2Et → 1. 3 EtMgBr, THF 2. aq.H^+

(g) Br → 1. Li, ether 2. 0.5 CuI 3. butanoyl chloride

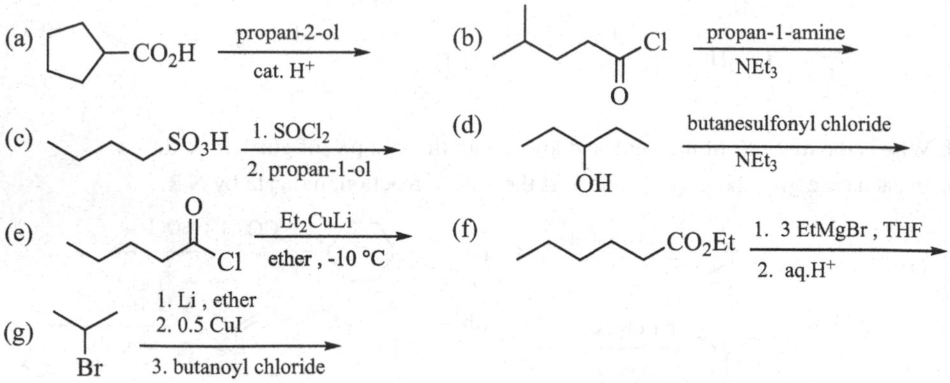

14. When ethyl butanoate is treated with one equivalent of butylmagnesium bromide, why is it difficult to obtain octan-4-one as the final major product?

15. In each case give the major product. If there is no reaction, indicate by N.R.

(a) cyclohexyl–OH → 1. CrO_3, aq. H^+ 2. $SOCl_2$

(b) acid chloride (O, Cl) → 1. NH_3 2. P_4O_{10}

(c) CO_2H → 1. NaH, DMF 2. heat, Et_2HC(C=O)Cl

(d) cyclic anhydride (O, O, O) → 1. aq. NaOH 2. pH 7

(e) cyclohexyl–OH → triethylamine, acid chloride (Cl, O)

(f) Br → 1. KCN, DMF 2. H_3O^+, 20°C

(g) cyclopentyl–OH → Ac_2O, NEt_3

(h) lactone (O, O) → EtOH, cat. H^+

(i) OH → EtCOOH, cyclohexyl–N=C=N–cyclohexyl

(j) CO_2Et → MeOH, cat. H^+

(k) cyclopentyl–NHEt → acid chloride (O, Cl), triethylamine

(l) cyclic anhydride (O, O, O) → MeOH, cat. H^+

(m) anhydride (O, O, O) → CH_3NH_2, NEt_3

(n) lactone (O, O) → 1. $LiAlH_4$, THF 2. H_3O^+

(o) CO_2Et → NH_3, heat

(p) amide (O, NH_2) → 1. $LiAlH_4$, THF 2. H_3O^+

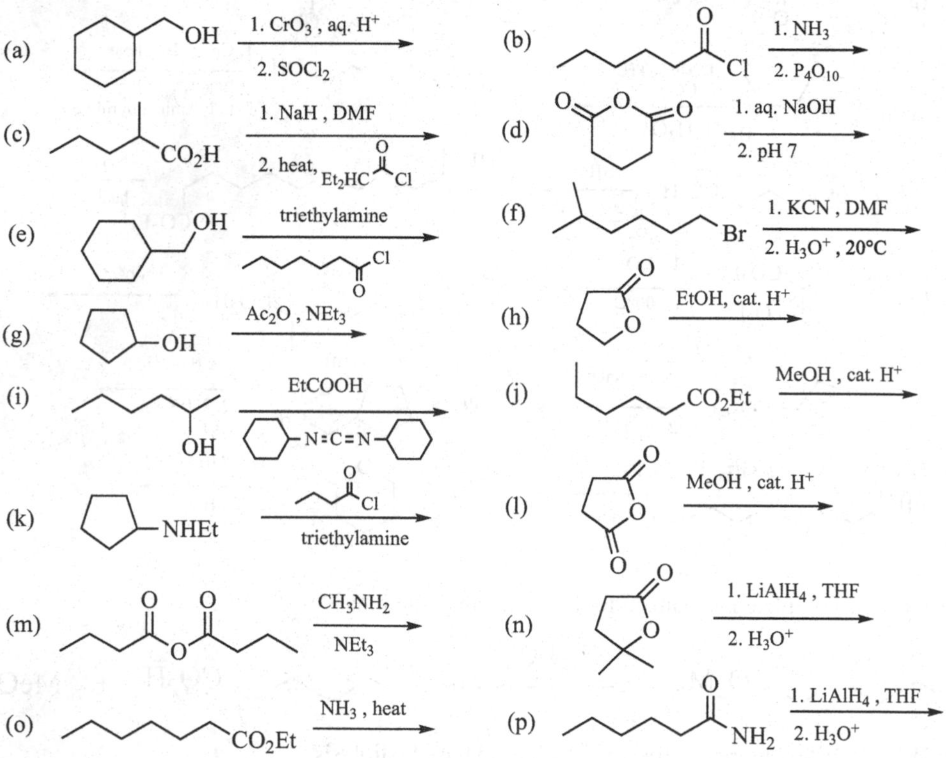

16

Benzene, Aromaticity, and Benzene Derivatives

Benzene is one of the most important organic molecules known and it is representative of a wide variety of molecules known as aromatic compounds. The special stability called aromaticity that is associated with its structure leads to special types of reactions.

16.1 BENZENE AND NOMENCLATURE OF AROMATIC COMPOUNDS

What is the empirical formula of benzene?

The formula is C_6H_6.

Hydrogenation of cyclohexene is a process that releases 28.6 kcal mol^{-1} of energy. For two double bonds in cyclohexadiene, 55.4 kcal mol^{-1} is released (roughly twice the value of 28.6). When benzene is hydrogenated, however, only 49.8 kcal mol^{-1} is released, not the 3 × 28.6 (85.8) kcal mol^{-1} expected for "cycloheptatriene." Why?

If the C=C units in benzene were the same as in cyclohexene and cyclohexadiene, 3 × 28.6 kcal mol^{-1} would be expected. The fact that less energy is liberated suggests that benzene is inherently more stable than either the alkene or the diene. This "extra stability" is about 36 kcal mol^{-1} and is due to the special lowering of energy that occurs when the p-orbitals are parallel, contiguous (every p-orbital has a p-orbital neighbor on every adjacent carbon), and able to share electron density with their neighboring p–orbitals. In other words, *benzene is stabilized by resonance.*

What is a picture that represents the electron delocalization in benzene due to resonance?

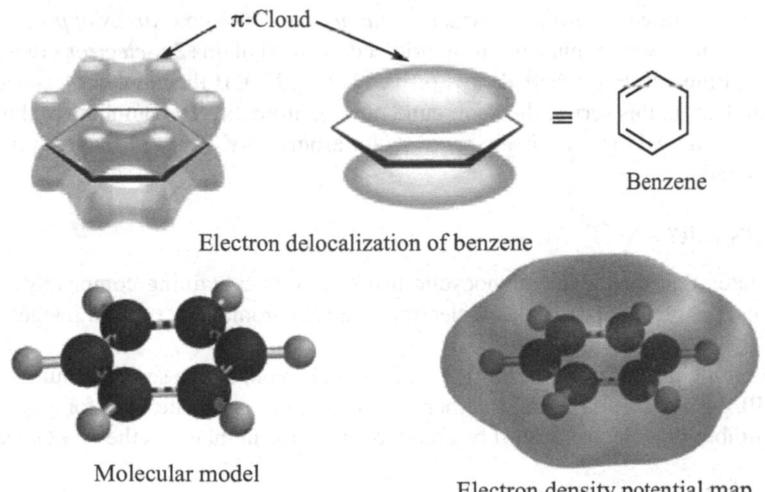

Benzene is a planar molecule consisting of six sp^2 hybridized carbons connected in a ring, with six p-orbitals perpendicular to the plane of the carbons). There are six π-electrons in the six contiguous orbitals that are delocalized over all six orbitals. The delocalization is apparent in the electron density potential map, which clearly shows higher electron density (the light gray shaded area) on the top (and also on the bottom) of the six-membered ring.

Cyclohexene and cyclohexadiene both react with HCl, but benzene does not. What can be concluded about the stability and reactivity of benzene from this observation?

The π-bond of both cyclohexene and cyclohexadiene are electron donors in the presence of HCl. In other words, they both react as Brønsted–Lowry bases in the presence of a Brønsted–Lowry acid. This chemistry is described in Section 7.3. Benzene has π-bonds, but benzene does not react with HCl as a Brønsted–Lowry base. In other words, it is a poor electron donor: it has poor reactivity and greater stability. This extra stability, manifested by the fact that it is a poor Brønsted–Lowry base, is due to the aromaticity of benzene. If the π-electrons are "tied up" in the aromatic cloud they are not available for donation without disrupting the special stability that arises from aromaticity.

What are the Kekulé structures?

Kekulé structures are representations of benzene where the bonds are localized, and different structures are used to show that the bond positions "change." These structures are meant to represent delocalization of the electrons and to represent the fact that the structure does not have true double or single bonds, but rather a bond that is "in between" (shorter than a normal single bond but longer than a normal double bond).

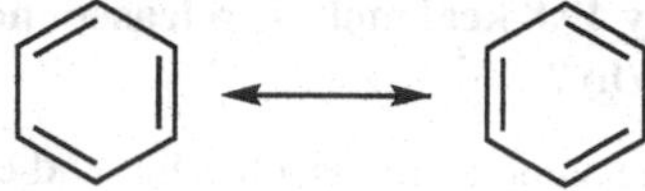

What are π-electrons?

A π-electron is an electron that resides in the π-bond(s) of a double bond or a triple bond, or in conjugated p-orbitals. The six electrons in a benzene ring are π-electrons because they reside in three contiguous π-bonds, with six p-orbitals.

What are the necessary structural features required for aromaticity?

Several criteria are required for aromaticity: a *continuous* and contiguous *array of p-orbitals in a cyclic system* are required (every atom must be sp^2-hybridized). A total of *4n+2 π-electrons* (where n is a series 0, 1, 2, 3... generating a new series $4n+2$ = 2, 6, 10, 14, 18, 22...). If the number of π-electrons is equal to one of the numbers in this series, the compound may be aromatic. The numbers in this series are the result of *Hückel's rule*. All the criteria are *required* for aromaticity. If one of them is missing, the compound is not aromatic.

What is Hückel's rule?

Hückel's rule states that for planar, monocyclic hydrocarbons containing completely conjugated sp^2-hybridized atoms, the presence of ($4n$+2) π-electrons leads to aromaticity (n is an integer in the series 0, 1, 2, 3, etc.).

As the value on n changes in the series 0, 1, 2, 3, 4, and so on, a new series of numbers is generated by $4n+2$: 2, 6, 10, 14, 18, 22, and so on. In other words, Hückel's rule states that for a hydrocarbon to be aromatic, the number of π-electrons must be equal to one of the numbers in the $4n+2$ series.

Can a cation or anion be aromatic?

Yes! As long as the criteria given above are met, a cationic or anionic molecule can be aromatic.

Are (a)–(j) aromatic or non-aromatic?

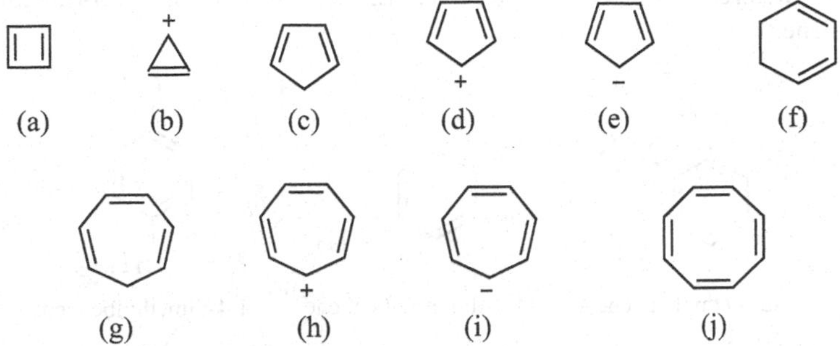

In (a) cyclobutadiene has only four π-electrons and is not aromatic. In (b) the cyclopropenyl cation has two π-electrons and is aromatic. In (c) cyclopentadiene does not have a continuous array of p-orbitals and is not aromatic. In (d) the cyclopentadienyl cation has only four π-electrons and is not aromatic. In (e) the cyclopentadienyl anion has six π-electrons and is aromatic. In (f) cyclohexadiene does not have a continuous array of p-orbitals and is not aromatic. In (g) cycloheptatriene does not have a continuous array of p-orbitals and is not aromatic. In (h) the cycloheptatrienyl cation has six π-electrons and is aromatic whereas the cycloheptatrienyl anion (i) has eight π-electrons and is not aromatic. Likewise, in (j) cylooctatetraene has eight π-electrons and is not aromatic.

Are there molecules with more than one ring that are considered to be aromatic?

Yes! There are many examples of molecules of this type of molecule that are aromatic. As long as the criteria listed in preceding questions are met, a molecule with more than one ring may be aromatic. Typical examples are naphthalene (a), anthracene (b), and phenanthrene (c).

(a) (b) (c)

What is a list of functional groups that are commonly attached to a benzene ring?

Virtually any functional group can be attached, but some appear more often. Several of the common functional groups are halogen, hydroxyl, amino, cyano, carboxylic acid, ester, aldehyde, ketone, methoxy, ethoxy, sulfonic acid, alkene, alkyne, and nitro. In addition, alkyl groups can be attached to a benzene ring such as methyl or ethyl.

What is a representative structure for each of the functional groups from the preceding question when attached to a benzene ring? Name each one!

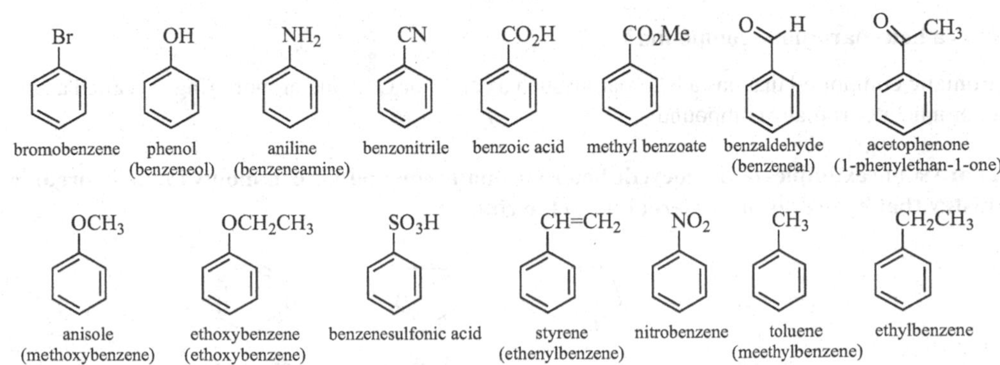

How many isomers are possible if two methyl groups are attached to a benzene ring?

A total of three different isomers are possible, 1,2-dimethylbenzene; 1,3-dimethylbenzene; and 1,4-dimethylbenzene.

CH_3 CH_3 CH_3 CH_3 CH_3 CH_3

1,2-dimethylbenzene 1,3-dimethylbenzene 1,4-dimethylbenzene

What are the common names of the three isomers presented in the preceding question?

The common name for dimethylbenzene is xylene. The common name of 1,2-dimethylbenzene is ortho-xylene; for 1,3-dimethylbenzene is meta-xylene; for 1,4-dimethylbenzene is para-xylene.

What do the terms ortho, meta, and para- signify?

The terms refer to the relative positions of groups on a benzene ring. The term ortho- signifies a 1,2- relationship of the substituents; meta- a 1,3- relationship, and para- signifies a 1,4- relationship.

When a benzene ring is attached to a molecule, it is treated as a substituent. What is the nomenclature designation?

A benzene ring that is treated as a substituent is given the name *phenyl.*

If a benzene ring is attached to a long chain alkane, is it an alkylbenzene or phenyl alkane?

The general "rule" is that if the alkyl chain is greater than six carbons, the benzene ring is treated as a substituent and it is a phenylalkane. If the chain is less than six carbons, it is named as a benzene derivative (alkyl benzene such as ethyl benzene).

What is the name of (a), (b), and (c)?

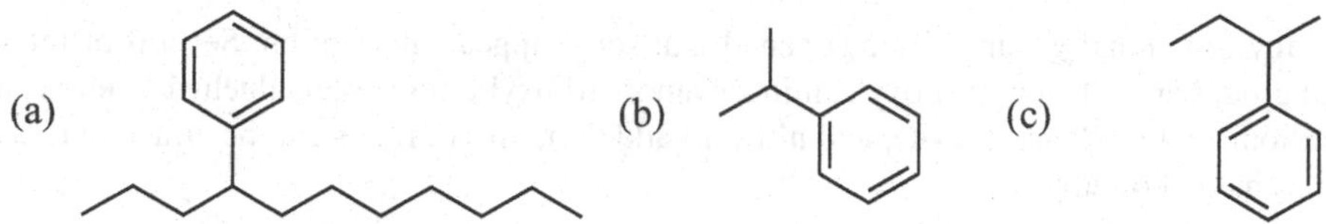

Compound (a) is 4-phenylundecane, (b) is 1-methylethylbenzene (isopropylbenzene), and (c) is 1-methylpropylbenzene.

What is a heteroaromatic compound?

An aromatic compound that has a heteroatom such as N, S, or O in one or more rings is called a heterocycle, or a heteroaromatic compound.

What are some examples of monocyclic heteroaromatic compounds commonly found in organic chemistry that have only one heteroatom in the ring?

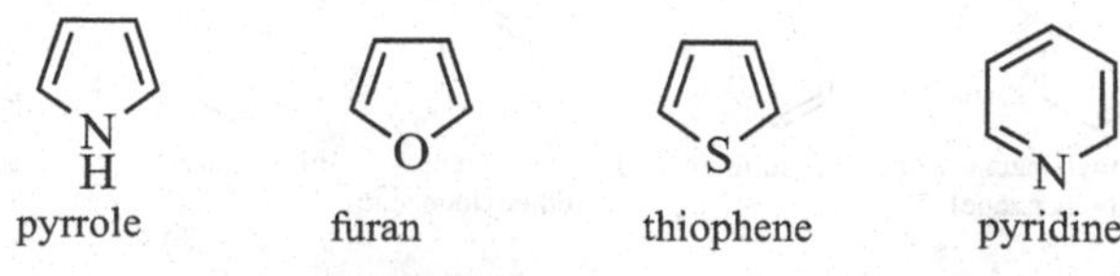

Simple examples are the nitrogen-containing heterocycles pyrrole and pyridine, the oxygen containing heterocycle named furan, and the sulfur-containing heterocycle called thiophene.

16.2 ELECTROPHILIC AROMATIC SUBSTITUTION

What is electrophilic aromatic substitution?

When benzene reacts with a suitable electrophilic species (X) that group replaces a hydrogen on the benzene ring (Ph-H ⟶ Ph-X). If the X group is electrophilic and/or cationic, replacement of H by X is a substitution and benzene is aromatic. This process is called *electrophilic aromatic substitution.*

What is the designation for electrophilic aromatic substitution?

This type of reaction is a S_EAr reaction.

Does benzene react with HBr? With Br_2 without any other additive?

No! Benzene does not react with HBr, HCl, or HI, and it does not react with Br_2, Cl_2, or I_2 without another additive present in the reaction medium. The fact that benzene is aromatic indicates that it is a poor electron donor since the electrons are tied up in the aromatic cloud. In other words, donation of electrons by benzene would disrupt the aromatic stability and such reactions are disfavored.

Why does benzene not react with HBr or Br_2 unless other reagents are added?

Benzene is a very poor Brønsted–Lowry base, and a weak Lewis base when it reacts with molecules such as Br_2. To function as a base benzene must donate the aromatic π-electrons, but these electrons are "tied up" in the aromatic cloud that gives benzene its special stability. Both HBr and Br—Br are insufficiently strong Lewis acids to react. The loss of resonance energy associated with donation of electrons by benzene precludes its reaction.

If benzene is too weak a base to react with Br_2, is it a strong enough electron donor to react with a cationic species such as Br^+?

Yes! Benzene reacts quickly with a suitable cation to form a highly reactive, resonance-stabilized carbocation.

How is Br^+ generated? Cl^+?

Bromine and chlorine are polarizable so when mixed with a good Lewis acid such as $AlCl_3$ or BF_3, with a strongly electrophilic atom (aluminum or boron), the halogen in close proximity to the Lewis acid takes on a negative dipole and reacts in a Lewis acid–Lewis base reaction. The product of the reaction of Br_2 and $AlCl_3$ is $Br^+AlCl_3Br^-$. Similar reaction of Cl_2 gives $Cl^+AlCl_4^-$. The Lewis acid–Lewis base reaction of halogens with BF_3 proceeds to give $Br^+BF_3Br^-$ or $Cl^+BF_3Cl^-$.

$$Cl_3Al \quad \overset{\delta-}{Br}—\overset{\delta+}{Br} \longrightarrow Cl_3Br\overset{-}{Al}\ Br^+$$

What does polarizable mean?

Polarizability is the ability of a bond to be polarized by distortion of the electron cloud when that bond is close to a polarizing atom or group. The ability of a molecule to distort its electron cloud will occur when in close proximity to a charged or polarized species. In other words, a polarizable atom will assume a δ^+ in the presence of a highly electronegative species and it will assume a δ^- dipole in the presence of an electropositive dipole.

What is a mechanistic rationale for the reaction of benzene with the cation, Br^+?

Benzene donates a pair of electrons to Br^+, generated by reaction with a Lewis acid such as $AlCl_3$, forming a C—Br bond and leaving a positive charge on the ring, as in ***A***. This carbocation intermediate, called an *arenium ion*, is resonance-stabilized since the positive charge can be delocalized by the adjacent π-bonds. A total of three resonance forms can be drawn, representing the delocalization of the charge and the relative stability of the cationic intermediate. A proton is lost from ***A*** to regenerate the aromatic ring in the final product, bromobenzene. The driving force for loss of the hydrogen is generation of the very stable aromatic ring from the reactive intermediate. This overall process involves cationic intermediates and leads to substitution of the hydrogen by X. It is therefore called *electrophilic aromatic substitution.*

$Br^+AlCl_3Br^-$; $-H^+$; H, Br ; Br

A (an arenium ion)

What is the name given to the resonance-stabilized intermediate (A) in the reaction shown in the preceding question?

The arcane name for this intermediate is a *Wheland intermediate* but nowadays such a species is called an *arenium ion*. The latter term will be used in this book.

Although this reaction is called *electrophilic aromatic substitution*, it is in reality two sequential reaction types. What are they?

The initial reaction of the benzene ring with Br^+ is a Lewis acid–Lewis base reaction, and loss of a proton from a carbocation is called an E1 reaction (see Section 9.2). Therefore, electrophilic aromatic substitution is a combination of an acid–base reaction followed by an E1 reaction.

Why does the resonance-stabilized intermediate lose a proton to give the substitution product?

To form an arenium ion such as ***A*** in the question above (from the reaction of benzene and Br^+), the aromatic character of benzene must be disrupted. The hydrogen is easily lost from ***A*** because regeneration of the aromatic ring is an exothermic process.

What is halogenation in electrophilic aromatic substitution?

Halogenation is the replacement of a hydrogen atom on a benzene ring with a halogen atom. Benzene reacts with halogens, in the presence of a suitable Lewis acid, to give a halobenzene (chlorobenzene, bromobenzene, or iodobenzene).

What is the product when diatomic bromine reacts with ferric bromide ($FeBr_3$)? With aluminum chloride ($AlCl_3$)?

When $FeBr_3$ comes in close proximity to diatomic bromine, the closest bromine takes on a negative charge (an induced dipole), inducing a positive charge on the other bromine (polarizability). The bromine (behaving as a Lewis base) attacks the electrophilic iron in $FeBr_3$, which is a Lewis acid, generating the usual "ate" complex. This Lewis acid–Lewis base complex contains an electrophilic bromine, Br^+.

$$FeBr_3 + \overset{\delta-}{Br}-\overset{\delta+}{Br} \longrightarrow Br^+ \; FeBr_4^-$$

How are phenyl halides named by the IUPAC system?

They are named as benzene derivatives using the chloro, bromo, iodo, and fluoro substituent terms. The names are, therefore, fluorobenzene, chlorobenzene, bromobenzene, and iodobenzene.

What is the structure of 1,4-dibromo-3-chlorobenzene?

The structure is shown, *but this is an incorrect name.* The substituents are numbered to give the smallest numbers. The correct name is, therefore, *1,4-dibromo-2-chlorobenzene.*

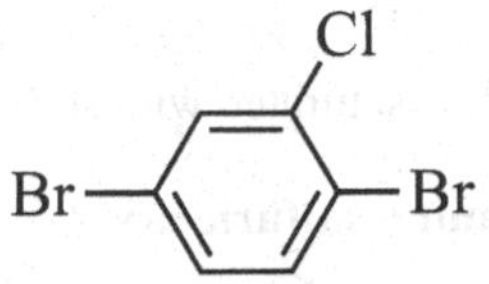

What is the isolated product when benzene reacts with Cl_2 and BF_3?

Formation of Cl^+ when Cl_2 reacts with BF_3 allows reaction with benzene to give an arenium ion, and loss of a proton gives the aromatic product, chlorobenzene.

Why does the reaction of bromine and $AlCl_3$ with benzene give bromobenzene and not chlorobenzene?

The initial product of the reaction between bromine and aluminum chloride is $Br^{+-}AlCl_3Br$, where the electrophilic species is Br^+. Since Br^+ is the species that reacts with benzene to form an arenium ion, the final product is bromobenzene. The chlorine atoms are associated with the counterion, $^-AlCl_3Br$ which does not react with benzene, so chlorine never appears in the product.

What product is formed when benzene reacts with nitric acid and sulfuric acid?

A mixture of nitric acid and sulfuric acid converts benzene to *nitrobenzene.*

What is the electrophilic species (the cation) formed when nitric acid reacts with sulfuric acid?

The electrophilic species is the *nitronium ion*, NO_2^+.

$$HNO_3 + H_2SO_4 \rightleftharpoons H_2NO_3^+ + HSO_4^-$$

$$H_2NO_3^+ + H_2SO_4 \rightleftharpoons NO_2^+ HSO_4^- + H_3O^+$$

In the reaction of nitric acid and sulfuric acid, which is the acid and which is the base?

Since nitric acid accepts the proton from sulfuric acid, an oxygen of nitric acid functions as a base and sulfuric acid is the acid (sulfuric acid is the stronger acid).

What is the reaction that includes the arenium ion of benzene with HNO_3/H_2SO_4?

Initial reaction with NO_2^+ generates the arenium intermediate, ***A***. Loss of a proton generates the final substitution product, nitrobenzene.

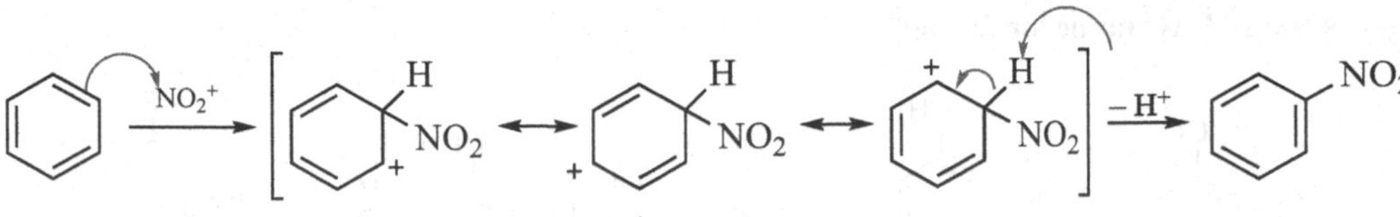

A

What is the product when benzene reacts with fuming sulfuric acid?

Benzenesulfonic acid is produced when benzene reacts with fuming sulfuric acid.

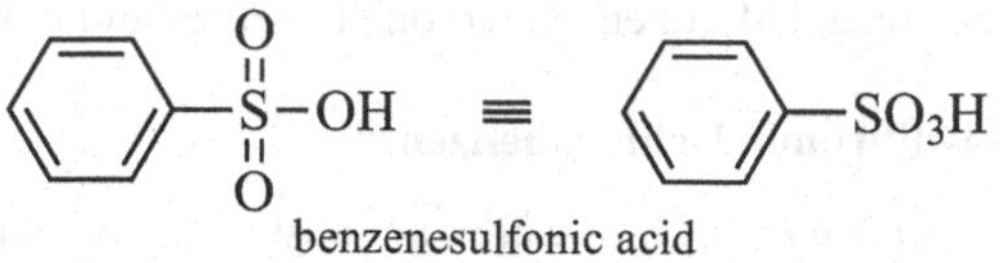

benzenesulfonic acid

What is fuming sulfuric acid?

Fuming sulfuric acid is sulfuric acid that is saturated with sulfur trioxide, SO_3.

What is the electrophilic species in fuming sulfuric acid?

Both SO_3 and HSO_3^+ are electrophilic species in this medium, but SO_3 is taken to be the reactive entity.

What is the reaction and the arenium ion intermediate of benzene with fuming sulfuric acid?

The benzene ring attacks the sulfur of SO_3 to generate arenium ion *A*. Loss of hydrogen in the usual manner regenerates the aromatic ring with transfer of a hydrogen to the oxygen of the SO_3^- moiety, forming benzenesulfonic acid.

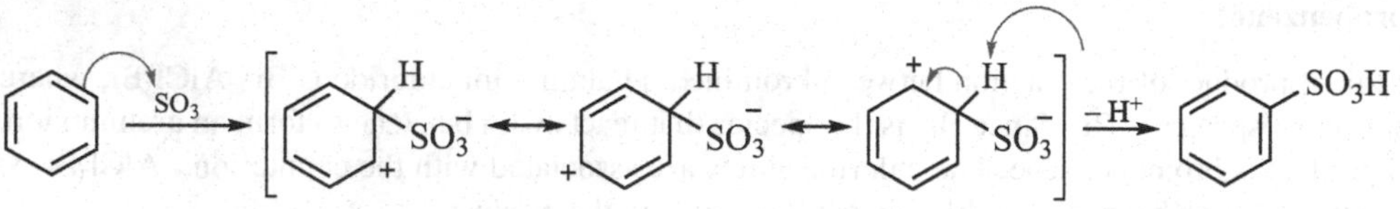

A

Is an electrophilic aromatic substitution (S_EAr) reaction possible when the benzene ring has substituents?

Yes!

What products are possible when a S_EAr reaction is done with a molecule that has one substituent attached to a benzene ring?

For a monosubstituted benzene ring, three products are possible. The new group can be attached to C2, C3, or C4 relative to the benzene carbon that bears the substituent, which is C1.

What is the common name of two substituents that are situated on a benzene ring in a: (a) 1,2 fashion; (b) 1,3-fashion; (c) 1,4-fashion?

The common name for (a) 1,2-substitution is *ortho*; (b) for 1,3-substitution is *meta*; and (c) for 1,4-substitution is *para*.

Is the ortho, meta, para- nomenclature used if the substituents are not the same?

No! These terms are usually used only when the substituents are the same.

What is the IUPAC name for (a)–(e)?

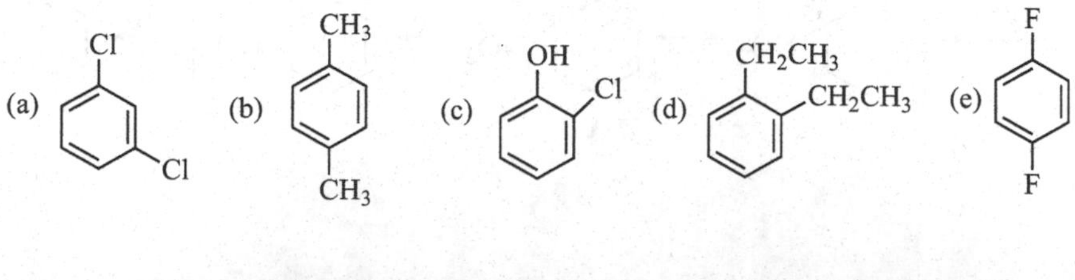

(a) (b) (c) (d) (e)

The ring is numbered to give the substituents the lowest possible number. Compound (a) is 1,3-dichlorobenzene; (b) is 1,4-dimethylbenzene; (c) is 2-chlorophenol; (d) is 1,2-diethylbenzene; (e) is 1,4-difluorobenzene.

Using the ortho, meta, and para- nomenclature what is the name of (a)–(e) in the preceding question?

Compound (a) is ortho-dichlorobenzene; (b) is para-dimethylbenzene (the common name is para-xylene). In (c) the two groups are not the same and the ortho/meta/para- nomenclature is not used. In this case the name is 2-chlorophenol. Compound (d) is ortho-diethylbenzene and (e) is para-difluorobenzene.

Using the IUPAC nomenclature, what is the name of each of the following?

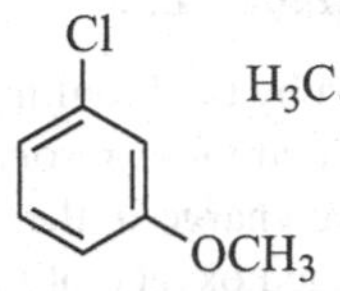

(a) 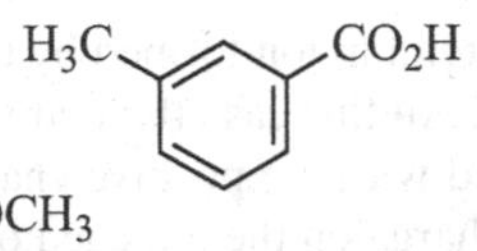 (b) 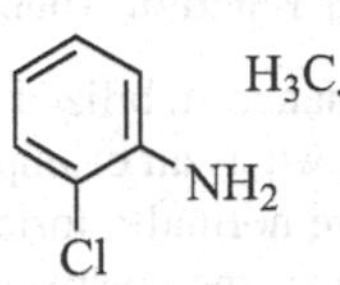 (c) 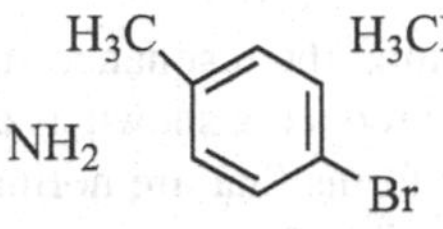 (d) 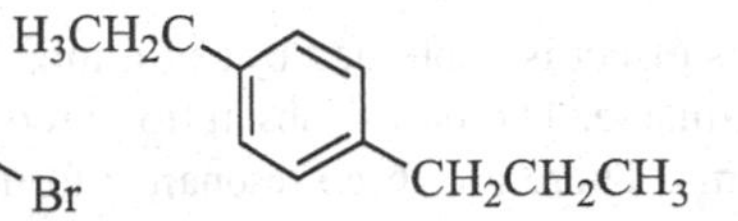 (e)

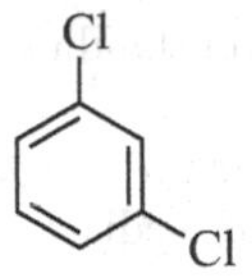

(f) 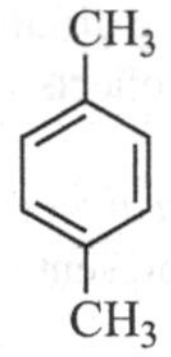 (g) 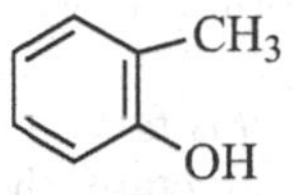 (h) 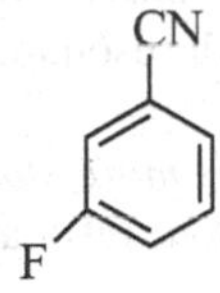 (i) 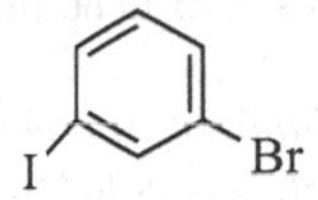 (j)

Compound (a) is 3-chloroanisole (3-chloromethoxybenzene); (b) is 3-methylbenzoic acid; (c) is 2-chloroaniline (2-chlorobenzenamine); (d) is 4-bromotoluene (4-bromomethylbenzene); (e) is 4-ethylpropylbenzene; (f) is 1,3-dichlorobenzene; (g) is 1,4-dimethylbenzene; (h) is 2-methylphenol (2-methylbenzenol); (i) is 3-fluorobenzonitrile; and (j) is 3-bromoiodobenzene.

Why is (h) in the preceding question named 2-methylbenzenol and not 2-hydroxy-1-methylbenzene?

The OH group has a higher priority than a methyl group. Recall the Cahn–Ingold–Prelog selection rules from Section 6.3: O > C. For this reason, benzenol is the priority name, and the methyl group is a substituent. However, the common name of phenol is commonly used and (h) would be 2-methylphenol using this nomenclature.

What is an electron releasing substituent on benzene?

An electron-releasing group is one that has a negative charge or a δ^- dipole when attached to a benzene ring.

Is a benzene ring electron rich or electron poor with respect to substituents?

Benzene has six π-electrons and is considered to be electron rich.

What is a list of activating groups in the order of their activating power?

The activating substituents in an approximate order of reactivity is $-NH_2$, $-NR_2$ > -OH, -OR > -NHCOR > $-CH_3$ and other alkyl groups. Note that alkyl groups are considered to be electron releasing. Also note that amides are less electron donating because of the proximity of the electron-withdrawing carbonyl. A similar argument can be made for esters, which are more electron donating than the amide but less than an ether.

Why are electron releasing groups referred to as activating groups?

When an electron releasing group is attached to a benzene ring, the rate of electrophilic aromatic substitution is greatly increased. Phenol, for example, undergoes bromination about 6×10^{11} times faster than benzene and toluene undergoes chlorination about 340 times faster than benzene. The fact that the methyl group in toluene increases the rate of the reaction relative to benzene causes it to be placed among the activating substituents.

Which molecule reacts faster with bromine/$FeBr_3$, anisole or benzene?

As mentioned, anisole reacts much faster because it contains the strongly electron-releasing OMe group. Bromination of anisole, for example is 1.79×10^5 times faster than the bromination of benzene.

Why does an activating group lead to a faster reaction when attached to a benzene ring?

This effect is explained by examining the resonance-stabilized arenium ion formed by the bromination of anisole. The para- substitution product is shown as an example. In this case there are four resonance forms. There are three resonance forms that are normally formed with the positive charge in the ring, but a fourth resonance form is possible that places the positive charge on the attached oxygen of OMe, and the unshared electrons on oxygen are donated to the electrophilic center, generating $C{=}O^+{-}CH_3$. This "extra" resonance form represents the increased stability realized by delocalization of the positive charge out to the oxygen. For substitution reactions that have an activating group with electron pairs such as O or N as a substituent, the fourth resonance form is possible that reflects the extra stability of that intermediate.

If the arenium ion intermediate is more stable, it is formed more easily and accelerates the overall rate of reaction. It is noted that the four resonance structures shown represent *one* intermediate.

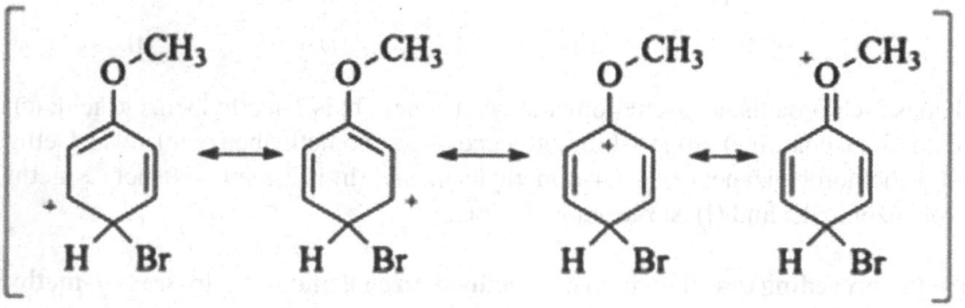

What are all resonance forms for the arenium ion formed by the bromination of anisole at the meta- position.

The three resonance forms for bromination at the meta- position are shown. Note that the positive charge of the arenium is *never* on the carbon bearing the electron-releasing methoxy group, so a fourth resonance contributor as observed in the preceding question can never form. In other words, there are only three resonance forms and the arenium ion for meta- bromination is *less stable* than the arenium ions for ortho- or para- bromination, and ortho- and para- bromination are therefore faster than meta- bromination.

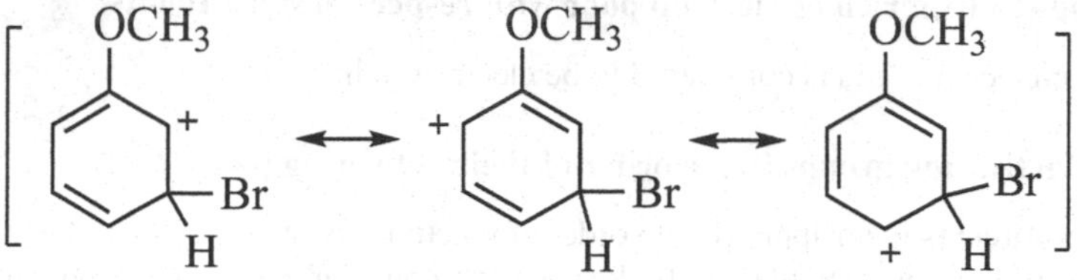

Is ortho- bromination of anisole more or less rapid than meta- bromination?

As with para- bromination, the positive charge of the arenium ion will be on the carbon bearing the methyl group (Me) in one resonance form, so the extra stability due to formation of the fourth resonance form is possible. The four resonance forms are shown in the figure. The arenium ion from ortho- bromination is about as stable as that for para- bromination and should form as quickly, and both ortho- and para- bromination are therefore faster than meta- bromination.

OMe Br H + ⟷ OMe Br H + ⟷ OMe + Br H ⟷ + OMe Br H

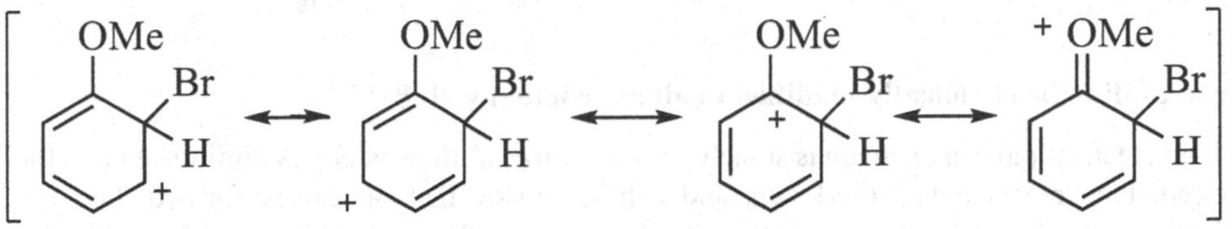

If ortho- and para- bromination occur much faster than meta- bromination, what is the expected ratio of ortho- and para- products?

In the absence of other factors, a 1:1 ratio of ortho- and para- products are formed. In some cases, coordination of the bromine cation with the group on the ipso carbon can lead to more ortho- product. Conversely, steric hindrance leads to more para- product. In general, however, close to a 1:1 ratio of products can be assumed.

What name is given to the carbon atom bearing a substituent in electrophilic aromatic substitution?

That carbon atom is called the ipso carbon. For the arenium ions shown in preceding questions, the carbon that bears the positive charge and is attached to the substituent is called the ipso carbon.

What products are formed by the reaction of anisole with Br_2 and $FeBr_3$?

About 90–95% of this reaction gives 2-bromoanisole and 4-bromoanisole, in about the same proportion, with 5% of less of the product being 3-bromoanisole. In general, there is an equal amount of the ortho- and para- products and a very minor amount of the meta- product, but steric interactions may favor the formation of more of the para- product than the ortho- product. However, in the absence of additional information it is appropriate to assume that the products are close to a 1:1 mixture.

Why are ortho- and para- bromoanisole the major products of the preceding reaction?

The extra resonance stability of the ortho- and para- arenium ions relative to the arenium ion formed by reaction at the meta- position means that formation of the ortho- and para- arenium ions is much faster than formation of the meta- arenium ion. Formation of the ortho- and para- arenium ions means that the ortho- and para- bromination products are formed faster and account for the major products of this reaction.

Will the major products of the electrophilic substitution reaction of benzene with activating substituents always be the ortho- and para- products?

Yes! Formation of the more stable arenium ion, where the positive charge of one resonance form will always be on the ipso carbon and will be stabilized by the electron-releasing substituent on that carbon, will always give the ortho- and para- products as the major products.

Although NH_2 is a powerful activating group, the reaction of bromine/$AlCl_3$ and aniline does not give a bromoaniline derivative. Why?

The NH_2 group is a good Lewis base and reacts rapidly with $AlCl_3$ to form *A before* $AlCl_3$ can react with bromine, which is a weaker Lewis base than aniline. In other words, the acid–base reaction is faster than the reaction of Br_2 + $AlCl_3$. For this reason, the cation Br^+ is not formed and the electrophilic bromination cannot occur.

$$PhNH_2 \xrightarrow{AlCl_3} PhN^+H_2{-}Al^-Cl_3 \;\; (\textbf{A})$$

How can aniline be chemically modified to allow reaction with Br^+?

If the lone electron pair on nitrogen is somehow "delocalized," the basicity is diminished and the Lewis acid–Lewis base reaction with the Lewis acid will be so slow that Br^+ can be formed. The most common method for doing this is to *protect* the nitrogen as an amide (see Sections 15.3 and 15.6). Indeed, if the aniline group of aniline is reacted with acetyl chloride, the acetamide derivative (*N*-acetyl aniline; acetanilide, ***A***) is formed. If ***A*** is treated with bromine and $AlCl_3$, a mixture of ortho- and para- bromo derivatives (***B*** and ***C***, respectively) is formed via the usual electrophilic aromatic substitution reaction. Treatment with aqueous acid or 1. NaOH, 2. H_3O^+ will remove the acetyl group, regenerating the NH_2 group, giving 2-bromoaniline and 4-bromoaniline.

$$PhNH_2 \xrightarrow{H_3C{-}C(=O){-}Cl} PhNHC(=O)CH_3\ (\textbf{A}) \xrightarrow{Br_2,\ AlCl_3} \text{2-Br-}C_6H_4NHC(=O)CH_3\ (\textbf{B}) + \text{4-Br-}C_6H_4NHC(=O)CH_3\ (\textbf{C})$$

$$\xrightarrow[\text{or 1. aq. KOH; 2. } H_3O^+]{H_3O^+} \text{2-bromoaniline} + \text{4-bromoaniline}$$

What is (are) the major product(s) for the reactions of (a), (b), and (c)?

(a) $PhOMe \xrightarrow{Cl_2,\ AlCl_3}$

(b) $PhNHC(=O)CH_3 \xrightarrow{HNO_3,\ H_2SO_4}$

(c) $PhCH_2CH_3 \xrightarrow{SO_3,\ H_2SO_4}$

In (a) the reaction of anisole and $Cl_2/AlCl_3$ generates a mixture of 2-chloroanisole and 4-chloroanisole. *N*-Acetyl aniline undergoes nitration in (b) to give a mixture 2-nitro-*N*-acetylaniline and 4-nitro-*N*-acetylaniline. Note that Ac is an abbreviation for acetyl. In (c) sulfonation of ethylbenzene generates a mixture of 2-ethylbenzenesulfonic acid and 4-ethylbenzene-sulfonic acid. In all cases the meta- product is a minor product.

(a) 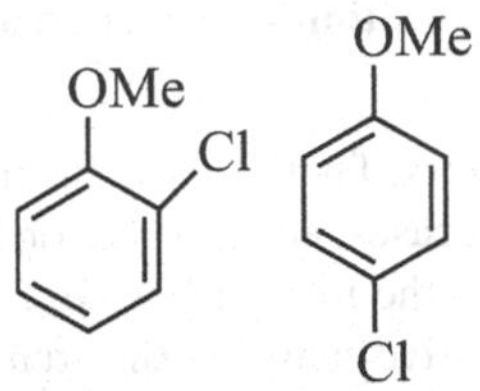 OMe, Cl; OMe, Cl (b) 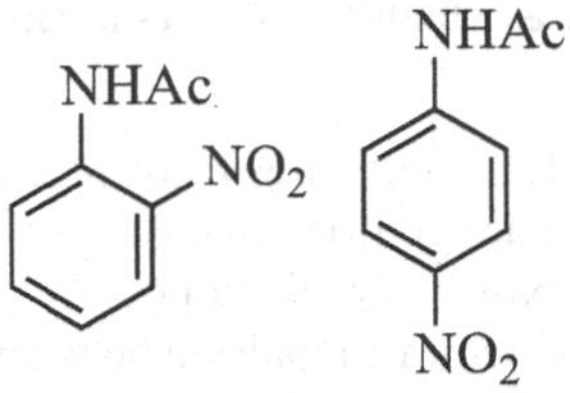 NHAc, NO_2; NHAc, NO_2 (c) 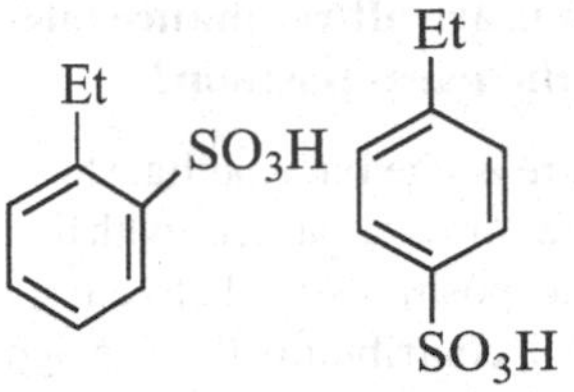 Et, SO_3H; Et, SO_3H

What is an electron-withdrawing group when attached to benzene?

An electron-withdrawing group is one that has a positive or δ^+ charge directly attached to the benzene ring.

Why are electron-withdrawing groups referred to as deactivating groups?

When the benzene ring attacks an electrophilic species (X^+), the resonance-stabilized intermediate has a positive charge in the ring. If this positive charge is adjacent to a + or δ^+ charge of an electron-withdrawing group substituent (i.e., on the ipso carbon), the electrostatic repulsion of like charges destabilizes the intermediate and slows down formation of that arenium ion intermediate.

Are each of the following activating or deactivating: -NO_2, OEt, CH_3, CH_2CH_3, Me_2S^+, Me_3N^+, -CO_2Et, Ph, NH_2?

The activating groups are OEt, CH_3, CH_2CH_3, Ph, and NH_2. The deactivating groups are -NO_2, Me_3N^+, ketones and aldehydes, and -CO_2Et.

What the relative order of deactivating substituents?

The relative order is: -NO_2, -$^+NR_3$ > -CN, -SO_3H, R_2C=O, RCO_2R'.

When compared with nitrobenzene, does benzene react faster or slower with bromine and aluminum chloride?

Benzene reacts faster than nitrobenzene in electrophilic aromatic substitution reactions.

Why does an electron-withdrawing group slow electrophilic aromatic substitution?

The nitro group is an example of an electron-withdrawing group and it has a positive charge on the nitrogen. When the arenium ion positive chare is on the ipso carbon, repulsion of this charge with the + or δ^+ charge of the substituent raises the energy of that intermediate and makes the intermediate less stable and slows the overall reaction.

Why is nitro a more powerful deactivating group than the carbonyl of a ketone (as in acetophenone)?

The nitrogen of nitro has a formal charge of +1 ($O=N^+–O^-$) whereas the carbon of a carbonyl is part of polarized bond and has a δ^+ charge. The greater the electrophilic character of the atom (the larger the positive charge), the greater will be its deactivating ability.

What is the major product or products formed when nitrobenzene reacts with bromine/Lewis acid?

The major product is 3-bromonitrobenzene.

Is the reaction in the preceding question faster or slower than the bromination of benzene using the same Lewis acid?

The nitro group is strongly deactivating, so the bromination of nitrobenzene is much slower than the bromination of benzene.

What are all resonance intermediates when Br^+ reacts at the ortho- position of nitrobenzene? At the para- position?

There is one intermediate for ortho- attack, with three resonance contributors. There is also one intermediate for para- attack, with three resonance contributors. Note that in both cases, attack at the ortho- and para- positions leads to a resonance contributor with a positive charge on the ipso carbon. In the resonance contributors there is significant electronic repulsion between the positive charge of the arenium ion and the positive chare on the nitrogen of the nitro group. Such repulsion is very destabilizing and these arenium ions are very unstable and difficult to form. In other words, the electronic interaction destabilizes formation of the arenium ion intermediates and slows their formation.

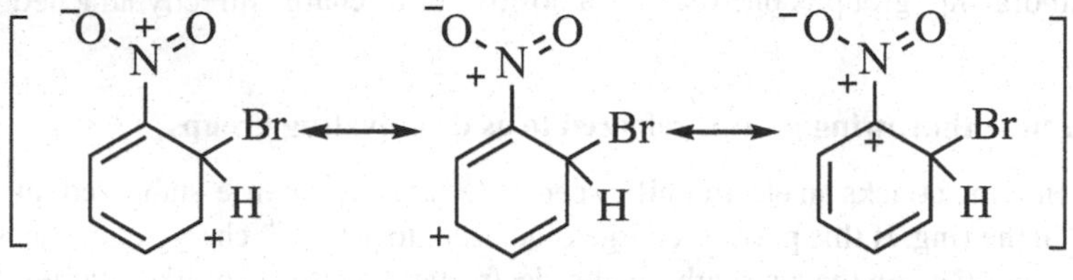

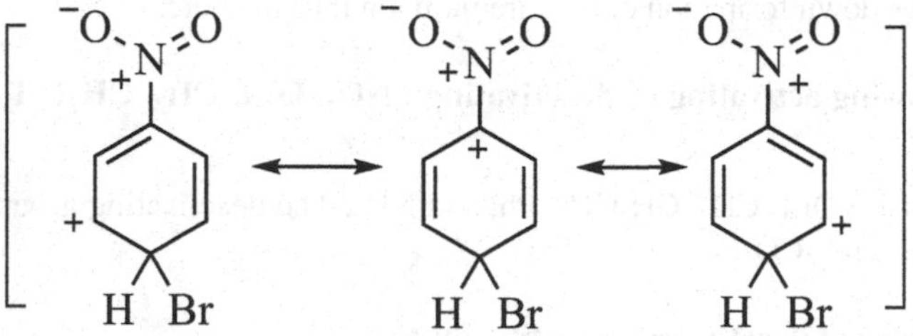

What are all resonance intermediates when Br^+ reacts at the meta- position of nitrobenzene?

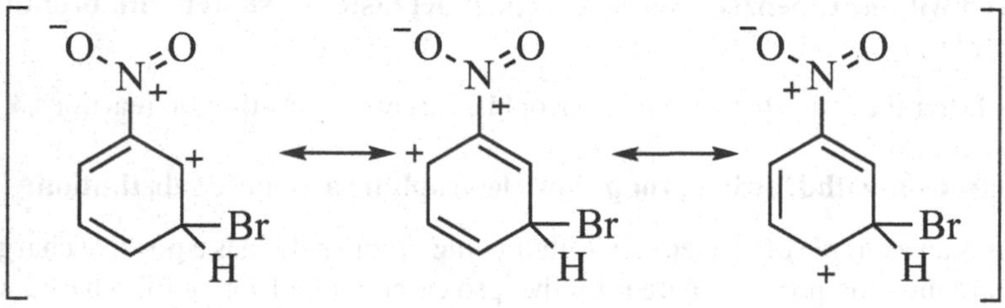

Reaction with Br^+ at the meta- position generates one intermediate with three resonance contributors. Note that with reaction at the meta- position, the charge of the arenium ion is never on the ipso carbon, which makes this intermediate more stable than the arenium ions formed from reaction at the ortho- and para- positions.

In reactions of nitrobenzene, what is the lowest energy intermediate: ortho, meta-, or para- attack? Why?

The lowest energy intermediate arises from meta- attack. The positive charge on the ring is never adjacent to the positive charge on the nitrogen. In the intermediates resulting from ortho- and para- attack, at least one contributor is on the ipso carbon and places the two charges on adjacent atoms.

Is the arenium ion formed by reaction at the meta- position of nitrobenzene higher or lower in energy than the arenium ion formed by reaction at the meta- position of methylbenzene? Is the reaction faster or slower?

The arenium ion formed by reaction at the meta- position of nitrobenzene is much higher in energy than that formed by reaction at the meta- position of methylbenzene. Remember that the nitro group is very destabilizing and even though the arenium ion formed from nitrobenzene is more stable than the ortho-/para- arenium ions, it is still high in energy. All of this discussion means that formation of the arenium ion from reaction at the meta- position of methylbenzene is *faster* than formation of the arenium ion from reaction at the meta- position of nitrobenzene.

What is (are) the major product(s) for the reactions of (a), (b), and (c)?

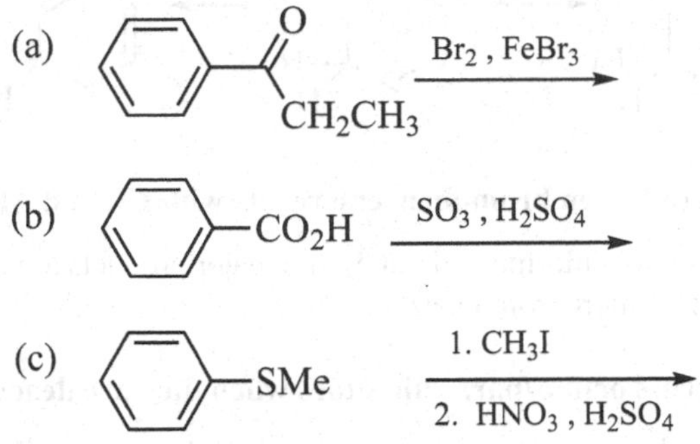

The carbonyl of the ketone in (a) is deactivating and a meta- director. The product is, therefore, [1-(3-bromophenyl)propan-1-one]. The carboxyl group in (b) is also deactivating and the major product is benzenesulfonic acid-3-carboxylate. Initial reaction of (c) with iodomethane generates a dimethylsulfonium ion (a deactivating group whereas -SMe is activating). The product of nitration is, therefore, 3-(dimethylsulfonium)nitrobenzene.

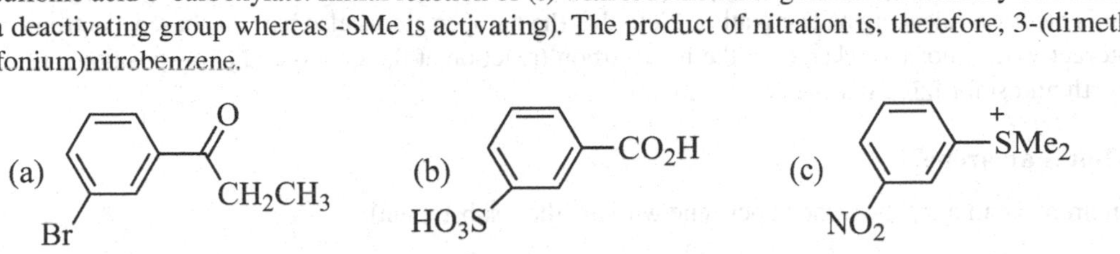

Does bromobenzene react faster or slower than benzene in electrophilic aromatic substitution reactions?

Since bromine is polarizable, the Br takes a δ^+ dipole when attached to the electron rich benzene ring. Bromobenzene therefore reacts *slower* than benzene in electrophilic aromatic substitution. Other aryl halides (fluorobenzene, chlorobenzene, and iodobenzene) also react slower than benzene.

Is Br an activating or a deactivating group?

Since the bromine atom takes a δ^+ dipole, bromine is a deactivating group. The other halogens (fluorine, chlorine, iodine) are also deactivating.

What are all resonance intermediates when Br^+ reacts at the ortho- position of bromobenzene?

There are a total of four resonance contributors to the intermediate resulting from ortho- attack. Similarly, para- attack leads to four resonance contributors. In one resonance contributor the positive charge on the ring is on the ipso carbon. The charge can be therefore be delocalized onto bromine, which contains electrons that can be donated to the positive center, leading to the additional resonance form. The presence of this fourth resonance contributor indicates that reaction at the ortho- and at the para- positions leads to a positive charge on the ipso carbon, and are stabilized more than reaction at the meta- position.

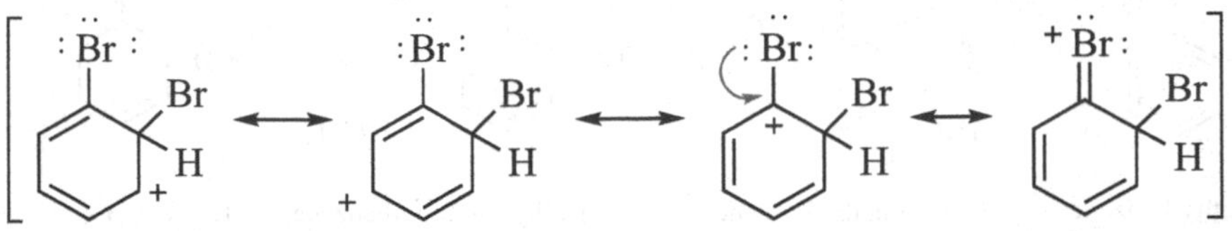

What are all resonance intermediates when Br^+ reacts at the meta- position of bromobenzene?

Reaction at the meta- position generates one intermediate with only three resonance contributors. It is, therefore, less stable than the arenium ions generated by reaction at the ortho- and at the para- positions.

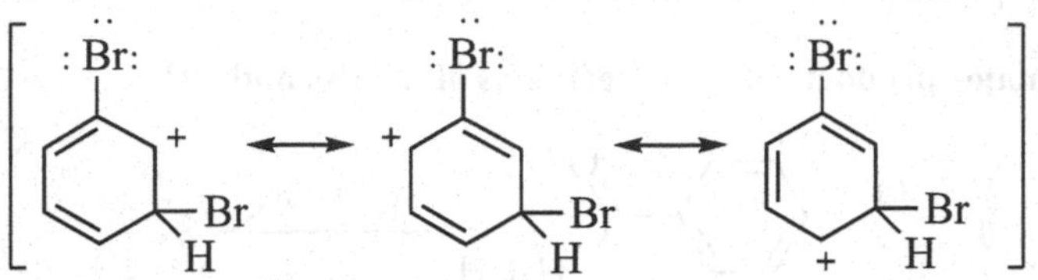

What is the major product(s) when bromobenzene reacts with Cl_2 and $AlCl_3$?

When bromobenzene reacts with chlorine and $AlCl_3$, the major products are a roughly equal mixture of 2-chlorobromobenzene and 4-chlorobromobenzene.

Why are halogen substituents ortho-/para- directors when they are deactivating?

First, realize that the halogens are polarizable. When attached to a neutral and electron-rich benzene ring, the halogen assumes a δ^+ dipole, which makes halogen atoms deactivating in the initial reaction with X^+. However, once the arenium ion is formed, the charge on the ion is +, and the halogen on the ipso carbon adopts a δ^- dipole due to the polarizability of the halogen. Therefore, the halogen in the arenium ion is electron releasing and activating. Note that the halogen atoms also have unshared electrons, which interact with a positive charge on the ipso carbon (reaction at the ortho- and para- positions) to form a fourth and stabilizing resonance contributor.

What is an arene?

An arene is an alkyl benzene (a benzene with an alkyl substituent).

What is the common name of 1,2-dimethylbenzene? Of 1,3-dimethylbenzene? Of 1,4-dimethylbenzene?

Common names are often used for these compounds. A dimethylbenzene is referred to as a *xylene.* 1,2-Dimethylbenzene is called ortho-xylene. 1,3-Dimethylbenzene is called meta-xylene and 1,4-dimethylbenzene is called para-xylene.

What is the IUPAC name of each of (a), (b), (c), and (d)?

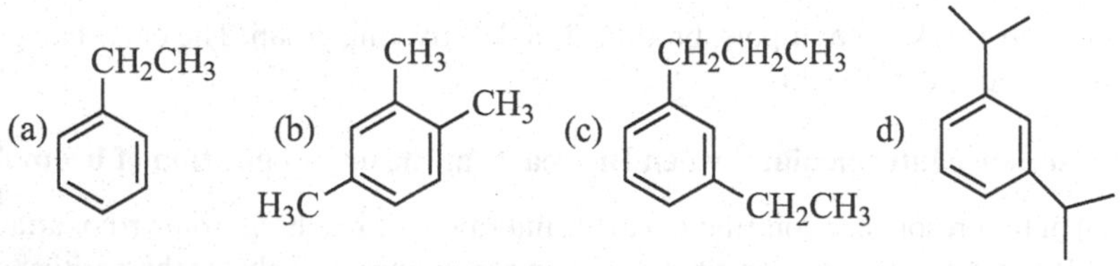

The IUPAC name of (a) is ethylbenzene. Arene (b) is 1,2,4-trimethylbenzene; (c) is 1-ethyl-3-propylbenzene, and (d) is 1,3-diisopropylbenzene, as well as 1,3-di(1-methylethyl)benzene.

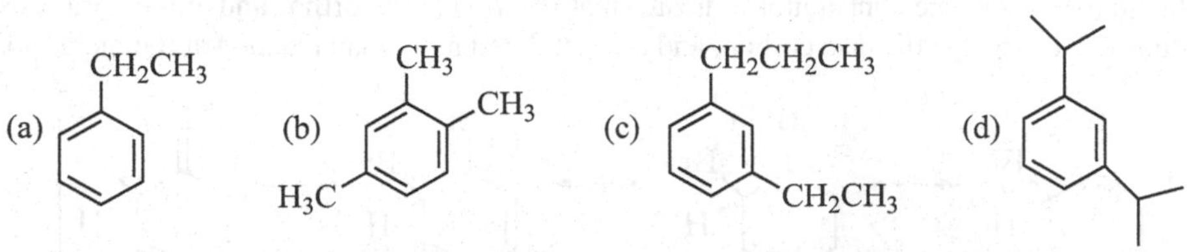

ethylbenzene 1,2,4-trimethylbenzene 1-ethyl-3-propylbenzene 1,3-diisopropylbenzene

What is the intermediate product when 2-bromopropane reacts with $AlCl_3$?

The intermediate of this reaction is a carbocation. When 2-bromopropane reacts with $AlCl_3$ the product is $Me_2CH^+ AlCl_4^-$.

What is the product when 1-chloro-2,2-dimethylpropane reacts with $AlCl_3$?

The product is the tertiary carbocation, ***A***.

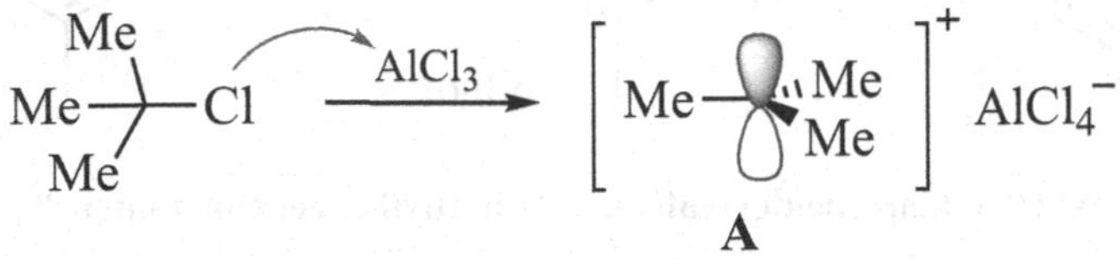

What is the product when 1-chlorobutane reacts with $AlCl_3$?

The initial product of this reaction is a primary carbocation (***A***), but this rearranges to the more stable secondary carbocation (***B***), as expected with any carbocation.

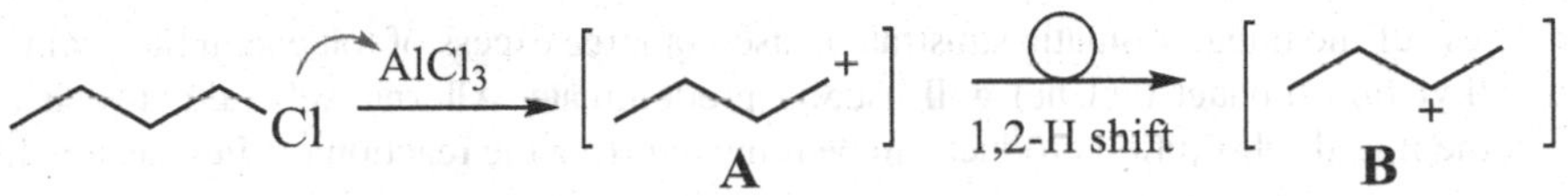

What is the major product when benzene reacts with 1-chloropropane and $AlCl_3$?

The initially formed primary carbocation ($CH_3CH_2CH_2$+) *rearranges* to the secondary carbocation ***A***, which reacts with benzene to give (1-methylethyl)benzene (isopropylbenzene) via the usual resonance-stabilized arenium ion intermediate, ***B***.

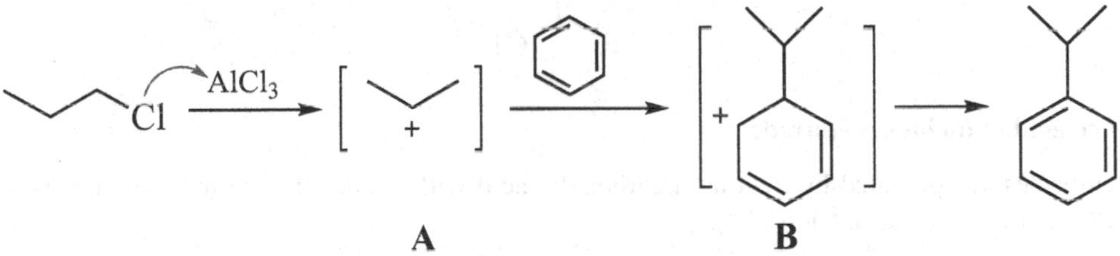

What is the name of the reaction of alkyl halides and aromatic compounds with a Lewis acid catalyst?

The reaction is called *Friedel–Crafts alkylation* and is useful for the preparation of arenes.

Why is formation of linear 1-phenylalkanes [$Ph(CH_2)_nCH_3$] virtually impossible via Friedel–Crafts alkylation?

Although primary halides will react with the Lewis acid to give a primary carbocation, this unstable intermediate almost always rearranges to a more stable secondary or tertiary carbocation. The aromatic substitution product of the Friedel–Crafts reaction will therefore be the arene derived from reaction of benzene with the secondary or tertiary carbocation. Due to rearrangement, the relative population of primary carbocation is very low, and few or no substitution products arise from that species (no linear arenes).

If para-xylene and ortho-xylene are formed by the reaction of toluene and iodomethane/$AlCl_3$, explain how 1,2,4-trimethylbenzene is also formed in the reaction.

Toluene (methylbenzene) reacts with iodomethane to give a new methyl group at the ortho- and para-positions, as with para-xylene, which is shown) Alkyl groups are activating (see above) and since xylene has two alkyl groups, the benzene ring is more activated than toluene, which has only one methyl group. Therefore, xylene reacts faster with unreacted MeI, $AlCl_3$ reagent than does toluene. The third methyl group will be incorporated ortho- to the methyl groups, which are both ortho-/para- directors.

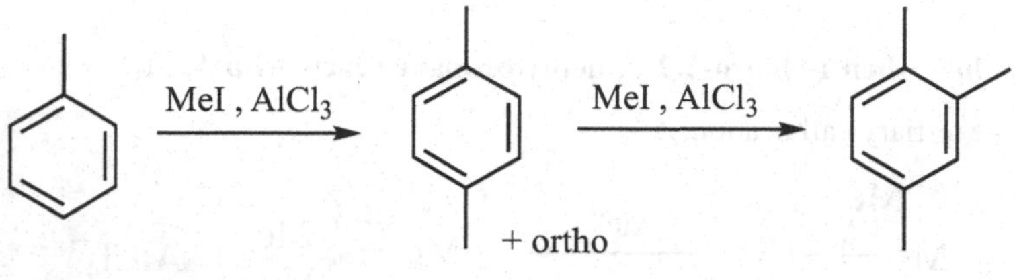

MeI , $AlCl_3$ → (+ ortho) MeI , $AlCl_3$ →

Which is the more reactive benzene derivative, 1,2-diethylbenzene or toluene?

As noted in the preceding question 1,2-diethylbenzene has two more activating methyl groups than toluene, which has only one. Therefore, the dimethylbenzene will react faster in electrophilic aromatic substitution reactions.

How can polyalkylation be suppressed in electrophilic aromatic substitution?

If a large excess of the initial aromatic substrate is used (a large excess of toluene in the example cited), the mono- alkylation product (xylene) will usually predominate. Alternatively, although it is usually impractical, the initial substitution product can be removed from the reaction medium as it is formed.

What is the structure of an acid chloride?

An acid chloride is a derivative of carboxylic acids where the –OH group has been replaced with Cl, as shown (see Sections 15.3 and 15.4).

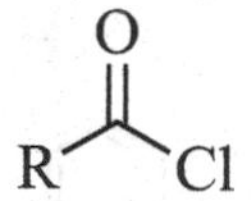

O R Cl

How are acid chlorides prepared?

Acid chlorides are prepared by treating a carboxylic acid with a halogenating reagent such as $SOCl_2$, PCl_3, PCl_5, or $POCl_3$ (see Section 15.4).

What is the major product when propanoyl chloride reacts with $AlCl_3$?

When propanoyl chloride reacts with $AlCl_3$, the chlorine attacks Al to form $AlCl_3^-$ and a resonance-stabilized cation called an *acylium ion, **A***.

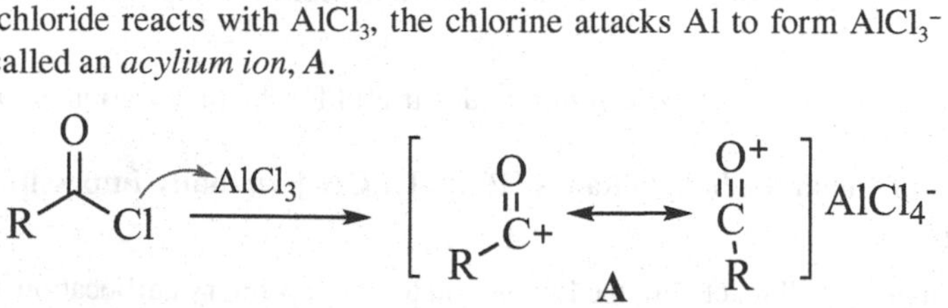

O R Cl $AlCl_3$ → [O R C+ ⟷ O+ C R] $AlCl_4^-$ **A**

Does an acylium ion rearrange as a normal carbocation does?

No! An acylium ion is stabilized by the oxygen atom to give the resonance contributors shown in the preceding question. This additional stabilization prevents cationic rearrangement before reaction with benzene or other aromatic compounds.

What is the name of this reaction?

The reaction of acyl halides and aromatic compounds is called *Friedel–Crafts acylation*.

What is the product when propanoyl chloride reacts with $AlCl_3$ and benzene?

When propanoyl chloride reacts with benzene and $AlCl_3$, the product is 1-phenylpropan-1-one. The initial reaction generates the arenium ion ***A***, which loses a proton to give the ketone product.

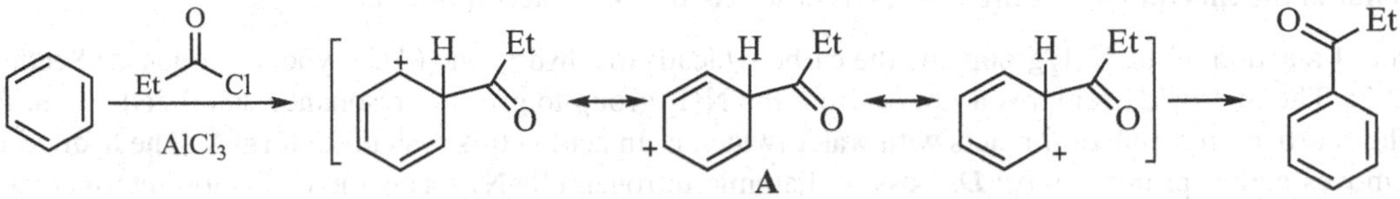

What is the product when anisole reacts with propanoyl chloride and $AlCl_3$?

The OMe group of anisole is strongly activating and an ortho- /para- director. The products are, therefore, a mixture of (2-methoxyphenyl)propan-1-one and (4-methoxyphenyl)-1-propan-1-one.

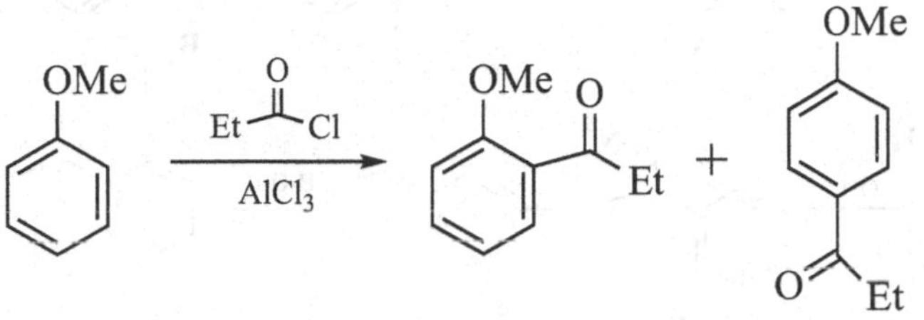

What is the product when nitrobenzene reacts with propanoyl chloride and $AlCl_3$?

In this case, the NO_2 group strongly deactivates the ring and Friedel–Crafts acylation does *not* occur. In general, *Friedel–Crafts acylation does not occur with deactivated aromatic rings* because the acyloin ion is much less reactive than a normal cation.

Is the ketone product of a Friedel–Crafts acylation more reactive or less reactive than benzene?

The product is a ketone and the C=O group is deactivating (due to the δ^+ charge on the carbonyl carbon). This makes the ketone product *less* reactive than benzene.

Is polyacylation a problem in Friedel–Crafts acylation?

No! Since the carbonyl is a deactivating group, the product is generally less reactive than the starting material. Further acylation is not, therefore, a problem.

Can primary arenes be formed using Friedel–Crafts acylation?

Yes, indirectly! Primary arenes cannot be formed by Friedel–Crafts alkylation, but they can be formed by Friedel–Crafts acylation, if the C=O (carbonyl) group is removed from the molecule by conversion into a methylene (-CH_2-) group in a subsequent chemical step.

What is the product when 1-phenylpropan-1-one is treated with hydrazine and KOH?

The reduction of a ketone C=O to a -CH_2- with hydrazine (NH_2NH_2) under basic conditions is called the *Wolff–Kishner Reduction.* When 1-phenylpropan-1-one is treated with KOH and NH_2NH_2, the product is propylbenzene. Note that propylbenzene is a primary arene.

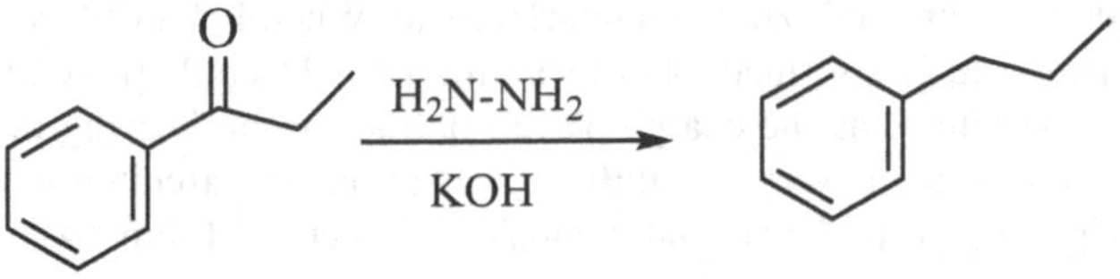

What is the name of this reaction?

This reaction is called *Wolff–Kishner reduction.*

What is the mechanism of the Wolff–Kishner reduction of acetophenone?

Initial reaction of the NH_2 group and the carbonyl leads to a hydrazone (***A***), a type of imine (see Section 12.2). The hydroxide removes a proton from the NH_2 group to give the resonance-stabilized anion, ***B***. The "carbanion form" of ***B*** reacts with water (which is an acid in this system) to form ***C***. The hydroxide removes anther proton to give ***D***. Loss of diatomic nitrogen (N≡N) forms the carbanion intermediate, which reacts with water to complete the reduction, producing ethylbenzene.

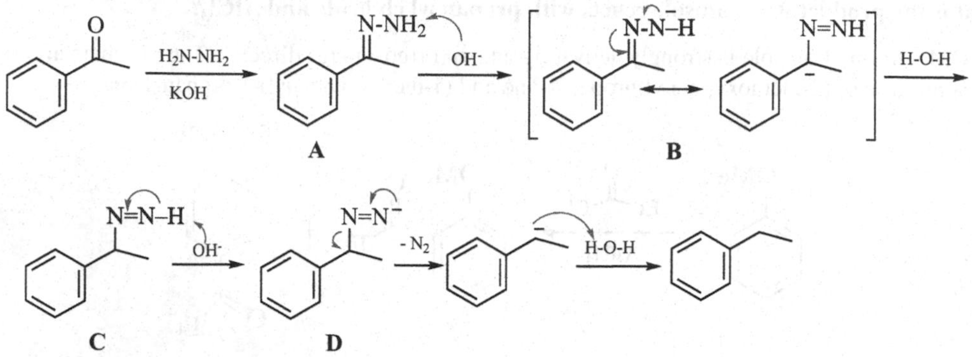

What is the product when acetophenone is treated with zinc amalgam and HCl?

When acetophenone is treated with HCl and zinc amalgam the product is ethylbenzene. This reaction process is called *Clemmensen reduction* and is the acid medium compliment of the basic medium Wolff–Kishner reduction. Ethanol is often used as a solvent in this reaction.

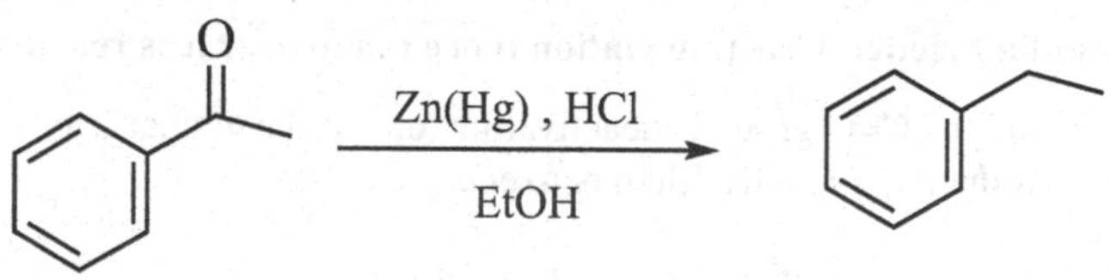

What is zinc amalgam?

An amalgam is an element compounded with mercury, and zinc amalgam is zinc compounded with mercury. Zinc amalgam is usually written as Zn(Hg).

What is the name of this reaction?

The *Clemmensen reduction.*

What is the resonance intermediate formed when Br^+ reacts at C2 of 4-nitroanisole? At C3?

There are two sites of reaction, the carbon adjacent to the carbon bearing OMe and the carbon adjacent to the carbon bearing NO_2. Reaction of 4-nitroanisole with bromonium ion at the carbon adjacent to the methoxy generates a resonance-stabilized arenium ion with four resonance contributors, ***A***. In one of the resonance contributors, the positive charge is placed on the carbon bearing the OMe where the charge is dispersed to the oxygen, further stabilizing this intermediate. When Br^+ attaches to C3 next to the nitro group, resonance intermediate ***B*** is formed, but this arenium ion has only three resonance contributors. Since one resonance contributor has the charge placed on the carbon bearing the positive nitrogen of the nitro group, this intermediate is very destabilized. Therefore, the arenium ion from reaction at C2, adjacent to the methoxy group, is preferred and the major product is 2-bromo-4-nitroanisole.

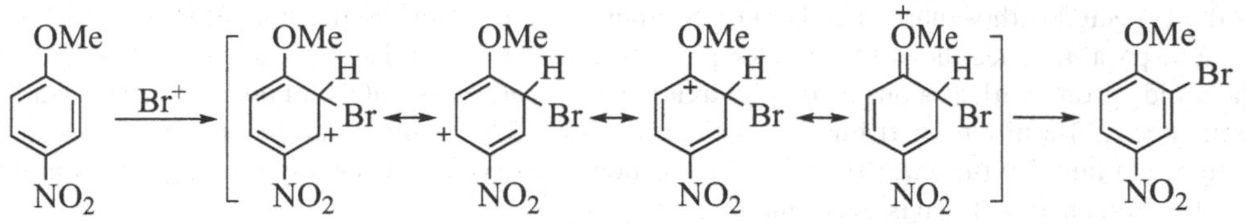

OMe OMe OMe OMe OMe OMe
H H H H Br
Br^+ Br Br Br Br
NO_2 NO_2 NO_2 NO_2 NO_2 NO_2
A

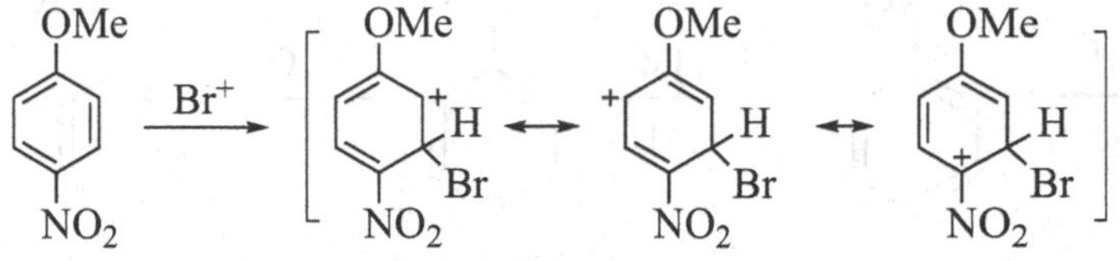

OMe OMe OMe OMe
Br^+ H H H
Br Br Br
NO_2 NO_2 NO_2 NO_2
B

What is the major product of this reaction?

The major product of this reaction is 2-bromo-4-nitroanisole.

If an activating and a deactivating group are in a molecule, which dominates the electrophilic substitution reaction? Why?

By definition, an activating group increases the rate of electrophilic aromatic substitution whereas a deactivating group diminishes the rate of the reaction. If both are in the same molecule, electrophilic aromatic substitution will be directed by the reaction with the faster rate, dictated by the activating group. If there are two activating groups, the product will be determined by the most activating. If there are two deactivating groups, the product will be directed by the least deactivating group.

16.3 SYNTHESIS VIA AROMATIC SUBSTITUTION

What is synthesis?

Synthesis is a progression of chemical steps that begins with a molecule (the starting material) and adds functional groups and/or carbon–carbon bonds via chemical reactions until a new molecule (the target or product) is constructed. Note that all of the chemical reactions in preceding (and also the subsequent) chapters may be used in solving synthesis problems.

What is a suitable synthesis for the conversion of benzene to (4-aminophenyl)-butan-1-one?

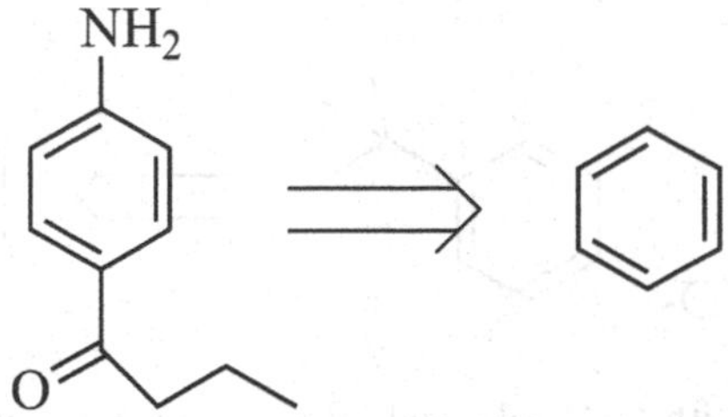

NH_2

O

Since the carbonyl is a meta- director and deactivating, the target is most likely formed by first incorporating the amine unit, an ortho-/para- director. To incorporate nitrogen, the first reaction is a nitration to give nitrobenzene (Section 15.4). The nitro group is *reduced* with hydrogen and a palladium catalyst (see Sections 14.1 and 14.4) to give aniline. Before a Friedel–Crafts reaction can be done, the basic amino group must be protected as the amide. Treatment of aniline with acetic anhydride leads to *N*-acetyl aniline (Section 15.4) and subsequent reaction with butanoyl chloride and $AlCl_3$ leads to the ketone, along with the expected ortho- substituted ketone (Section 16.2). To complete the synthesis, separation of the ortho- and para- ketones allows the targeted para- product is isolated. The last chemical step is hydrolysis of the amide group with aqueous acid or by treatment with aqueous NaOH followed by neutralization to give the target, 4-aminophenyl)-butan-1-one (see Section 15.5). In this sequence, not only the reactions are important but also the *order* in which the reactions are performed. This synthesis requires planning before the first chemical step is performed.

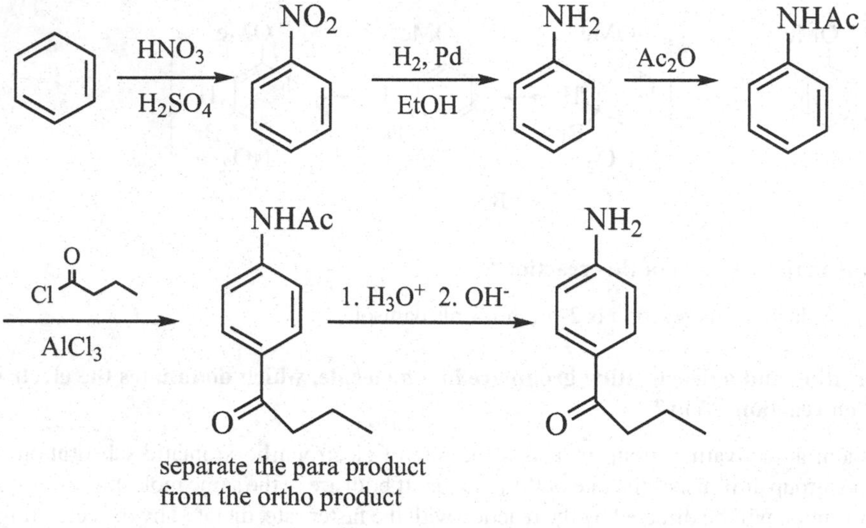

NO_2 HNO_3 H_2SO_4 H_2, Pd EtOH NH_2 Ac_2O NHAc

NHAc O Cl $AlCl_3$ 1. H_3O^+ 2. OH^- NH_2 O O

separate the para product
from the ortho product

What is a complete synthesis for (a), (b), and (c) from the indicated starting material?

(a) OEt Br NO_2 ⟹ OH

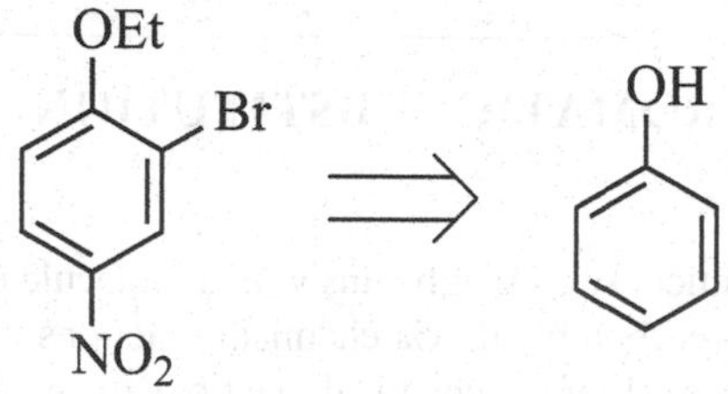

(b) Br SO_3H ⟹

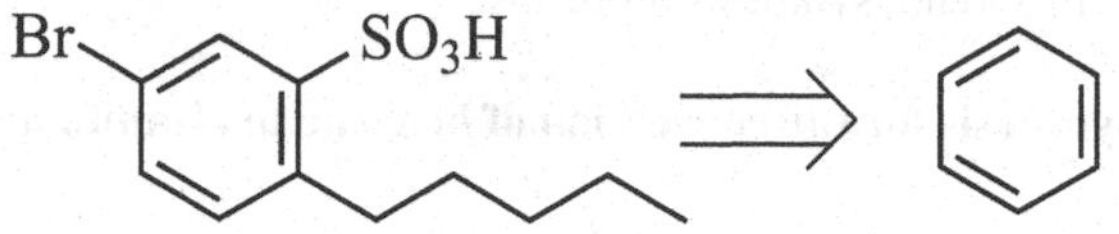

(c) NO_2 ⟹

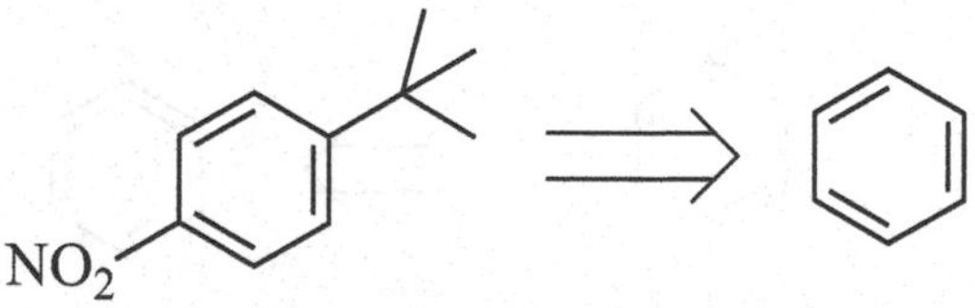

In (a), the reaction of phenol with NaH followed by a S_N2 reaction with bromoethane gives ethoxybenzene (see Section 8.2). Nitration of the activated benzene ring gives a mixture of ortho- and para- nitro compounds (Section 16.2). Separation of the isomers allows isolation of the para- product. Bromination puts the bromine ortho- to the OEt activating group (Section 16.2) to give the targeted 2-bromo-4-nitroethoxybenzene.

In (b) Friedel–Crafts acylation of benzene with pentanoyl chloride gives 1-phenylethan-1-one (Section 16.2). A Wolff–Kishner reduction (Section 16.2) gives pentylbenzene. Bromination of the activated benzene ring gives a mixture of the ortho- and para- products (Section 16.2) and the targeted para- product is isolated by separation from the ortho- product. Sulfonation occurs ortho- to the activating alkyl group (Section 16.2) to give the target, 5-bromo-2-pentylbenzenesulfonic acid.

In (c) Friedel–Crafts alkylation with the tertiary halide gives *tert*-butylbenzene (Section 16.2). Nitration of the activated ring gives the ortho- and para- nitro compounds (Section 16.2) and separation from the ortho- product allows isolation of the targeted product, 4-nitro-*tert*-butylbenzene.

(a) OH → a → OEt → b → OEt, NO_2 + ortho → c → OEt, Br, NO_2

separate the para product from the ortho product

(a) i. NaH ii. EtBr (b) HNO_3 , H_2SO_4 (c) Br_2, $AlCl_3$

(b) → a → O → b →

5-bromo-2-pentylbenzenesulfonic acid

→ c → Br + ortho → d → Br, SO_3H

separate the para product from the ortho product

(a) pentanoyl chloride , $AlCl_3$ (b) NH_2NH_2 , KOH (c) Br_2 , $FeBr_3$ (d) H_2SO_4 , SO_3

(c) → a → → b → NO_2 + ortho

separate the para product from the ortho product

(a) Me_3CCl , $AlCl_3$ (b) HNO_3 , H_2SO_4

16.4 NUCLEOPHILIC AROMATIC SUBSTITUTION

What is the definition of nucleophilic aromatic substitution?

When a leaving group on a benzene ring (such as a halogen) is displaced by a nucleophile, the reaction is known as nucleophilic aromatic substitution. In general, such a reaction is less facile than electrophilic aromatic substitution because an electron rich nucleophile must attack an electron rich benzene ring.

What is an aryl halide?

Aryl halides are benzene derivatives, Ar–X, where the X group is Cl, Br, I, and sometimes F. Aryl halides are common reaction partners in nucleophilic reactions of benzene derivatives.

Can a nucleophile displace halogen of an aryl halide in a substitution reaction?

Yes, but the reaction requires very vigorous conditions.

What is the name of the substitution reaction in which a nucleophile displaces the halogen of an aryl halide?

Nucleophilic aromatic substitution.

What is the designation for nucleophilic aromatic substitution?

This type of reaction is a S_NAr reaction.

What is the product when chlorobenzene reacts with KOH or NaOH in aqueous media at ambient temperatures?

There is no reaction. Neither KOH nor NaOH are sufficiently nucleophilic to attack an electron-rich benzene ring and displace the chlorine. High temperatures and pressures are required to force the nucleophile to attack the benzene ring and complete this reaction.

What is the product when chlorobenzene reacts with aqueous KOH at 350°C and 2000–3000 psi?

When chlorobenzene reacts with KOH at elevated temperature and pressure, the resulting product is phenol.

Cl
aq. NaOH , 350 °C
2500 psi
OH

What is the mechanism of the reaction in the preceding question?

The initial reaction involves collision of the negatively charged hydroxide with the chlorine-bearing carbon of electron-rich benzene ring of chlorobenzene, the ipso carbon. The π-bond is broken, dumping the electrons into the ring to give the resonance-stabilized intermediate ***A***. The electrons in the ring displace the chlorine, which is a leaving group, in the final step to generate phenol. However, the reaction is done in aqueous hydroxide and phenol is acidic (pK_a, 10). Therefore, the phenol product reacts with hydroxide to give the phenoxide anion, ***B***. A second reaction with aqueous acid is required to regenerate phenol so it can be isolated. This S_NAr reaction has a high activation energy for the initial attack of hydroxide since the negatively charged species must attack a benzene ring that is rich in electron density. Therefore, the high reaction temperature and pressure are required for the substitution reaction. At much lower temperatures and pressures, no reaction occurs.

Cl
$^-$OH
Cl OH
Cl OH
Cl OH
– Cl$^-$
aq. NaOH
O$^-$
H_3O^+
OH
A
B

Can this reaction be used for a general synthesis for phenols?

The high reaction temperatures and pressures make it unattractive for the synthesis of all but the *simplest* phenol derivatives. It is very useful in industrial labs, however, for the production of phenol.

Why do electron-withdrawing substituents increase the facility of S_NAr reactions?

The resonance-stabilized intermediate for S_NAr reactions has a negative charge that is stabilized by electron-withdrawing substituents.

Under what conditions will 2-chloronitrobenzene react with hydroxide?

The reaction involves treatment with aqueous NaOH at about 150–175°C, and the product is 4-nitrophenol. Note that a lower reaction temperature is required relative to the reaction with chlorobenzene due to the stabilizing influence of the nitro substituent.

Under what conditions will 2-chloro-1,5-dinitrobenzene react with hydroxide?

The reaction involves the use of aqueous sodium carbonate (or hydroxide) at about 125–150°C, and the product is 2,4-dinitrophenol.

Under what conditions will 2-chloro-1,3,5-trinitrobenzene react with hydroxide?

In this case, heating with warm water converts the chloride to 2,4,6-trinitrophenol. Clearly, the presence of three nitro groups has a great stabilizing effect for formation of the intermediate and the overall S_NAr reaction.

Why are the reaction conditions for phenol formation milder as more nitro groups are added to the benzene ring?

Nitro is an electron-withdrawing group with a positive charge on the nitrogen. The reaction of hydroxide with the chlorine-bearing carbon of 4-chcloronitrobenzene gives resonance-stabilized carbanion intermediate ***A***. Examination of intermediate ***A*** reveals that the negative charge in one resonance contributor is on the carbon that is adjacent to the positively charged nitrogen of the nitro group. The proximity of the two charges allows delocalization of the charge onto the nitro group, formation of another resonance form, and increased stability for the intermediate. This stability allows the overall reaction to proceed faster; e.g., under milder reaction conditions.

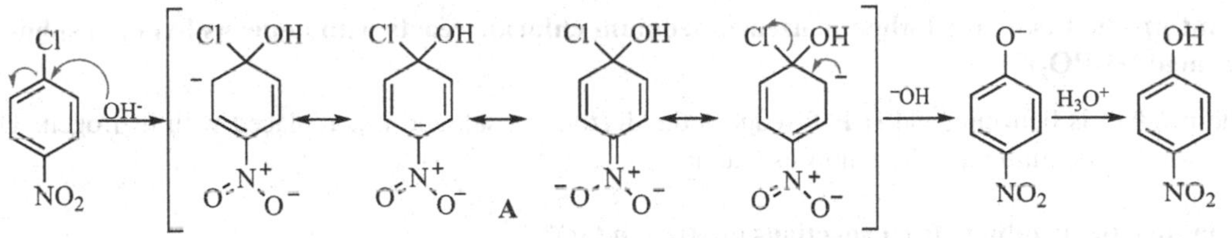

Cl OH OH⁻ A ⁻OH H_3O^+ NO_2 O⁻

What are the reaction conditions for the reaction of NaOH with 2,4,6-trinitrochlorobenzene in aqueous media?

The S_NAr reaction is so facile with the three nitro groups that reaction occurs to give 2,4,6-trinitrophenol in hot water, without the need for added hydroxide.

What is the product when 4-chloroanisole reacts with hydroxide?

There is no reaction. The electron-releasing methoxy group makes the nucleophilic attack even more difficult than in chlorobenzene and, in general, no reaction occurs, or the reaction is very sluggish with low yields at the usual reaction conditions for S_NAr reactions.

What product is formed when $NaNO_2$ (sodium nitrite) reacts with HCl?

The product is nitrous acid, HONO.

What is the product when HONO, formed by reaction of $NaNO_2$/HCl, reacts with aniline?

The product is benzenediazonium chloride. Note that the diazonium moiety has a N≡N unit that is highly reactive since it is essentially the N_2 leaving group for substitution reactions.

$$\text{PhNH}_2 \xrightarrow{\text{NaNO}_2\text{, HCl}} \text{PhN}_2^+\ \text{Cl}^- \equiv \text{Ph}-\overset{+}{\text{N}}\equiv\text{N}\ \ \text{Cl}^-$$

What product is formed when benzenediazonium chloride is heated with CuCl? With CuBr?

The product of this reaction is chlorobenzene via displacement of the diazonium unit by chloride. The reaction with CuBr is bromobenzene, formed in the same manner.

What is the name of the reactions in the preceding question?

The *Sandmeyer reaction.*

What reaction product is formed in the reaction of benzenediazonium chloride with CuCN?

The product is benzonitrile.

What product is formed when benzenediazonium chloride reacts with H_3PO_2, hypophosphorus acid?

Hypophosphorus acid reduces the diazonium unit, replacing it with hydrogen (deamination). In other words, benzenediazonium chloride reacts to give benzene as the final product.

What product is formed when benzenediazonium chloride reacts with water heated to reflux?

The product is phenol.

What product is formed when benzenediazonium chloride reacts with aqueous hypophosphorus acid (H_3PO_2)?

The product is benzene, and H_3PO_2 reduces the diazonium salt and it is replaced with hydrogen. This reaction is essentially a hydrogenolysis reaction.

What are the products from reactions (a), (b), and (c)?

(a) $\text{PhNH}_2 \xrightarrow[\text{2. CuBr}]{\text{1. NaNO}_2\text{, HCl}}$

(b) $\text{C}_6\text{H}_6 \xrightarrow[\text{3. HONO; 4. CuCN}]{\text{1. HNO}_3\text{, H}_2\text{SO}_4\text{; 2. H}_2\text{, Ni}}$

(c) NO_2, CO_2Me, MeO_2C-substituted benzene $\xrightarrow{\text{1. H}_2\text{, Ni; 2. NaNO}_2\text{, HCl; 3. H}_3\text{PO}_2}$

In (a), conversion of the amine unit to the diazonium salt is followed by reaction with CuBr to give bromobenzene. In (b), nitration of benzene and reduction of nitrobenzene to the aniline is followed by conversion to the diazonium's salt with HONO, and reaction with CuCN gives benzonitrile. In (c), reduction of the nitro group to the amino group allows reaction with HONO and then reaction with hypophosphorus acid leads to deamination to give the 1,4-diester.

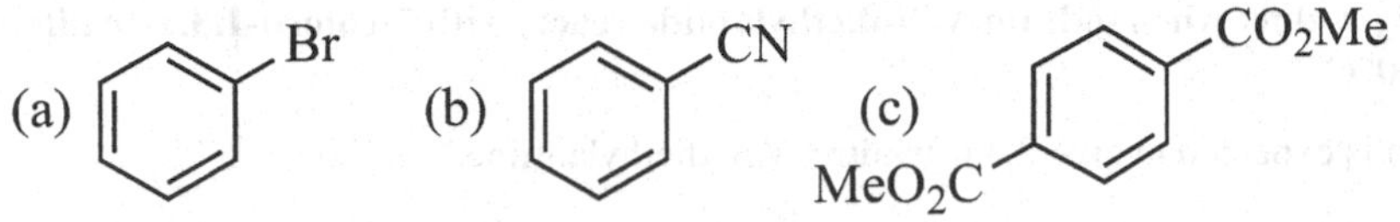

(a) Br (b) CN (c) CO_2Me MeO_2C

What is an azo dye?

An azo dye is typically a brightly colored solid with the structure Ar-N=N-Ar', where Ar are aromatic rings.

How is an azo dye prepared?

The reaction of an aryl diazonium salt with an activated aromatic ring generates the ortho- or para- substituted azo dye.

What product is formed when benzenediazonium chloride reacts with aniline?

The reaction of benzenediazonium chloride and aniline gives the diazo compound, (*E*)-4-(phenyldiazenyl) aniline, otherwise known as *aniline yellow*, which is an orange powder in solid form. Aniline yellow was first produced in 1861 and is believed to be the first commercial azo dye.

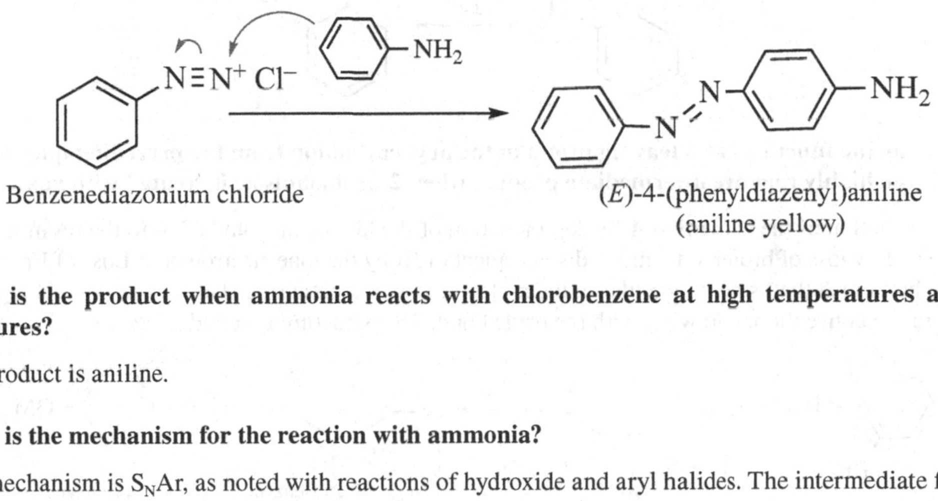

$N{\equiv}N^+ Cl^-$ NH_2 N N NH_2

Benzenediazonium chloride (*E*)-4-(phenyldiazenyl)aniline (aniline yellow)

What is the product when ammonia reacts with chlorobenzene at high temperatures and pressures?

The product is aniline.

What is the mechanism for the reaction with ammonia?

The mechanism is S_NAr, as noted with reactions of hydroxide and aryl halides. The intermediate for the reaction of chlorobenzene and ammonia is, **A**.

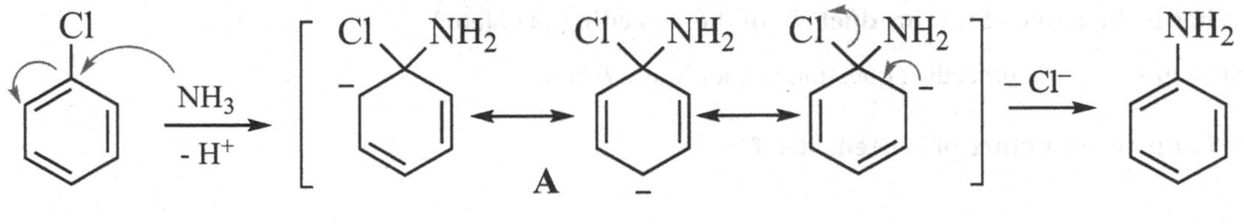

Cl NH_3 - H^+ Cl NH_2 Cl NH_2 Cl NH_2 **A** $- Cl^-$ NH_2

What is the product when methylamine reacts with 4-chloronitrobenzene in ethanol at reflux?

The reaction product is expected to be *N*-methylaniline, if the reaction is done at high temperatures and pressures.

What is the product when sodium amide ($NaNH_2$) reacts with chlorobenzene at high temperatures and pressures?

The reaction produces aniline as the product, but the mechanism may not be the same as in nucleophilic aromatic substitution (see below).

What is the product when sodium *N,N*-diethylamide reacts with 2-chloro-1,3,5-trinitrobenzene at about 100°C?

The reaction is expected to give 2,4,6-trinitro-*N,N*-diethylaniline.

What is the approximate pK_a of the ortho- hydrogen of chlorobenzene?

The pK_a of the ortho- hydrogen of chlorobenzene is approximately 40. A very powerful base is required for its removal as an acid.

What bases are strong enough to remove this ortho- hydrogen?

Suitable bases for removal of the ortho- hydrogen are organolithium reagents such as *n*-butyllithium and amide bases such as sodium amide ($NaNH_2$).

What is the initial product if the ortho- hydrogen is removed from chlorobenzene?

Deprotonation of chlorobenzene leads to a phenyl carbanion. This carbanion is a highly unstable and reactive intermediate.

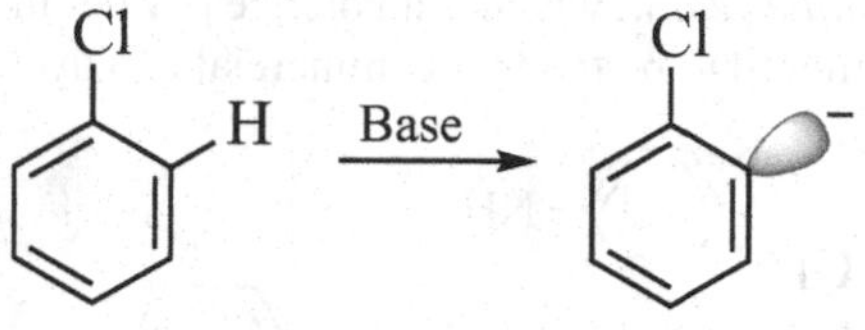

If the chlorine functions as a leaving group in the aryl carbanion from the preceding question, what is the highly reactive intermediate product when 2-bromoanisole is treated with base?

Initial formation of the carbanion ***A*** by deprotonation of the hydrogen atom ortho- to the bromine atom is followed by loss of bromine from via displacement of Br by the lone electron pair. Loss of Br leads to a triple bond in ***B*** that is perpendicular to the π-cloud of the aromatic ring. This new π-bond is shown in ***B*** and in the conventional drawing with the triple bond. This structure is called a *benzyne*.

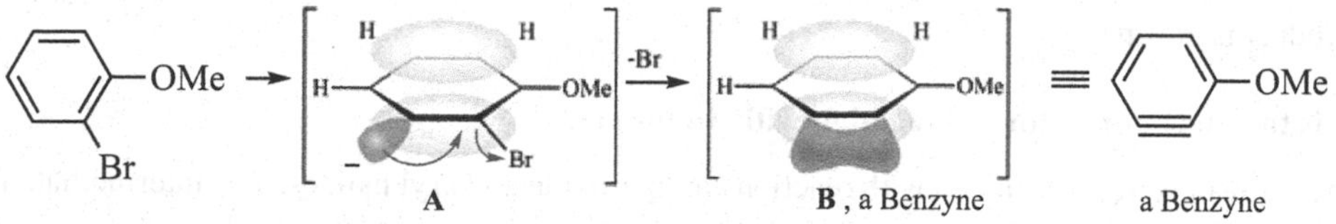

What is the name of this product (*B*) in the preceding problem?

Structure ***B*** in the preceding question is known as a *benzyne*.

What is the structure of benzene itself?

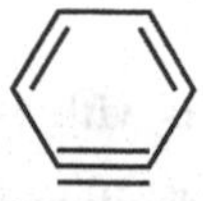

What amide bases are commonly used to generate a benzyne?

The sodium, lithium, or potassium salts of ammonia or simple primary and secondary amines such as methylamine, ethylamine, diethylamine, or diisopropylamine.

What is the product when potassium amide reacts with chlorobenzene in liquid ammonia?

The product is aniline.

What is the mechanism of the reaction in the preceding question?

The reaction proceeds via a benzyne intermediate. The amide base deprotonates the ortho- proton to give carbanion ***A***. Loss of chloride in leads to the triple bond in benzyne. Benzyne is very reactive with nucleophiles and the amide anion adds to the triple bond to form a new carbanion (***B***), which reacts with the ammonia solvent in an acid–base reaction to give aniline.

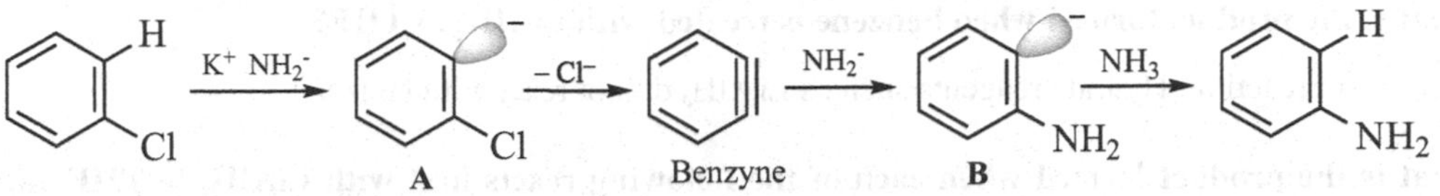

What is the product when sodium amide reacts with 2-bromoethylbenzene? Discuss the formation of two major products?

The two products are 2-ethylaniline and 3-ethylaniline. The initial deprotonation of 2-chloroethylbenzene gives ***A*** and loss of chloride ion gives the benzyne intermediate, ***B***. When the benzyne reacts with the amide anion nucleophile, there are two sites of reaction, C2 and C3, relative to the ethyl group. When the benzyne intermediate reacts at the C2 position, the product is carbanion ***C*** whereas reaction at C3 gives carbanion ***D***. The electron-releasing ethyl group is expected to destabilize the proximal carbanion at C2 (***D***) relative to the distal carbanion at C3 (***C***) and ***C*** is therefore slightly favored. This reaction usually gives a 40–50:50–60 ratio of 2-ethylaniline and 3-ethylaniline favoring 3-ethylaniline.

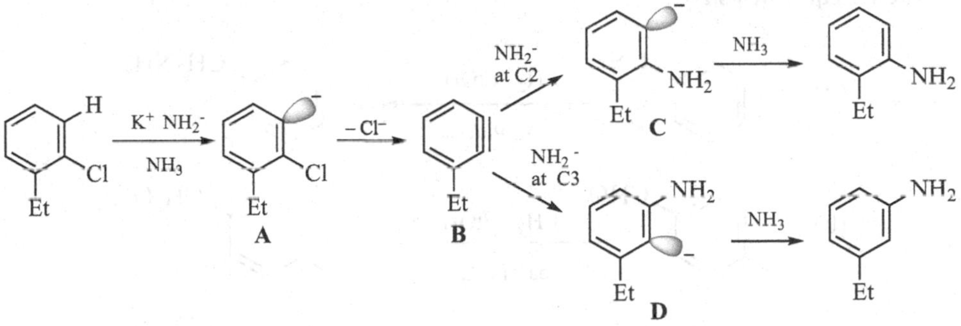

What is the major product (or products) the reactions of (a), (b), and (c)?

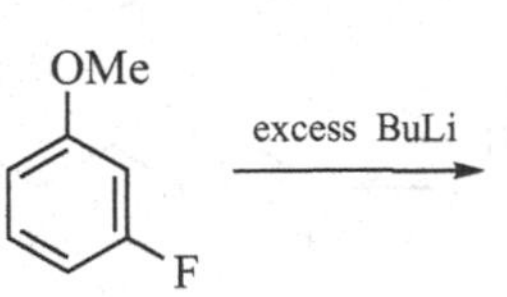

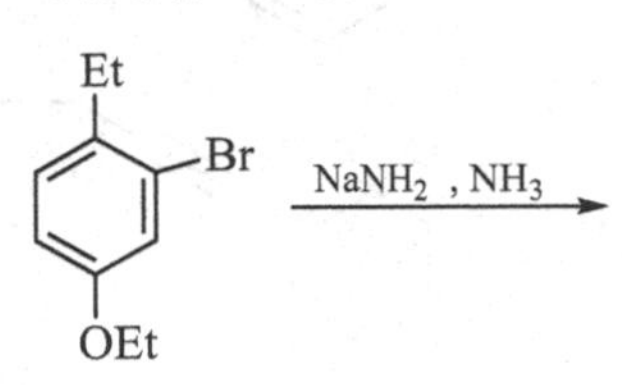

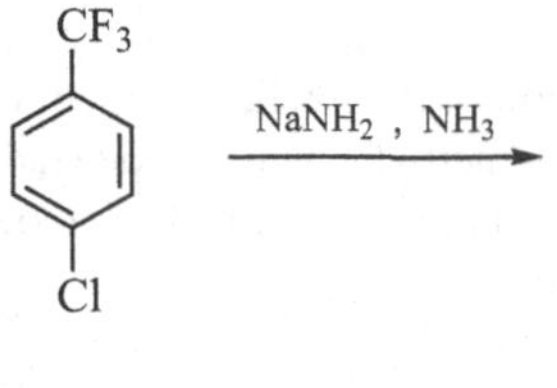

The reaction in (a) generates a mixture of 2-butylanisole and 3-butylanisole. The reaction in (b) gives a mixture of 4-ethyl-3-aminophenetole and 4-ethyl-2-aminophenetole. The final reaction (c) leads to a mixture of 4-trifluoromethylaniline and 3-rifluoromethylaniline.

(a) OMe, Bu; OMe, Bu (b) Et, NH_2, OEt; Et, NH_2, OEt (c) CF_3, NH_2; CF_3, H_2N

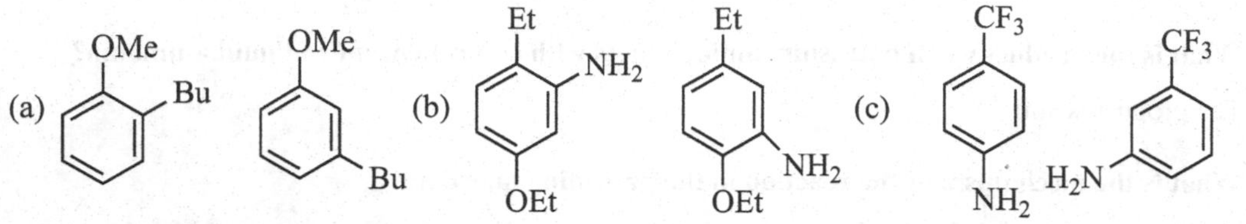

16.5 REDUCTION OF BENZENE AND BENZENE DERIVATIVES

What is the product formed when benzene is treated with $LiAlH_4$ in THF?

There is no reaction. Hydride reagents such as $LiAlH_4$ do not react with benzene.

What is the product formed when each of the following reacts first with $LiAlH_4$ in THF and then with dilute aqueous acid? (a) ethyl benzoate; (b) benzophenone; (c) N-methylbenzamide; (d) phenol.

The reduction of ethyl benzoate in (a) gives benzyl alcohol ($PhCH_2OH$) and ethanol. The reduction of benzophenone in (b) gives 1-phenylethan-1-ol, $PhCH(OH)CH_3$. The reduction of N-methylbenzamide in (c) gives N-phenylmethanamine ($PhNHCH_3$). The reaction of phenol with $LiAlH_4$ gives only the acid–base reaction and the product is phenoxide, PhO^-Li^+.

What is the product in the following reactions when each is reacted with hydrogen gas in ethanol in the presence of a palladium on carbon catalyst: (a) benzonitrile + 2 equivalents H_2; (b) 4-methylbenzaldehyde + 1 equivalent H_2; (c) 3-bromostyrene + 1 equivalent H_2; (d) 1-phenylbut-1-yne + 2 equivalents H_2?

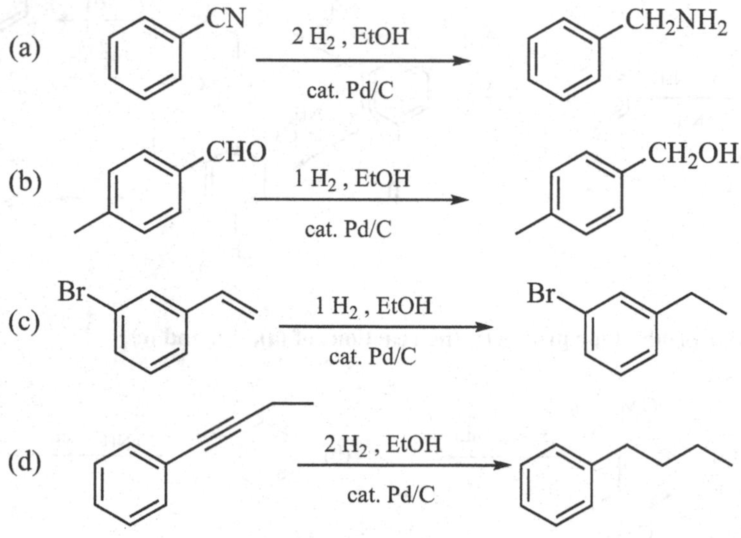

(a) CN —(2 H_2, EtOH; cat. Pd/C)→ CH_2NH_2

(b) CHO —(1 H_2, EtOH; cat. Pd/C)→ CH_2OH

(c) Br —(1 H_2, EtOH; cat. Pd/C)→ Br

(d) —(2 H_2, EtOH; cat. Pd/C)→

The hydrogenation of benzonitrile in (a) leads to reduction of the nitrile group and the product is benzylamine. In (b) selective reduction of the aldehyde unit of 4-methylbenzaldehyde leads to 4-methylbenzyalcohol. In (c) the alkene unit is selective hydrogenation and the product is 3-bromoethlbenzene. Selective reduction of the alkyne unit in (d) leads to butylbenzene.

What is the product when benzene reacts with an excess of hydrogen gas in ethanol in the presence of a palladium on carbon catalyst? What is the product when 1,3-dimethylbenzene reacts with an excess of hydrogen gas in ethanol in the presence of a palladium on carbon catalyst?

The hydrogenation of benzene with an excess of hydrogen leads to cyclohexane. Similar hydrogenation of 1,3-dimethylbenzene leads to 1,3-dimethylcyclohexane.

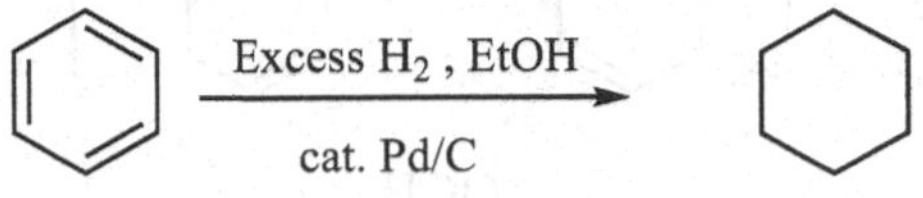

Excess H_2 , EtOH

cat. Pd/C

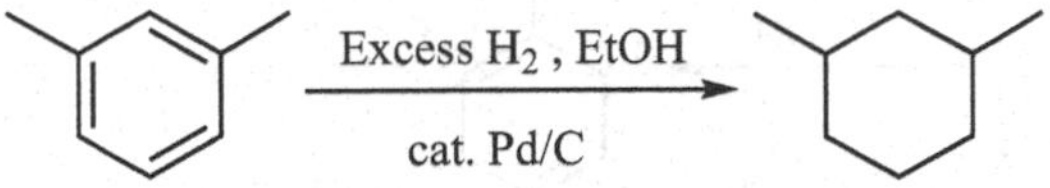

Excess H_2 , EtOH

cat. Pd/C

What is the product when benzene reacts with sodium metal in liquid ammonia and ethanol?

The product is cyclohexa-1,4-diene as shown.

Na , liquid NH_3

EtOH

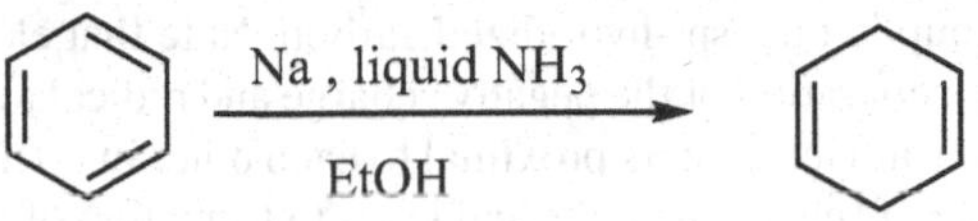

Why is liquid ammonia used?

Ammonia is a gas at ambient temperature. To liquify ammonia so it can be used in this reaction, the reaction is cooled to at least –33°C where it condenses to a blue liquid. In all of these reactions, liquid ammonia is used so the reaction is done at or below –33°C.

What name is associated with this reaction?

This reaction is known as a *dissolving metal reduction*, but the common name associated with this reduction is *Birch reduction*. Also see Sections 14.2 and 14.4.

Why is ethanol added to this reaction?

The ethanol is more acidic than ammonia in this system where a radical carbanion is formed as the intermediate. The ethanol is there to facilitate the required acid–base reaction of the carbanion intermediate.

What is the product when anisole reacts with sodium metal in liquids ammonia and ethanol?

The product is 1-methoxycyclohexa-1,4-diene, as shown.

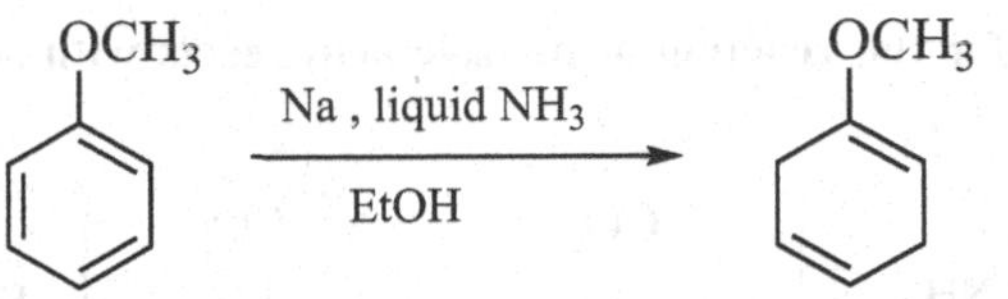

OCH_3

Na , liquid NH_3

EtOH

OCH_3

What is the product when benzoic acid reacts with sodium metal in liquids ammonia and ethanol?

The product is 1-carboxycyclohexa-2,5-diene, as shown.

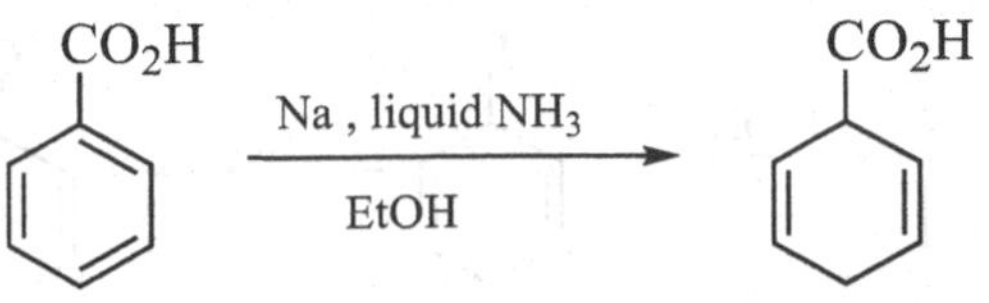

CO_2H

Na , liquid NH_3

EtOH

CO_2H

What is the mechanism for the reaction of anisole reacts with sodium metal in liquids ammonia and ethanol?

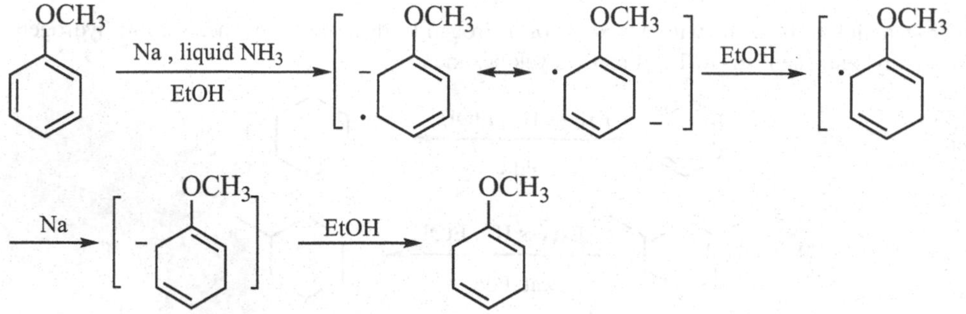

Initial reaction with sodium leads to a one-electron transfer and formation of a resonance-stabilized radical anion. Two resonance contributors are shown with the negative charge and radical *not* on the carbon bearing the electron rich oxygen of the OCH_3 group. In other words, these resonance contributors are formed so that the OCH_3 group is on a sp^2-hybridized carbon. Note that electronic repulsion of the two electron-rich centers leads to separation of the negative charge and radical to the more stable 1,4-position rather than having those electron-rich centers proximal to each other in a 1,2-position. This charge separation sets the 1,4-relationship of the alkene units and leads to formation of the final cyclohexa-1,4-diene product. An acid–base reaction with ethanol, which is a strong acid in the medium, leads to protonation of the carbanion and formation of the radical shown. A second reaction with sodium leads to another carbanion, which rapidly reacts with ethanol to give the final product, 1-methoxycyclohexa-1,4-diene.

Why does the OCH_3 group in the preceding question reside on a sp^2-carbon in the final product?

In the radical anon intermediate required for conversion to the methoxy derivative with the OCH_3 group on a sp^3-carbon, the negative charge is on the carbon that bears the electron releasing (δ–) oxygen. The proximity of the two like-charges is very destabilizing relative to the radical anion shown in the mechanism, so the final product is 1-methoxycyclohexa-1,4-diene rather than 1-methoxyccylcohexa-2,5-diene, with the OCH_3 group on a sp^2-hyridized carbon.

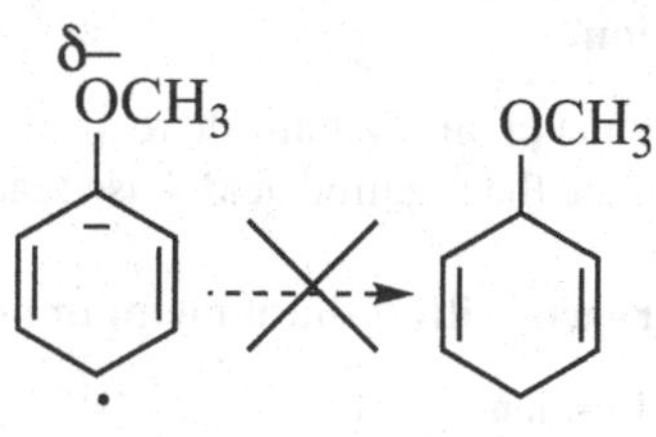

What is the mechanism for the reaction of benzoic acid reacts with sodium metal in liquids ammonia and ethanol?

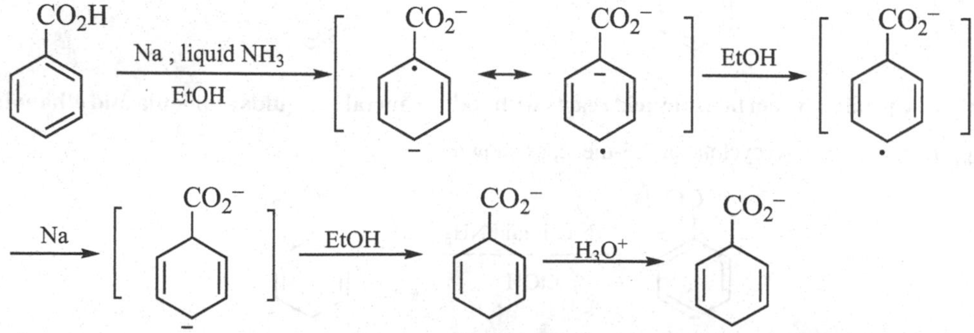

The first reaction is an acid–base reaction to deprotonate the carboxylic acid unit to give the carboxylate anion (CO_2^-). Note that at the end of the reaction treatment with dilute aqueous acid is required to regenerate the carboxylic acid. Initial reaction with sodium leads to a one-electron transfer and formation of a resonance-stabilized radical anion. Two resonance contributors are shown with the negative charge and radical on the carbon bearing the electrophilic carbon of the CO_2^- group. In other words, these resonance contributors are formed so that the CO_2^- group is on a sp^3-hybridized carbon. Note that electronic repulsion of the two electron-rich centers leads to separation of the negative charge and radical to the more stable 1,4-position rather than having those electron rich centers proximal to each other in a 1,2-position. This charge separation sets the 1,4-relationship of the alkene units and leads to formation of the final cyclohexa-1,4-diene product. An acid–base reaction with ethanol, which is a strong acid in the medium, leads to production of the carbanion and formation of the radical shown. A second reaction with sodium leads to another carbanion, which rapidly reacts with ethanol to give the final product, 1-carboxycyclohexa-2,5-diene.

Why does the CO_2H group in the preceding question reside on a sp^3-carbon in the final product?

In the radical anon intermediate required for conversion to the carboxylate derivative with the COO^- group on a sp^3 carbon, the negative charge is on the carbon that bears the electron-withdrawing (δ^+) carboxyl carbon. The proximity of the two opposite charges is much less stabilizing relative to the radical anion shown in the mechanism where the two opposite charges have the maximum attraction when they are adjacent to one another. Therefore, the final product is 1-carboxycyclohexa-2,5-diene rather than 1-carboxycyclohexa-1,4-diene, with the COOH group on a sp^3-hybridized carbon.

$\delta+$ CO_2^- CO_2^-

16.6 POLYCYCLIC AROMATIC COMPOUNDS AND HETEROAROMATIC COMPOUNDS

What are the structures of naphthalene, anthracene, and phenanthrene?

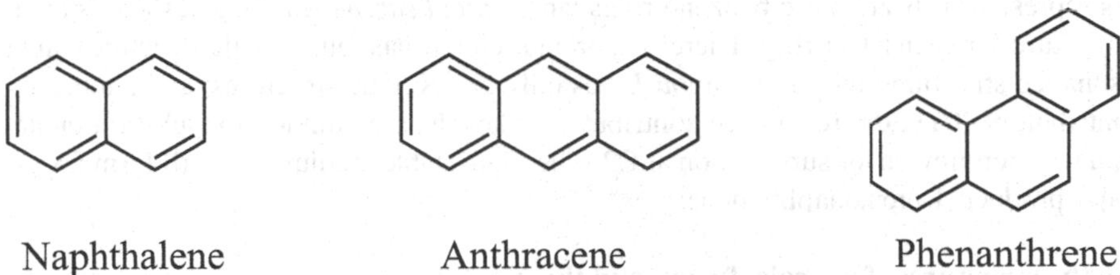

Naphthalene Anthracene Phenanthrene

Do polycyclic aromatic compounds react via S_EAr reactions?

Yes!

What is the major product when naphthalene reacts with $Br_2/FeBr_3$?

The major product is 1-bromonaphthalene. There are only two possible products, bromination at C1 or at C2, and C1 bromination is strongly referred.

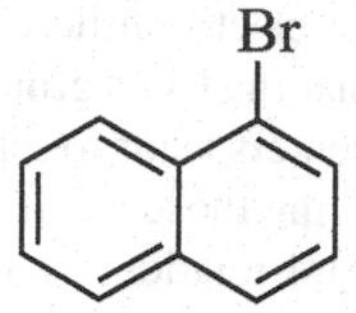

Br

1-Bromonaphthalene

Why does the reaction in the preceding question give 1-bromonaphthalene rather than 2-bromonaphthalene as the major product?

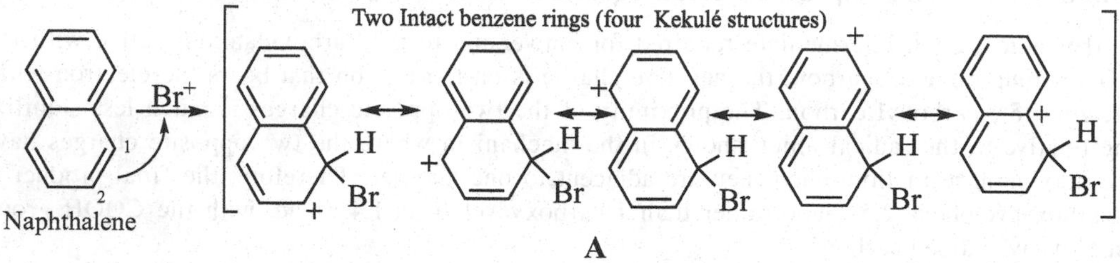

Two Intact benzene rings (four Kekulé structures)

Naphthalene

A

One Intact benzene ring (two Kekulé structures)

Naphthalene

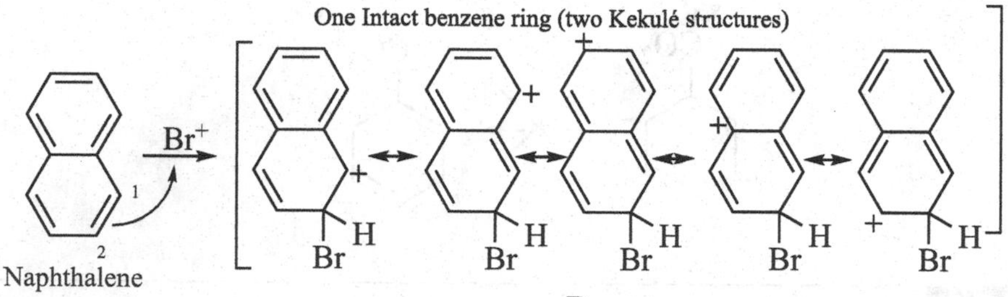

B

Bromination of naphthalene at C1 leads to arenium ion ***A*** with five resonance structures. A similar reaction at C2 yields arenium ion ***B***, which also has the five resonance structures shown. However, note that arenium ions ***A*** and ***B*** each have one or two Kekulé structures as resonance contributors. These Kekulé structures represent fully aromatic benzene rings (an "*intact benzene ring*"), and there is an additional Kekulé structure for each intact ring. Therefore, arenium ion ***A*** has four Kekulé structures and a total of seven resonance structures, but arenium ion ***B*** has only two Kekulé structures, and a total of six resonance contributors. The extra resonance contributor makes the arenium ion for substitution at C1 more stable than the arenium ion for substitution at C2. The more stable arenium ion will form faster and lead to the major product, 1-bromonaphthalene.

What are the structures of pyrrole, furan, and thiophene?

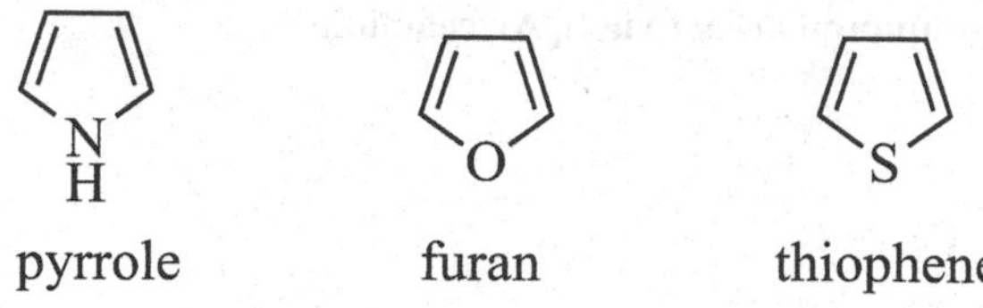

The nitrogen atom of pyrrole is not very basic. Why?

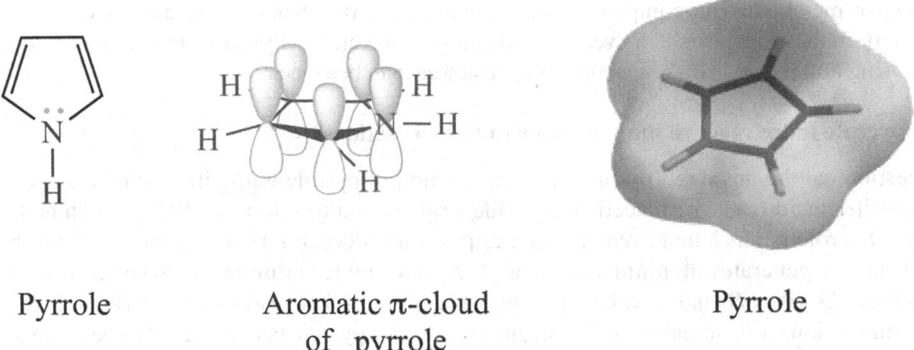

Pyrrole Aromatic π-cloud of pyrrole Pyrrole

Pyrrole is a secondary amine, but it is not very basic. The nitrogen of pyrrole must donate its electron pair to a proton to react as a Brønsted–Lowry base, but that electron pair is "tied up" in the aromatic π-cloud, and so are not available for donation. If pyrrole reacts as a base and donates two electrons, the aromaticity of the ring must be disrupted. The electron density map for pyrrole shows the concentration of electron density (dark gray shaded area) above and below the ring, and *not* on the nitrogen atom. The hydrogen atom on the nitrogen of pyrrole is actually somewhat acidic, with a pK_a of 17.5 in water. Note the light gray color to the left, which indicates low electron density.

Can the basicity of pyrrole be compared with furan and thiophene?

In furan, one of the two electron pairs on oxygen is involved in the aromatic π-cloud (those two electrons are needed to make a total of six), but the other lone electron pair is perpendicular to the π-cloud. Therefore, furan can function as a base and it should be a *stronger* base than pyrrole because of the availability of those electrons. A similar argument can be made for thiophene, but the lessened electron density of sulfur makes thiophene a weaker base than furan.

What is the structure of pyridine? How basic is pyridine?

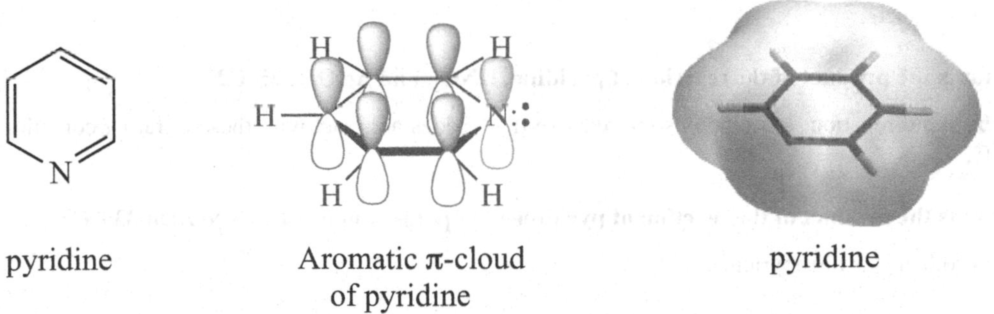

pyridine Aromatic π-cloud of pyridine pyridine

Pyridine is aromatic, so it is a planar compound with an aromatic π-cloud above and below the plane of the ring. The nitrogen atom is sp^2-hybridized, but the lone electron pair on nitrogen is *not* part of the aromatic π-cloud. That electron pair is perpendicular to that π-cloud, as shown, so it is available for donation in acid–base reactions. This fact means that, unlike pyrrole, pyridine is a good Brønsted–Lowry and Lewis base because the electron pair is readily available for donation without disrupting the aromaticity. The electron density map of pyridine clearly shows a high concentration of electron density (dark shaded area) on the nitrogen.

Can the heterocyclic compounds in the preceding questions be evaluated as more or less reactive than benzene in S_EAr reactions?

Yes! The five-membered ring compounds are much more reactive than benzene and are considered to be *activated* aromatic rings. Pyrrole is very reactive in S_EAr reactions. Pyridine, however, is a *deactivated* aromatic ring and reacts in S_EAr reactions much slower than benzene.

Why is pyrrole more reactive than benzene in S_EAr reactions?

This question can be answered by the nitration reaction of pyrrole with nitric acid/acetic anhydride. Note that nitric acid reacts with acetic anhydride to give the nitronium ion, NO_2^+, which is the nitrating agent. Pyrrole is much more reactive and requires a milder nitration reagent relative to benzene. Reaction at C2 generates arenium ion ***A***, with a very stable iminium ion resonance contributor. Reactions at C3 gives ***B***, and also has a very stable iminium ion resonance contributor. These very stable iminium ions are, arguably, a significant reason why pyrrole is considered to be more activated than benzene. The ability to form stable arenium ions contributes to the electron-donating ability of pyrrole in S_EAr reactions, making pyrrole very reactive and activated. Note that reaction at C2 generates an arenium ion with three resonance contributors (***A***) whereas reaction at C3 gives an arenium ion with only two resonance contributors (***B***). Therefore, pyrrole is expected to give the C2 substituted product as the major product.

What is the major product of the reaction of pyrrole with nitric acid/acetic anhydride?

The product is 2-nitropyrrole.

Is C2 substitution in S_EAr reactions also expected with furan and thiophene?

Yes! Pyrrole, furan, and thiophene all react in S_EAr reactions to give the C2 substituted product as the major product.

What is the product of the reaction of pyridine, HNO_3, and Ac_2O at 25°C?

There is no reaction. Pyridine is so unreactive that it does not react with these nitrating conditions at 25°C.

What is the product of the reaction of pyridine with potassium nitrate (KNO_3) at 330°C?

The product is 3-nitropyridine.

Why does a S_EAr reaction with pyridine gives the 3-substitued product?

Potassium nitrate is a nitrating agent, and reaction with pyridine at C2 gives arenium ion ***A***. Likewise, reaction at C2 gives ***B*** and reaction at C4 gives ***C***. Note that reaction at C2 and C4 generates a resonance contributor with the positive charge on nitrogen, which is particularly unstable. Reaction at C3 generates an arenium ion, ***B***, with a positive charge in the ring but it is not possible to form a stable iminium ion, though this ion is much more stable than ***A*** or ***C***. Therefore, the more stable arenium ion ***C*** is formed faster and leads to the product, 3-nitropyridine. *Note that all S_EAr reactions of pyridine give the 3-substituted product.*

pyridine $\xrightarrow[330\ °C]{KNO_3}$ [A] [B] [C] → 3-Nitropyridine

What products are formed in reactions (a), (b), (c), and (d)?

(a) pyrrole $\xrightarrow{SOCl_2}$

(b) furan $\xrightarrow{HNO_3,\ Ac_2O}$

(c) thiophene $\xrightarrow{N\text{-bromosuccinimide}}$

(d) pyridine $\xrightarrow[300\ °C]{Br_2}$

In (a) thionyl chloride is a chlorinating reagent, which gives 2-chloropyrrole. In (b) the nitrating reagent gives 2-nitrofuran. (c) *N*-bromosuccinimide reacts to give 2-bromothiophene. At 300°C, pyridine react with bromine to give 3-bromopyridine.

(a) 2-chloropyrrole (b) 2-nitrofuran (c) 2-bromothiophene (d) 3-bromopyridine

What is the product formed when pyridine reacts with $NaNH_2$ at 100°C?

The product is pyridine-2-amine (2-aminopyridine).

pyridine $\xrightarrow{NaNH_2,\ 100\ °C}$ pyridin-2-amine

What is the mechanism of the reaction given in the preceding question?

The mechanism is S_NAr, and it is the only S_NAr reaction that will be discussed for heterocyclic compounds in this book. Reaction with ammonia generates the intermediate ***A***, and loss of the leaving group bromine gives the product, pyridine-2-amine

2-Bromopyridine $\xrightarrow{NH_3}$ [**A**] $\xrightarrow[-\ H^+]{-\ Br^-}$ Pyridin-2-amine (2-aminopyridine)

What is the name of the reaction in the preceding question?

This reaction is known as the *Chichibabin reaction.*

What is the structure of indole? Of quinoline? Of isoquinoline?

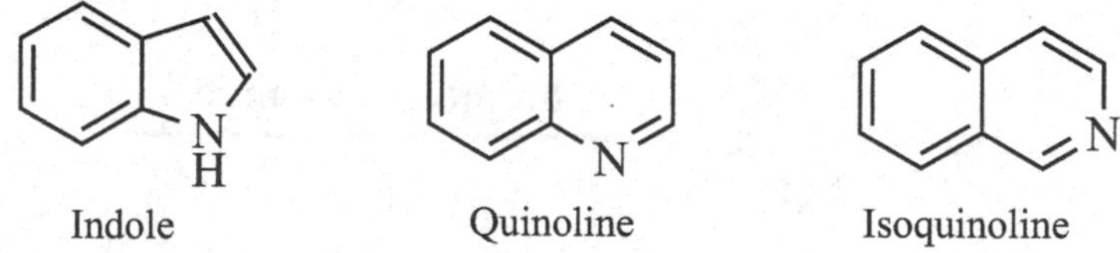

Indole Quinoline Isoquinoline

For a S_EAr reaction of indole, does substitution occur in the five-membered ring or the six-membered ring?

Reaction will occur in the activated five-membered ring, at C3.

Why does reaction occur at the five-membered ring unit of indole?

The pyrrole unit is more reactive (more activated) than the benzene ring unit of indole.

END OF CHAPTER PROBLEMS

1. Which of the following are aromatic?

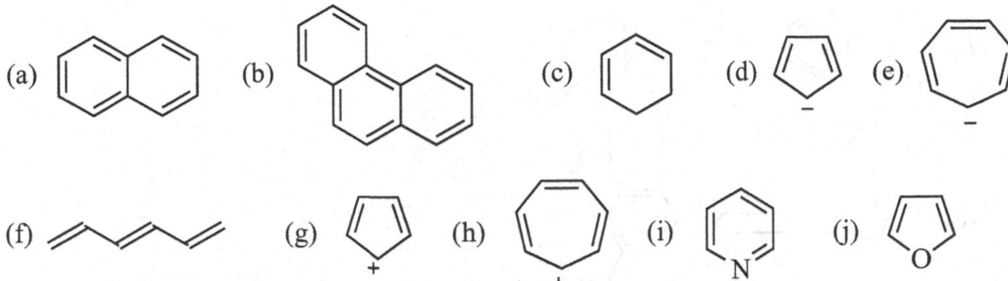

2. Draw all Kekulé structures for the following molecules:

(a) —CH_3 (b) (c)

3. Give the correct IUPAC name for each of the following:

(a) OH, Cl, Cl (b) NO_2, NO_2 (c) (d) CO_2H

(e) Cl, Cl, Cl, Cl, Cl, Cl (f) OH (g) $NHCH_3$ (h) Br, SO_3H

4. Why is methyl considered to be an activating group in electrophilic aromatic substitution?
5. Draw all resonance contributors for the reaction product of Br^+ and *N* acetylaniline when the aromatic ring reacts to place Br+ at the ortho- position.
6. How can a pure sample of ortho-chlorotoluene be obtained from the reaction of chlorine, toluene, and aluminum chloride?
7. Give the IUPAC name for each of the following:

(a) CO_2H, C_4H_9, C_4H_9 (b) CO_2Me (c) O, Cl, Ph, Ph (d) O, NH_2, Br

8. Why does the nitration of anisole give more ortho- product than does the nitration of toluene under similar reaction conditions?

9. Provide a suitable synthesis for each of the following. Give all intermediate products and show all reagents. Do not give mechanistic intermediates.

(a) 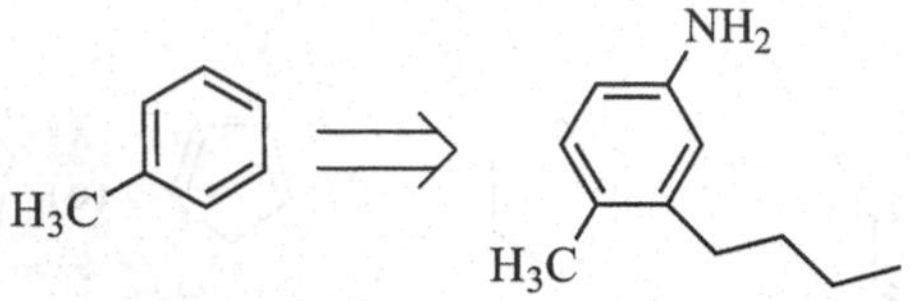 H_3C ⟹ NH_2 H_3C

(b) 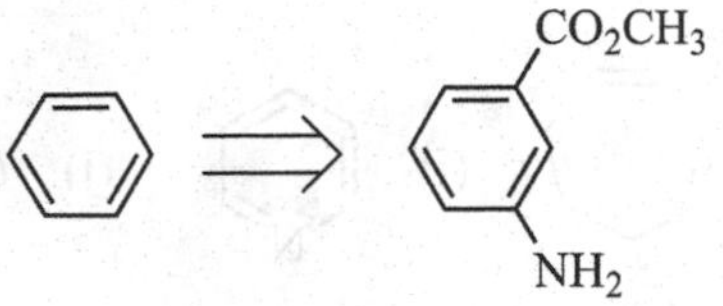 ⟹ CO_2CH_3 NH_2

(c) 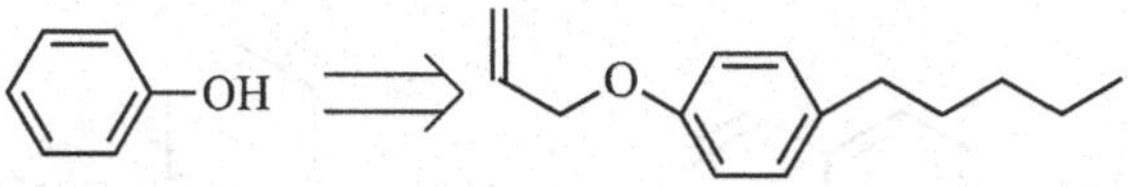 OH ⟹ O

10. For each reaction give the major product. If there is no reaction, indicate by N.R.

(a) 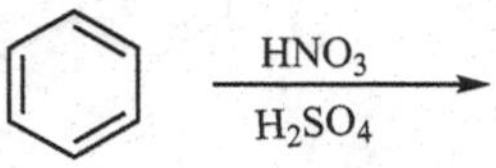 $\xrightarrow[H_2SO_4]{HNO_3}$

(b) $\xrightarrow[AlCl_3]{Et_3CCl}$

(c) $\xrightarrow{Cl_2\text{ , }FeBr_3}$

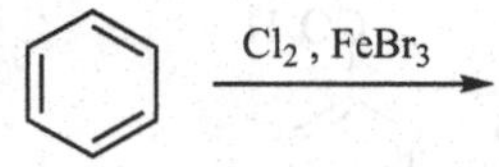

(d) Br $\xrightarrow[AlCl_3]{}$

(e) OCH_3 $\xrightarrow[H_2SO_4]{HNO_3}$

(f) C_3H_7 OCH_3 $\xrightarrow[SO_3]{H_2SO_4}$

(g) NH_2 $\xrightarrow[\text{2. }Br_2\text{ , }FeBr_3]{\text{1. }Ac_2O\text{ , }NEt_3}$

(h) $\xrightarrow[AlCl_3]{\text{pentanoyl chloride}}$

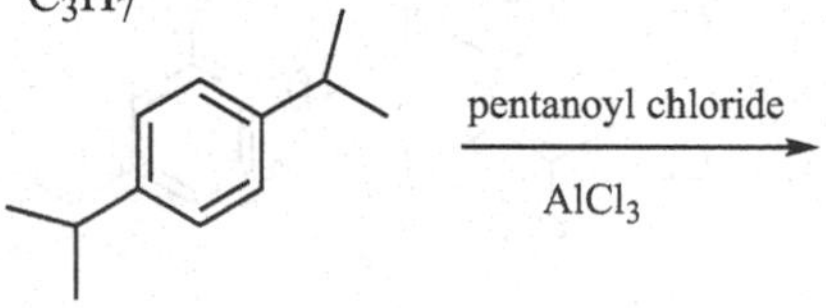

(i) 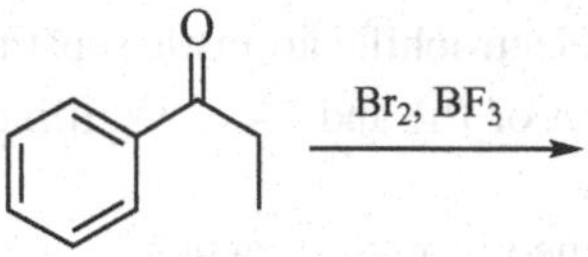 O $\xrightarrow{Br_2\text{, }BF_3}$

(j) 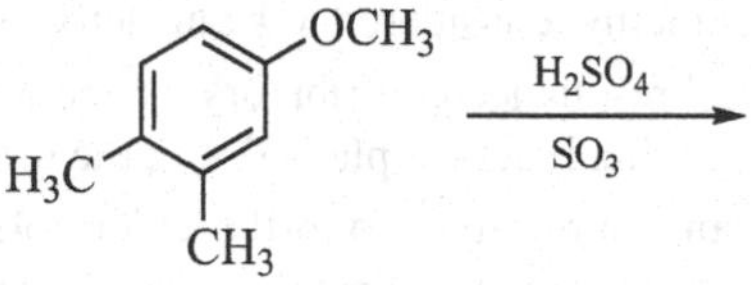 OCH_3 H_3C CH_3 $\xrightarrow[SO_3]{H_2SO_4}$

(k) 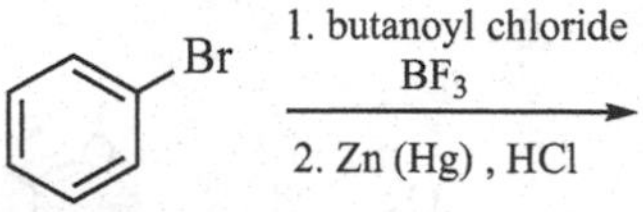 Br $\xrightarrow[\text{2. Zn (Hg) , HCl}]{\text{1. butanoyl chloride } BF_3}$

(l) 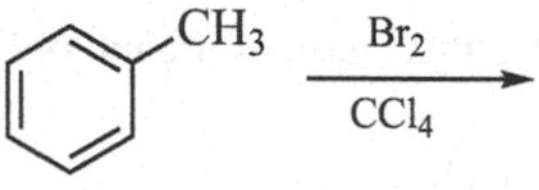 CH_3 $\xrightarrow[CCl_4]{Br_2}$

(m) 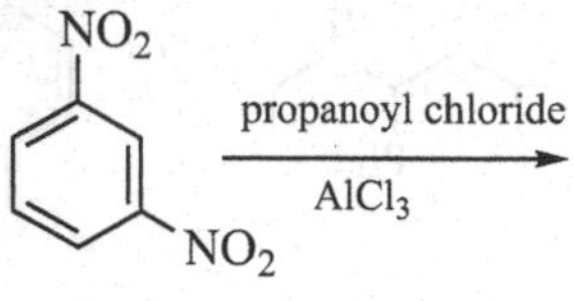 NO_2 NO_2 $\xrightarrow[AlCl_3]{\text{propanoyl chloride}}$

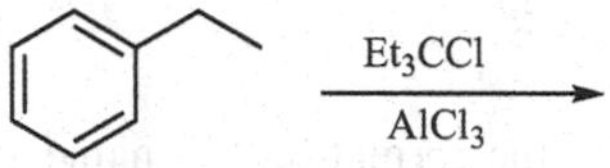

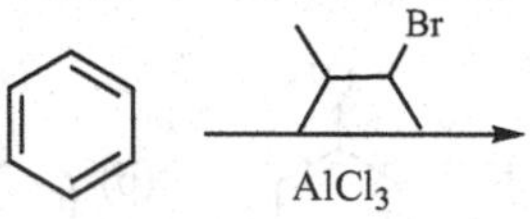

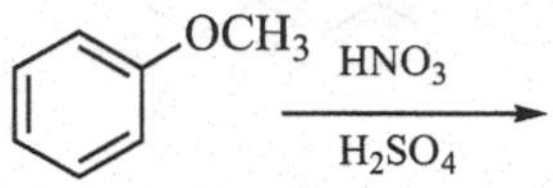

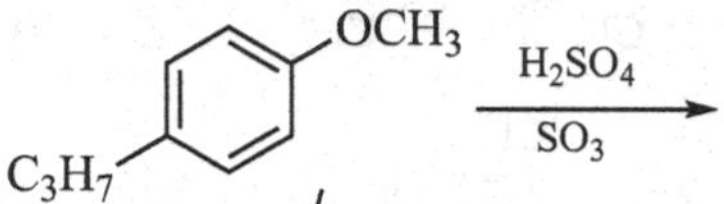

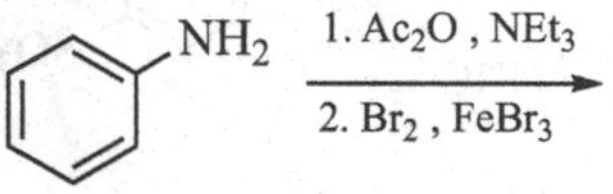

(n) 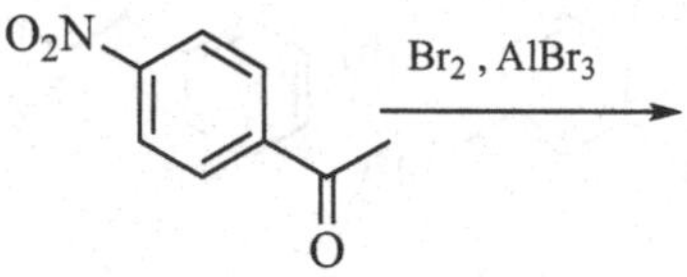 O_2N O $\xrightarrow{Br_2\text{ , }AlBr_3}$

11. What is the product of this reaction? Explain.

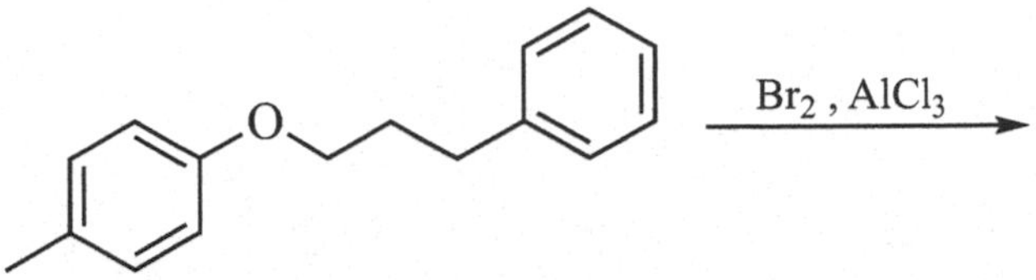

Br_2, $AlCl_3$ →

12. Draw all resonance contributors to the intermediate of the reaction of KOH and 1-bromo-2,4,6-trinitrobenzene.

13. Give a suitable synthesis for each of the following. In each case give all intermediate products and show all reagents that are used.

(a) NHAc, O_2N ⟹

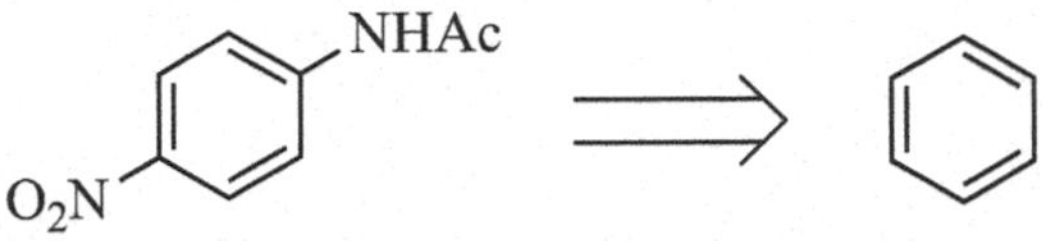

(b) C_4H_9, C_4H_9 ⟹ Br

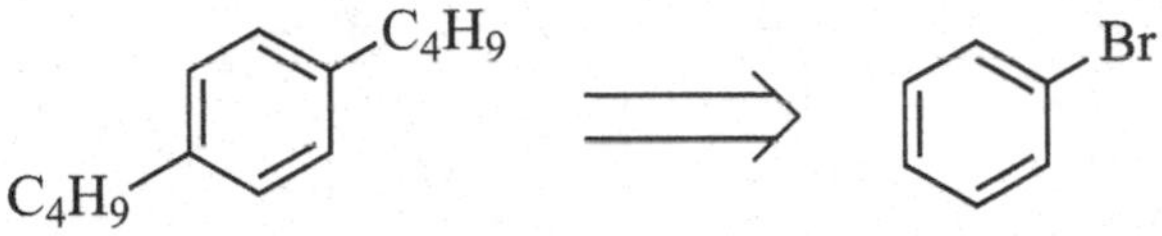

14. Give the major product of each of the following reactions. If there is no reaction, indicate by N.R.

(a) NH_2 —$AlCl_3$→

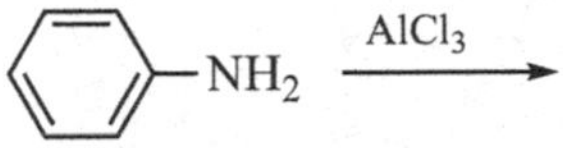

(b) NH_2 —1. $NaNO_2$, HCl; 2. H_2O, reflux→

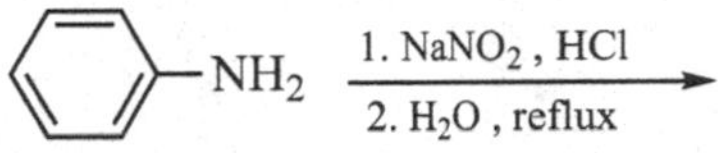

(c) O —$SOCl_2$→

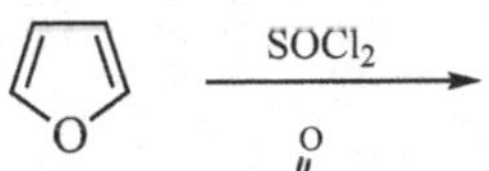

(d) NH_2 —1. Ac_2O; 2. $AlCl_3$, butanoyl chloride; 3. saponification→

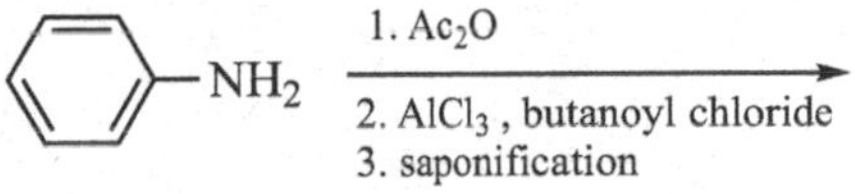

(e) S —N·Cl (O, O); hv→

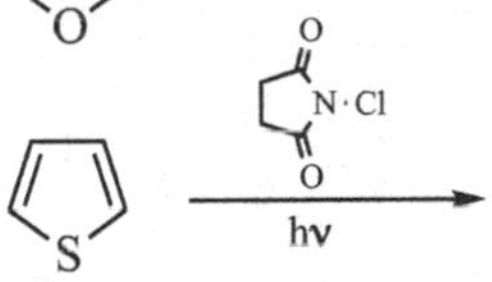

(f) N_2^+ Cl^- —CuBr→

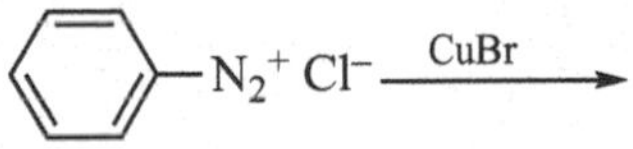

(g) C_4H_9, NO_2 —1. H_2, Pd-C; 2. Ac_2O, pyridine→

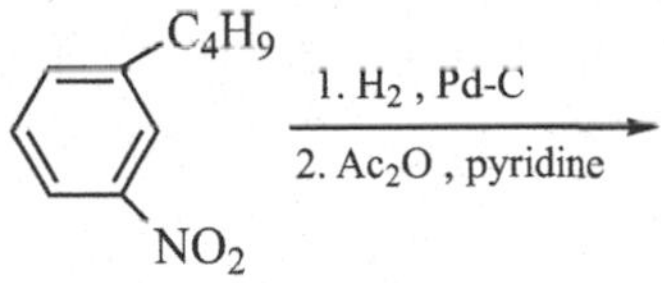

(h) NH_2 —1. $NaNO_2$, HCl; 2. H_3PO_2→

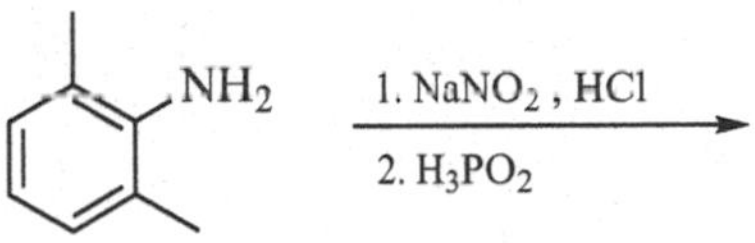

(i) N —Br_2; 300 °C→

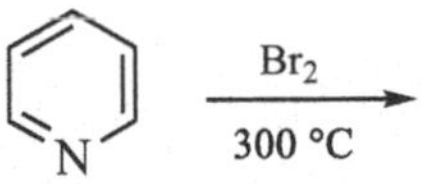

(j) Me, Me, Me, Me, N, Me —Cl_2, AcOH→

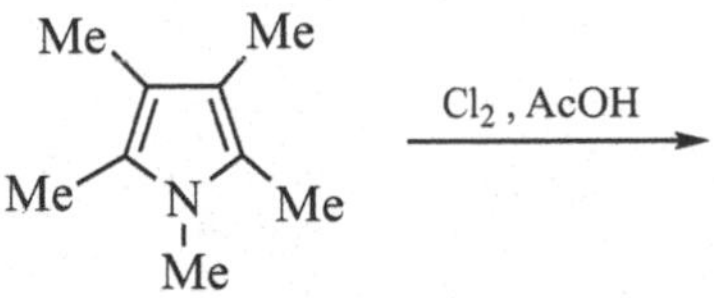

(k) N, Me —HNO_3, AcOH→

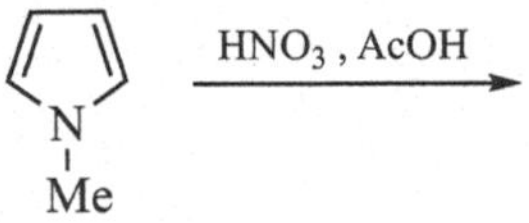

(l) N, H —HNO_3, Ac_2O→

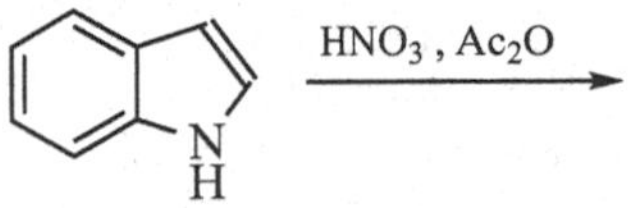

17

Enolate Anions and Condensation Reactions

The carbonyl of ketones, aldehydes, and acid derivative makes the α-hydrogen acidic. This hydrogen can be removed by a suitable base to form an enolate anion, which can react with alkyl halides in an alkylation reaction or with carbonyl derivatives in a condensation reaction.

17.1 ALDEHYDES, KETONES, ENOLS, AND ENOLATE ANIONS

What is the α-carbon in a ketone or aldehyde?

The α-carbon is the carbon adjacent to a carbonyl group. An α-hydrogen is a hydrogen atom attached to the α-carbon. The α-hydrogen is polarized δ^+ due to the electron-withdrawing effects of the carbonyl oxygen.

What is the pK_a of the hydrogen on the carbon attached to a carbonyl?

The pK_a of this hydrogen is generally in the range 19–22.

Why is this hydrogen acidic?

The electron-withdrawing carbon group of the carbonyl induces a δ^+ charge on the α-hydrogen, making it susceptible to attack by a base. In addition, most ketones and aldehydes are in equilibrium with an enol (see the following question), which has an acidic O—H moiety.

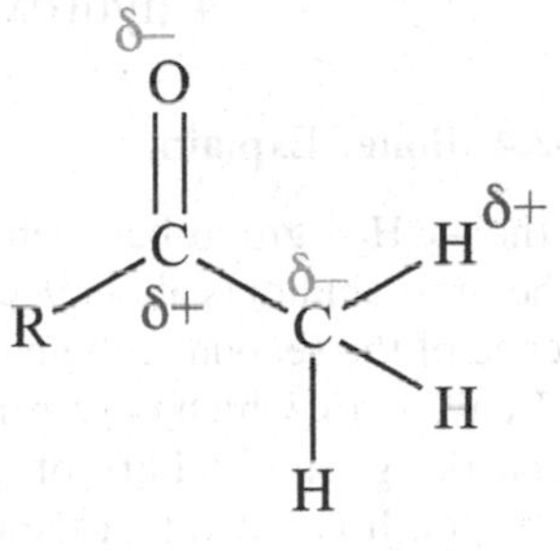

δ–
O
C
δ+
R
δ–
C
H δ+
H
H

What is an enol?

An enol is a molecule that has an OH group directly attached to a carbon–carbon double bond, as shown.

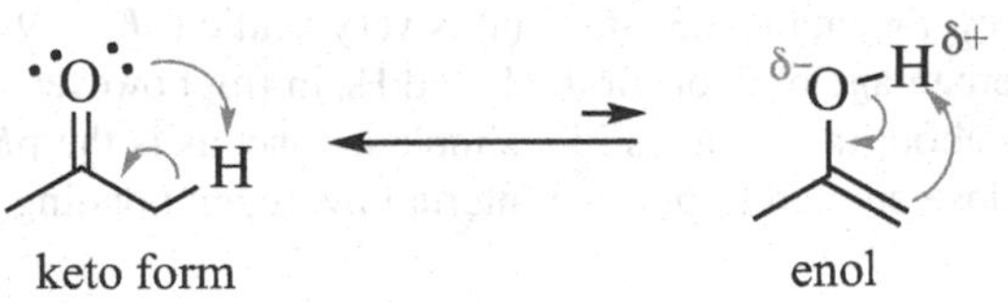

O
H
keto form
δ- O-H δ+
enol

What is keto-enol tautomerism?

Most ketones and aldehydes (the carbonyl form) are in equilibrium with an enol form shown in the preceding question. Indeed, the keto form and the enol form are in equilibrium in what is known as *keto-enol tautomerism.* In most aldehydes and ketones that are not functionalized the equilibrium favors the carbonyl partner to a very great extent (often >99% of the keto form). In other words, a ketone or aldehyde is expected to exist primarily in the carbonyl form. This equilibrium occurs when the acidic α-hydrogen is removed by the basic carbonyl oxygen, forming the enol. The reverse reaction has the less basic alkene π-bond removing the acidic hydrogen from the O—H, regenerating the carbonyl.

When the α-carbon is substituted, what is the effect on the acidity of that α-proton?

Since a carbon group is electron-releasing, its presence makes the α-hydrogen less acidic (larger pK_a) by about one pK_a unit for each alkyl substituent.

What is the pK_a of propan-2-one (acetone)?

The pK_a of acetone is about 19.3, and it is known that acetone has an enol content of about 1.5×10^{-4} % enol.

What is the pK_a of pentane-3-one?

The pK_a of pentan-3-one is about 20, less acidic than acetone due to the electron-releasing methyl group at is attached to each α-carbon.

What structural features can lead to greater percentages of enol?

If the enol form is stabilized by internal hydrogen bonding, a higher percentage of the enol form will result. This shift occurs primarily when an atom capable of hydrogen bonding (such as an oxygen) is located at the position β-to the carbonyl carbon, as in 1,3-dicarbonyl compounds such as pentane-2,4-dione.

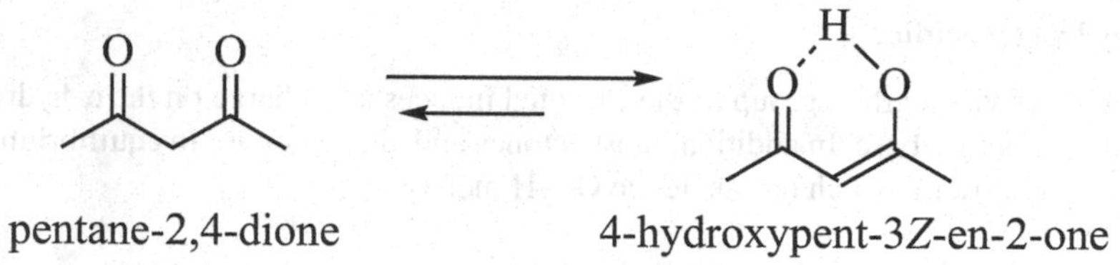

pentane-2,4-dione ⇌ 4-hydroxypent-3*Z*-en-2-one

What is the relative pK_a of pentane-2,4-dione? Explain.

The pK_a of the hydrogen atoms on the $-CH_2-$ group between the carbonyls (the presence of two C=O groups make these hydrogens the most acidic) is about 9, compared with 19.3 for acetone. This increase in acidity is due to the presence of the second carbonyl group that stabilizes the enol tautomer of this ketone (4-hydroxypent-3Z-en-2-one), which is present in >90% in hydrocarbon solvents. Indeed, there is a correlation between the greater acidity of a carbonyl compound and a greater percentage of the enol form at equilibrium. It is noted that the common name of pentane-2,4-dione is acetylacetone.

What is the acidity of H_a in (a) and (b)?

The proton marked H_a in cyclopentane-1,3-dione (a) is very acidic (pK_a ≈ 9–10 due to its proximity to two carbonyls the high percentage of enol. Both H_a and H_b in (b), however, have the same pK_a (≈ 20). The enol content of (b) is about the same as in a simple ketone, as is the pK_a, due to the fact that the carbonyl groups are not close enough to provide internal hydrogen bonding which would stabilize the enol form.

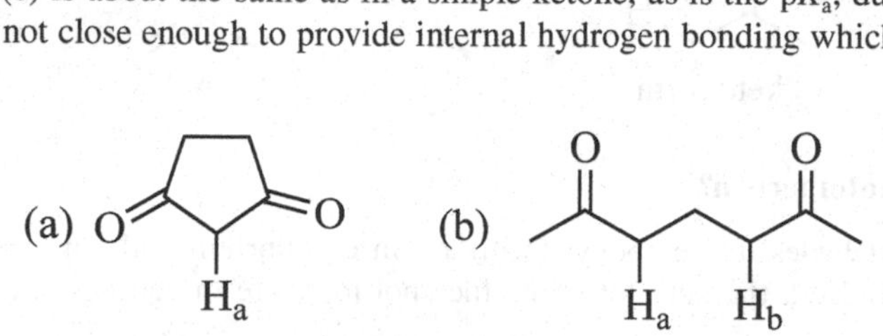

(a) (b)

When the acidic α-proton of a ketone is removed by a suitable base, what is the product?

If one assumes the hydrogen is removed from the enol form of the ketone, the product is an enolate anion, which is a resonance-stabilized anion. There are two resonance contributors to the enolate anion, the carbanion form ***A*** and the alkoxide form ***B***.

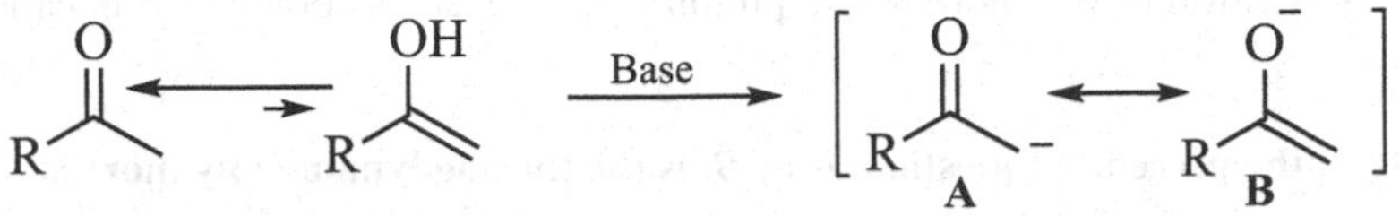

enolate anion

Why is the enolate anion particularly stable and how does this fact contribute to acidity?

Enolate anions are resonance-stabilized, as shown with ***A*** and ***B*** in the preceding question. This stability enhances the equilibrium by shifting the acid–base equilibrium toward the product, the enolate anion, as the proton is removed by base.

What bases are used to remove this acidic proton?

Since the α-proton is a weak acid, the base used to remove that proton must be rather strong. A variety of bases can be used, including NaOEt, NaOH, NaOMe, KO*t*-OBu, and amide bases such as $NaNH_2$, $NaNR_2$ $LiNH_2$, and $LiNR_2$. Note that the conjugate acids of all of these bases (EtOH, MeOH, NH_3, R_2NH, etc.) are relatively weak acids, weaker than the α-proton of a ketone or aldehyde.

What are "non-nucleophilic" bases?

Non-nucleophilic bases are usually amide bases ($^-NR_2$) where the R groups are bulky, and the conjugate acid is much weaker (large pK_a) than the proton of the aldehyde or ketone. The bulky groups cause steric hindrance as the nitrogen approaches a carbon (behaving as a nucleophile) but does not hinder approach to a hydrogen (behaving as a base). Lithium diisopropyl amide [$LiN(iPr)_2$], often abbreviated LDA, is probably the most commonly used non-nucleophilic base.

What is the product when pentane-2,4-dione is reacted with LDA? With sodium ethoxide?

In both cases, the product is the same, enolate ***A*** (as the Li or Na salt, respectively). The presence of the second carbonyl group allows the formation of a third resonance contributor that makes this enolate anion even more stable than that shown of acetone.

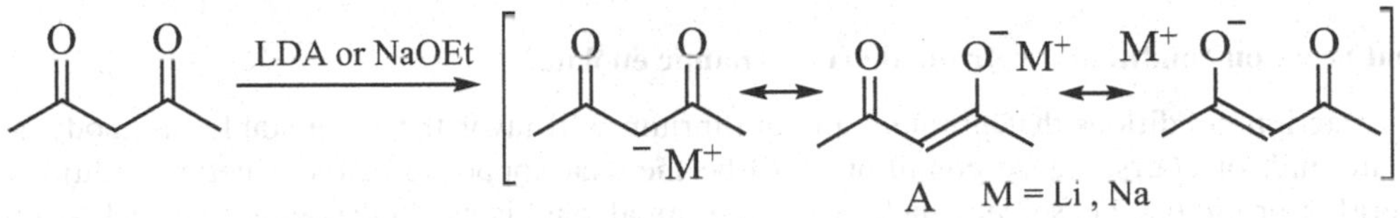

A M = Li , Na

Two different enolate anions are possible from the reaction of butan-2-one and a suitable base. What are they?

Note that butan-2-one is an unsymmetrical ketone. There are two acidic α-protons, H_a and H_b. Removal of H_a generates ***A*** and removal of H_a generates ***B***. When these isomeric enolate anions react, isomeric products can result by reaction of both ***A*** and ***B***.

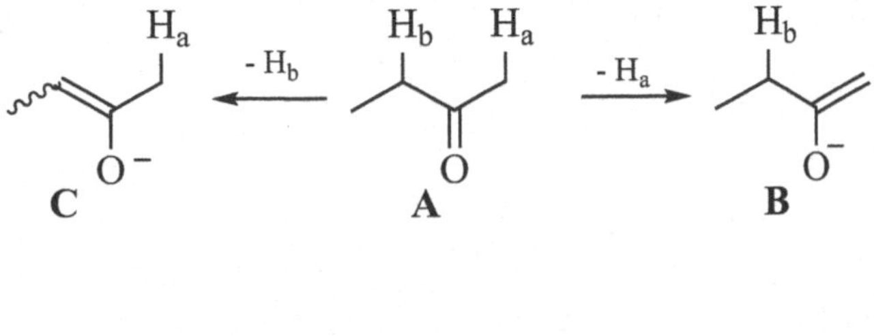

In the preceding question, which enolate is formed by removing the most acidic hydrogen?

Since an alkyl group is electron-releasing, its presence will make the α-proton *less* acidic. The most acidic hydrogen will, therefore, be attached to the *less-substituted carbon*. In the case of butan-2-one, H_a is on the less-substituted carbon and it is the most acidic, leading to enolate anion ***B***. The enolate anion formed by removal of the more acidic proton is the faster reaction and it is called the *kinetic enolate.*

Which enolate in the preceding question, *A* or *B*, is the thermodynamically more stable?

The most stable enolate is the one with the most substituents. In the case of butan-2-one removal of H_b leads to enolate ***C*** with three substituents whereas enolate anion ***B*** by removal of H_a has only two substituents. In this case ***C*** is the most stable enolate. The enolate anion that is the more stable due to greater substitution on the C=C unit is called the *thermodynamic enolate.*

If the most acidic hydrogen is always removed faster and first in an acid–base reaction, how can the thermodynamic enolate ever form?

In the case of butan-2-one, the only way to generate the thermodynamic enolate from the initially formed kinetic enolate is to establish an equilibrium between ***B***, butan-2-one, and ***C***. Since removal of H_a or H_b is an acid–base reaction, which is inherently an equilibrium process, reaction conditions that promote this equilibrium will lead to a preponderance of the thermodynamic enolate, ***C***.

What reaction conditions favor the kinetic enolate?

Since the kinetic enolate is formed faster (and first), and an equilibrium is required for the kinetic enolate to be converted into the thermodynamic enolate, conditions that *disfavor* an equilibrium will favor formation of the kinetic enolate as the major product. In general, these conditions are: a polar, aprotic solvent (no acidic proton is available to reprotonate the enolate once it is formed); low temperatures (0 to −78°C are typical, which makes the proton transfer required for an equilibrium much slower); a strong base such as LDA which removes the proton in a fast reaction and, most importantly, that *does not produce a conjugate acid with an acidic proton that is more acidic than the proton on the aldehyde or ketone.* If NaOEt is used, EtOH is the conjugate acid ($pK_a \approx 17$), which is a stronger acid than the starting carbonyl compound, so it is strong enough to reprotonate the enolate. If LDA is used, however, the conjugate acid is diisopropylamine ($pK_a \approx 25$), which is a weaker acid that the starting carbonyl compound, so it is not a strong enough acid to quickly reprotonate the enolate anion. Short reaction times also favor the kinetic enolate.

What reaction conditions favor the thermodynamic enolate?

Any reaction conditions that promote an equilibrium will favor the more stable thermodynamic enolate and, of course, those conditions will be the exact opposite of the kinetic conditions. In general, a protic (acidic) solvent such as water or an alcohol is used (also an amine such as ethylamine or ammonia) since these compounds are more acidic than the starting carbonyl compound, so the acidic proton can react with the enolate anion to regenerate the starting carbonyl compound, which promotes the equilibrium. A base that generates a conjugate acid that is stronger than the acidic proton of the aldehyde or ketone (NaOEt, NaOH, etc.) will also favor thermodynamic control. Higher reaction temperatures (heating to reflux for example) will promote the equilibrium, and longer reaction times also favor the equilibrium and formation of the thermodynamic enolate anion.

What is the major enolate anion product from the reactions of (a), (b), and (c)? Are each of the reactions under kinetic or thermodynamic control?

(a) NaOEt , EtOH / reflux

(b) LDA , THF / -78 °C

(c) NaOMe , MeOH / reflux

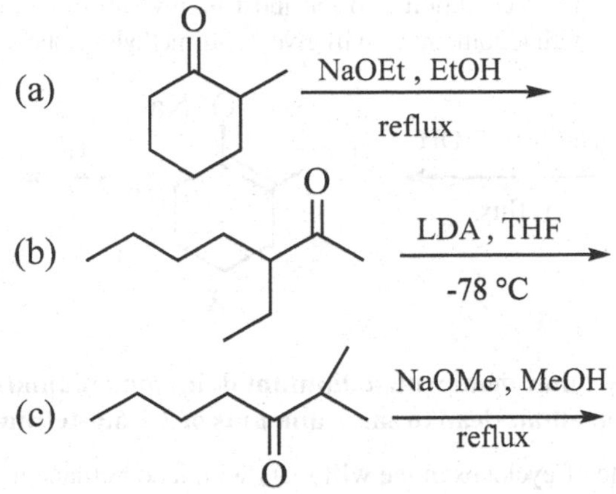

The thermodynamic conditions in (a) lead to the more highly substituted enolate anion, the thermodynamic enolate anion. The kinetic control conditions of (b) give the kinetic enolate anion but the thermodynamic control conditions of (c) give the thermodynamic enolate anion.

(a) O^-Na^+ (b) O^-Li^+ (c) O^-Na^+

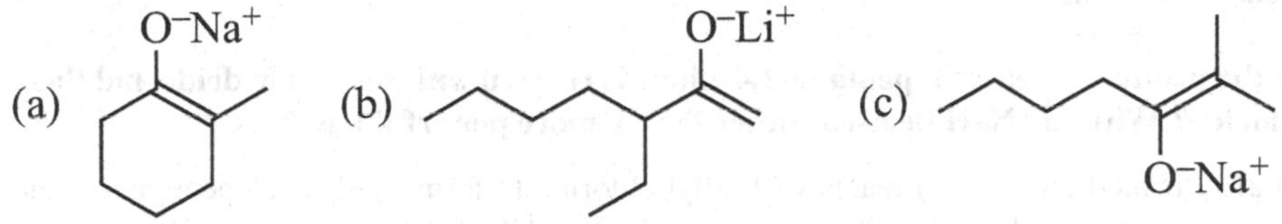

17.2 ENOLATE ALKYLATION

What type of reagents are enolate anions expected to react with?

Both the carbon and the oxygen of an enolate anion are nucleophilic and expected to react with suitable electrophilic electrophiles. For the most part, enolate anions react at carbon with the electrophilic carbon of alkyl halides, epoxides, or carbonyl compounds to give the α-coupling product.

Are there substrates that react with enolate anions at the oxygen rather than the carbon?

Yes! Enolate anions react at oxygen with the silicon of silyl halides (e.g., R_3SiCl) or the acyl carbon of anhydrides to give the vinyl alkoxy product. These reactions will not be discussed further in this book.

When the kinetic enolate derived from pentan-2-one is reacted with bromobutane, what is the major product?

The product is nonan-4-one. The reaction with LDA generates the less-substituted, kinetic enolate anion shown, and a S_N2 reaction with bromobutane gives the product, nonan-4-one.

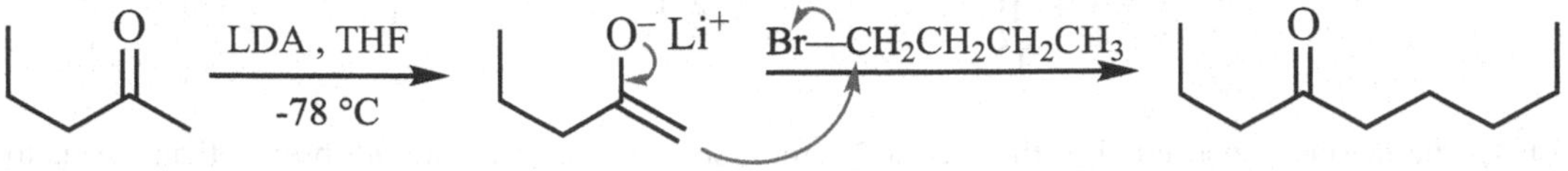

LDA , THF / -78 °C → $O^-\ Li^+$ — $Br\text{—}CH_2CH_2CH_2CH_3$ →

When 2-methylcyclohexanone reacts with sodium ethoxide in ethanol and then with iodomethane, what is the expected major product?

These are thermodynamic control conditions, so the most highly substituted enolate will form, enolate anion *A*. Subsequent reaction with iodomethane will give 2,2-dimethylcyclohexanone as the major product.

NaOEt , EtOH reflux → **A** (O⁻ Na⁺) → CH_3I →

How does the reaction of cyclohexanone with sodium amide in ammonia and subsequent treatment with a large excess of iodomethane lead to small amounts of 2,2,6,6-tetramethylcyclohexanone?

The initially formed enolate of cyclohexanone will react with iodomethane to form 2-methylcyclohexanone. This ketone can react with more $NaNH_2$ to form the thermodynamic enolate anion and subsequent reaction with iodomethane will give 2,2-dimethylcyclohexanone. Since there are additional α-protons, deprotonation-methylation can occur sequentially to produce 2,2,6,6-tetramethylcyclohexanone. This over-methylation will occur only with excess iodomethane and under thermodynamic control conditions with a relatively strong base.

What is the product when cyclopentane-2,4-dione is reacted with sodium hydride and then with allyl chloride? Why can NaH be used rather than a more powerful base?

The initially formed enolate (*A*) reacts with allyl chloride to form 2-allylcyclopentane-1,3-dione. The presence of two carbonyls makes the proton on the "middle" $-CH_2-$ moiety very acidic ($pK_a \approx 9$). Therefore, a much weaker base such as NaH can be used for the deprotonation. Note that NaH reacts as a base to give 0.5 equivalents of H_2 and the enolate anion, *A*.

NaH , THF → **A** → allyl chloride (Cl) →

What is the major product from the reactions of (a) and (b)?

(a) 1. NaOMe , MeOH reflux 2. EtBr

(b) 1. LDA, THF, -78 °C 2. D_2O

In (a), the ketone is converted to the thermodynamic enolate and reaction with bromoethane leads to the highly substituted product, 1-(1-ethylcyclopentyl)ethan-1-one. In (b), the diketone has four acidic positions. Since the two carbonyls have a 1,4-relationship rather than a 1,3-relationship, there is no special acidity of the "inside" protons nor special stability for those enolates. These are kinetic control conditions and quenching with deuterium oxide will transfer a D (^{2}H) to the less-substituted carbon to give heptane-2,5-dione-1-*d*.

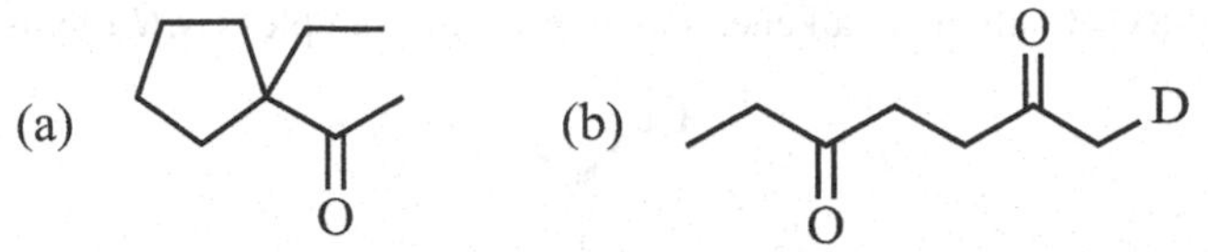

(a) (b)

Why are epoxides highly reactive to nucleophiles when simple ethers are relatively unreactive?

The three-membered ring ethers are under a great deal of strain and the carbon atoms attached to oxygen are polarized with a δ^+ dipole. The combination of these two prosperities makes reaction with nucleophiles facile, and ring-opening is facile due to relief of the strain of a three-membered ring.

What is the product formed when NaOH reacts with 2-ethyloxirane in THF?

The reaction of the epoxide with hydroxide leads to a diol but the ring-opened oxygen from the epoxide is an alkoxide, which requires an acid hydrolysis step to give the diol. Therefore, the final product is butane-1,2-diol.

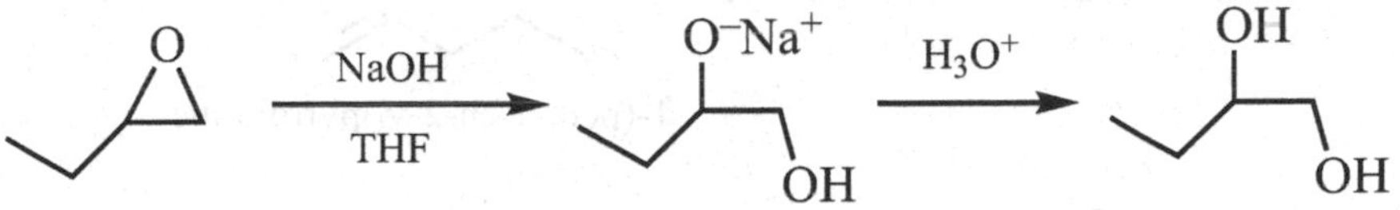

NaOH, THF → O^-Na^+, OH → H_3O^+ → OH, OH

What is the product when the sodium salt of prop-1-yne reacts with 2-ethyloxirane in THF?

The reaction of the epoxide with the alkyne anion leads to the alkoxide, and aqueous hydrolysis gives the final product, hept-5-yn-3-ol.

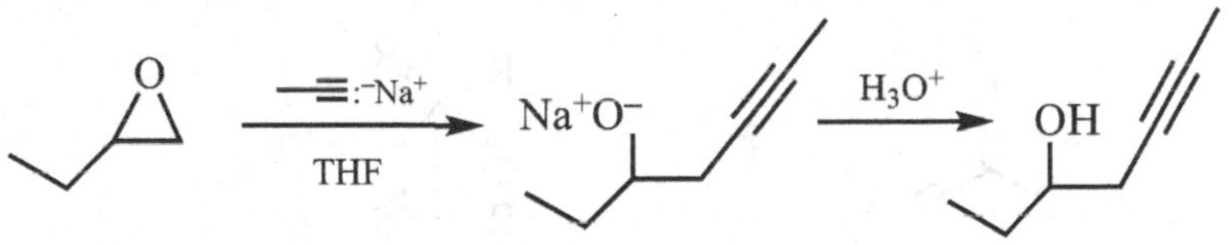

$\equiv$:$^-$Na$^+$, THF → Na^+O^- → H_3O^+ → OH

Why does the alkyne anion react preferentially with the less-substituted carbon atom of 2-ethyloxirane in the preceding question?

The reaction of an epoxide with a nucleophile is a S_N2-like reactions, and the less sterically hindered (less-substituted) carbon is the site of reaction.

What is the product when the kinetic enolate of hexan-2-one reacts with 1-ethyloxirane followed by hydrolysis?

The electropositive carbon of an epoxide is subject to attack by a nucleophile such as an enolate. The nucleophile generally attacks the less sterically hindered (less-substituted) carbon of the epoxide. In this case, the enolate anion of hexane-2-one reacts with the epoxide and the resulting alkoxide is subjected to hydrolysis to give the product, 8-hydroxydecan-5-one.

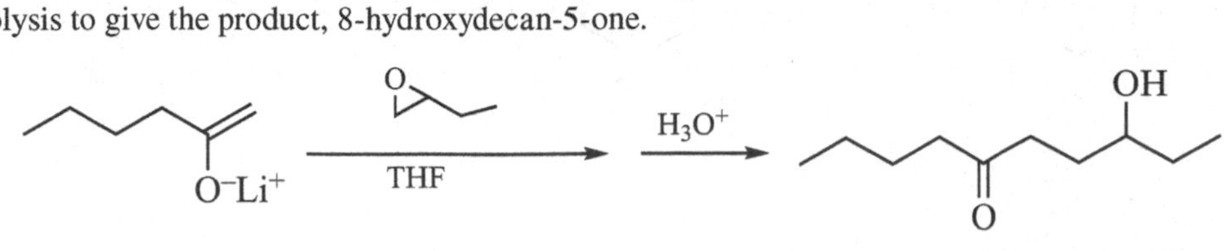

O^-Li^+ → THF → H_3O^+ → OH, O

8-hydroxydecan-5-one

What is an enamine?

An enamine is literally an alkene-amine. In other words, it is a molecule that has an amine moiety directly attached to the C=C unit of an alkene: R_2N–C=C. An example is *N,N*-diethylpent-1-en-2-amine.

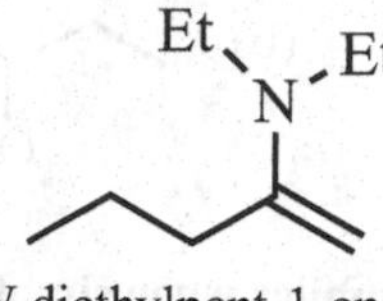

N,N-diethylpent-1-en-2-amine

How are enamines formed?

Some aldehydes and most ketones react with secondary amines to give the enamine. An example is the reaction of pentan-2-one with pyrrolidine to give 1-(pent-1-en-2-yl)pyrrolidine.

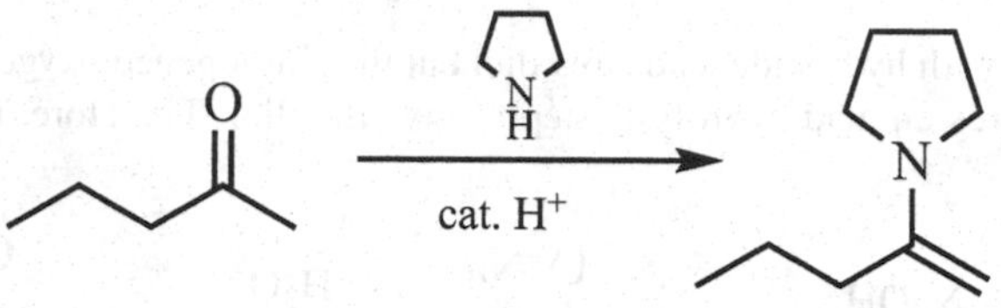

cat. H^+

1-(pent-1-en-2-yl)pyrrolidine

How are enamines related to enolate anions?

An enolate anion can donate electrons from oxygen to an electrophile (E^+) via the π-bond of the C=C unit, making the α-carbon nucleophilic. Similarly, electrons can be donated from the nitrogen of an enamine via the π-bond of the C=C unit, again making the α-carbon nucleophilic. In a very practical sense, an enamine can be considered as a nitrogen analog of an enolate anion.

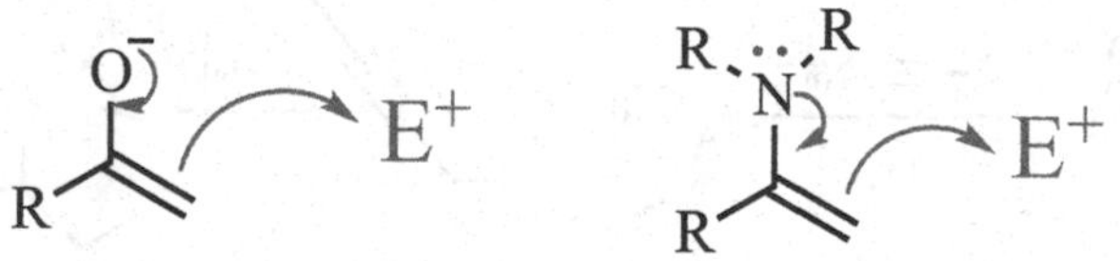

What is the initial product when the pyrrolidine enamine of cyclohexanone reacts with bromopropane?

When the α-carbon of the enamine attacks the electropositive carbon of bromopropane the initial product is an iminium salt, *A*. Hydrolysis of iminium salt *A* gives the ketone product, 2-propylcyclohexanone.

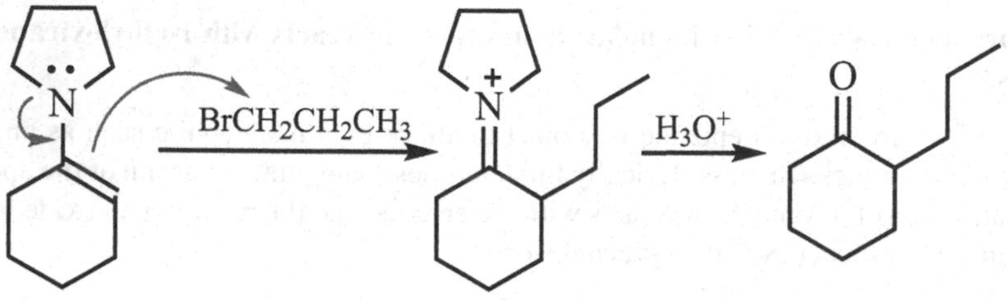

$BrCH_2CH_2CH_3$ → **A** → H_3O^+

Is *A* the only product of the reaction in the preceding question?

Not necessarily. There is an equilibrium between iminium salt ***A*** and the enamine form of this product, ***B***. This equilibrium is known as *imine-enamine tautomerism* and the position of this equilibrium depends on the solvent to a large extent. In problems such as this one encountered in this book, assume that the alkylation reaction of an enamine generates the iminium salt, ***A***. In general, due to steric interactions between the amine unit and the alkyl group, the equilibrium favors the less-substituted enamine form (***B***) due to diminished steric hindrance.

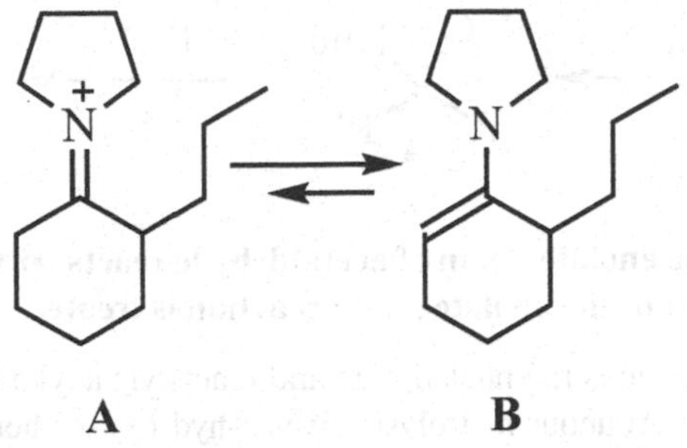

A **B**

What is the product when *A* in the preceding question is treated with aqueous acid?

As noted, when an iminium salt such as ***A*** is treated with aqueous acid, the final product is a ketone, in this case 2-propylcyclohexanone.

What is the mechanism for the hydrolysis reaction of *A* in the preceding question?

The carbon of the iminium salt is susceptible to attack by the nucleophilic oxygen of water, transferring electrons to nitrogen and forming ***A***. Loss of a proton gives ***B*** and transfer of a proton to the more basic nitrogen gives ***C***. This transfer of a proton from oxygen in ***A*** may occur intramolecularly directly to ***C*** without formation of ***B***. Once protonated, pyrrolidine becomes a good leaving group and its loss gives the protonated carbonyl, oxocarbenium ion ***B***, and simple loss of a proton gives the final product, 2-propylcyclohexanone.

OH_2, H^+ → **A** → $-H^+$ → **B** → $+H^+$ → **C** → $-$ pyrrolidine → **D** → $-H^+$ →

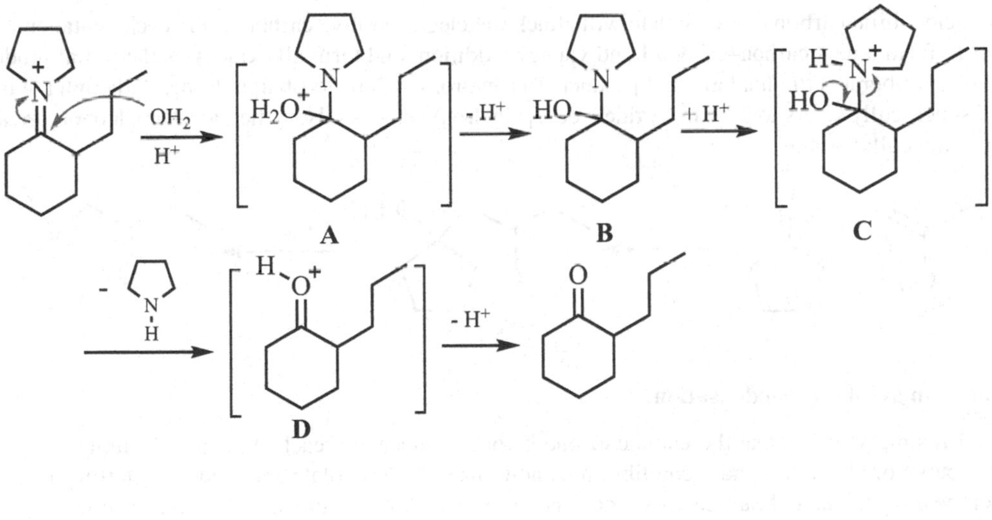

17.3 CONDENSATION REACTIONS OF ENOLATE ANIONS AND ALDEHYDES OR KETONES

What is an acyl addition reaction of a ketone?

A nucleophile (Nuc) is electron-rich and donates electrons to the δ^+ carbon of the carbonyl to give alkoxide *A*. Hydrolysis gives an acid–base reaction that leads to protonation of the alkoxide to give the final alcohol product.

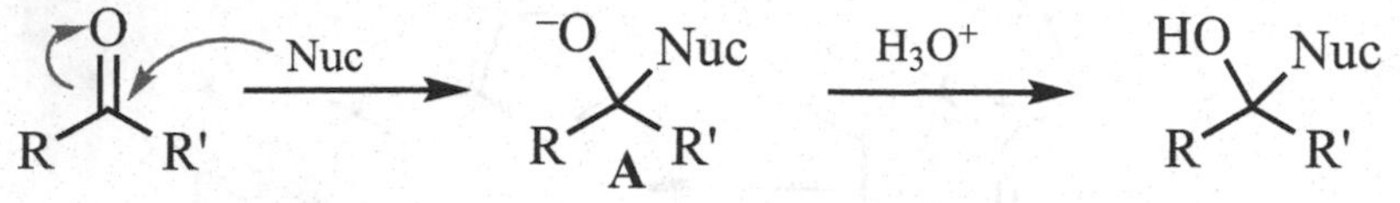

What is the product when the enolate anion of acetaldehyde reacts with benzaldehyde? What is the product when the product of the enolate anion reaction is treated with dilute aqueous acid?

The enolate anion of acetaldehyde is the nucleophile and reacts via acyl addition with the carbonyl carbon of benzaldehyde to give *A*. Aqueous hydrolysis gives 2-hydroxy-3-phenylacetaldehyde. The product is a β-hydroxy aldehyde, which has the common name of an *aldol.*

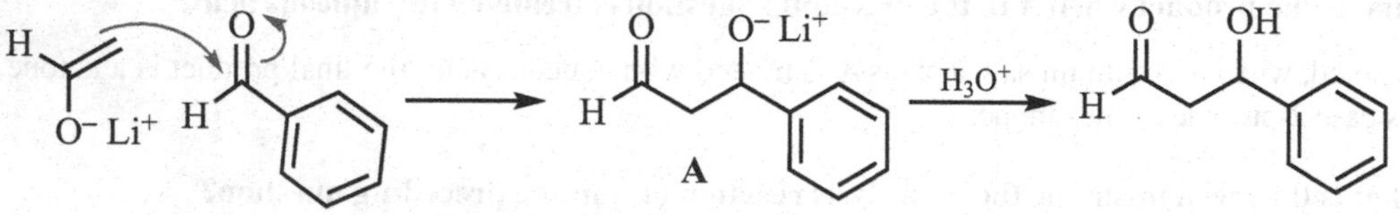

What is the name of the reaction in the preceding question?

This reaction is called the *aldol condensation.*

What is the product of the reaction between the kinetic enolate of butan-2-one and cyclopentanone?

The nucleophilic carbon of the enolate will attack the electropositive carbon of the cyclopentanone carbonyl to form a new carbon–carbon bond via acyl addition, and form alkoxide *A* as the initial product. Hydrolysis liberates the final alcohol product, 1-(1-hydroxycyclopentyl)butan-2-one. Although the term aldol specifically refers to β-hydroxyaldehydes, β-hydroxyketones (also called a β-ketoalcohol) are also commonly called aldols.

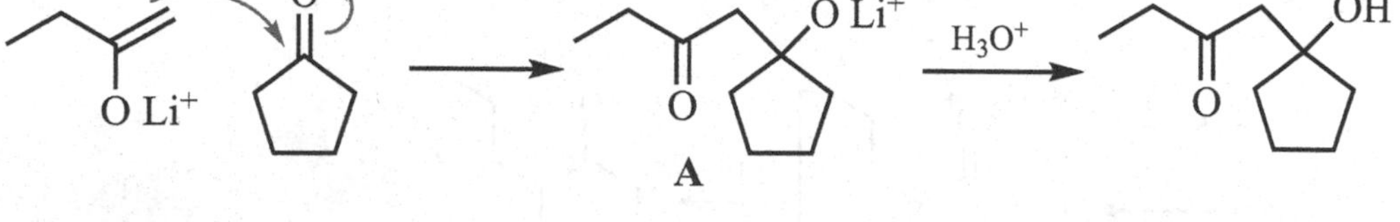

What is an aldol self-condensation?

The term simply means that the enolate of one ketone or aldehyde reacts with another molecule of the same ketone or aldehyde. Under equilibrium conditions both the enolate anion and the starting aldehyde or ketone are present and can react with one another in an aldol reaction, a "self-condensation."

What is a "mixed" aldol condensation?

Formation of 1-(1-hydroxycyclopentyl)butan-2-one by condensing butan-2-one and cyclopentanone in the preceding question is an example of a mixed aldol. The term simply means that the enolate of one ketone or aldehyde is reacted with a different ketone or aldehyde.

Why are thermodynamic conditions not used very often in mixed aldol reactions?

If two different ketones are present in a reaction under thermodynamic control, two different enolates can be formed, and each enolate can react with either ketone. In other words, both enolate anions and both unreacted ketones remain in solution as part of the equilibrium with the base, and cross reactions lead to four different aldol condensation products. As an example, the enolate of butan-2-one could react with both butan-2-one and cyclopentanone. Alternatively, the enolate of cyclopentanone could react with both butan-2-one and cyclopentanone. If only one aldol is the target, it must be separated from the other products, which may not be easy and certainly will lead to a diminished yield of the target.

What is the advantage of using kinetic control in forming mixed aldol products?

Under kinetic control conditions, the enolate anion is formed essentially irreversibly. A second carbonyl partner is then added, giving a single "mixed aldol" product. Under thermodynamic control conditions, both carbonyls must be present at the same time. This mixture is not present when kinetic control conditions are used.

What is the reaction product when butan-2-one is treated with sodium ethoxide in ethanol?

When butan-2-one is converted to the thermodynamic enolate, significant amounts of base *and unreacted butan-2-one* are present in the equilibrium mixture. The enolate of butan-2-one can and does react with unchanged butan-2-one in a condensation reaction that produces the alkoxide as the product. Hydrolysis gives the aldol, 4-hydroxy-3,4-dimethylhexan-2-one.

NaOEt , EtOH; O Na$^+$; H_3O^+; HO; O; heat or H^+; $-H_2O$; O

Why are conjugated ketones or aldehydes often isolated from this reaction when the product is treated with aqueous acid or is heated?

Loss of water (dehydration) can be facile since the final product is a β-hydroxy carbonyl compound and the product is a conjugated carbonyl compound. An unconjugated carbonyl derivative such as 4-hydroxy-3,4-dimethylhexan-2-one in the preceding question is less stable than the conjugated carbonyl derivative, 3,4-dimethylhex-3*E*-en-2-one. Dehydration can be induced thermally (by heating the aldol product) or during the aqueous acid workup (H^+/H_2O under vigorous conditions will induce dehydration, as shown in the preceding question). It is important to note, however, that dehydration does *not* occur in all cases with the usual acid workup, and isolation of the aldol product is often straightforward unless a stronger acid concentration is used in the hydrolysis and/or the aldol is heated.

What is the major product of the reactions (a) and (b)?

(a) O; 1. NaOMe , MeOH, reflux; 2. H_3O^+

(b) O; LDA , THF, -78 °C; 1. O; 2. H_3O^+

In (a), under thermodynamic conditions, cyclohexanone is expected to react with itself, (self-condensation) to give the aldol product 2-(1-hydroxycyclohexyl)cyclohexanone (after hydrolysis). In (b), conversion to the kinetic enolate anion of 4-methylhexan-3-one under kinetic control conditions. No self-condensation can occur since all of the ketone was converted to the enolate and the equilibrium reaction is suppressed under kinetic control conditions. In order for the condensation to occur, 4-methylhexan-3-one is added to the enolate solution, and condensation gives the aldol product, 6-ethyl-6-hydroxy-3,5,7-trimethyloctan-4-one (after mild hydrolysis).

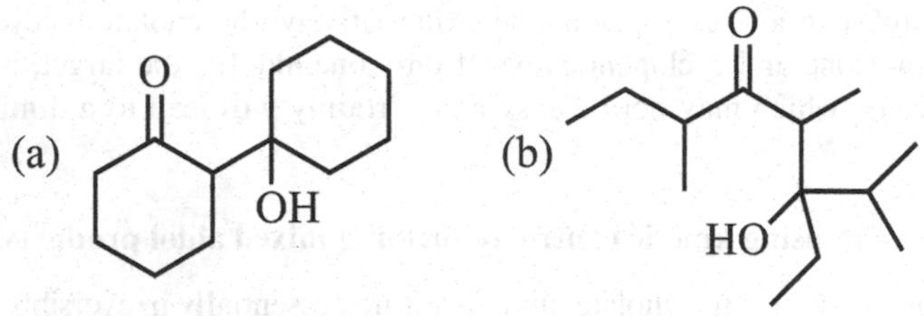

(a) O OH (b) O HO

What is an intramolecular aldol condensation?

The term simply means that an enolate anion generated on one side of a molecule reacts with a carbonyl partner that is part of the same molecule, but distal to the enolate anion. The aldol condensation is an intramolecular acyl addition.

What is the product when hexane-2,5-dione reacts with LDA and the product is hydrolyzed?

Aldol condensation reactions can occur intramolecularly as well as intermolecularly. The kinetic enolate of one of the two identical methyl ketone moieties of hexane-2,5-dione (***A***) will attack the carbonyl at the other end of the molecule (as shown) to form the cyclic alkoxide, ***B***. Note that the conformational change shown is likely in order to facilitate the intramolecular acyl addition. Hydrolysis then gives the alcohol product, 3-hydroxy-3-methylcyclopentan-1-one. In general, intramolecular attack is faster than intermolecular attack for formation of five-, six- and seven-membered rings.

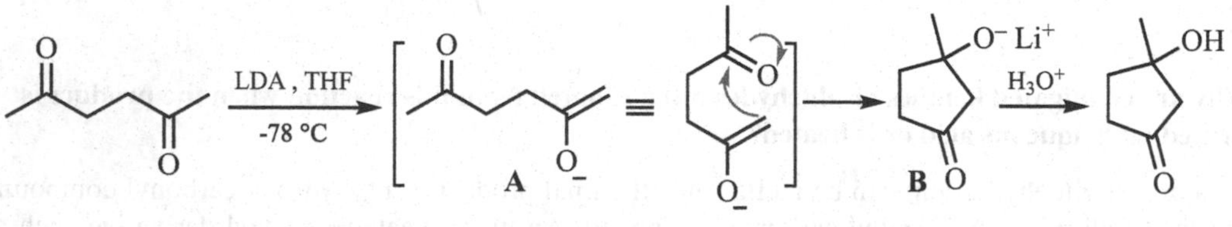

O O LDA, THF -78 °C O A O^- ≡ O O^- O^- Li^+ B O H_3O^+ OH O

What is the product when hexane-2,5-dione is treated with sodium methoxide in methanol and then hydrolyzed?

The major product is the cyclopentanone derivative, 3-hydroxy-3-methylcyclopentan-1-one. Under thermodynamic conditions, enolates ***A*** and ***C*** are in equilibrium with hexane-2,5-dione. The intramolecular aldol condensation of enolate ***A*** would generate a three-membered ring aldol (***B***), which is energetically unfavorable when compared to formation of the five-membered ring derivative from enolate ***C***. In other words, the activation energy (Section 3.2) to form the strained three-membered ring is high in energy relative to the lower activation energy barrier required to form the five-membered ring. Under equilibrium conditions, both the kinetic and the thermodynamic enolate are present, but the thermodynamic enolate anion cannot lead to an acyl addition product. The kinetic enolate anion, however, leads to more stable and easily formed five-membered ring product. The equilibrium conditions allow the reaction to proceed to product due to formation of both kinetic and thermodynamic enolate anions.

NaOMe, MeOH; **A**; very slow; H_3O^+; **B**; **C**; H_3O^+

3-hydroxy-3-methylcyclopentan-1-one

What is 1,4-addtion, otherwise known as conjugate addition?

In a conjugated carbonyl system, C=C—C=O, a nucleophile can react at the acyl carbon (1,2-addition) or at the end of the conjugated system, on the C=C moiety (1,4-addition). Due to bond polarization, the carbon that is β- to the carbonyl has a δ^+ dipole and is susceptible to reaction with a nucleophile. This 1,4-addition is also called conjugated addition.

What is vinylogy?

Vinylogy is the extension of points of reactivity by conjugating π-bonds. Therefore, the carbon β- to the carbonyl carbon in C=C—C=O is susceptible to reaction with a nucleophile due to vinylogy.

What is a Michael addition?

Michael addition is another term for 1,4-addition or conjugate addition of a nucleophile with a conjugated (α,β-unsaturated) ketone or aldehyde (usually a ketone) where the nucleophile adds to the π-bond of the alkene rather than to the carbonyl carbon.

What is the initial product when a nucleophile reacts with methyl vinyl ketone?

Reaction of methyl vinyl ketone (but-3-en-2-one) and a nucleophile will produce an enolate anion (***A***) via Michael addition. When the enolate anion reacts with aqueous acid, protonation gives the enol, and tautomerization (Sections 7.6 and 17.1) gives the β-substituted ketone. Amines are typical nucleophiles in the Michael reaction, but an enolate anion can add in a 1,4-addtion, as well as Grignard reagents (Section 10.2) and organocuprate reagents (Section 10.6).

What is the product when methyl vinyl ketone reacts with methylamine?

The product is enolate anion ***A***, and reaction with dilute aqueous acid gives the Michael addition product, 4-(methylamino)butan-2-one.

What are the products of the reactions of (a), (b), and (c)?

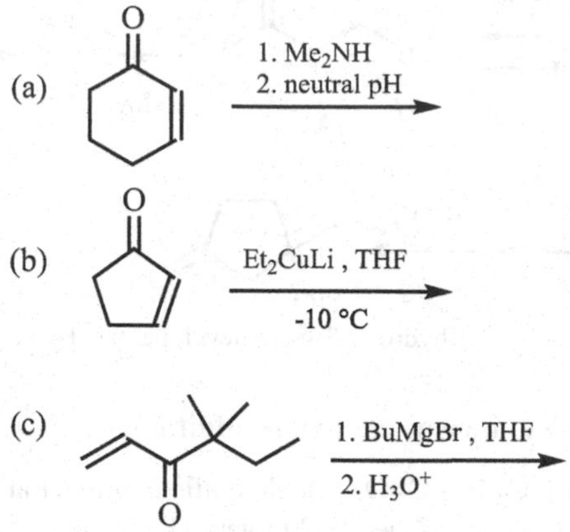

(a) 1. Me_2NH 2. neutral pH

(b) Et_2CuLi, THF, -10 °C

(c) 1. BuMgBr, THF 2. H_3O^+

In (a), a Michael addition occurs with cyclohexenone to give the 3-dimethylamino product, 3-(dimethylamino)cyclohexan-1-one, after careful neutralization of the amino ketone product. These *Michael adducts* are often unstable and are usually sensitive to heat and acid, losing the amine to regenerate the conjugated ketone. In (b), the cuprate reacts with cyclopentenone to give 3-ethylcyclopentan-1-one. In (c), the Grignard reagent adds to the double bond of 4,4-dimethylhex-1-en-3-one primarily because the approach to the carbonyl is hindered by the adjacent methyl substituents. Michael addition leads to 3,3-dimethyldecan-4-one.

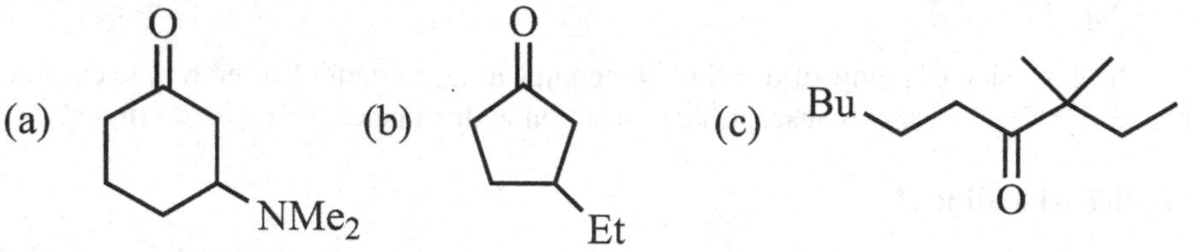

(a) NMe_2 (b) Et (c) Bu

What is the Robinson annulation?

The *Robinson annulation* is a cyclization reaction that combines an initial Michael addition followed by an intramolecular aldol condensation. When cyclopentenone is treated with cyclopentane-1,3-dione under thermodynamic conditions, the product after hydrolysis is ***A*** (2,3,7,7a-tetrahydro-1*H*-indene-1,5(6*H*)-dione). This reaction to form the bicyclic product is an example of the Robinson annulation.

+ 1. NaOEt, EtOH reflux 2. H_3O^+ → **A**

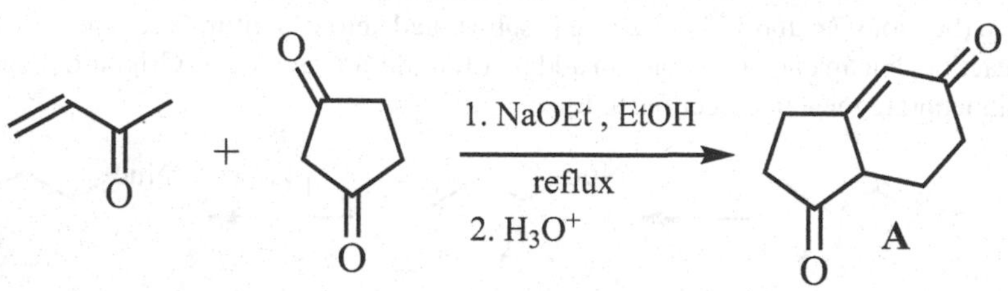

What is a mechanistic rationale for why the Robinson annulation leads to a six-membered ring?

The initially formed enolate from cyclopentane-1,3-dione (***A***) adds to methyl vinyl ketone in a Michael reaction to give enolates ***B*** and ***C*** under equilibrium conditions. Under the thermodynamic conditions, both are in equilibrium and ***B*** is favored since it is the more highly substituted enolate anion. However, an intramolecular aldol condensation from ***B*** would lead to a higher energy four-membered ring and is disfavored due to the high energy transition state for this reaction. Since under equilibrium conditions the kinetic enolate ***C*** is in equilibrium with the diketone and the initially formed thermodynamic enolate anion, an intramolecular aldol of *C* forms a six-membered ring since this cyclization has a relatively low energy transition state and the reaction is facile. The product is alkoxide (*D*), which is protonated by hydrolysis to give *E*. In many cases *E* is the isolated product. Heating or hydrolysis with strong aqueous acid will induce dehydration to give the conjugated ketone, 2,3,7,7a-tetrahydro-1*H*-indene-1,5(6*H*)-dione.

NaOEt A B C D H_3O^+ E $- H_2O$ F

What is the Cannizzaro reaction?

The *Cannizzaro reaction* is a condensation reaction of aromatic aldehydes (or other aldehydes that do not have an α-hydrogen), induced by reaction with aqueous hydroxide. Two products are formed, an oxidation product (an acid) and a reduction product (an alcohol). This *"self-oxidation-reduction"* type of reaction is known as *disproportionation.* An example is the conversion of benzaldehyde to benzoic acid and benzyl alcohol upon treatment with aqueous hydroxide, followed by neutralization.

$$PhCHO \xrightarrow[2.\ H_3O^+]{1.\ aq.\ NaOH,\ heat} PhCO_2H + PhCH_2OH$$

What is a mechanistic rationale for the Cannizzaro reaction?

Hydroxide attacks the carbonyl of benzaldehyde to produce an alkoxide intermediate, *A*, via acyl addition. This acyl addition is a reversible process but given sufficient energy, the alkoxide reacts with another molecule of benzaldehyde, as shown. Transfer of hydrogen to the carbonyl (as a *hydride*), generates the anion of benzoic acid and an alcohol. The carboxylate is converted to benzoic acid upon hydrolysis.

OH^- A H_3O^+ CO_2H + CH_2OH

What are the limitations on the carbonyl partner of the Cannizzaro Reaction?

This only works if the aldehyde does not have an α-hydrogen. If it does, deprotonation leads to the enolate anion. Ketones do not give this reaction. Only aldehydes have the hydrogen that is transferred.

Do enamines react with aldehydes and ketones?

Since enamines behave as "nitrogen enolates" they will react with both aldehydes and ketones to produce iminium salts. Hydrolysis will then produce aldol-like products.

What is the major product for the reaction of (a) and (b)?

(a) [1-(diethylamino)cyclohexene] 1. cyclopentanone; 2. H_3O^+ →

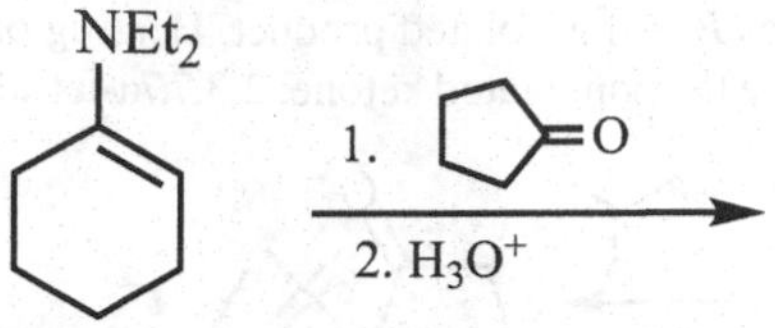

(b) [morpholine enamine] 1. CHO (butanal); 2. H_3O^+ →

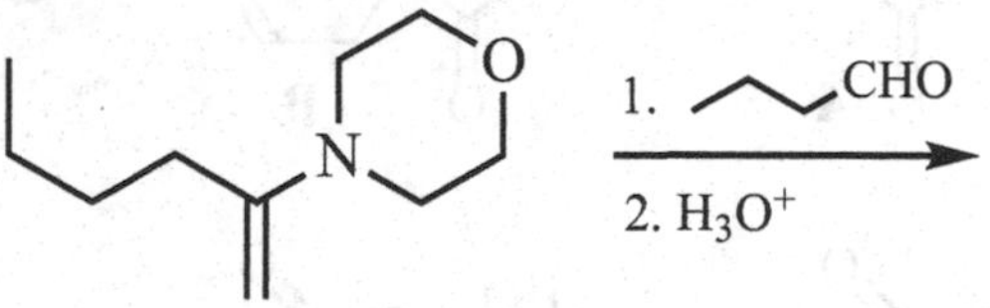

In (a) the diethylamino enamine of cyclohexanone is condensed with cyclopentanone to give, after hydrolysis, 2-(1-hydroxycyclopentyl)cyclohexan-1-one. In (b) the enamine is condensed with butanal and gives, after hydrolysis, 7-hydroxydecan-5-one.

(a) [2-(1-hydroxycyclopentyl)cyclohexan-1-one: O, OH] (b) [7-hydroxydecan-5-one: O, OH]

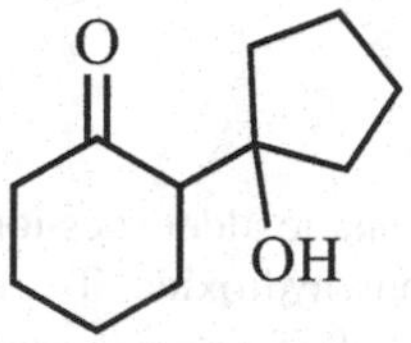

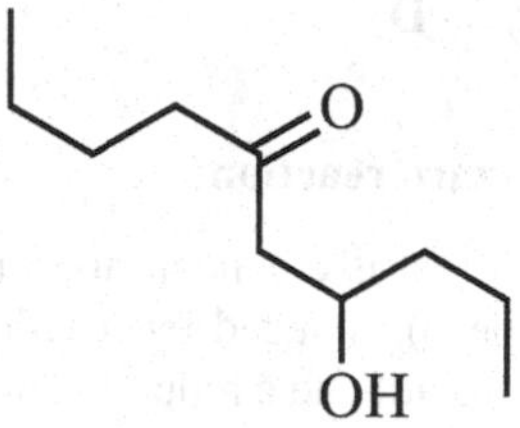

17.4 ENOLATE ANIONS FROM CARBOXYLIC ACIDS AND DERIVATIVES

Can esters react with a suitable base to form an enolate anion?

Yes! Esters have a carbon next to the carbonyl, an α-carbon, and if that carbon has attached hydrogen atoms (α-hydrogens) then reaction with a suitable base will give an ester enolate anion.

What is the product when butanoic acid reacts with sodium ethoxide?

Since sodium ethoxide is a strong base, the acidic hydrogen (O—H) of butanoic acid is removed to form the sodium salt of the acid, sodium butanoate.

What is the most favorable reaction when ethyl butanoate reacts with sodium methoxide in methanol?

The most electropositive atom is the carbonyl carbon. It is, therefore, reasonable to assume that sodium methoxide will attack the carbonyl via a reversible nucleophilic acyl addition reaction to give the tetrahedral intermediate ***A***. It is also possible that ethoxide can be lost from ***A*** to form the methyl ester, which is also a reversible reaction. An excess of methoxide will lead to the methyl ester and an excess of ethoxide will lead to the ethyl ester.

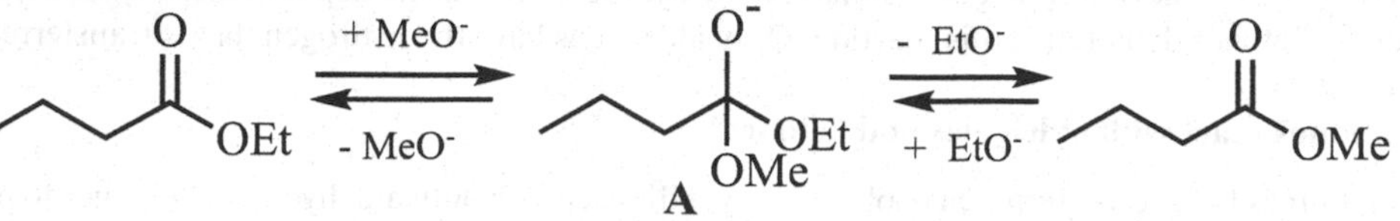

[ethyl butanoate: O, OEt] $\underset{-\,MeO^-}{\overset{+\,MeO^-}{\rightleftharpoons}}$ [O^-, OEt, OMe] **A** $\underset{+\,EtO^-}{\overset{-\,EtO^-}{\rightleftharpoons}}$ [methyl butanoate: O, OMe]

If thermodynamic conditions are used to deprotonate an ester, what are the limitations on the base that can be used?

Examination of *A* shows that OMe and OEt are present in the preceding question, which shows that a transesterification reaction can occur if the alkoxide base is different from the alcohol portion of the ester. In other words, if OEt is lost from *A*, a methyl ester is formed whereas if OMe is lost, the ethyl ester is formed. For this reason, NaOEt is used with ethyl ester, NaOMe with methyl esters, etc.

What is the product when ethyl butanoate reacts with lithium diethylamide in THF, at -78 °C?

Lithium diethylamide is a powerful and non-nucleophilic base. The usual nucleophilic attack at the carbonyl is, therefore, slow. The hydrogen on the carbon adjacent to the carbonyl (the α-carbon) is acidic and can be removed by this strong base. The product is the enolate anion., ***A***.

$LiNEt_2$, ether
-78 °C
A

What is the relative pK_a of the α-hydrogen of ethyl butanoate when compared to the two acidic protons of butan-2-one?

The α-hydrogen of an ester is less acidic than the α-hydrogen of a ketone or aldehyde. The α-hydrogen atoms of butan-2-one have a pK_a of 20 and 21 (for C1 and C3, respectively). The α-hydrogen of ethyl butanoate (the carbon next to the carbonyl, *not* next to the oxygen of the alcohol portion of the ester) has a pK_a of about 24–25.

What are the enolate anions derived from ethyl butanoate under both kinetic and thermodynamic control conditions?

In both cases there is only one possible enolate anion as shown. Under kinetic control (aprotic solvents, low temperature, strong non-nucleophilic base) *A* is formed in an effectively irreversible manner. Under thermodynamic control (protic solvent, alkoxide bases, higher reaction temperatures) the reaction is reversible, and *A* is in equilibrium with the starting ester.

Base
A

Can ester enolate anions participate in alkylation reactions?

Yes! Ester enolate anions react as carbon nucleophiles. Just as with the enolates derived from aldehydes and ketones, ester enolates are nucleophilic and react with alkyl halides to give the substitution product.

What is the product when methyl propionate is reacted first with sodium methoxide in methanol and then with iodomethane?

The initial reaction gives the enolate (*A*), which reacts with iodomethane to give methyl 2-methylpropionate

NaOMe , MeOH
reflux
A
MeI

What is the product when the isopropyl ester of phenylacetic acid (2-phenyl ethanoic acid) reacts first with LDA (-78°C, THF) and then with benzyl bromide?

Formation of the enolate is followed by alkylation with benzyl bromide to give isopropyl 2,3-diphenylpropanoate.

1. $LiN(iPr)_2$, THF -78 °C
2. $PhCH_2Br$

What is the acidity of the α-hydrogen of a dibasic acid ester such as diethyl malonate?

The hydrogens on the carbon between the two carbonyl groups have a pK_a of 12.9. The inductive effects of two carbonyl groups greatly enhance the acidity of those hydrogens.

What is the relative stability of the enolate derived from dimethyl malonate?

The presence of the second carbonyl in the enolate anion of dimethyl malonate leads to three resonance structures, ***B***, and ***A,A'*** which are identical due to the symmetry of the molecule. The three resonance contributors impart greater stability when compared to enolate derived from a monocarboxylic acid. Note that the extra stability of the malonate anion leads to diminished reactivity for the nucleophile.

NaOMe, MeOH
reflux

A B A'

Are ester enolate anions derived from dibasic acids more or less reactive than ester enolates derived from monobasic acids? Explain.

These enolate anions are more stable, due to the resonance stability of the anion (see, the enolate of dimethyl malonate in the preceding question), which makes them *less reactive*.

What is the product when diethyl malonate is reacted with: 1. NaOEt, EtOH; 2. $PhCH_2Br$? If this product is then reacted with 1. NaOEt; 2. CH_3I, what is the final product?

The first product is the 2-alkylated product, diethyl 2-benzylmalonate (***A***). If ***A*** is treated with additional base, a new enolate is formed (***B***), which then reacts with iodomethane to form diethyl 2-benzyl-2-methyl malonate, ***C***. This "double alkylation" of malonate derivatives is particularly attractive.

1. NaOEt
2. $PhCH_2Br$

NaOEt

MeI

A B C

How can malonic acid be converted into 2-ethyl-2-propyl malonic acid? What is the IUPAC name of this compound?

The first step is to convert diethyl malonate (or another ester) into the 2-ethyl derivative (*A*) by treatment with NaOEt followed by bromoethane. Repetition of this base-halide sequence to form enolate anion B followed by reaction with iodopropane leads to incorporation of the propyl group at C2. When this ester is saponified (1. aq. NaOH 2. aq. H^+), the corresponding malonic acid derivative (***C***) is produced. The IUPAC name of ***C*** is 2-ethyl-2-propyl-1,3-propanedioic acid.

CO_2Et / CO_2Et —(1. NaOEt; 2. CH_3CH_2Br)→ **A** —(NaOEt)→ **B** —(1. $CH_3CH_2CH_2Br$; 2. i. aq. NaOH ii. aq. H^+)→ **C**

If 2-ethyl-2-propyl-1,3-propanedioic acid is heated, what is the resulting product?

Since this malonic acid derivative is a 1,3-dicarbonyl acid, heating 2-ethyl-2-propyl-1,3-propanedioic acid will lead to decarboxylation (loss of CO_2) and the product will be 2-ethylpentanoic acid. See Section 15.6.

CO_2H / CO_2H —(200 °C, $-CO_2$)→ CO_2H

What is the name of this overall transformation?

The reaction sequence that converts malonic acid into a mono carboxylic acid via alkylation-decarboxylation is called the *malonic ester synthesis.* This reaction sequence is very powerful for the synthesis of highly substituted carboxylic acids.

What is a suitable synthesis for the transformation shown?

Ph — CHO ⇒ CO_2H / CO_2H

In this synthesis, malonic acid is esterified and then alkylated with benzyl bromide to give methyl 2-benzylmalononate. A second alkylation sequence is required, giving methyl 2-benzyl-2-(3-methylbutyl)malonate. Hydrolysis to the diacid (Sections 15.5 and 15.7) followed by decarboxylation gives the mono acid, 2-benzyl-5-methylhexanoic acid. In this case, the carboxylic acid must be transformed into an aldehyde. One way to do this is to first reduce the acid to an alcohol (2-benzyl-5-methylhexan-1-ol) with $LiAlH_4$ (Section 14.3) Subsequent treatment with PCC (pyridinium chlorochromate, Section 13.5) gives the final aldehyde target, 2-benzyl-5-methylhexanal.

CO_2H / CO_2H —(1. H_3O^+, MeOH; 2. NaOMe; 3. $PhCH_2Br$)→ Ph, CO_2Me / CO_2Me —(1. NaOMe; 2. Br; 3. H_3O^+)→ Ph, CO_2H / CO_2H —(200 °C)→ Ph — CO_2H

—(1. $LiAlH_4$; 2. H_2O)→ Ph — CH_2OH —(PCC)→ Ph — CHO

What is acetoacetic acid? What is the IUPAC name?

Acetoacetic acid is a β-keto acid and has the structure shown. The IUPAC name is 3-oxobutanoic acid.

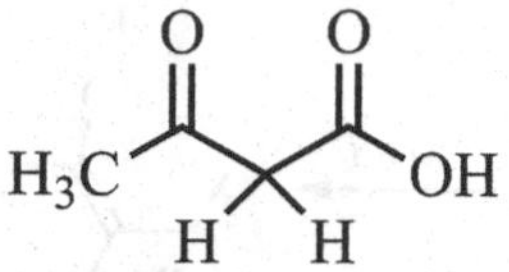

acetoacetic acid
(3-oxobutanoic acid)

What is the pK_a of the most acidic hydrogen in the ethyl ester of this molecule? Identify that hydrogen.

The most acidic hydrogen atoms are those between the two carbonyl groups, as in malonic acid esters. The pK_a of the hydrogen atoms in 3-oxobutanoic acid is about 11.

What is the product if ethyl acetoacetate is treated with 1. LDA, THF, -78°C; 2. bromoethane; 3. aq. KOH; 4. aq. H⁺ 5. heat to 250°C?

The final product is a ketone, pentan-2-one. The initial reaction generates the enolate anion (*A*) and alkylation with bromoethane gives the 2-ethyl product. Saponification of the ester leads to the acid, 2-ethyl-3-oxobutanoic acid. Since 2-ethyl-3-oxobutanoic acid is a 1,3-dicarbonyl compound, it can be decarboxylated to give the ketone as the final product, pentan-2-one.

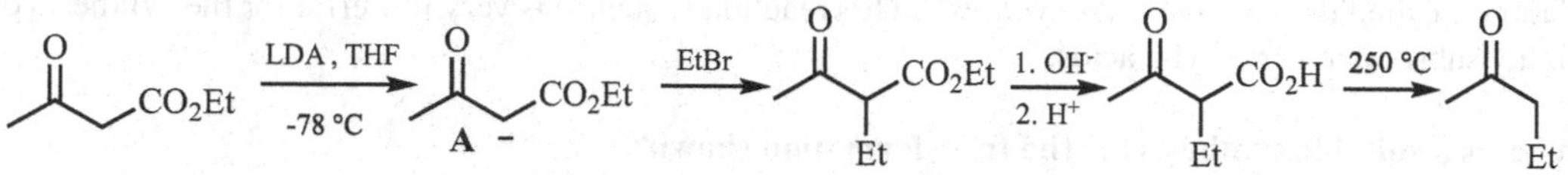

Is the initial product of the preceding question the ketone?

The initially formed product of the decarboxylation is an enol, which tautomerizes to the ketone.

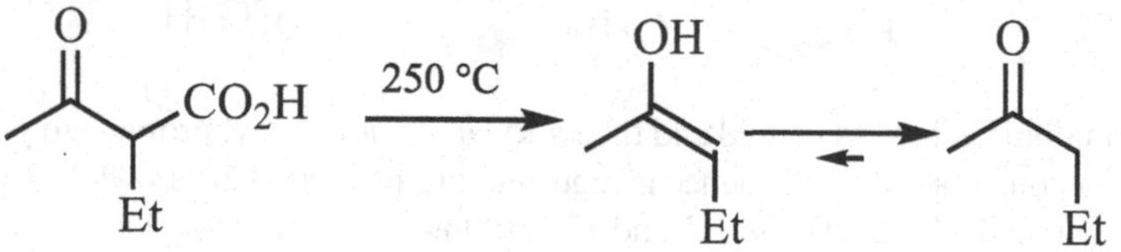

What is the name of the overall process in the preceding question?

This synthetic sequence is known as the *acetoacetic ester synthesis.*

What is a suitable synthesis for the preparation of the targeted ketone from the indicated starting material

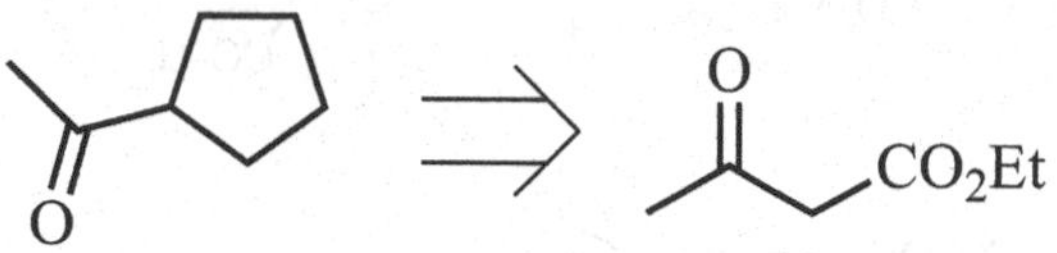

In this case, a ring is formed. Initial alkylation of the enolate, under thermodynamic conditions, with 1,4-dibromobutane gives ***A***. In a subsequent step under thermodynamic control conditions ***A*** is converted to its enolate (***B***) and an intramolecular S_N2 reaction displaces the bromine to give the keto-ester product (***C***). Saponification and decarboxylation give the final ketone product, 1-cyclopentylethan-1-one.

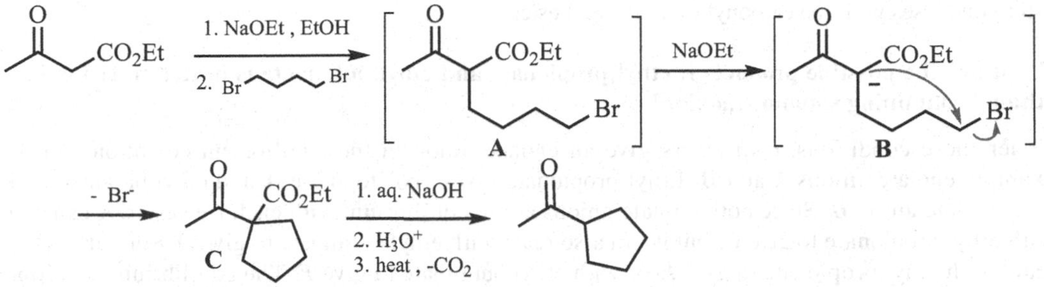

1. NaOEt, EtOH; 2. Br⌒⌒Br → A; NaOEt → B; - Br⁻ → C; 1. aq. NaOH; 2. H_3O^+; 3. heat, $-CO_2$

Is it possible for an ester enolate to react with aldehydes, ketones, or another ester?

Yes! It is also possible for an ester enolate anion to react with another ester. Just as the enolate anions of aldehydes and ketones react with other aldehydes and ketones in the aldol condensation, ester enolates react with a variety of carbonyl derivatives.

What is the product when ethyl propanoate is reacted with 1. LDA, THF, -78°C; 2. ethyl propanoate?

The product is a β-keto-ester, ethyl 2-methyl-3-oxopentanoate.

1. $LiN(iPr)_2$, THF, -78 °C; 2. ethyl propanoate (CO_2Et)

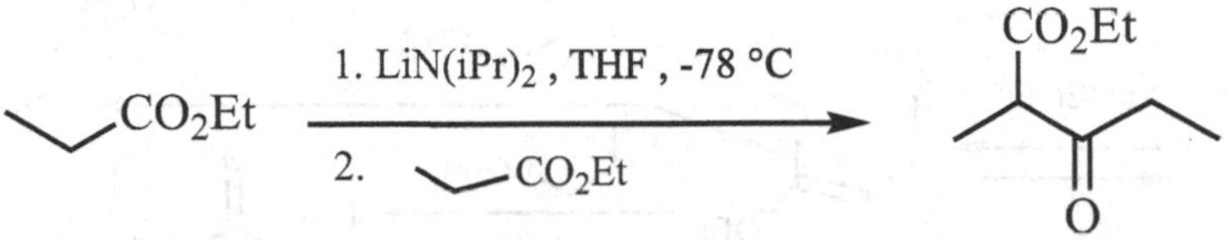

How and why does the reaction in the preceding question work?

Initial reaction of ethyl propanoate with NaOEt gives the ester enolate. Under thermodynamic conditions the enolate anion and unreacted ester are present at equilibrium, and the carbanionic carbon of the enolate anion attacks the carbonyl of the second molecule of ethyl propionate in an acyl substitution reaction (Sections 15.4 and 15.5) to give the tetrahedral intermediate *A*. Displacement of the ethoxy moiety by the alkoxide moiety generates the ketone group in the final keto-ester product, ethyl 2-methyl-3-oxopentanoate.

NaOEt, EtOH → A

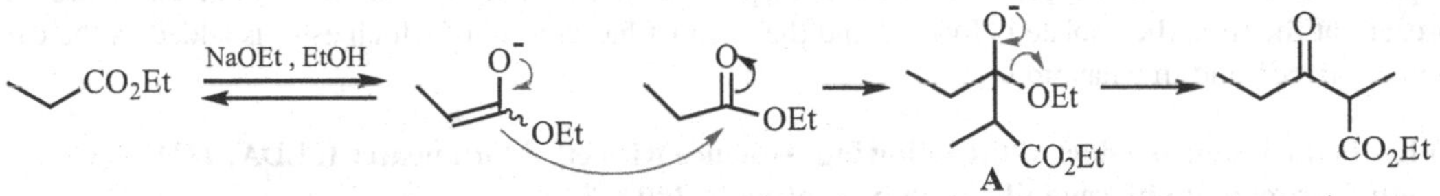

What is the name of the reaction in the preceding questions?

This reaction is called the *Claisen condensation*.

What is a Claisen self-condensation?

The reaction of two molecules of the same ester, which is possible under thermodynamic (equilibrium) conditions will produce the Claisen product via self-condensation. Both the enolate of one molecule and the ester form of another ester molecule are present at equilibrium, and the enolate anion reacts with the carbonyl of the ester to give the Claisen self-condensation product.

What is a "mixed" Claisen condensation?

The reaction of two different esters to produce the Claisen product is a mixed Claisen. The enolate of one ester condenses with the carbonyl of a different ester.

What are the possible products if ethyl propionate and ethyl butanoate is heated to reflux in ethanol containing sodium ethoxide?

Under these conditions, *both* esters give an enolate anion in the equilibrium conditions, in this example enolate anions ***A*** and ***B***. Ethyl propionate gives enolate anion ***A*** and ethyl butanoate will give enolate anion ***B***. Since both enolate anions are in equilibrium with each free ester, ***A*** can react with ethyl propionate to give ***C***, but it can also react with ethyl butanoate to give ***D***. Similarly, ***B*** can react with ethyl propionate to give ***E*** or with ethyl butanoate to give ***F***. The equilibrium conditions with two different esters therefore lead to four possible ester products. If the target is only one of these condensation products, the yield will be low and separation from the other keto-esters may be problematic.

CO_2Et — NaOEt, EtOH ⇌ **A** (O^-, OEt); **A** + CO_2Et → **C** (CO_2Et); **A** + CO_2Et → **D** (CO_2Et)

CO_2Et — NaOEt, EtOH ⇌ **B** (O^-, OEt); **B** + CO_2Et → **E** (CO_2Et); **B** + CO_2Et → **F** (CO_2Et)

Which are the better conditions for a mixed Claisen condensation, kinetic control or thermodynamic control conditions? Explain!

Although both conditions will generate the same enolate, kinetic control conditions are better for mixed Claisen condensations. Reaction of ethyl propionate with LDA, for example, will give ***A*** as the only enolate (see preceding problem) and either ethyl propionate or ethyl butanoate can be added to give the appropriate mixed Claisen product (***C*** or ***D***, respectively). Under these conditions both esters are not present at the time the enolate is formed and the chemist has control of which ester is added as the carbonyl partner, and in what order.

What is the major product of the following sequence with ethyl butanoate: 1. LDA, THF, -78°C; 2. ethyl propionate iii. saponification iv. heating to 200°C?

Under these kinetic control conditions, the initially formed enolate anion (***B***) condenses with ethyl propanoate to give the Claisen product, ***E***. Saponification liberates the free carboxylic acid and heating leads to decarboxylation (this is a 1,3-dicarbonyl compound) to give the ketone product, hexan-3-one.

CO_2Et — LDA, THF, - 78 °C → **B** (O^-, OEt) — CO_2Et → **E** (CO_2Et) — 1. i. aq. NaOH, ii. aq. H^+; 2. 200 °C → hexan-3-one

What is the product or products when ethyl butanoate is treated with sodium methoxide in methanol?

Transesterification can occur under these conditions, so ethyl butanoate is in equilibrium with methyl butanoate. In the presence of the base, ethyl butanoate will be converted to enolate anion ***B*** and methyl butanoate will be converted to enolate anion ***G***. Under these equilibrium conditions, enolate ***B*** will react with both ethyl butanoate and methyl butanoate to give keto-esters ***E*** and ***H***. Similarly, enolate anion ***G*** will react with both ethyl butanoate and methyl butanoate, also to give ***F*** and ***H***. Therefore, the result is a mixture of keto-esters that will complicate isolation and identification of the product of interest. However, saponification to the keto-acid will give the same product, 2-ethyl-3-oxohexanoic acid.

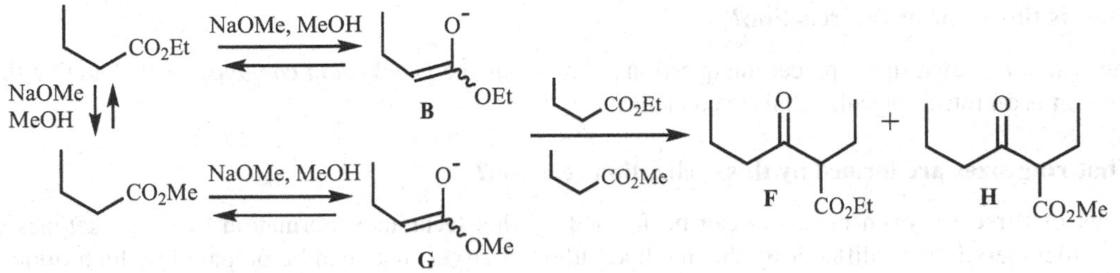

CO_2Et NaOMe, MeOH ⇌ O^- OEt **B**

NaOMe MeOH ⇅

CO_2Me NaOMe, MeOH ⇌ O^- OMe **G**

CO_2Et / CO_2Me → O **F** CO_2Et + O **H** CO_2Me

What is the lesson of the preceding question?

If thermodynamic conditions are used, the solvent (ROH) and the base (RO^-) should be the same as the alcohol portion of the ester in the reaction to avoid the transesterification problems shown in the preceding question.

What is the major product of the reactions of (a) and (b)?

(a) 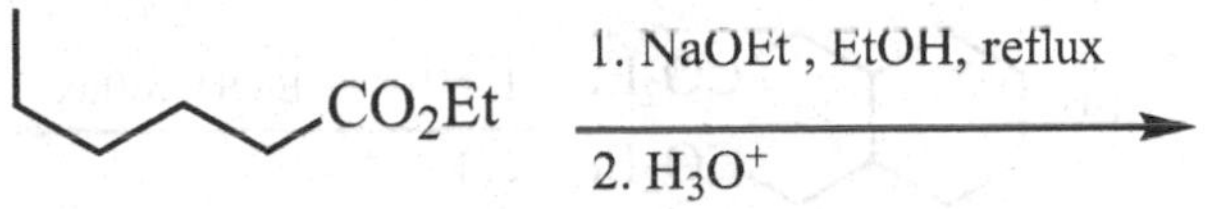 CO_2Et — 1. NaOEt, EtOH, reflux; 2. H_3O^+ →

(b) 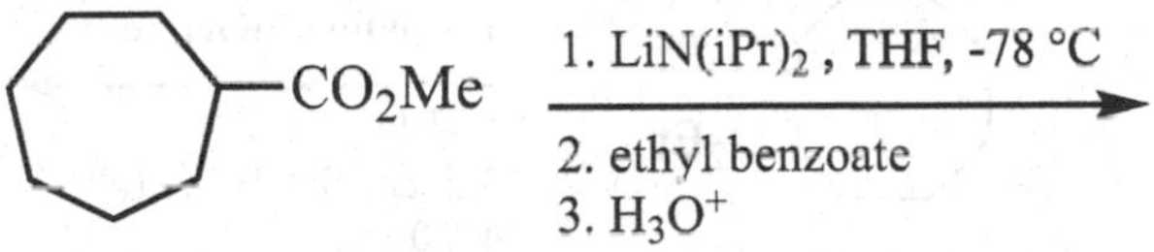 CO_2Me — 1. $LiN(iPr)_2$, THF, -78 °C; 2. ethyl benzoate; 3. H_3O^+ →

In (a), ethyl hexanoate condenses with itself under thermodynamic conditions to give the "symmetrical" Claisen product, ethyl 2-butyl-3-oxooctanoate. In (b), the enolate from ethyl cycloheptane carboxylate reacts with ethyl benzoate ($PhCO_2Et$) to give the "mixed" Claisen product, methyl 1-benzoylcycloheptane-1-carboxylate.

(a) 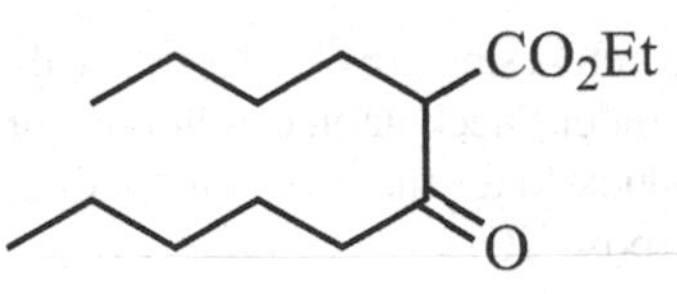 CO_2Et O (b) 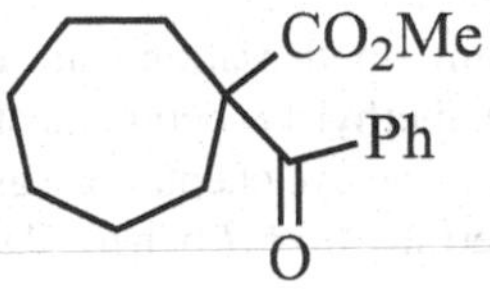 CO_2Me Ph O

What is the major product when the diethyl ester of 1,6-hexanedioic acid reacts with sodium ethoxide in ethanol?

This transformation is an intramolecular Claisen condensation and the product is the cyclic keto-ester, ethyl 2-oxocyclopentane-1-carboxylate.

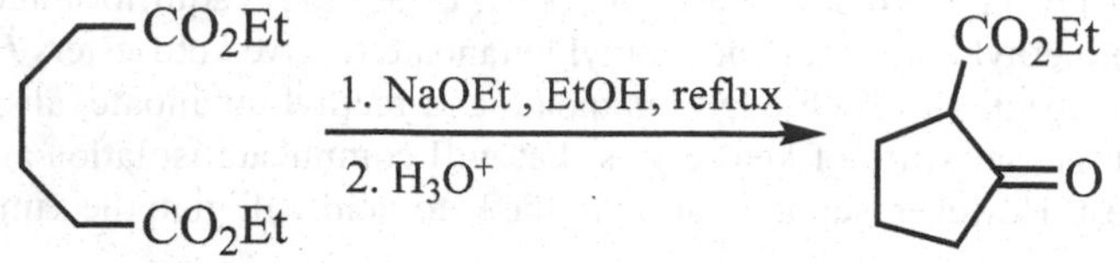

CO_2Et / CO_2Et — 1. NaOEt , EtOH, reflux; 2. H_3O^+ → CO_2Et, =O

What is the name of this reaction?

The reaction shown in the preceding question is known as the *Dieckmann condensation.* Note that this reaction is an intramolecular Claisen condensation.

What ring sizes are formed by this cyclization reaction?

Rings of three to seven members can be formed by this technique. Formation of cyclic ketones of 8–13 members is very difficult by this method although larger rings can be prepared by high dilution techniques.

What is the major product of the following sequence with the diethyl ester of 1,7-heptanedioic acid: 1. LDA, THF, -78°C; 2. saponification; 3. heating to 200°C?

The Claisen product is the keto-ester but saponification and decarboxylation will lead to the final product, cyclohexanone.

What is the major product of the reactions of (a), (b), and (c)?

(a) CO_2Et, CO_2Et — 1. NaOEt , EtOH, reflux; 2. H_3O^+ →

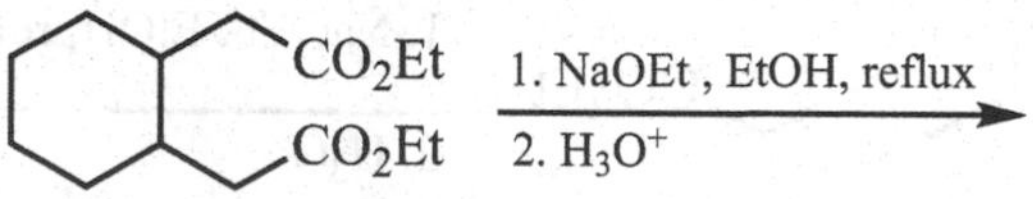

(b) CO_2Et, CO_2Et — 1. NaOEt , EtOH, reflux; 2. H_3O^+; 3. i. aq. NaOH ii. H_3O^+; 4. 200 °C →

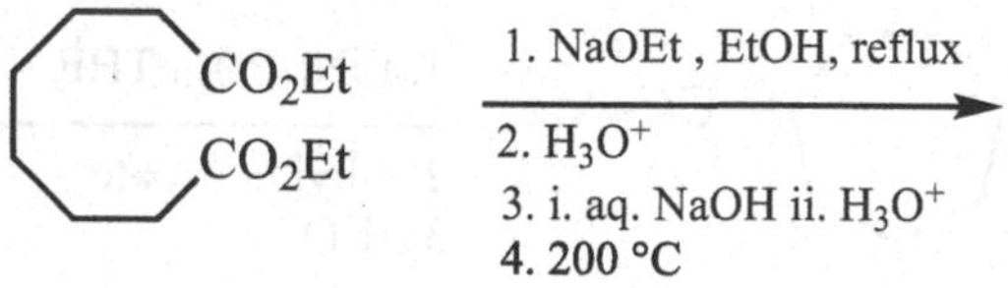

(c) CO_2Et, CO_2Et — 1. NaOEt , EtOH, reflux; 2. H_3O^+ →

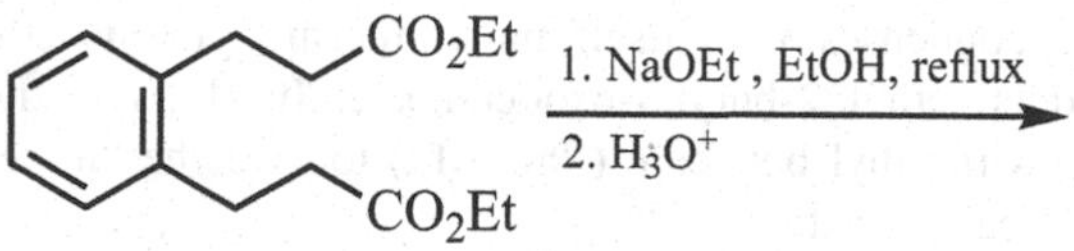

In (a), Dieckmann condensation leads to the bicyclic keto-ester, ethyl 2-oxooctahydro-1*H*-indene-1-carboxylate. In (b), diethyl 1,8-octanedioate is cyclized under Dieckmann conditions but saponification and decarboxylation give cycloheptanone as the final product. In (c), the diester is cyclized to keto-ester ethyl 7-oxo-6,7,8,9-tetrahydro-5*H*-benzo[7]annulene-6-carboxylate.

(a) CO_2Et, =O (b) =O (c) CO_2Et, =O

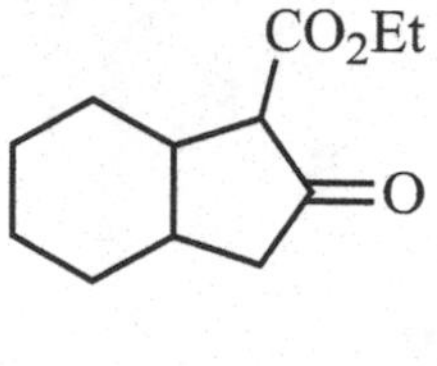

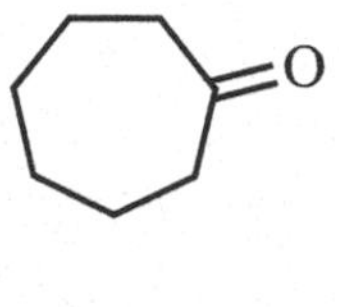

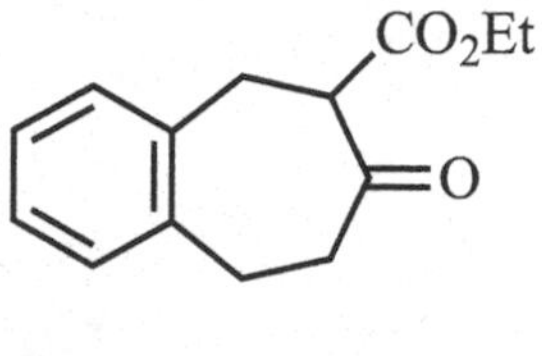

If the enolate of methyl 2-phenylethanoate is treated with cyclohexanone, what is the major product after hydrolysis?

Ethyl 2-phenylethanoate is converted to the ester enolate (*A*). Subsequent reaction with cyclohexanone followed by hydrolysis gives β-hydroxy-ester, ethyl 2-(1-hydroxycyclohexyl)-2-phenylacetate.

Ph CO2Et → Ph OEt A O⁻ → (cyclohexanone) → H_3O^+ → Ph CO2Et OH

Which is better for the condensation of an ester enolate and an aldehyde, kinetic control conditions or thermodynamic control conditions?

In order to prevent a Claisen condensation of the ester, kinetic control conditions are better. Under thermodynamic control conditions, especially when both aldehyde or ketone and the ester are present in the same reaction, an aldol condensation could also compete with the Claisen condensation, in addition to the "mixed" condensation.

With what type of aldehyde can thermodynamic control conditions best be utilized?

If an aldehyde does not have an α-carbon with acidic hydrogens (such as benzaldehyde), it can be added directly into the flask with the ester, under thermodynamic control conditions.

What is the major product of the following sequence with ethyl butanoate: 1. LDA, THF, -78°C; 2. 5-methylhexan-2-one; 3. saponification; 4. heating to 200°C?

The product is 4,7-dimethyloctan-4-ol.

What is the Reformatsky reaction?

The *Reformatsky reaction* is the condensation of a *zinc enolate* of an ester formed from an α-halo ester and an aldehyde.

What is an example of the Reformatsky reaction?

When ethyl 2-bromoacetate reacts with zinc, the zinc enolate is formed (*A*). This nucleophilic enolate anion reacts with benzaldehyde via *B* to give the hydroxy-ester (ethyl 3-hydroxy-3-phenylpropanoate) after hydrolysis.

Br CO2Et —Zn°→ [$BrZn^+ {}^-CH_2CO_2Et$ ↔ $O^- {}^+ZnBr$ OEt] A —PhCHO→

[Br Zn⁺ ⁻O O Ph H H_2C OEt] B → —H_2O→ Ph OH CO2Et

In what ways is the Reformatsky reaction similar to the enolate reactions described above?

The Reformatsky is an enolate condensation reaction of an ester with an aldehyde. It is a zinc-enolate anion rather than a lithium or sodium enolate anion, as in the usual Claisen-type condensations. The reaction with aldehydes is typically more facile than reaction with ketones.

How are α-halo esters prepared?

A common method for the preparation of α-halo acids is the reaction of an acid such as acetic acid with phosphorus and chlorine or bromine (P, Cl_2 or P, Br_2). Under these conditions, PCl_3 or PBr_3 is formed and reacts to give 2-chloroacetyl chloride or 2-bromoacetyl chloride, which is hydrolyzed to the corresponding acid. Such α-halo acids are converted to the corresponding ester by the usual methods. The conversion of an acid to an α-halo acid chloride is called the *Hell–Volhard–Zelinsky* reaction (see below).

$$ClCH_2CO_2Cl \xleftarrow{P,\ Cl_2} CH_3CO_2H \xrightarrow{P,\ Br_2} BrCH_2COBr$$

What is the major product when ethyl malonate is treated with 1. NaOEt; 2. acetone; 3. H_3O^+?

The initially formed malonate anion (***A***) reacts with acetone to give the alkoxide (***B***). Aqueous hydrolysis gives the alcohol (***C***) but the alcohol usually dehydrates under these conditions to the alkylidene derivative, ***D*** [diethyl 2-(propan-2-ylidene)malonate]. Note that the great acidity of the malonic ester often allows the use of a weaker base.

$$(EtO_2C)_2CH_2 \xrightarrow{NaOEt} (EtO_2C)_2CH^- \ (\textbf{A}) \xrightarrow{H_3C(C{=}O)CH_3} (EtO_2C)_2CH{-}C(O^-)Me_2 \ (\textbf{B}) \xrightarrow{H_3O^+} (EtO_2C)_2CH{-}C(OH)Me_2 \ (\textbf{C}) \xrightarrow{H_3O^+} (EtO_2C)_2C{=}CMe_2 \ (\textbf{D})$$

Why is the major product usually an alkene?

The proximity of the alcohol moiety to two carbonyl groups allows extensive hydrogen bonding and a hydroxyl group β- to two carbonyl groups allows facile loss of water under the acidic conditions of the workup. In other words, elimination of water leads to the alkene moiety.

What is the name of this type of condensation?

This transformation is known as the *Knoevenagel condensation.*

Why can an amine be used for the base for the Knoevenagel reaction rather than NaOEt?

The pK_a of the proton on the -CH_2- moiety of malonic ester is about 11. With such a strong acid, pyridine or triethylamine be used as a base, rather than the stronger NaOEt.

What is the product of the reaction between bromine and butanoic acid?

The reaction of a carboxylic acid and bromine or chlorine is usually very slow. There is usually only a little reaction since a halogen must react with the enol form of the acid, which is present in very small concentration. If the percentage of enol can be increased, halogenation is more viable.

What is the enol form of a carboxylic acid?

An enol is C=C—OH and is usually present with a carbonyl compound as a minor tautomer. With carboxylic acids, the enol form is $C{=}C(OH)_2$.

What is tautomerism?

Tautomers are two or more isomers of a compound that exist together in equilibrium and are readily interchanged by migration of an atom or group within the molecule. Tautomerism is the ability of some compounds to exist as a mixture of two interconvertible isomers that are in equilibrium

What is the Hell–Volhard–Zelinsky Reaction?

The *Hell–Volhard–Zelinsky* reaction is the conversion of a carboxylic acid to an α-halo acid by treatment with a halogen (usually bromine) and a halogenating agent such as PCl_3. An example is the conversion of butanoic acid to 2-bromobutanoic acid. Initial reaction with PCl_3 gives the acid chloride, which has a relatively high enol content (*A*). The π-bond of the enol will attack the bromine, as shown, which is polarizable and in the presence of the alkene exists as $^{\delta+}Br—Br^{\delta-}$. Displacement of bromide leads to the α-bromo acid chloride (***B***). This acid chloride usually reacts with the starting acid to produce the final product, α-bromobutanoic acid and the acid chloride, which can be recycled. For this reason, only a catalytic amount of PCl_3 is required.

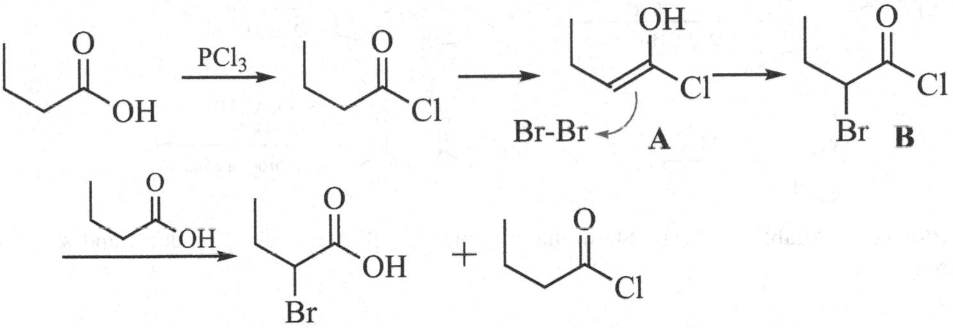

O OH PCl3 O Cl OH Cl Br-Br A O Cl Br B

O OH O OH Br + O Cl

2-bromobutanoic acid butanoyl chloride

END OF CHAPTER PROBLEMS

1. What is the most acidic hydrogen in each of the following molecules?

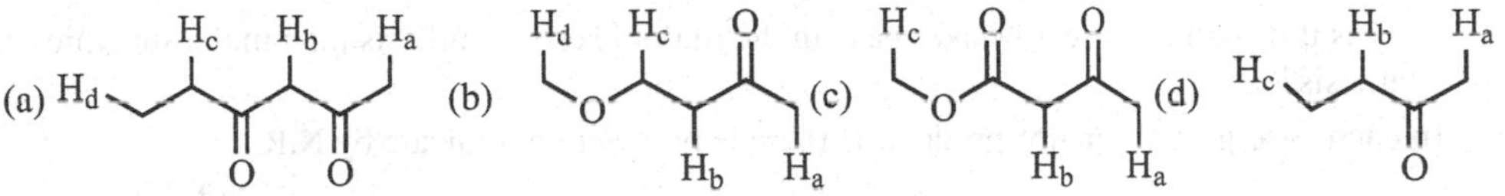

(a) Hd Hc Hb Ha O O (b) Hd Hc O O Hb Ha (c) Hc O O O Hb Ha (d) Hc Hb Ha O

2. Which of the following has the highest enol content? Explain.

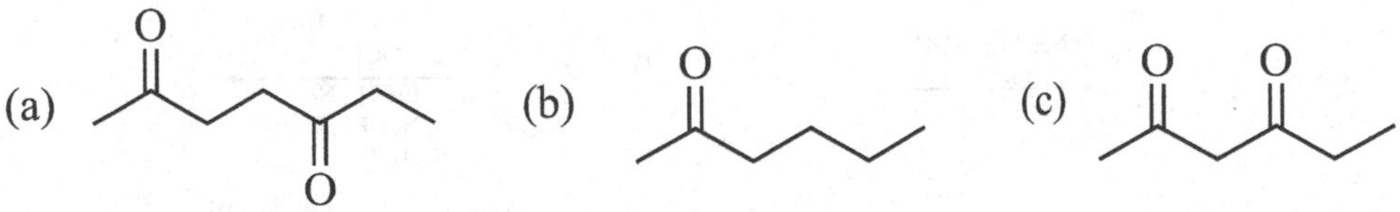

(a) O O (b) O (c) O O

3. What reaction conditions favor kinetic control in forming an enolate anion from butan-2-one?
4. Give all aldol products that are possible from the following reaction.

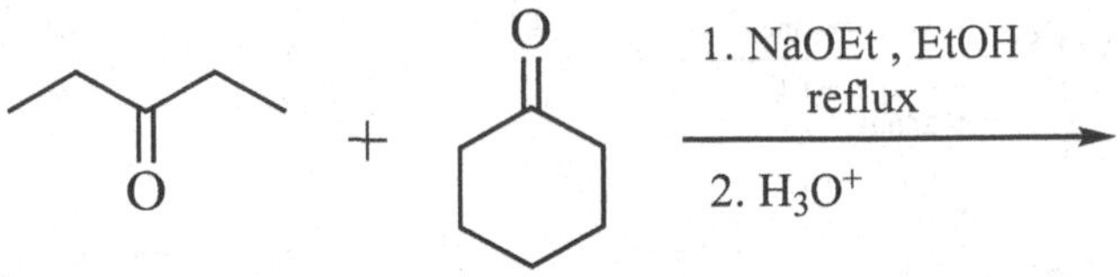

O + O 1. NaOEt , EtOH reflux 2. H_3O^+

5. Predict the product from the reaction of but-3-en-2-one and lithium dibutylcuprate.
6. In each case, give the major product. Remember stereochemistry where appropriate and if there is no reaction, indicate by N.R.

(a) 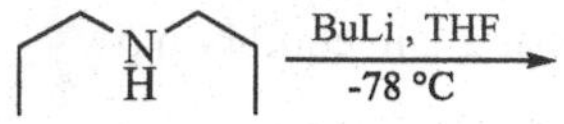 N H — BuLi, THF / -78 °C →
(b) 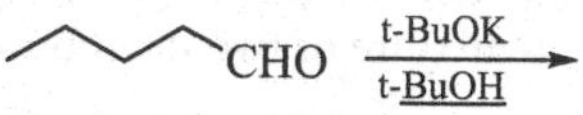 CHO — t-BuOK / t-BuOH →
(c) 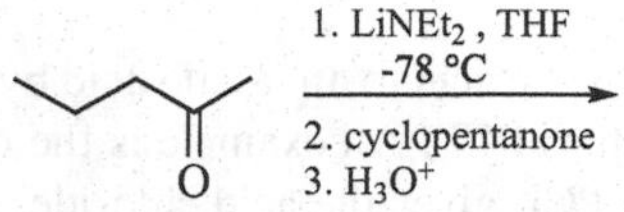 O — 1. $LiNEt_2$, THF -78 °C / 2. cyclopentanone 3. H_3O^+ →
(d) 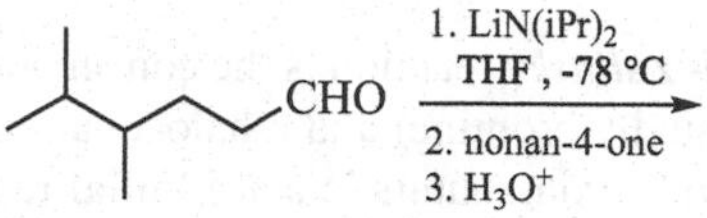 CHO — 1. $LiN(iPr)_2$ THF, -78 °C / 2. nonan-4-one 3. H_3O^+ →
(e) 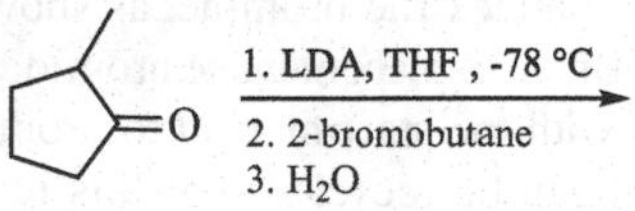 O — 1. LDA, THF, -78 °C / 2. 2-bromobutane 3. H_2O →
(f) 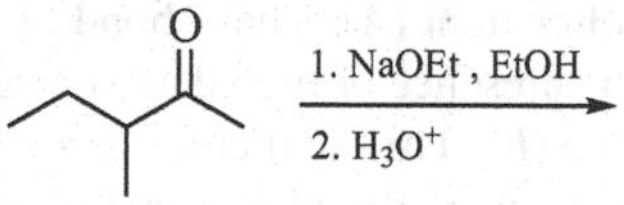 O — 1. NaOEt, EtOH / 2. H_3O^+ →
(g) 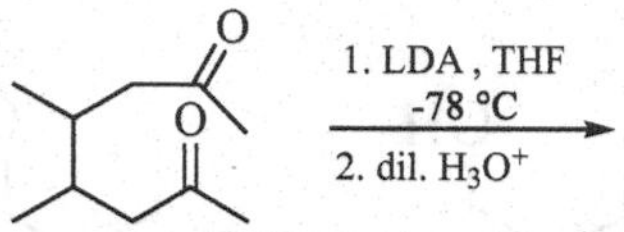 O O — 1. LDA, THF -78 °C / 2. dil. H_3O^+ →
(h) 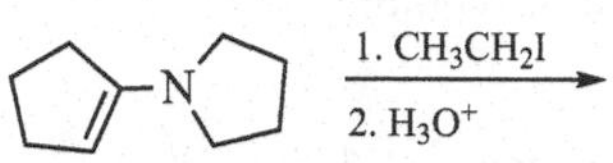 N — 1. CH_3CH_2I / 2. H_3O^+ →
(i) 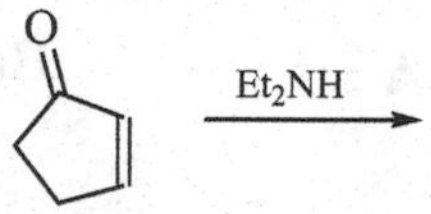 O — Et_2NH →
(k) 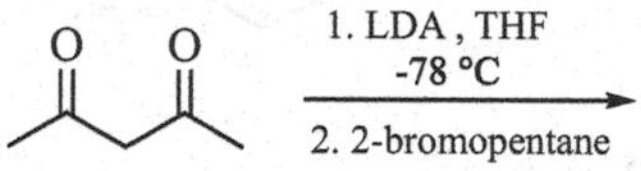 O O — 1. LDA, THF -78 °C / 2. 2-bromopentane →

7. Provide a suitable synthesis. Show the structure of all intermediate products and show all reagents.

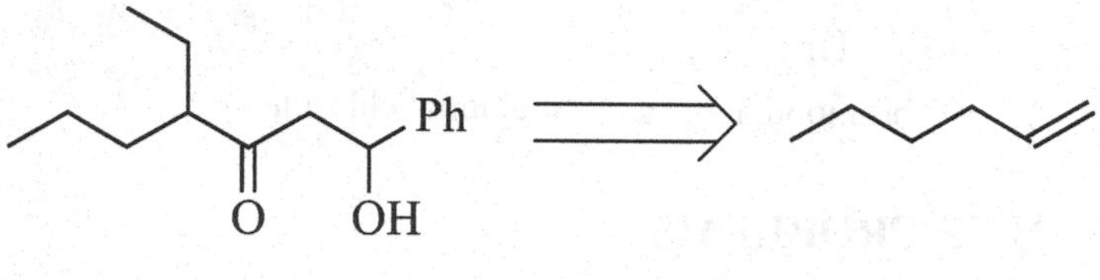

Ph O OH ⟹

8. Why is it important to use sodium ethoxide with an ethyl ester rather than sodium methoxide when forming an enolate anion to do a reaction?
9. Why is it possible to use a weaker base in the malonic ester synthesis than in the succinic ester synthesis?
10. In each case give the major product. If there is no reaction, indicate by N.R.

(a) 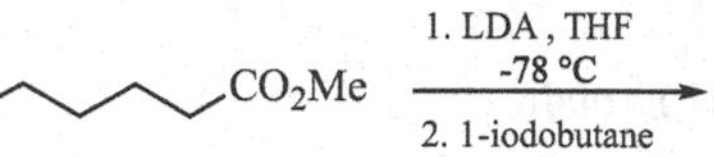 CO_2Me — 1. LDA, THF -78 °C / 2. 1-iodobutane →
(b) 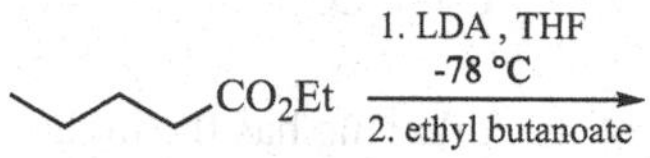 CO_2Et — 1. LDA, THF -78 °C / 2. ethyl butanoate →
(c) 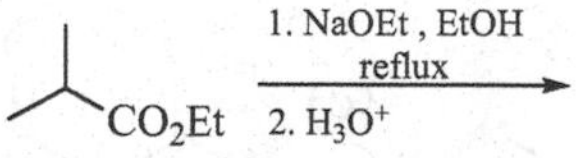 CO_2Et — 1. NaOEt, EtOH reflux / 2. H_3O^+ →
(d) 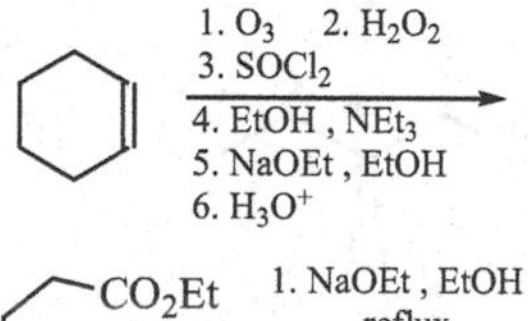 — 1. O_3 2. H_2O_2 3. $SOCl_2$ / 4. EtOH, NEt_3 5. NaOEt, EtOH 6. H_3O^+ →
(e) 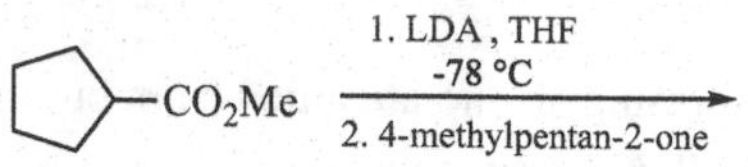 CO_2Me — 1. LDA, THF -78 °C / 2. 4-methylpentan-2-one →
(f) 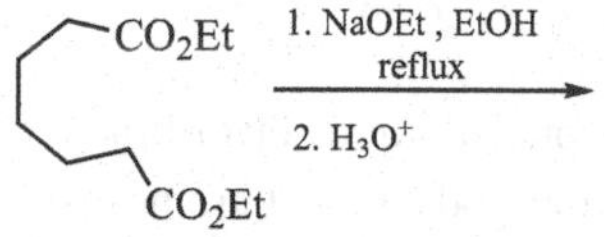 CO_2Et CO_2Et — 1. NaOEt, EtOH reflux / 2. H_3O^+ →
(g) 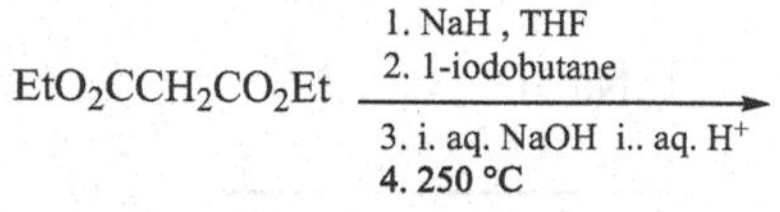 $EtO_2CCH_2CO_2Et$ — 1. NaH, THF 2. 1-iodobutane / 3. i. 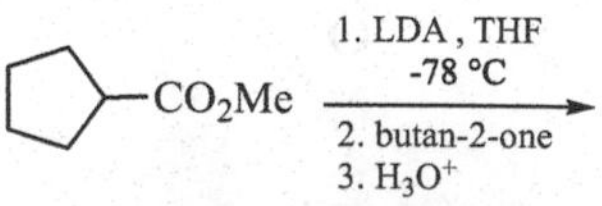 aq. NaOH i.. aq. H^+ 4. 250 °C →
(g) 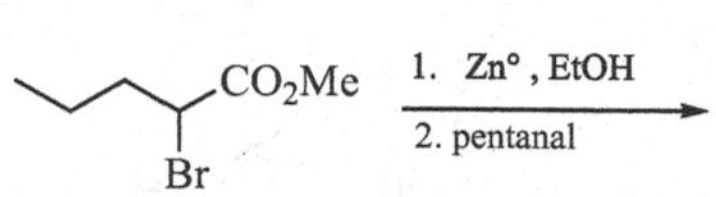 CO_2Me Br — 1. Zn°, EtOH / 2. pentanal →
(h) 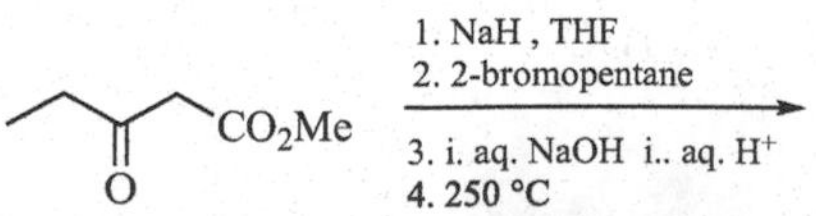 CO_2Me O — 1. NaH, THF 2. 2-bromopentane / 3. i. aq. NaOH i.. aq. H^+ 4. 250 °C →
(i) CO_2Me — 1. LDA, THF -78 °C / 2. butan-2-one 3. H_3O^+ →

18

Conjugation and Reactions of Conjugated Compounds

When a π-bond is directly attached to another π-bond, each influences the reactivity and properties of the other. One π-bond of an alkene is directly connected to another alkene moiety (forming a diene), a carbonyl (giving α,β-unsaturated ketones, aldehydes and acid derivatives), or part of other π-bond containing functional groups such as imines, nitro compounds, or nitriles. When the π-bonds are directly connected, the arrangement is called *conjugation*. The important properties of conjugation include the interaction of these molecules with ultraviolet light (and other light such as infrared light) and the changes in chemical reactivity that are induced, relative to unconjugated molecules. The idea of competing reactions, 1,2- vs. 1,4-addition with conjugated π-bonds, will be discussed.

18.1 CONJUGATED MOLECULES

What is the electron distribution when a π-bond is adjacent to a p-orbital?

When a π-bond is adjacent to a p-orbital, as in the allylic cation, the three p-orbitals (two from the π-bond and the third one) will share electron density, as shown. The electrons are, therefore, delocalized over all three orbitals rather than localized on a single atom, and the positive charge will be dispersed to the two termini (shown by δ^+). This is represented as two structures and is called *resonance*. The allylic cation is represented by two resonance contributors, which makes this cation easier to form and more stable once it has been formed. The allylic cation is said to be *resonance stabilized.*

δ+ δ+

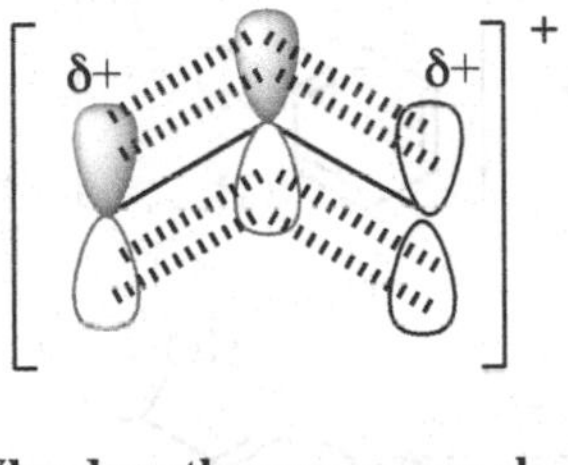

$$\left[CH_2{=}CH{-}\overset{+}{C}H_2 \longleftrightarrow \overset{+}{C}H_2{-}CH{=}CH_2 \right]$$

Why does the resonance shown for $CH_2{=}CH{-}CH_2^+$ not occur in $CH_2{=}CHCH_2CH_2CH_2^+$?

In $CH_2{=}CHCH_2CH_2CH_2^+$ the p-orbitals of the π-bond are not connected to the p-orbital of the positive charge and they are too far away from the p-orbital containing the positive charge to share electron density. It is, therefore, impossible to disperse the charge; there is no resonance and the charge is localized on a single carbon.

What is the initially formed intermediate for the reaction of prop-2-en-1-ol with H^+?

When 2-prop-2-en-1-ol ($CH_2{=}CHCH_2OH$) reacts with an acid, an oxonium salt is formed ($CH_2{=}CHCH_2OH_2^+$), which loses water to form the resonance-stabilized allyl cation.

What is the intermediate for the reaction of pent-3-en-2-ol with H^+?

The alcohol (pent-3-en-2-ol) is an *allylic* alcohol and will form an allylic cation. Initial reaction with acid generates oxonium ion ***A***. Subsequent loss of water gives the resonance-stabilized allylic cation ***B***.

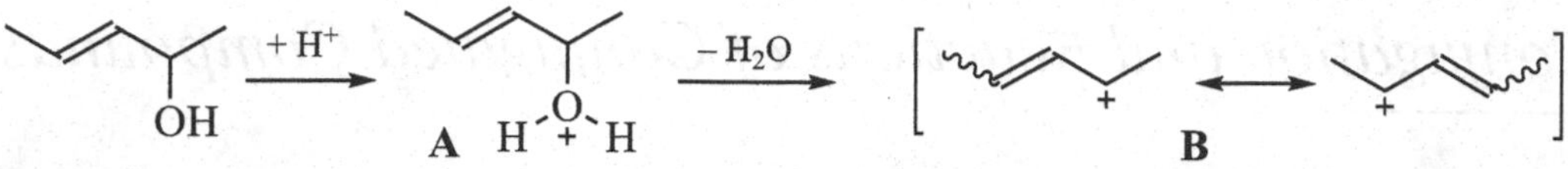

What are the resonance contributors of the benzylic carbocation?

The benzyl carbocation is a CH_2^+ unit that is attached to a benzene ring. This cation is resonance stabilized as shown, with the charge dispersed into the benzene ring. The extensive charge delocalized of the benzyl cation makes it very stable, and the activation barrier to formation of the benzyl cation is low.

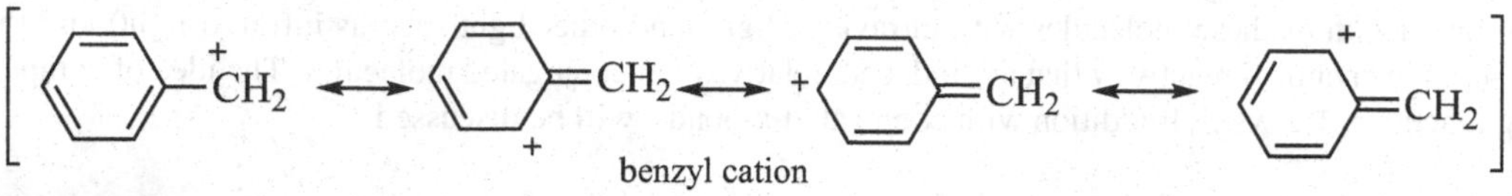

benzyl cation

What is the intermediate when 1-phenylpropan-2-ol is treated with aqueous acid? What is the final product of this reaction?

The initial reaction of the alcohol with aqueous acid generates oxonium ion ***A***, which loses water to give carbocation ***B***. Note that carbocation ***B*** is a secondary carbocation. A rearrangement (1,2-hydrogen shift) will generate a resonance stabilized benzylic carbocation, ***C***, where the charge is delocalized into the benzene ring. The increased stability of ***C*** relative to secondary carbocation ***B*** provides the energetic driving force for the rearrangement. The final product is generated by reaction of ***C*** with water to give oxonium ion ***D***. Loss of a proton gives the final product, 1-phenylpropan-1-ol.

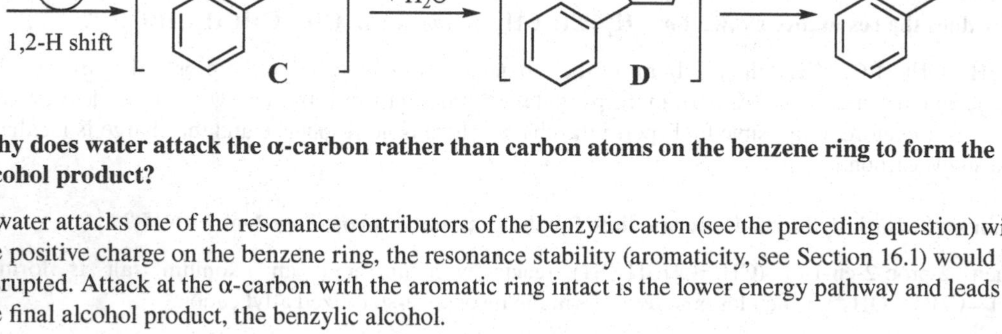

Why does water attack the α-carbon rather than carbon atoms on the benzene ring to form the alcohol product?

If water attacks one of the resonance contributors of the benzylic cation (see the preceding question) with the positive charge on the benzene ring, the resonance stability (aromaticity, see Section 16.1) would be disrupted. Attack at the α-carbon with the aromatic ring intact is the lower energy pathway and leads to the final alcohol product, the benzylic alcohol.

What is (are) the major product(s) when but-2-en-1-ol is treated with HCl?

But-2-en-1-ol reacts with aqueous HCl to give an oxonium ion, which loses water to give a resonance stabilized allylic cation, ***A***. Note that there are two sites of electrophilic reactivity, at a primary carbon and also at a secondary carbon. Subsequent reaction with the chloride counterion leads to two products via reaction with both resonance contributors. Therefore, the products are (*E* + *Z*) 1-chlorobut-2-ene and 3-chlorobut-1-ene. Note that 1-chlorobut-2-ene is a mixture of *E*- and *Z*-isomers (denoted by the squiggle line). There are, therefore, a total of three products.

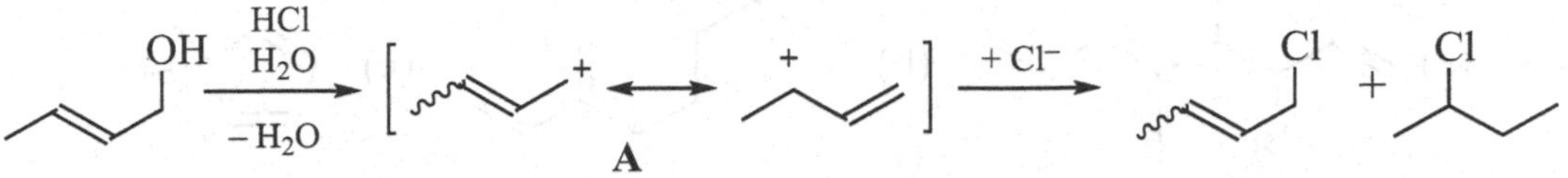

OH —HCl, H_2O / $-H_2O$→ [+ ⟷ +] **A** —$+Cl^-$→ Cl + Cl

When benzyl alcohol (phenylmethanol) is treated with HCl the product is benzyl chloride (chlorophenylmethane). Explain why no products are isolated with a chlorine attached to the benzene ring.

The benzyl carbocation is generated by protonation of the OH unit to give an oxonium ion and subsequent loss of water. The benzyl carbocation is resonance stabilized and has the charge delocalized on the benzene ring. The chlorine attaches to the benzylic carbon to give the major product, benzyl chloride, which retains the aromatic character of the benzene ring. If chlorine were to attach to the benzene ring, however, the final product would lose the resonance stability inherent to the benzene ring (see Section 16.1), making that reaction too high in energy to compete with attachment at the benzylic position.

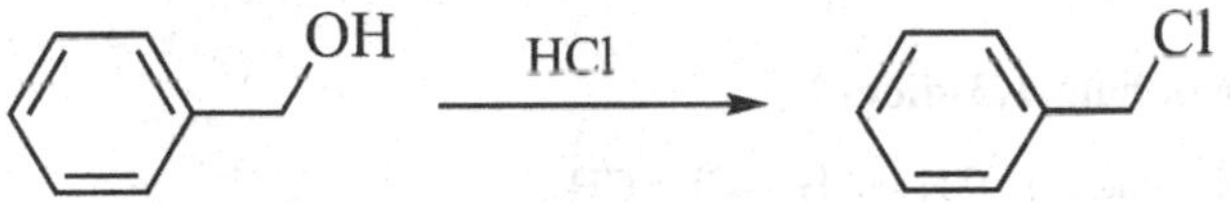

OH —HCl→ Cl

What is the major product when hex-5-en-1-ol reacts with HCl?

The product is 6-chlorohex-1-ene. No resonance-stabilized intermediate is possible if the alkene reacts with HCl. In this case, the oxygen of the hydroxyl group is more basic than the π-bond and reacts preferentially with HCl. Formation of the oxonium ion and displacement by chloride give the product.

What is the product when 2-phenylethan-1-ol reacts with HBr?

The product is 1-bromo-1-phenylethane

18.2 STRUCTURE AND NOMENCLATURE OF CONJUGATED SYSTEMS

When two double bonds are present in a molecule, what is the IUPAC rule for naming such compounds?

The prefix *di*- is used for two functional groups of the same kind (diene). *Tri*- is used for three groups (triene) and *tetra*- is used for four groups (tetraene). A molecule with two carbon–carbon double bonds is, therefore, a *diene* and numbers are used to denote the first carbon of each double bond. The double bonds should be given the lowest possible numbers and *both* double bonds must be part of the longest continuous chain.

What is the structure of (a) hepta-1,4*E*-diene (b) cyclopentadiene (c) cycloocta-1,5-diene

(a) 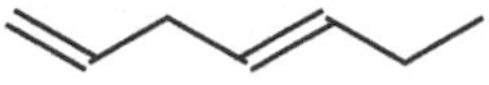 hepta-1,4*E*-diene (b) cyclopentadiene (c) cycloocta-1,5-diene

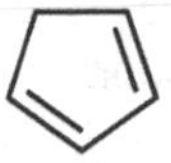

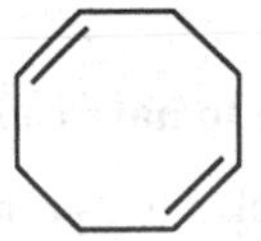

What is the structure for: (a) 3-bromo-4,5-dimethylocta-1,6*E*-diene (b) 1,4-diethylcyclohexa-1,3-diene (c) 5,5-dimethylcyclopenta-1,3-diene (d) hepta-2*E*,4*E*-diene (e) hepta-2*E*, 4*Z*-diene?

(a) 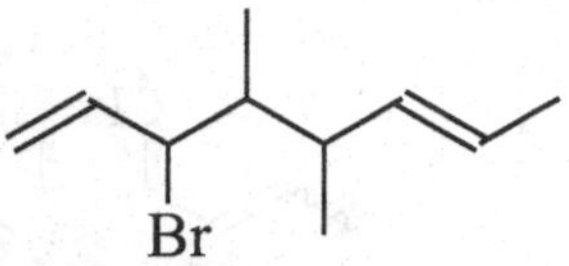 Br

3-bromo-4,5-dimethyl-octa-1,6*E*-diene

(b)

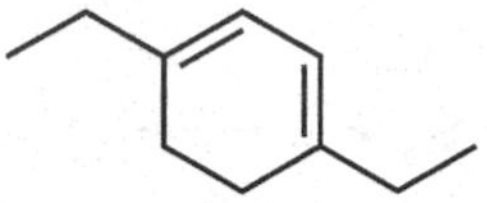

1,4-diethylcyclo-hexa-1,3-diene

(c)

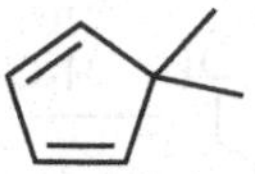

5,5-dimethylcyclo-penta-1,3-diene

(d)

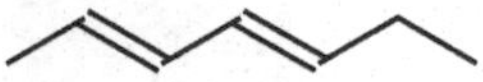

hepta-2*E*,4*E*-diene

(e)

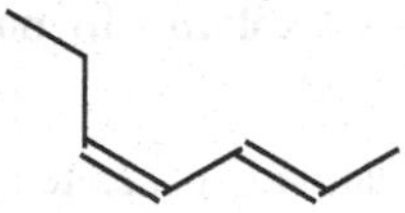

hepta-2*E*, 4*Z*-diene

Is hexa-1,5-diene considered to have a conjugated double bond?

No! The double bonds are separated by two -CH_2 groups and they are not conjugated.

What is the structure of buta-1,3-diene?

The structure of buta-1,3-diene is CH_2=CH—CH=CH_2.

Is buta-1,3-diene resonance stabilized?

Buta-1,3-diene is *not* resonance stabilized. Each double bond has the π-bond localized between the two carbons.

Is the C2–C3 bond length of buta-1,3-diene shorter or longer than the C2–C3 bond of but-1-ene? Explain.

There is some overlap of the p-orbitals on the C2 and C3 carbons of buta-1,3-diene. For this reason, the bond length for the C2–C3 bond of buta-1-3-diene is 146 pm, which is shorter than the C—C single bond found between C2 and C3 in but-1-ene, which is about 150 pm. This overlap does not constitute resonance, however. Note that the C—C bond distances of sp^3–sp^3 atoms is about 1.54 pm.

What is the structure of hexa-2*E*,4*Z*-diene and hexa-1,4*E*-diene? Which is a conjugated molecule?

The C=C unit in hexa-2*E*,4*Z*-diene is directly connected to and therefore conjugated to the C=C unit and it is a conjugated molecule. The C=C unit in hexa-1,4*E*-diene is separated from the other C=C unit by a sp^3 carbon atom so it is *not* conjugated.

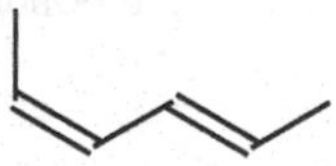

hexa-2*E*,4*Z*-diene 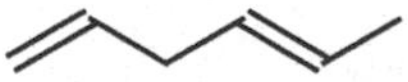 hexa-1,4*E*-diene

Is it possible to have conjugated triple bonds?

Yes! Two triple bonds constitute a diyne, and there are triynes, tetraynes, etc.

What is the structure of: (a) hexa-1,3-diyne (b) nona-2,6-diyne (c) hepta-2,4-diyne (d) hepta-2*E*-en-4-yne

(a) hexa-1,3-diyne (b) 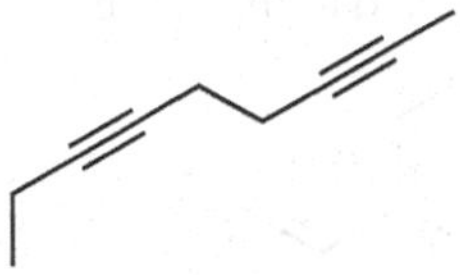 nona-2,6-diyne (c) 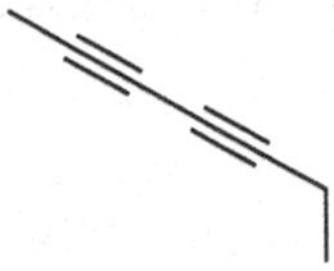 hepta-2,4-diyne (d) 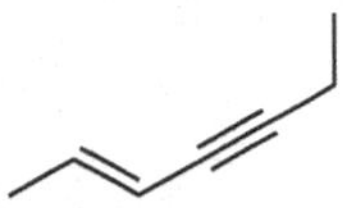 hepta-2*E*-en-4-yne

In the preceding question, which, if any, of these compounds are conjugated?

The conjugated compounds are (a) hexa-1,3-diyne; (c) hepta-2,4-diyne; and (d), hepta-2*E*-en-4-yne. In (a) and (c) the triple bonds are conjugated to each other, whereas in (d) the double bond is conjugated to the triple bond. The triple bonds in (b) are not conjugated.

Can a C=C unit be conjugated to a carbonyl? To a benzene ring?

Yes, to both questions! The examples shown are pent-3-en-2*E*-one, where the C=C unit is conjugated to a carbonyl. In 2-phenylbut-1-ene, the C=C unit is conjugated to a benzene ring.

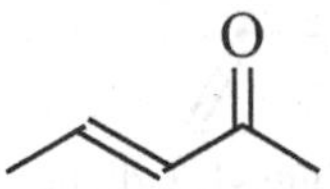

O

pent-3-en-2*E*-one 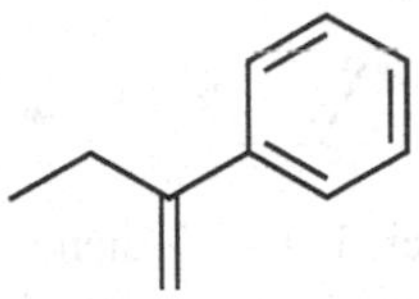 2-phenylbut-1-ene

What is the structure of hex-4*Z*-ene-2-one and hex-3*E*-en-2-one? Which is a conjugated molecule?

The C=C unit in hex-3*E*-en-2-one is conjugated to the C=O unit so it is a conjugated molecule. The C=C unit in hex-4*Z*-ene-2-one is separated from the C=O unit by a sp^3 carbon atom so it is *not* conjugated.

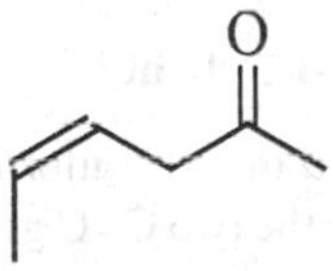

O O

hexa-4*Z*-ene-2-one 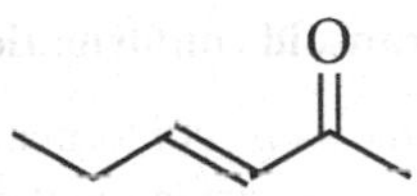 hexa-3*E*-en-2-one

What is the structure of: (a) but-3-en-2-one (b) cyclohex-2-en-1-one (c) cyclohex-3-en-1-one (d) octadec-1,3-dien-5-one (e) hex-3-yn-2-one

(a) 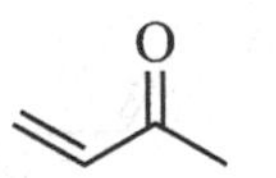 O but-3-en-2-one

(b) 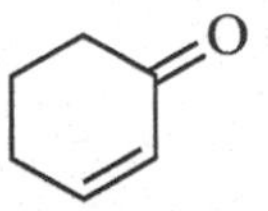 O cyclohex-2-en-1-one

(c) 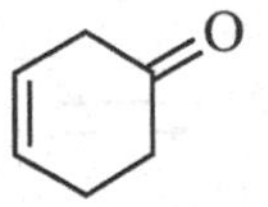 O cyclohex-3-en-1-one

(d) 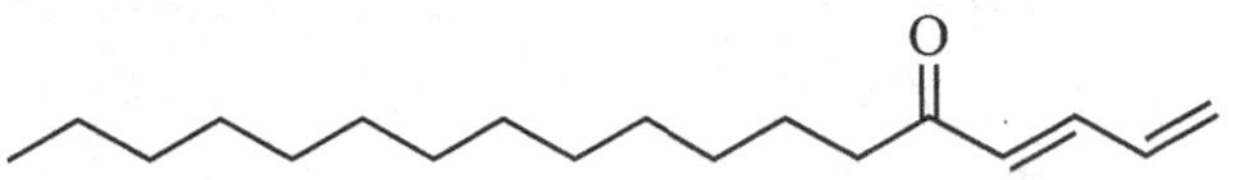 O octadec-1,3*E*-dien-5-one

(e) 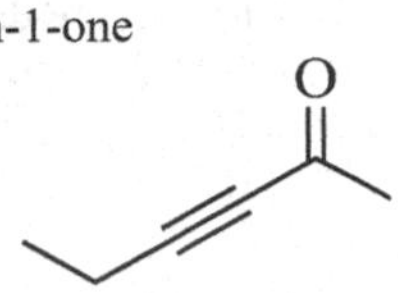 O hex-3-yn-2-one

What is the structure of styrene?

The molecule is shown, abbreviated $PhCH{=}CH_2$, and is named ethenylbenzene, with the common name of styrene. In this molecule the C=C unit is conjugated to the benzene ring.

ethenylbenzene
(styrene)

Is there rotation about the C—C bond of buta-1,3diene?

Yes! As a result of the rotation about this single bond, there are eclipsed and anti-conformation of buta-1,3-diene. See Section 5.1 for conformations about C—C single bonds.

What are the structures of the s-cis- and s-trans- conformations of buta-1,3-diene?

The two rotamers of interest for rotation about the C2–C3 bond are the s-cis- rotamer, where the two C=C units are eclipsed and the s-trans- rotamer where the two C=C units are anti.

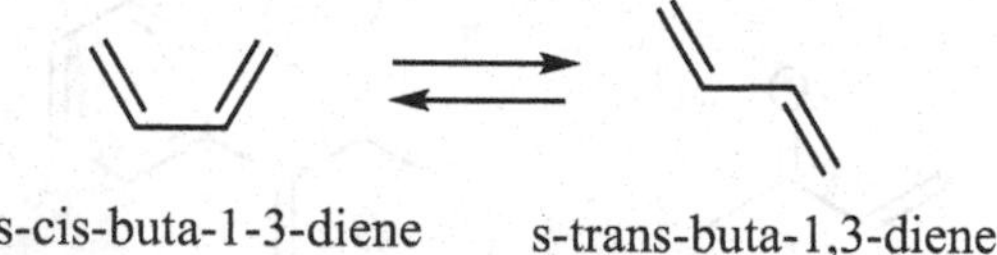

s-cis-buta-1-3-diene s-trans-buta-1,3-diene

Which is more stable, s-*cis*-buta-1,3-diene or s-*trans*-buta-1,3-diene?

As expected, the s-cis- and the s-trans- conformations of buta-1,3-diene are in equilibrium, and the less sterically hindered conformation is expected to be the lower energy and the more stable. The hydrogen atoms on the $C{=}CH_2$ groups sterically interact in the s-cis- conformation (see the figure in the preceding question), so it is higher in energy, making the s-trans- form more stable since there is less steric interaction. In other words, the steric interaction is not present in the s-trans- conformation.

What are the cisoid and transoid conformations of buta-1,3-diene?

The cisoid conformation is the s-cis- conformation and the transoid conformation is the s-trans- conformation. The s-cis- (the old term is *cisoid*) conformation has the two C=C groups on the same side of the molecule, whereas the s-trans- (the old term is *transoid*) conformation has the C=C groups on opposite sides These are rotamers generated by rotation around the C2–C3 bond of the diene.

What is the highest energy s-cis- rotamer of the three stereoisomers of hexa-2,4-diene? Which is the more stable s-trans- rotamer?

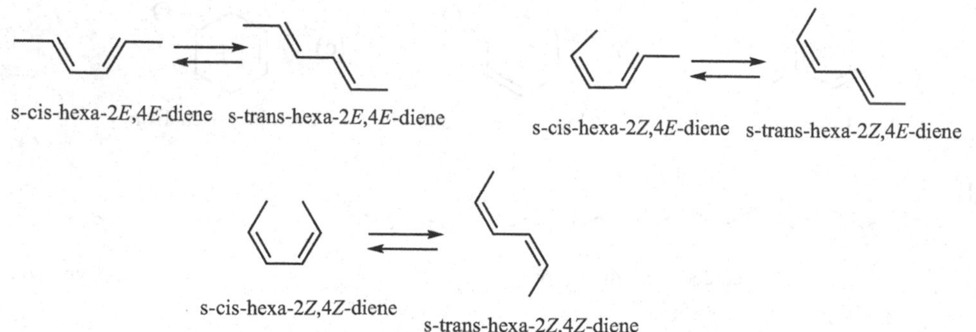

There are three stereoisomers of hexa-2,4-diene, the *EE*, *ZE*, and *ZZ* isomers. The s-trans- rotamer in each case is more stable than the s-*cis*-rotamer. The s-*cis*-hexa-2Z,4Z-diene isomer has two methyl groups in close spatial proximity, with greater steric interaction than the other s-cis- isomers. The s-*trans*-hexa-2*E*,4*E*-diene isomer has the methyl groups as far removed from one another as possible.

18.3 REACTIONS OF CONJUGATED MOLECULES

What is the intermediate when HCl reacts with buta-1,3-diene? What are the final products?

The reaction of the π-bonds of buta-1,3-diene with HCl generates the intermediate in this reaction, an allylic cation, ***A***. When the chloride counterion reacts with ***A***, reaction occurs at *both* cationic carbons, generating two products, 1-chlorobut-2-ene and 3-chlorobut-1-ene. However, since all resonance contributors of ***A*** react, including the E/Z isomers of the disubstituted C=C unit, both *E* and *Z* products are formed in the reaction with chloride ion. Therefore, there are actually three products, 1-chlorobut-2*E*-ene, 1-chlorobut-2*Z*-ene, and 3-chlorobut-1-ene.

HCl; A; Cl^-; Cl; Cl; Cl; 1-chlorobut-2*E*-ene; 3-chlorobut-1-ene; 1-chlorobut-2*Z*-ene

What products are formed when HCl reacts with penta-1,3-diene.

There are three products, 1-chloropent-2*E*-ene, 1-chloropent-2*Z*-ene, and 3-chloropent-1-ene.

When buta-1,3-diene reacts with HCl at -78°C, what is the major product? Explain.

At lower temperatures, the reaction generates the less substituted product and is said to be under *kinetic control*. The major product is the "1,2-addition" product, 3-chlorobut-1-ene. At low temperatures the reaction occurs fastest at the electrophilic secondary cationic position, which at low temperatures is more stable than the one with the positive charge on the primary carbon. Reaction with Cl^- generates 3-chlorobut-1-ene as the major product.

HCl; −78 °C; Cl; 3-chlorobut-1-ene

When buta-1,3-diene reacts with HCl at 30°C, what is the major product? Explain.

At higher temperatures, the reaction generates the more substituted product and is said to be under *thermodynamic control* At higher temperatures, both canonical forms of the resonance stabilized allylic cation ***A*** (see the preceding question) are present but the "primary" carbocation has a disubstituted double bond, whereas the "secondary" cation has a monosubstituted double bond. Under thermodynamic equilibration conditions (higher temperature) the more stable alkene product, which is the more substituted, is favored. In this case, the *major* products are 1-chlorobut-2*E*-ene and 1-chlorobut-2*Z*-ene.

HCl; 30 °C; Cl; Cl; 1-chlorobut-2*E*-ene; 1-chlorobut-2*Z*-ene

What are the products when hexa-2*E*,4*E*-diene reacts with aqueous acid?

This reaction is a hydration reaction (Section 7.4.1). The initial reaction of the acid catalyst with the diene generates an allylic cation ***A***. When ***A*** reacts with water, two oxonium ions ***B*** and ***C*** are formed by reaction at the two electrophilic carbon atoms of the allylic cation. Loss of a proton leads to the alcohol products, a mixture of 3*E*- and 3*Z* hex-3-en-2-ol (***B***) and 4*E*- and 4*Z* hex-4-en-3-ol (***C***).

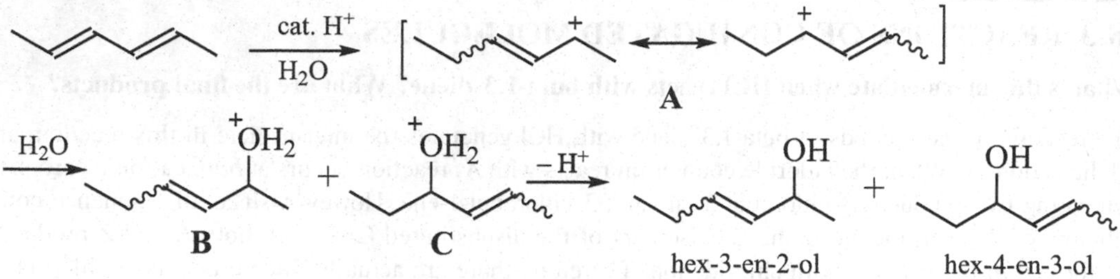

cat. H^+, H_2O — **A**; H_2O — **B** + **C**; $-H^+$ — hex-3-en-2-ol + hex-4-en-3-ol

What is the product of the reaction of cyclohexene and Br_2?

The π-bond reacts with bromine to give a bromonium ion intermediate, which reacts with the bromide counterion to give *trans*-1,2-dibromocyclohexane, as described in Section 7.4.

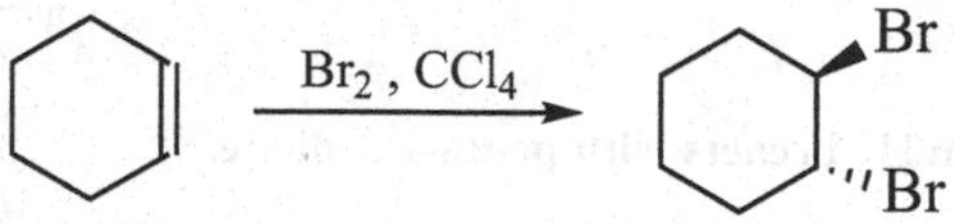

Br_2, CCl_4

trans-1,2-dibromocyclohexane

What is the intermediate of the bromination reaction in the preceding reaction?

The bromonium ion intermediate for the reaction of bromine and cyclohexene is shown: cation ***A***.

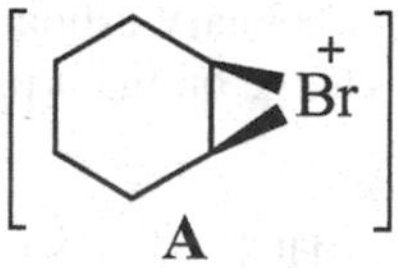

A

If bromine reacts with a diene, does one C=C unit react, or both?

With only one molar equivalent of Br_2, only one C=C unit reacts. However, two intermediates are possible from this reaction, an allylic cation and a bromonium ion with a pedant C=C unit. These structural features lead to different products than the simple reaction with a mono-alkene.

The reaction of bromine and buta-1,3-diene at -40°C gives what as the major product? Explain!

The major product is the "1,2-addition" product, 3,4-dibromobut-1-ene. The "1,4-addition" product (1,4-dibromobut-2-ene) arises by the bromide ion attacking the C=C moiety and opening the intermediate bromonium ion but this is a higher energy process that is very slow at this low temperature. At -40°C, 3,4-dibromobut-1-ene is formed first and faster and it is the kinetic control major product.

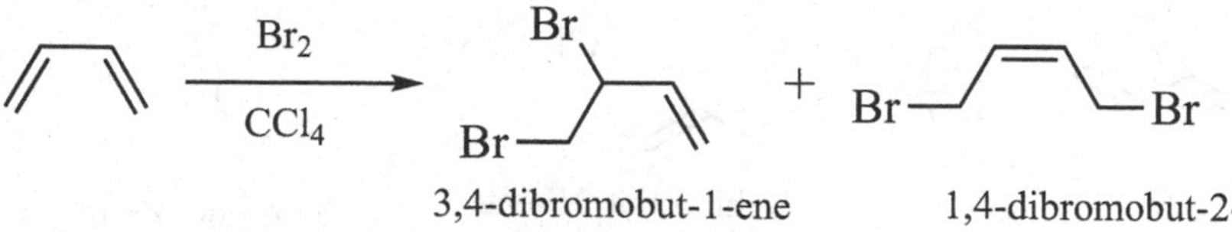

Br_2, CCl_4

3,4-dibromobut-1-ene + 1,4-dibromobut-2-ene

What is the product when bromine and buta-1,3-diene react at 30°C?

At higher temperatures, equilibration favors thermodynamic control and the "1,4-addition product," 1,4-dibromobut-2-ene is the major product, but there is a mixture of the 1,2-product and the 1,4-product.

If a bromonium ion is the intermediate in reactions of bromine buta-1,3-diene, how can 1,4-addition occur?

The bromonium ion formed in this reaction is shown. The initially formed bromonium ion can be attacked by Br^- in a vinylogous reaction at the attached C=C moiety, transferring electron density towards Br^+ and opening the three-membered ring. This vinylogous reaction is labeled an *S_N2' reaction* (nucleophilic substitution with allylic rearrangement) and generates the 1,4-product, 1,4-dibromobut-2-ene, directly. The 1,2-product, 3,4-dibromobut-1-ene, is formed by the normal reaction of the bromide ion with the bromonium ion formed at low temperature by the initial reaction.

At low temperatures the normal reaction of Br^- opens the bromonium ion to give the 1,2-product, 3,4-dibromobut-1-ene

Br^+

S_N2' reaction of Br^- opens the bromonium ion, which leads to the 1,4-product, 1,4-dibromobut-2-ene

Why do lower reaction temperatures favor 1,2-addition?

Attacking the C=C attached to the bromonium ion requires more energy. When the reaction is kept cold, this higher energy process is slower than direct opening of the bromonium ion to give the 1,2- or kinetic product, 3,4-dibromobut-1-ene.

18.4 THE DIELS–ALDER REACTION

What is a pericyclic reaction?

A pericyclic reaction is one in which electrons are transferred within a π-system to form new bonds. This type of reaction generally involves transfer of double bonds from one position to another within a molecule as well as formation of sp^3-hybridized carbon–carbon bonds.

What does the term [m+n] refer to in a pericyclic reaction?

The *m* and *n* refer to the number of π-electrons that are transferred during the reaction. Typical examples of [m+n] reactions are [2+2], [4+2], etc. The Diels–Alder reaction is an example of a [4+2] pericyclic reaction. A [2+2] reaction is one where a 2π system reacts with another 2π system. A [4+2] systems is one where a 4π system reacts with a 2π system, and so on.

What is frontier molecular orbital theory?

Frontier molecular orbital theory is a model that approximates reactivity by looking at the frontier orbitals, the highest occupied molecular orbital (HOMO) and the lowest unoccupied molecular orbital (LUMO). This theory is based on three main observations: occupied orbitals of different molecules repel each other; positive charges of one molecule attract the negative charges of the other; occupied orbitals of one molecule interact and attract the unoccupied orbitals of the other.

What are frontier molecular orbitals?

Frontier molecular orbitals are those molecular orbitals at the "frontier" of electron occupation in a π-system: the highest energy orbitals that contain electrons (HOMO) and the lowest energy orbitals that are empty, that is, they do not have electrons (LUMO).

What is a HOMO?

The term HOMO stands for Highest Occupied Molecular Orbital. It is the highest energy π-molecular orbital that contains valence electrons.

What is a LUMO?

A LUMO is the Lowest Unoccupied Molecular Orbital. It is the lowest energy orbital available to an electron if sufficient energy is added to the system, the lowest energy orbital that does not contain an electron. That orbital does not contain an electron in the ground state.

What is the HOMO of buta-1,3-diene?

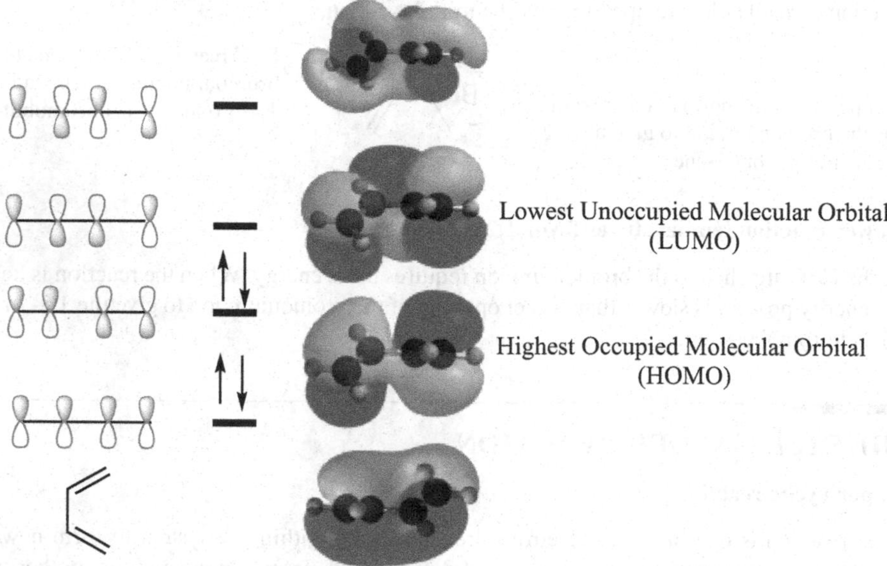

Buta-1,3-diene has four π-electrons and therefore it has four π-molecular orbitals, as shown in the figure. The actual shape of the four orbitals are also shown in the figure. Note the different symmetry of the orbitals with respect to the + lobes (marked in yellow) and the negative lobes (marked in white). The most symmetrical orbital is the lowest in energy in that all four of the + lobes are aligned, and the highest energy molecular orbital has the least amount of symmetry in that there is an alternating pattern, + - + -. Since buta-1,3-diene has a total of four π-electrons, the lowest energy filled orbital contains two electrons and the next highest energy filled orbital has the next two electrons. *The highest energy orbital that contains electrons is the HOMO.*

What is the LUMO of buta-1,3-diene?

Inspection of the diagram in the previous question shows that the LUMO is the third highest energy level for buta-1,3-diene and is the lowest energy molecular orbital that does not contain any electrons.

Experimentally, what is the HOMO?

The HOMO is the ionization potential for the π-electron, which is the energy required to remove a π-electron.

Experimentally, what is the LUMO?

The LUMO is the electron affinity, which is the energy required to promote the π-electron into the next available molecular orbital.

How many molecular orbitals are shown in the preceding question?

There are four molecular orbitals for the four π-electrons. Note that each molecular orbital has four "lobes" for the four contiguous p-orbitals, but each structure represents one molecular orbital.

What is a node?

A node is a point or plane of zero electron density in a molecular orbital. It is a point where the wave function for the orbital changes phase. Molecular orbitals are filled from lowest energy to the highest.

How are the number of nodes in the molecular orbitals correlated with energy?

The greater the number of nodes, the higher the energy of the molecular orbital; the fewer the nodes, the lower the energy. As shown in the preceding question for buta-1,3-diene, the lowest energy orbital has zero nodes, the HOMO has one node, the LUMO has two nodes, and the highest energy orbital as three nodes.

What is the energy of the HOMO and the LUMO of buta-1,3-diene in electron volts?

A HOMO and a LUMO represent energy levels. Their relative energy is expressed in terms of electron volts. The HOMO energy of buta-1,3-diene is -9.07 eV (electron volts) and the LUMO energy is +1.0 eV.

What is the correlation between electron volts and kcal? Between electron volts and kJ?

The correlation is that 1 eV = 1.8293×10^{-23} kcal and 1 eV = 1.602×10^{-22} kJ. Alternatively, 1 kcal = 2.611 $\times 10^{22}$ eV and 1 kJ = 6.242×10^{21} eV. As a practical matter, energy is measured in kcal mol^{-1} or kJ mol^{-1}. Therefore, *1 eV = 23.06 kcal* mol^{-1} *and 1 eV = 96.485 kJ* mol^{-1}.

Does a simple alkene have a HOMO?

Yes! There are two π-electrons and two molecular orbitals as shown in the figure. The two electrons are in the lowest, symmetrical molecular orbital, the HOMO. As shown in the figure, the HOMO is symmetrical and the higher energy LUMO has two lobes since it contains one node.

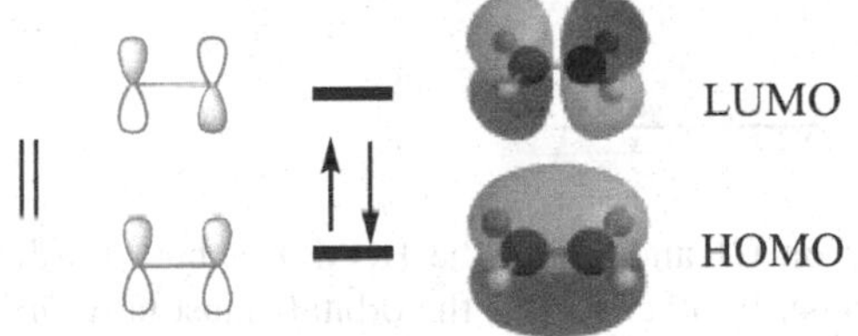

What is the value of HOMO of ethene in electron volts? Of methyl acrylate? Of methyl vinyl ether?

A HOMO represents an energy level. The relative energy is expressed in terms of electron volts. The HOMO of ethene appears at –10.52 eV, that of methyl acrylate (CH_2=$CHCO_2Me$) is at –10.72 eV, and that of methyl vinyl ether (CH_2=CHOMe) is at –9.05 eV. On this scale, –10.52 eV is lower in energy than –9.05 eV.

What is the LUMO of ethene? Of ethyl acrylate? Of methyl vinyl ether?

A LUMO represents an energy level. The relative energy is expressed in terms of electron volts. The LUMO value for ethene is +1.5 eV, the value for methyl acrylate is 0 eV, and for methyl vinyl ether it is +2.0 eV. Of these alkenes, the higher energy LUMO is +2.0 eV.

When buta-1,3-diene is heated with ethene, what is the product?

The product is cyclohexene.

How do buta-1,3-diene and ethene react?

The diene and the alkene react via interaction of their π-bonds, and rearrangement of the electrons in the π-bonds to form the product.

Using the reaction of buta-1,3-diene and ethene, which orbitals can react?

Buta-1,3-diene reacts with ethene to give cyclohexene via interaction of the π-electrons of buta-1,3-diene with those of ethene. Formally, the electrons in the HOMO of buta-1,3-diene are donated to the empty LUMO of ethene. Only those orbitals that have the proper symmetry can react. The symmetry in this case is the + (yellow label) or – (white label) for the lobes of each orbital. High symmetry is taken to mean that more + lobes are aligned, as shown in the lower orbital of the diagram, which has the ++++ array. In reactions with other molecules, symmetry refers to the overlap or reactivity of + lobes of the orbitals of one molecule with a + lobe of the orbital of another molecule.

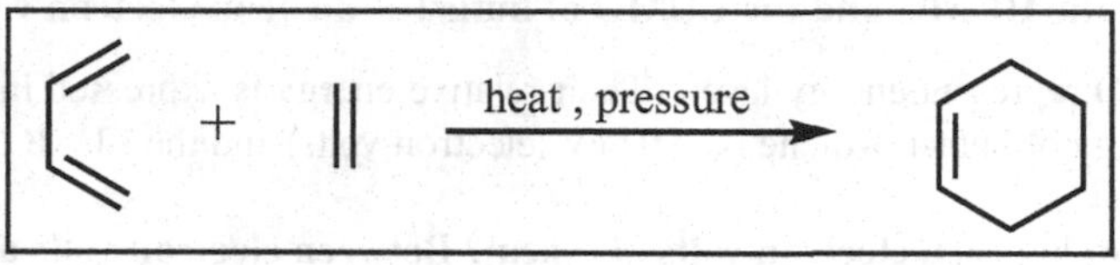

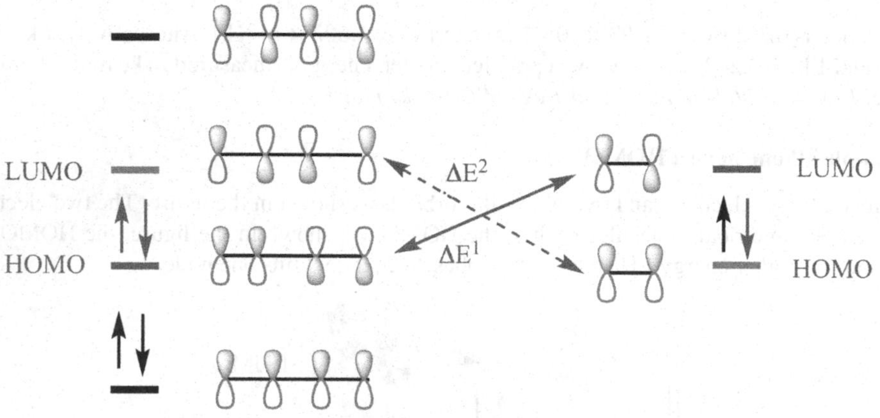

In this example, the orbitals on C1 and C4 of the HOMO of buta-1,3-diene can react with the two orbitals of the LUMO of ethene. In other words, the orbitals must have the correct symmetry to react. Therefore, only the HOMO of the diene can react with the LUMO of the alkene and the difference in energy between these orbitals is labeled ΔE^1. In principle, the LUMO of the diene can react with the HOMO of the alkene since these orbitals have the same symmetry, and the energy difference between these orbitals is labeled ΔE^2. In most cases, ΔE^1 is lower than ΔE^1 and the important interaction is ΔE^1 ($HOMO_{diene}$ – $LUMO_{alkene}$). This interaction is called *normal electron demand*. Note that ΔE^1 is essentially the activation energy (Section 3.2) for the reaction. The higher the activation energy, the slower or more difficult the reaction, and the lower the activation energy, the faster or the more facile reaction. As a practical matter, those Diels–Alder reactions with a small ΔE^1 (smaller activation energy) proceed at lower reaction temperatures and lesser reaction times.

How do the HOMO of buta-1,3-diene and the LUMO of ethene react?

The interaction of the $HOMO_{diene}$ and the $LUMO_{alkene}$ is shown in the figure. This figure clearly shows the interactions of the C1–C4 orbitals of the diene HOMO (– +) with the alkene LUMO (– +) that have like symmetry. The electron-rich HOMO can be thought of as donating electrons to the electron poor LUMO, if the ΔE is sufficiently small. This interaction initiates a reaction of six π-electrons (as shown), forming two new sigma bonds (shown as two light gray lines) and formation of a new π-bond. This reaction will generate cyclohexene.

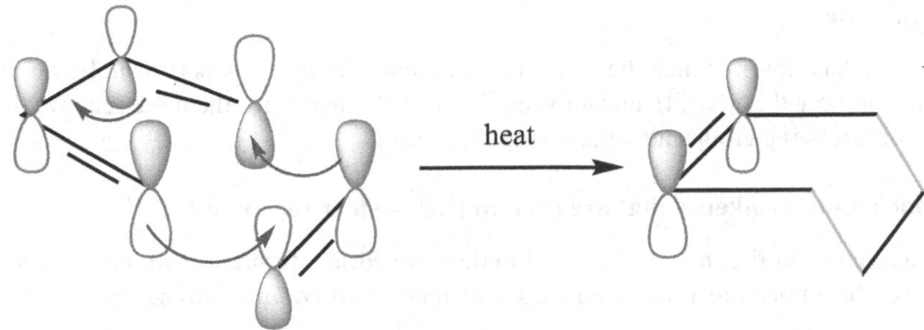

Which is more reactive, buta-1,3-diene and ethene or buta-1,3-diene and ethyl acrylate? Explain.

The HOMO of buta-1,3-diene is at –9.07 eV, which means the ΔE^1 for $\text{HOMO}_{\text{butadiene}}$–$\text{LUMO}_{\text{ethene}}$ is +1.5–[–9.07] or 10.57 eV. Similarly, the ΔE^1 for $\text{HOMO}_{\text{butadiene}}$–$\text{LUMO}_{\text{ethyl acrylate}}$ is 0–[–9.07] or 9.07 eV. Since ΔE^1 for ethyl acrylate is lower than for ethene, *ethyl acrylate will react faster* with buta-1,3-diene (or at a lower reaction temperature) than buta-1,3-diene will react with ethene.

Which is more reactive, buta-1,3-diene and ethene or buta-1,3-diene and methyl vinyl ether? Explain.

Using the same rationale as in the preceding question, the ΔE^1 for $\text{HOMO}_{\text{butadiene}}$–$\text{LUMO}_{\text{ethene}}$ is 10.57 eV, whereas the ΔE^1 for $\text{HOMO}_{\text{butadiene}}$–$\text{LUMO}_{\text{methyl vinyl ether}}$ is +2.0–[–9.07] or 11.07 eV. Since the ΔE^1 for methyl vinyl ether is larger than for ethene, *ethene will react faster* (i.e., at a lower temperature).

Why is ΔE^1 for important for reactivity in the Diels–Alder reaction?

The ΔE^1 represents the activation energy for the reaction (see Section 3.2). A lower ΔE^1 corresponds to a lower activation energy, so the reaction proceeds faster, or under milder conditions. A higher ΔE^1 corresponds to a higher activation energy, so the reaction is more difficult and requires harsher conditions.

What is the definition of a Diels–Alder reaction?

The reaction named was the work of Otto Diels and Kurt Alder, reported in the 1920s and 1930s, before the concept of molecular orbitals and cycloaddition reactions was developed. A Diels–Alder reaction is the [4+2]-cycloaddition of a 1,3-diene and an alkene to give a cyclohexene derivative. Buta-1,3-diene will react with ethene, for example, to give cyclohexene but only at high reaction temperatures and at high pressure (250°C and 2500 psi are typical reaction conditions).

What is the [*m*+*n*] designator for a Diels–Alder reaction?

A Diels–Alder reaction is a [4+2]-cycloaddition (four π-electrons from the diene and two π-electrons from the alkene).

What reactants are required for a Diels–Alder reaction?

A *1,3-diene* (called an *enophile*) and an *alkene* (an ene, called a *dienophile*).

What reaction conditions are common in Diels–Alder reactions?

The Diels–Alder reaction is a thermal reaction and temperatures in the range of 0°C to >300°C are common. Most uncatalyzed Diels–Alder reactions occur in the 60–180°C range at ambient pressure. Catalyzed reaction can proceed at ambient temperatures or temperatures below 0°C.

What is the product of a Diels–Alder reaction?

The product is a cyclohexene derivative.

What is an enophile?

An enophile is an "ene lover." Since the "ene" is the alkene, the enophile is that molecule which reacts with the alkene, namely the diene. In uncatalyzed Diels–Alder reactions, the more reactive dienes do not have electron-withdrawing groups attached to the diene unit.

What are some common alkenes that are used in Diels–Alder reactions?

Methyl acrylate, acrylonitrile, maleic acid and maleic anhydride, fumaric acid, acrolein, methyl vinyl ketone, and cyclohexenone are typical alkenes that react with common dienes under relatively mild conditions.

What is a s-cis- diene? A s-trans- diene?

A s-cis- diene is the rotamer of a 1,3-diene where the two C=C groups are syn- (the old term is cisoid), as shown. A s-trans- diene is the rotamer of a 1,3-diene where the two C=C groups are anti- (the old term is transoid), as shown. These two rotamers are in equilibrium and both are present in an acyclic diene but the s-trans- rotamer is lower in energy and is usually the more common rotamer in the equilibrium.

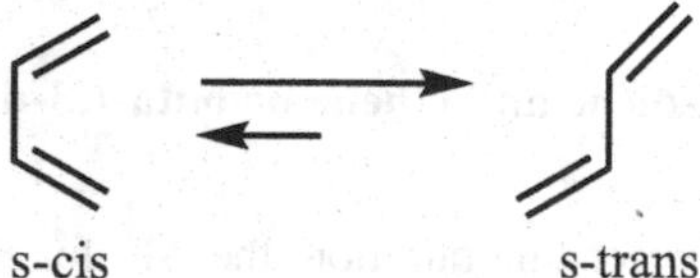

Which is more reactive in a Diels–Alder reaction, a s-cis- diene or a s-trans-diene?

Since it is the C1 and C4 carbons of the diene that undergo reaction, those carbons must *both* be in close proximity to the alkene orbitals. Only the *s-cis- conformation* brings all the reactive carbons of the alkene close enough to the C1 and C4 carbons of the diene.

Which of the dienes (a)–(f) can undergo a Diels–Alder reaction?

Of these dienes, (a) is *not* a conjugated diene and will not undergo the Diels–Alder reaction as a diene. Diene (e) is conjugated but is "locked" into a s-trans- conformation. It is, therefore, impossible for that diene to undergo the Diels–Alder reaction. In all other cases the diene reacts normally. Both cyclohexadiene (b) and furan (c) are "locked" in the s-cis- conformation and can react. Although diene (d) is drawn in the s-trans- conformation, it is acyclic and is not locked in that rotamer. The s-cis- rotamer will be in equilibrium with the s-trans- rotamer and the s-cis- rotamer will react normally.

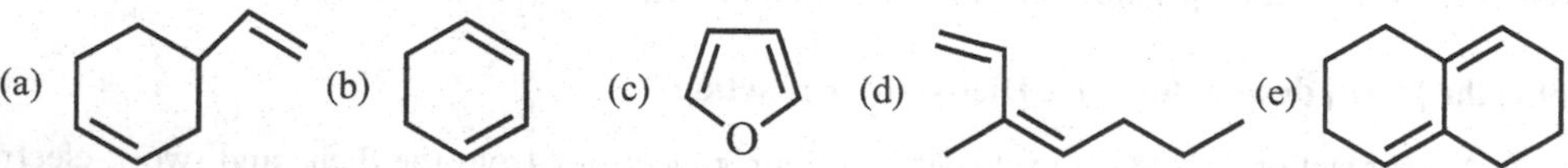

Which is more reactive, buta-1,3-diene or cyclopentadiene?

Since cyclopentadiene is locked into the s-cis- conformation, it is more reactive than buta-1,3-diene. When cyclopentadiene reacts with an appropriate alkene (such as ethyl acrylate) a mixture of two bicyclic products are formed, ***A*** and ***B***. In ***A*** the CO_2Et group is in the *exo* position whereas in ***B*** the CO_2Et is in the *endo* position. In other words, the CO_2Et group is on the same side (syn-) as the $-CH_2-$ bridge in ***A*** and the CO_2Et groups is anti- to the $-CH_2-$ bridge in B. In general, the endo product (***B***) is preferred by about 3:1.

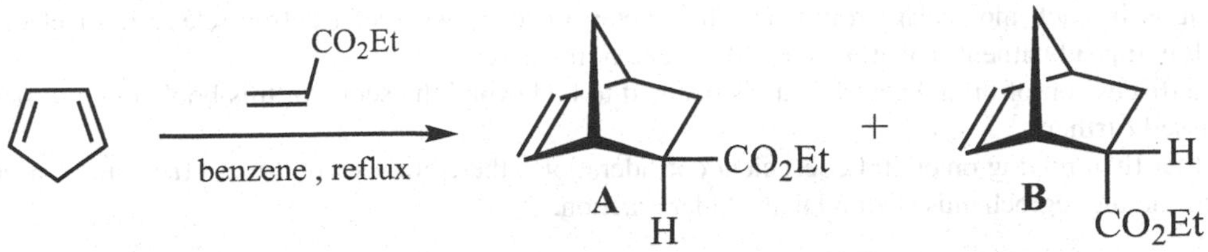

CO_2Et

benzene , reflux

A CO_2Et H + B H CO_2Et

What is the structure of the endo and exo products from the previous question but drawn as a planar cyclohexene ring with bridging substituents?

In this representation, the syn- vs. anti- relationship of the CO_2Et group with the $-CH_2-$ bridge is clear.

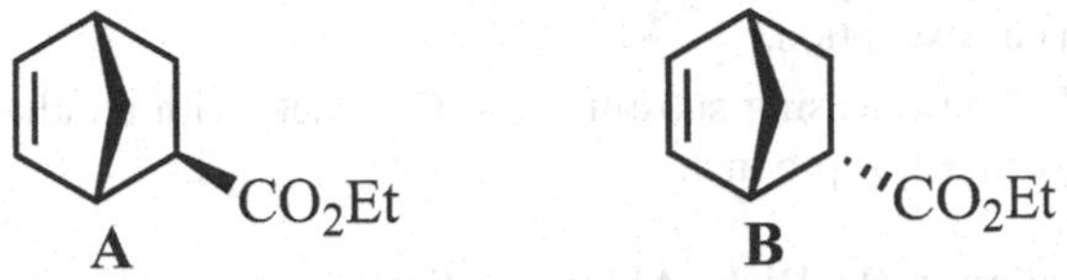

A CO_2Et B CO_2Et

What is a dienophile?

Dienophile means "diene loving" and refers to a molecule that reacts with the diene in a Diels–Alder reaction. This is, of course, the alkene (ene).

Which of the following dienophiles is the most reactive with buta-1,3-diene in a Diels–Alder reaction?
(a) $CH_2{=}CHCH_3$ (b) $CH_2{=}CHCO_2Et$ (c) $CH_2{=}CHOMe$

If these alkenes react in a Diels–Alder reaction such that ΔE^1 dominates the HOMO-LUMO interaction, ethyl acrylate (b) with an electron-withdrawing ester moiety will be the most reactive since it has the lowest energy LUMO to react with the HOMO of the diene.

Why does an alkene with an electron-withdrawing group react faster than a simple alkene or an alkene with an electron releasing group?

An electron-withdrawing substituent lowers the energy of the HOMO and the LUMO. If ΔE^1 is lower, the activation energy for that reaction is lower and the reaction is more favorable. If the ΔE^1 in a reaction with a diene is lower the reaction is faster.

What is an ortho- product in the Diels–Alder reaction? A meta- product? A para-product?

An ortho- Diels–Alder product has two substituents in a 1,2-position. Similarly, the meta- adduct has a 1,3 orientation of the substituents, and a para- product has a 1,4-relationship.

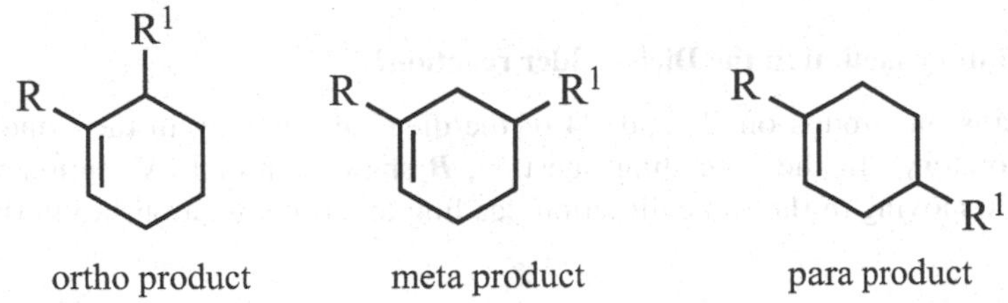

R^1 R R R^1 R R^1

ortho product meta product para product

Can the preferred regiochemical orientation for a given Diels–Alder product, ortho-, meta-, or para- as described in the previous question, be determined?

Yes! The overlap of the larger orbital coefficients for the HOMO and LUMO reaction partners in a Diels–Alder determines the regiochemical preference. The orbital coefficients are effectively the "size" of the p-orbitals in each molecular orbital, which is determined by whether electron-releasing or electron-withdrawing substituents are attached to the diene or the alkene.

The discussion of orbital coefficients is deemed to be beyond the scope of this book and will not be discussed further.

Rather than relying on orbital coefficient considerations, there are a set of "rules" that can be used to determine the regiochemistry of a Diels–Alder reaction.

1. A diene with a substituent at C1 (electron-withdrawing or releasing) reacts with an electron-rich alkene to give the ortho- product and it reacts with an electron-deficient alkene to yield the ortho- (1,2-) product.
2. A diene with a substituent at C2 (electron-withdrawing or -releasing) reacts with an electron-rich alkene to give the para- product and with an electron-deficient alkene to yield the para- (1,4-) product, with one exception.
3. A diene with an electron-releasing substituent at C2 reacts with an alkene with an electron-releasing group to yield a 1,3- product.

What is a disrotatory motion in the Diels–Alder reaction?

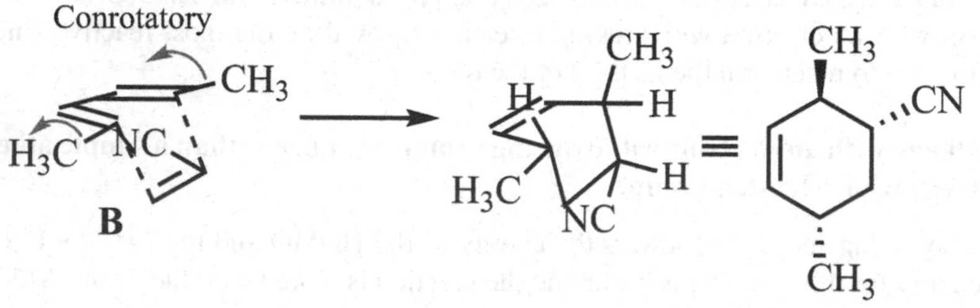

Disrotatory refers to the motion of the C1 and C4 groups of the diene during the Diels–Alder reaction. If the two methyl groups in *A* move in opposite directions, they either move toward each other as shown in the figure, or away from each other. This motion is referred to as *disrotatory motion*. This motion will lead to a cis- relationship of the two methyl groups in the final cyclohexene product in the example shown.

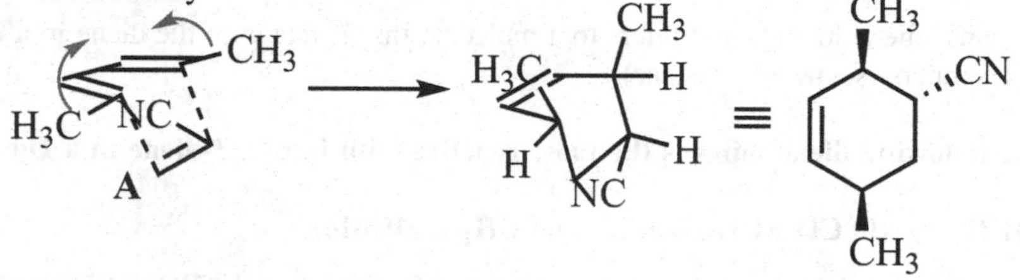

What is a conrotatory motion in the Diels–Alder reaction?

Conrotatory means the groups on C1 and C4 of the diene are moving in the same direction (the opposite of disrotatory). In the preceding question, *B* shows conrotatory motion where the two methyl groups are moving in the same direction, leading to a trans-relationship in the cyclohexene product.

Is conrotatory motion or disrotatory motion preferred in normal Diels–Alder reactions?

The relationship of the groups of C1 and C4 of the diene, and in the cyclohexene product result from *disrotatory* motion. Diels–Alder reactions are characterized by disrotatory motion.

What is the stereochemistry of the groups in the final product when penta-1,3-diene reacts with maleic anhydride?

The major product is ***B*** (the endo product). About 75% of ***B*** is produced, along with about 25% of the exo product (the anhydride moiety is on the same side of the molecule as the methyl group). The alkene portion of ethyl acrylate reacts with cyclopentadiene and the transition state with the C=O of ethyl acrylate "tucked under" the cyclopentadiene ring, as in **A**, leads to the endo product (***B***).

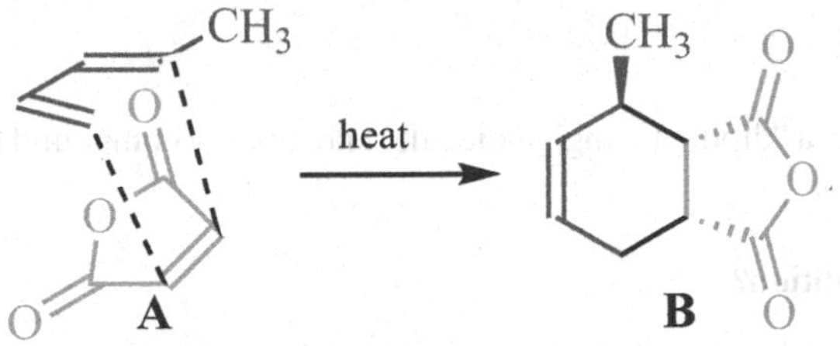

CH_3 heat CH_3 O O O O O O

A **B**

Why is the endo product preferred in this reaction?

Examination of ***A*** in the preceding question shows that the π-bonds of the carbonyl can interact with the π-bonds of the diene (π-stacking) in what is known as *secondary orbital interactions*. These interactions slightly increase the stability of the endo transition state at the expense of the exo transition state, leading to the endo product (***B***) as the major product. This secondary orbital interaction is not possible if the alkene approaches the diene with an exo approach, where the π-bonds of the carbonyls are not near the π-bonds of the diene.

What is the name associated with secondary orbital interactions?

The preference for the endo product in Diels–Alder reaction is known as the *Alder endo rul*e and it is the preference for an endo transition state that leads to an endo product. It is the result of the secondary orbital interactions discussed in the preceding question.

What is the stereochemistry of the groups in the final product when diethyl fumarate reacts with buta-1,3-diene?

The reaction of diethyl fumarate and buta-1,3-diene gives *trans*-diethyl cyclohex-4-ene-1,2-dicarboxylate. The trans- relationship of the two CO_2Et groups of the dienophile is retained during the Diels–Alder reaction and in the final cyclohexene product. In general, the *E*- or *Z*-stereochemistry of the alkene is retained in the cyclohexene Diels–Alder product.

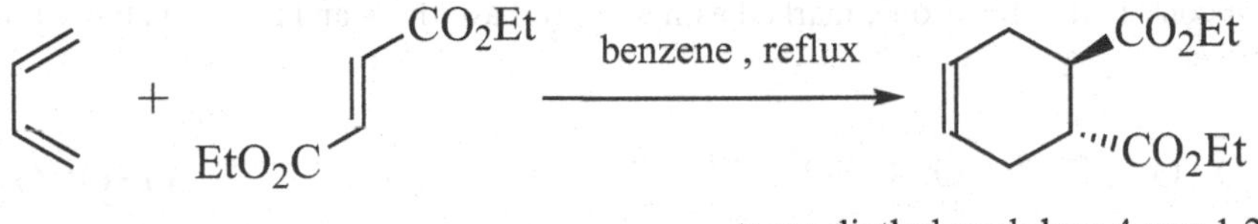

\+ CO_2Et EtO_2C benzene , reflux CO_2Et CO_2Et

trans-diethyl cyclohex-4-ene-1,2-dicarboxylate

18.5 [3+2]-CYCLOADDITION REACTIONS

What is a dipolar molecule?

Dipolar molecules contain a dipole (see Section 2.3). A *dipolar* compound is an electrically neutral molecule that has both a positive and a negative charge in at least one canonical structure.

What is a 1,3-dipole?

A *1,3-dipole* is a dipolar compound with delocalized electrons and a separation of charge over three atoms. A 1,3-dipole is an organic molecule that shares four electrons in the π-system over three atoms.

What are common 1,3-dipoles?

Ozone, diazo compounds, $KMnO_4$, and OsO_4.

What is a dipolarophile?

A *dipolarophile* is literally a "dipole loving" molecule, and it is any compound that react with 1,3-dipoles in a cycloaddition reaction.

What is a [3+2]-cycloaddition?

A cycloaddition reaction involves a molecule containing a π-bond (an alkene, alkyne, etc.) and a 1,3-dipole. It is a chemical reaction between a 1,3-dipole an a dipolarophile to form a five-membered ring.

Is there an intermediate in the [3+2]-cycloaddition reaction?

No! It is a concerted pericyclic reaction.

What is the mechanism of a [3+2]-cycloaddition?

The reaction is a concerted, pericyclic reaction in which the frontier molecular orbitals react; the HOMO of the 1,3-dipole reacts with the LUMO of the dipolarophile. The two π-electrons of the dipolarophile react with the four electrons of the dipolar compound. The product is a five-membered ring.

How are the HOMO and the LUMO orbitals involved in [3+2]-cycloaddition reactions?

The reaction is controlled by the interactions of the $HOMO_{dipole}$ and the $LUMO_{dipolarophile}$.

What are the resonance contributors of ozone?

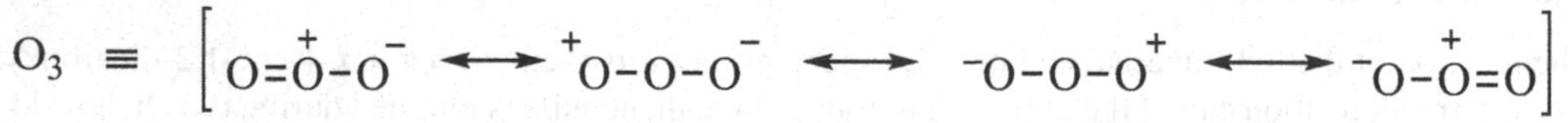

$$O_3 \equiv \left[O=\overset{+}{O}-\overset{-}{O} \longleftrightarrow \overset{+}{O}-O-\overset{-}{O} \longleftrightarrow \overset{-}{O}-O-\overset{+}{O} \longleftrightarrow \overset{-}{O}-\overset{+}{O}=O \right]$$

In what way is ozone considered to be a 1,3-dipole?

Two of the resonance contributors for ozone, marked as light gray, have the + and the – on atoms 1 and 3 of ozone; a 1,3-dipole.

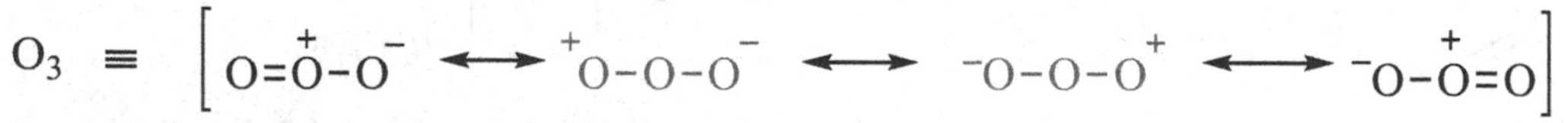

$$O_3 \equiv \left[O=\overset{+}{O}-\overset{-}{O} \longleftrightarrow \overset{+}{O}-O-\overset{-}{O} \longleftrightarrow \overset{-}{O}-O-\overset{+}{O} \longleftrightarrow \overset{-}{O}-\overset{+}{O}=O \right]$$

What is the initially formed product when ozone reacts with cyclopentene?

The initially formed cycloaddition product is a 1,2,3-trioxolane, as shown. This trioxolane is very unstable, however, and rapidly rearranges to the ozonide (a 1,2,4-trioxlane).

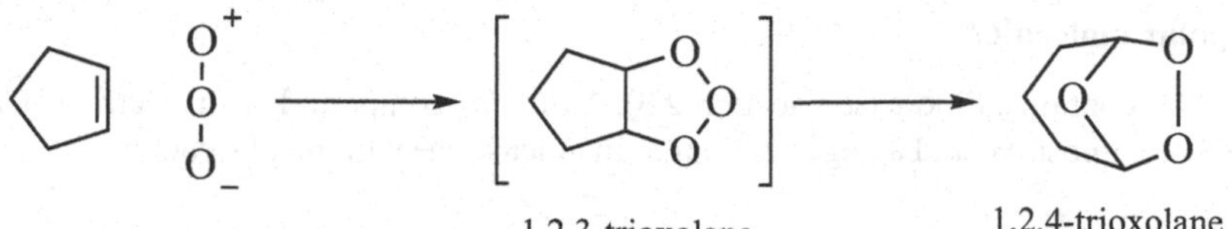

1,2,3-trioxolane

1,2,4-trioxolane
(an ozonide)

How is diazoethane considered to be a 1,3-dipole?

Diazoethane is CH_3CHN_2, with the resonance contributors shown. The two contributors marked as light gray are 1,3-dipoles since the charges are on atom 1 and atom 3.

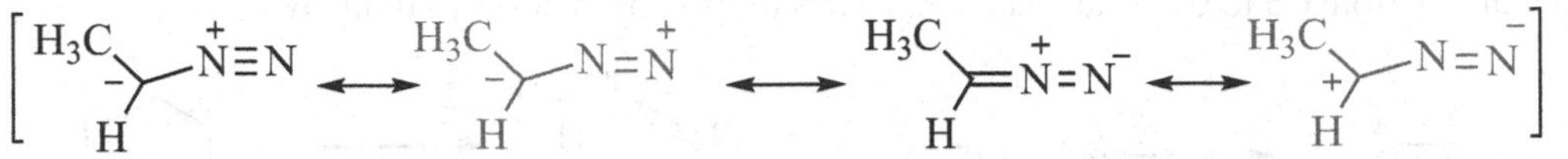

What is the product formed when cis-but-2-ene reaction with diazoethane?

The product is a five-membered ring with two nitrogen atoms called a pyrazoline (a dihydropyrazole).

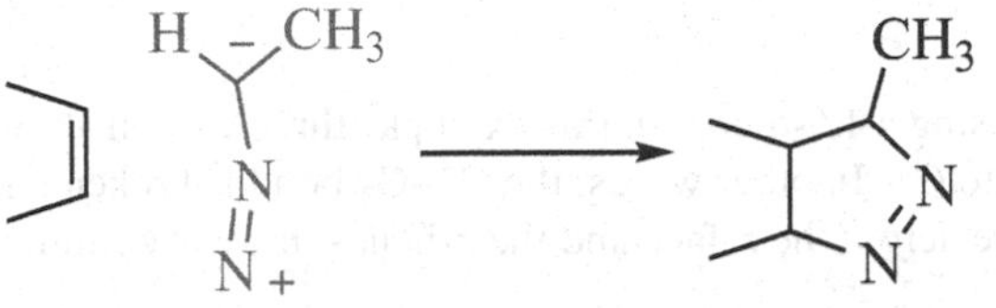

3,4,5-trimethyl-4,5-dihydro-3*H*-pyrazole

What is the product formed when cyclopentene reacts with $KMnO_4$?

A [3+2]-cycloaddition of permanganate and cyclopentene leads to the five-membered ring shown, a manganate ester.

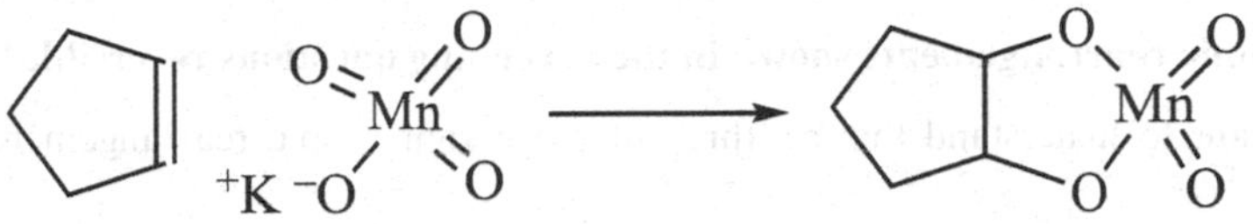

a manganate ester

What is the product formed when cyclopentene reacts with OsO_4?

A [3+2]-cycloaddition of osmium tetroxide and cyclopentene leads to the five-membered ring shown, an osmate ester.

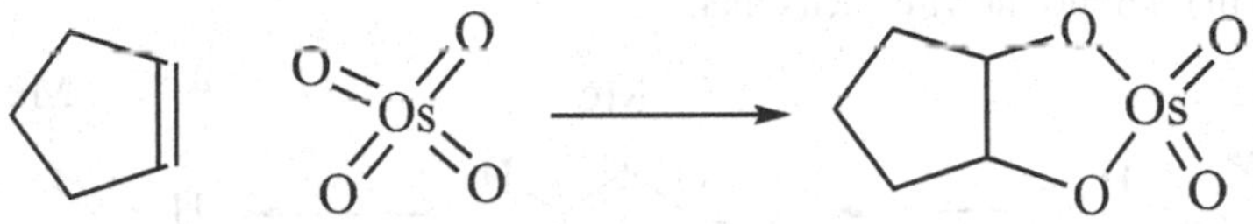

an osmate ester

What is the product when a manganate ester is formed in the presence of aqueous NaOH? What is the product when an osmate ester is formed in the presence of aqueous *tert*-butyl hydroperoxide?

In both cases the product is a 1,2-diol, as described in Section 7.4.3.

18.6 SIGMATROPIC REARRANGEMENTS

What is a sigmatropic rearrangement?

Sigmatropic rearrangements are defined as reactions in which a σ-bond to an atom or a substituent moves across a conjugated system to a new site. In other words, one fragment moves across another fragment.

What is a [1,3]-hydrogen shift? A [1,7]-hydrogen shift?

A putative [1,3]-hydrogen shift is illustrated using propene, where the hydrogen atom moves from C3 to C1, as marked. A putative [1,5]-hydrogen shift is illustrated using penta-1,3-diene, where a hydrogen atom moves from C5 to C1. Note that in both cases the π-bond(s) move accordingly.

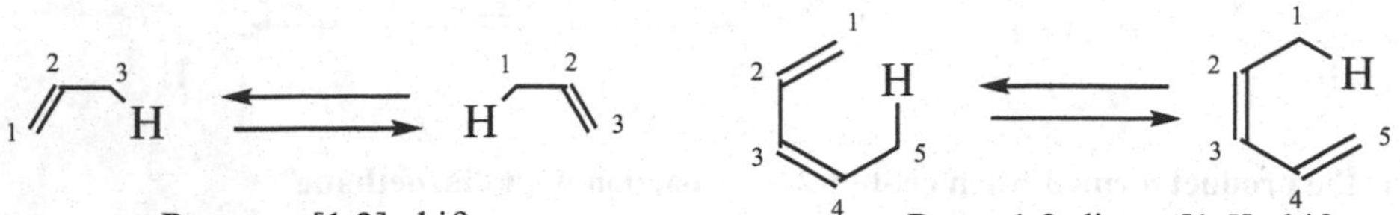

Propene: [1,3]-shift

Penta-1,3-diene: [1,5]-shift

What is a [3,3]-alkyl shift?

A [3,3]-alkyl shift is illustrated using a 1,5-diene. In this example, three carbon atoms (C1, C2, and C3) move across the π-face from C4 to C6. In other words, the C3–C4 bond is broken and a C1–C6 bond is formed as the three carbons move across the π-face and the π-bonds move accordingly.

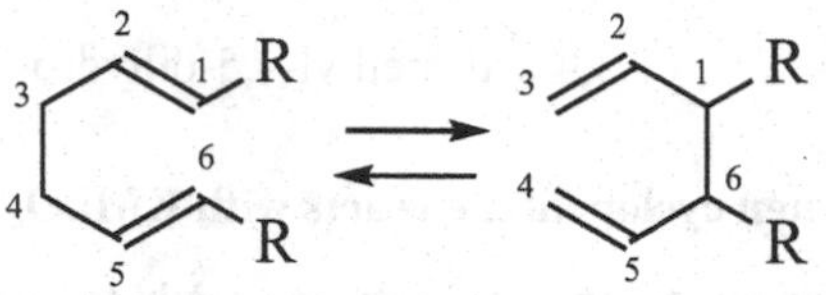

1,5-Diene derivatives: [3,3]-shift

Are the sigmatropic rearrangements shown in the preceding questions reversible?

Yes! It is important to understand that all three of these sigmatropic rearrangements are thermally reversible.

Are [1,5]-sigmatropic rearrangements possible with methylcyclopentadiene?

Yes! When 5-methylcyclopenta-1,3-diene is heated, the hydrogen marked in light gray moves from C1 to C5 to give 1-methylcyclopenta-1,3-diene via a [1,5]-sigmatropic shift. The hydrogen atom is a one-atom fragment and it moves across a five-carbon fragment (C1 to C5). Similarly, the hydrogen in 1-methylcyclopenta-1,3-diene moves to yield 2-methylcyclopenta-1,3-diene (from C5 to C4 as marked), and all of these isomers are in equilibrium with each other.

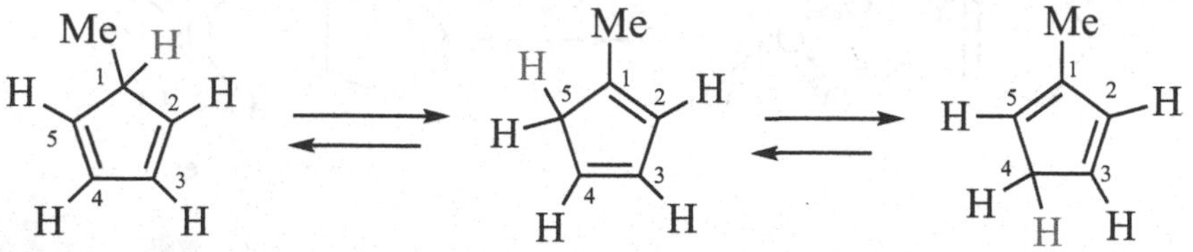

5-Methylcyclopenta-1,3-diene 1-Methylcyclopenta-1,3-diene 2-Methylcyclopenta-1,3-diene

What is a suprafacial shift?

A *suprafacial shift* is when the σ-bond to the hydrogen atom is made and broken on the same side of the conjugated system.

What is an antarafacial shift?

An *antarafacial shift* is when the σ-bond is broken on one side of the conjugated system but made on the opposite side of that system. Antarafacial shifts are generally not observed in systems found in this book.

What is the product of a [3,3]-sigmatropic rearrangement of hexa-1,5-diene?

The product is hexa-1,5-diene, as shown. There must be a substituent on the carbon atoms in order to distinguish the rearrangement product.

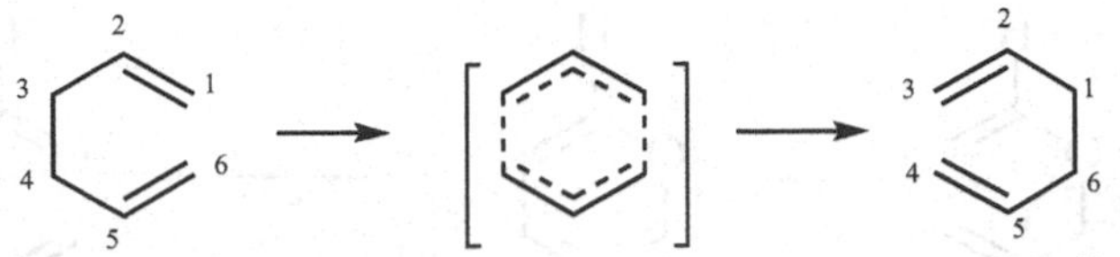

Hexa-1,5-diene A Hexa-1,5-diene

Is there an intermediate for [3,3]-sigmatropic rearrangements?

No! There is no intermediate for sigmatropic rearrangements since it is a pericyclic reaction.

What is the transition state for the [3,3]-sigmatropic rearrangement of hexa-1,5-diene in the preceding question?

The six-centered transition state is shown as ***A*** in the preceding answer.

What is the product of a [3,3]-sigmatropic rearrangement of 3,4-dimethylhexa-1,5-diene?

The product is octa-2,6-diene. The "squiggle" lines indicate a mixture of isomers.

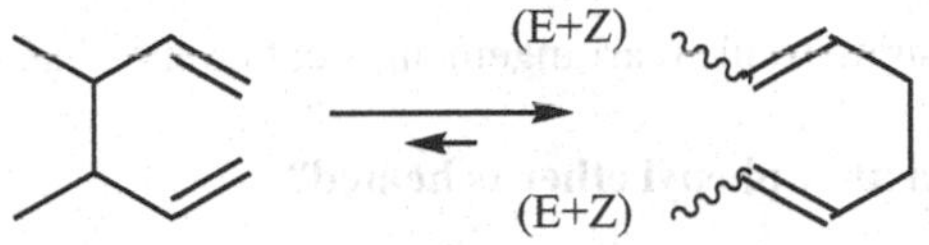

(E+Z)

(E+Z)

3,4-Dimethylhexa-1,5-diene octa-2,6-diene

The [3,3]-sigmatropic rearrangement is an equilibrium reaction. Is one of the dienes favored in the equilibrium?

Yes! These two dienes are in equilibrium, and the equilibrium favors the thermodynamically more stable diene. In this case, the more stable diene is octa-2,6-diene, where each C=C unit is disubstituted.

Does this particular [3,3]-sigmatropic rearrangement have a name?

Yes! This rearrangement is called the *Cope rearrangement*.

What is the main disadvantage of the Cope rearrangement?

The reaction is reversible and even if one diene is thermodynamically more stable than the other, the mixture of dienes must be separated. In many cases, the reaction is not practical for the preparation of a pure product in good yield.

What is a vinyl ether?

A vinyl ether has an OR group directly attached to a C=C unit: C=C–OR.

Do [3,3]-sigmatropic rearrangements occur with vinyl ethers?

Yes! Another variation of a [3,3]-sigmatropic rearrangement is particularly useful. If one —CH_2— unit of a 1,5-diene is replaced with an oxygen atom, the resulting structure is an allylic vinyl ether such as 3-(vinyloxy)prop-1-ene. This compound has two C=C units that constitute a 1,5-diene, and heating leads to a [3,3]-sigmatropic rearrangement reaction.

What is the final product and the transition state for a [3,3]-sigmatropic rearrangement of 3-(vinyloxy)prop-1-ene?

This rearrangement proceeds via transition state ***A*** to yield the aldehyde pent-4-enal as shown in the figure.

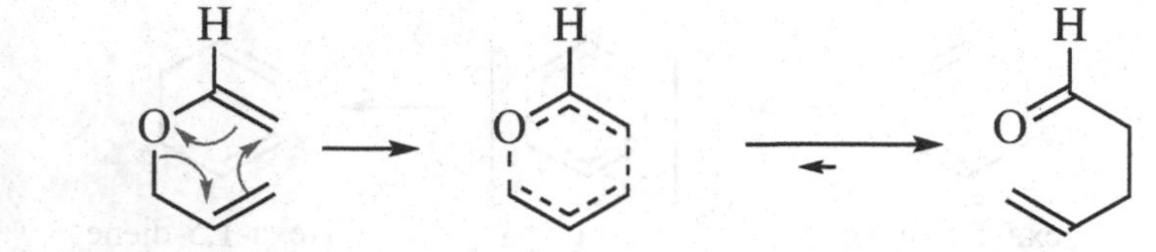

3-(vinyloxy)prop-1-ene **A** pent-4-enal

Does the reaction in the preceding question favor one compound over another?

Yes! The equilibrium in this reaction favors pent-4-enal because the C=O bond is favored over a C=C bond, so the equilibrium favors formation of the aldehyde. The presence of the oxygen leads to an acceleration of the rate of reaction, so the reaction temperature is relatively low when compared to the Cope rearrangement.

What structural features of the diene are required for the preceding reaction?

The 1,5-diene unit must be a vinyl allyl ether.

Does this variation of the [3,3]-sigmatropic rearrangements have a name?

Yes! This particular [3,3]-sigmatropic rearrangement is called the *Claisen rearrangement.*

What is the product when allyl phenyl ether is heated?

A Claisen rearrangement occurs since this molecule is a 1,5-diene if one counts the C=C unit of the benzene ring. The [3,3]-sigmatropic rearrangement disrupts the aromatic ring to give an intermediate, which tautomerizes to 2-allylphenol as the final product. Historically, this example is one of the first examples of the Claisen rearrangement.

heat

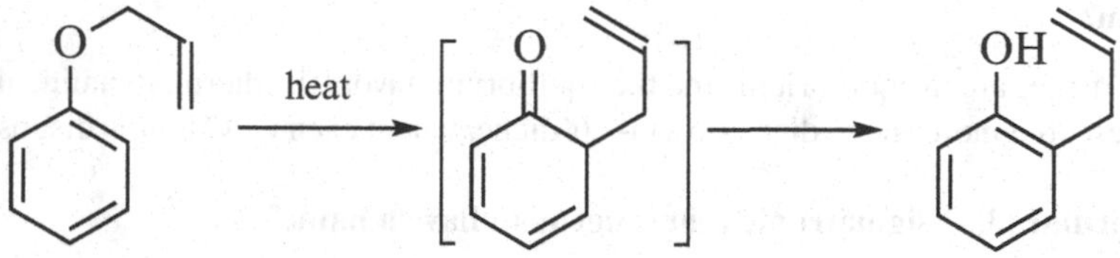

18.7 ULTRAVIOLET SPECTROSCOPY

What is the relative position (relative energy) of ultraviolet light in the electromagnetic spectrum?

From the portion of the electromagnetic spectrum shown, it is apparent that ultraviolet (UV) light is *higher* in energy than visible light or infrared light (≈ 71–143 kcal mol^{-1} for UV vs. 35–71.5 kcal mol^{-1} for visible).

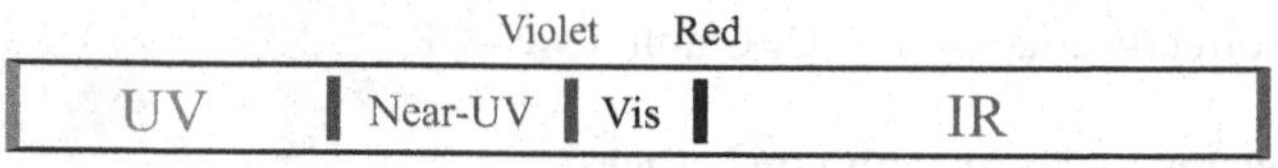

Violet Red

UV | Near-UV | Vis | IR

10	200	400	800	2860	28,600	ν (mμ = nm)
2860	143	71.5	35.75	10	1	E (kcal mol^{-1})
11,972	598.6	299.3	149.7	41.86	4.186	E (kJ mol^{-1})
100	2000	4000	8000	2.86×10^4	2.86×10^5	λ (Å)
1000×10^3	50×10^3	25×10^3	12.5×10^3	3530	353	ν (cm^{-1})

What functional groups absorb ultraviolet light?

The functional groups that best accept a photon of UV light are those that contain a conjugated π-bond or a polarized π-bond. Simple alkenes do not absorb UV light effectively, but conjugated dienes and conjugated carbonyls give strong absorption bands in the UV. The π-bond of the carbonyl group of ketones and aldehydes also absorbs UV light, as does benzene.

How does a photon of ultraviolet light react with the π-bond of an alkene?

As shown in the figure, a photon of light excites an electron in a valence, bonding molecular orbital, promoting that electron to an antibonding orbital, which generates a high energy species. This high energy species can dissipate energy in several ways, one of which is for the electron to cascade back to the lower energy orbital, with emission of heat and/or light. When a heteroatom with electrons and/or a π-bond is present, the electron is promoted from one of the vibrational levels to a higher energy antibonding orbital, $\pi \rightarrow \pi^*$, $n \longrightarrow \pi^*$, $\sigma \longrightarrow \pi^*$, or $n \rightarrow \sigma^*$. The energy difference between these energy levels (ΔE) is the energy for that absorption.

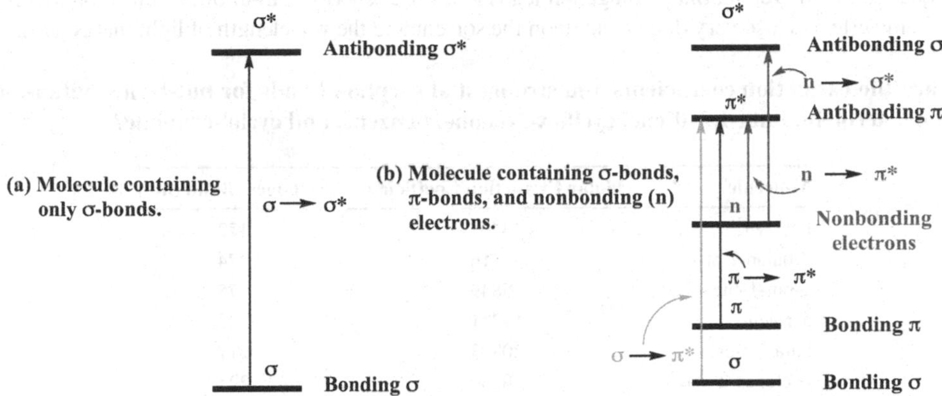

What is the extinction coefficient?

This term is also called the molar extinction coefficient. It is a measure of how strongly a substance absorbs light at a given wavelength, per molar concentration

What is λ_{max}?

This term is the maximum absorbance wavelength in the absorption UV spectrum. This term acts as a single quantitative parameter to compare the absorption range of different molecules.

Why is the UV absorption maximum for buta-1,3-diene shifted relative to that of an alkene such as but-1-ene?

For buta-1,3-diene (see the table below), the most intense absorption in the UV and appears at 217 nm (131.8 kcal mol^{-1} where 1 kcal = 28600 nm). For a simple alkene such as but-1-ene this signal appears at about 165 nm (173.3 kcal mol^{-1}). It takes more energy for the simple alkene to absorb the light than it does the conjugated diene. The interaction of the π-bonds in the conjugated diene makes absorption of the light easier (lower in energy), accounting for the difference in absorption maxima (see the following question).

For both alkenes and conjugated dienes, the orbital that accepts the photon is a π-orbital and the orbital that receives the electron after promotion is a high energy π-orbital, a π* orbital. The ΔE is, therefore, due to a $\pi \rightarrow \pi^*$ transition.

What is Beer's Law?

Also known as the *Beer–Lambert Law,* or *Beer's Law,* is: $A = \varepsilon \bullet l \bullet c$. Absorbance ($A$) is the amount of light absorption and is calculated by where ε is the molar extinction coefficient, a physical constant for each compound measured in liters mol^{-1} cm^{-1}, and l is the length of the sample cell in cm. The parameter c is the concentration in mol liter^{-1}.

Why is the absorption for a conjugated diene more intense than that of an alkene?

For both alkenes and conjugated dienes, there is a $\pi \rightarrow \pi^*$ transition but conjugated dienes have a *smaller* ΔE than simple alkenes. For this reason, it takes less energy for the absorption.

Why do conjugated molecules have greater absorption relative to non-conjugated molecules?

It is not a part of most undergraduate organic books, but $\pi \rightarrow \pi^*$ transitions can be classified as spin-*allowed* and spin-*forbidden.* Multiplicity is the sum of the spin quantum numbers of all the electrons in a species. If the multiplicity of the excited state is different from the multiplicity of the ground state, the transition is spin-forbidden. If they are the same, it is spin-allowed. In general, allowed transitions have larger extinction coefficients (more intense peaks) than forbidden processes. An overly simplistic way to give the answer to this question is, therefore, that conjugation leads to a lower energy spin-allowed transition that is more intense. This effect is also very dependent upon the solvent and the wavelength of light that is used.

What are the extinction coefficients and strongest absorption bands for but-1-yne, butan-2-ol, but-1-ene, acrolein, buta-1,3-diene, cyclhex-2-enone, benzene, and cyclohexanone?

Molecule	Molar Extinction Coefficient	Strongest Band (nm)
but1-yne	4467	172
2-butan-2-ol	316	174
1-but-1-ene	15849	175
acrolein	11221	207
buta-1,3-diene	20893	217
cyclohex-2-enone	8230	225
benzene	212	254
cyclohexanone	27	280

How can UV spectroscopy distinguish between buta-1,3-diene and hexa-1,5-diene?

Since buta-1,3-diene contains conjugated π-bonds it will have a λ_{max} at about 217 nm whereas hexa-1,5-diene (with only simple alkene units) will have a λ_{max} between 160-190 nm. In addition, the extinction coefficient for the conjugated diene will be much larger (more intense signal at the same concentration) than the unconjugated diene.

What is the λ_{max} for the carbonyl of acetone?

This question can be answered by the table of absorption spectra presented here.

Molecule	Transition	λ_{max} (nm)	E (kcal) (KJ)
C_4H_9-I	$n \longrightarrow \sigma^*$	224	127.7 (534.6)
CH_2=CH_2	$\pi \rightarrow \pi^*$	165	173.3 (725.4)
HC≡CH	$\pi \rightarrow \pi^*$	173	165.3 (691.9)
acetone	$\pi \rightarrow \pi^*$	150	190.7 (798.3)
	$n \rightarrow \sigma^*$	188	152.1 (636.7)
	$n \rightarrow \pi^*$	279	102.5 (429.1)
CH_2=CHCH=CH_2	$\pi \rightarrow \pi^*$	217	131.8 (551.7)
CH_2=CHCHO	$\pi \rightarrow \pi^*$	210	136.2 (570.1)
	$n \rightarrow \pi^*$	315	90.8 (380.1)
benzene	$\pi \rightarrow \pi^*$	180	158.9 (665.2)

Note that acetone has several absorption maxima and each different type of transition ($\pi \rightarrow \pi^*$ or $n \rightarrow \pi^*$, where n is an unshared electron) will have its own λ_{max}.

What is the λ_{max} for methyl vinyl ketone (but-3-en-2-one)?

The $\pi \rightarrow \pi^*$ maxima for this conjugated ketone is similar to that of the conjugated aldehyde (acrolein) shown: $\approx$ 210 nm. The $n \rightarrow \pi^*$ maxima is $\approx$ 315 nm.

What is the generic λ_{max} of a carbonyl group?

For unconjugated carbonyls, absorption occurs at 150 nm or lower, which is typically invisible to most ultraviolet spectrophotometers. A weak absorption appears at 260–290 nm which is typical of ketones and aldehydes. For conjugated carbonyls, a peak appears around 230 nm and around 300–310 nm.

What transitions are possible for a carbonyl?

The signal at 150 nm signal is due to a $\pi \rightarrow \pi^*$ transition. The 260–290 nm signal is weak and due to a $n \rightarrow \pi^*$ absorption. For conjugated carbonyls, the 230 nm absorption is the $\pi \rightarrow \pi^*$ absorption and the 300–310 signal is the weaker $n \rightarrow \pi^*$ transition.

How can UV spectroscopy distinguish between a ketone or aldehyde and an alkene?

Ultraviolet spectroscopy cannot distinguish between an aldehyde and a ketone, but alkenes show a $\pi \longrightarrow \pi^*$ transition at around 170–200 nm and no $n \rightarrow \pi^*$ transition.

What is the λ_{max} for benzene?

One absorption signal for benzene occurs at 254 nm (112.6 kcal mol^{-1}) in the UV and another appears at 204 nm (140.2 kcal mol^{-1}).

Is the UV absorption for benzene a strong signal or a weak signal?

The UV band at 254 nm is relatively weak (an extinction coefficient of only 212), but the signal at 204 nm is relatively strong (extinction coefficient of 7900).

What does the UV spectrum of methyl vinyl ketone (but-3-en-2-one) look like?

For but-3-en-2-one, the absorption maximum is at 212 nm with $\varepsilon = 7.125 \times 10^5$.

END OF CHAPTER PROBLEMS

1. Draw all resonance forms for each of the following:

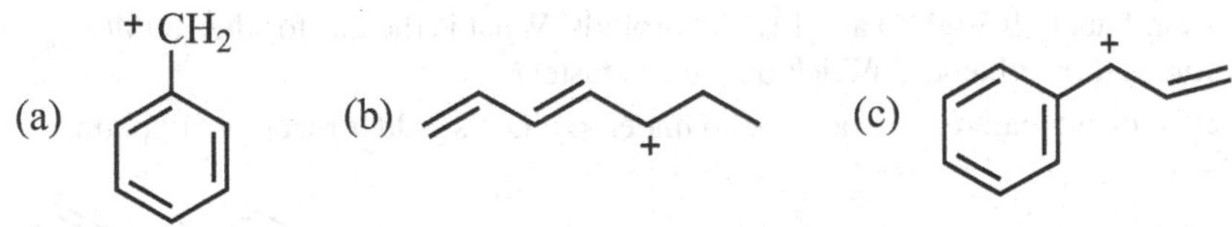

2. Which of the following contain a conjugated C=C bond?

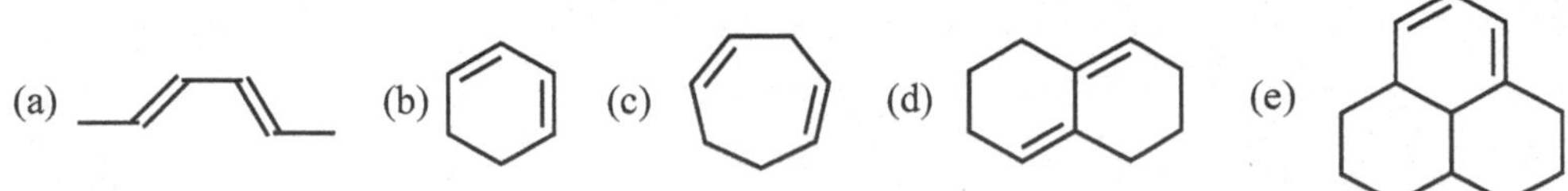

3. Identify each of the following as having a s-trans- conformation or a s-cis- conformation and indicate for which molecules the s-trans- and s-cis- rotamers are in equilibrium.

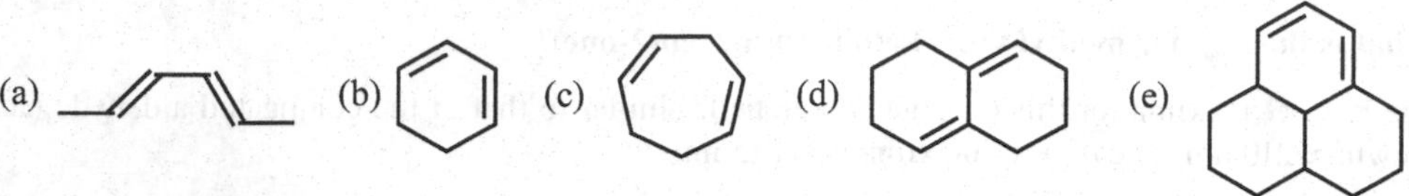

4. What are the products when HBr reacts with penta-1,3-diene at -78°C?
5. Correlate each of the following: (a) 83 kcal = __kJ = __cm^{-1} = __nm (b) 132 kJ = __ nm = __kcal (c) 0.45 nm = __kcal = __cm^{-1} (d) 2.4 kcal = __nm = __ Å = __ cm^{-1}
6. Which of the following are expected to give strong absorption bands in the UV?

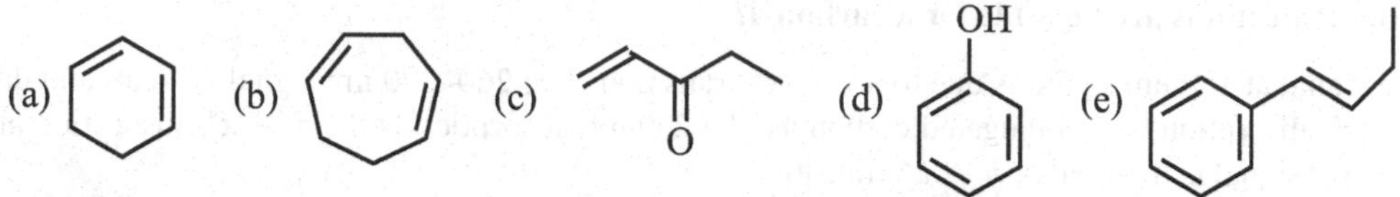

7. If the extinction coefficient of but-3-en-2-one is 6457 and the extinction coefficient of butan-2-one is 17, what is the absorbance of each one if the concentration is 0.3 M in a 5 cm cell?
8. Explain why the extinction coefficient of 1,4-diphenyl-1,3-butadiene is larger than the extinction coefficient for buta-1,3-diene.
9. For each reaction give the major product. If there is no reaction, indicate by N.R.

(a) 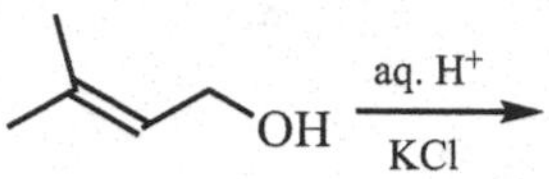 OH — aq. H^+, KCl →

(b) 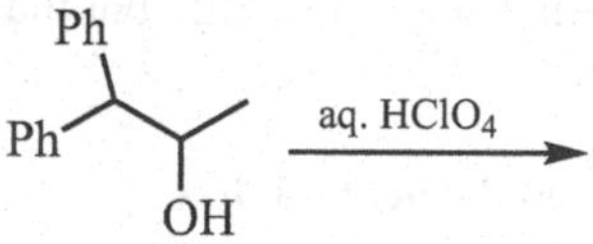 Ph, Ph, OH — aq. $HClO_4$ →

(c) 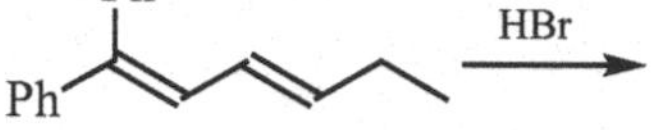 Ph, Ph — HBr →

(d) 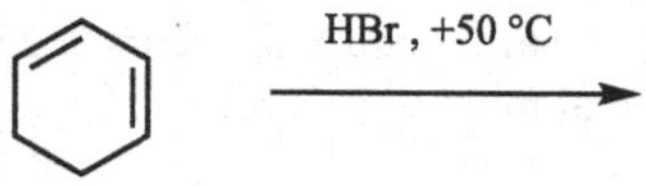 — HBr, +50 °C →

(e) 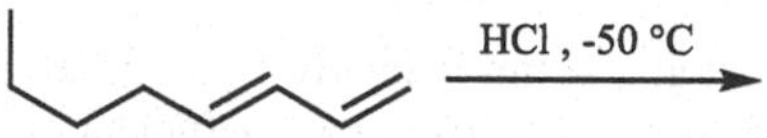 — HCl, -50 °C →

(f) 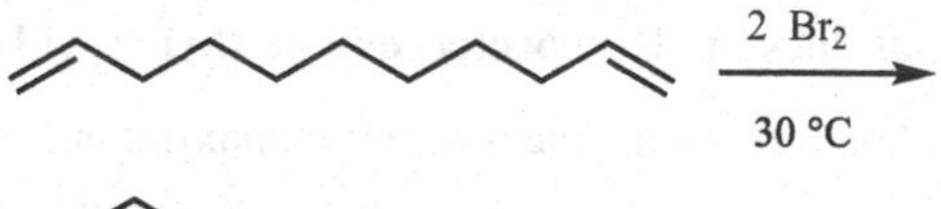 — 2 Br_2, 30 °C →

(g) 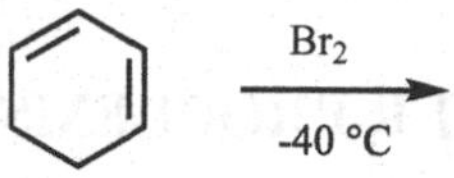 — Br_2, -40 °C →

10. Draw the molecular orbital diagram of buta-1,3-diene, of ethene, of maleic anhydride, and of ethyl vinyl ether. Label all HOMO and LUMO orbitals. What is the ΔE for the $HOMO_{butadiene}$–$LUMO_{alkene}$ for all three alkenes? Which one reacts faster?
11. Which of the following can react as a diene to undergo a Diels–Alder reaction? Explain.

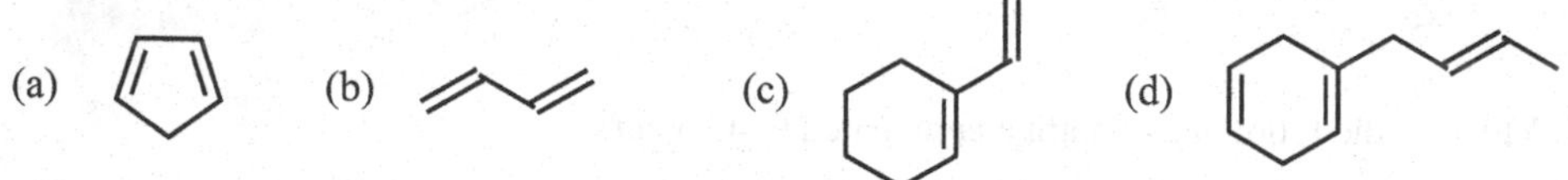

12. Predict the stereochemistry of each Diels–Alder product.

(a) 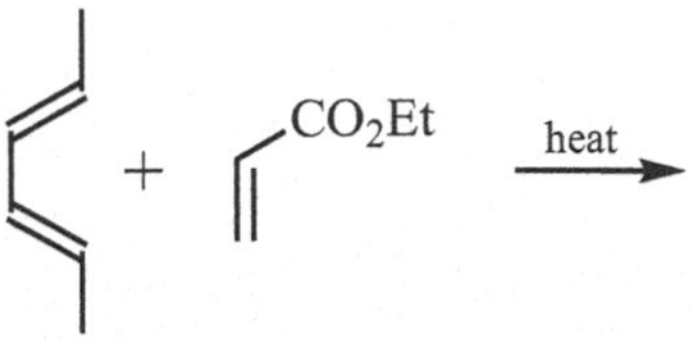 + CO_2Et heat (b) 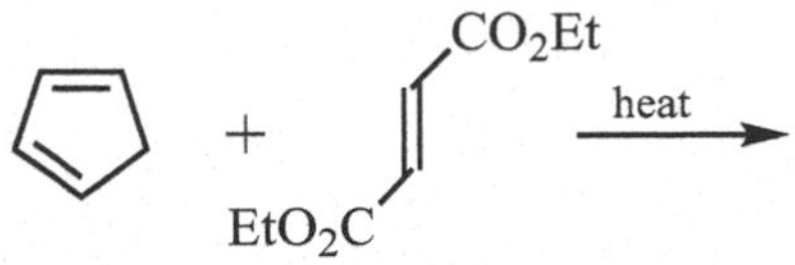 + CO_2Et EtO_2C heat

(c) 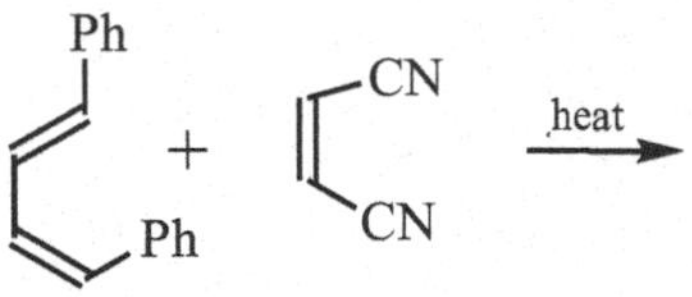 Ph Ph + CN CN heat (d) 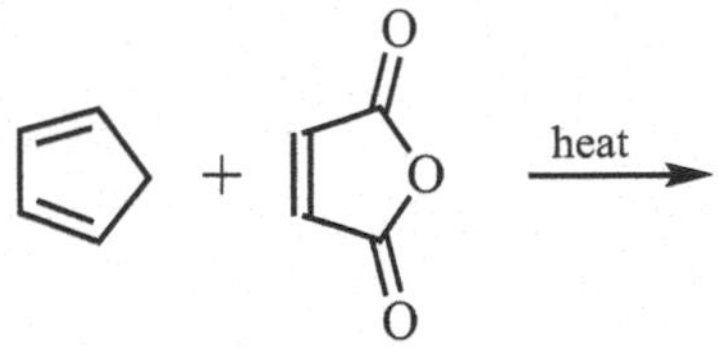 + O O O heat

13. In each case give the major product. Remember stereochemistry and if there is no reaction, indicate by N.R.

(a) 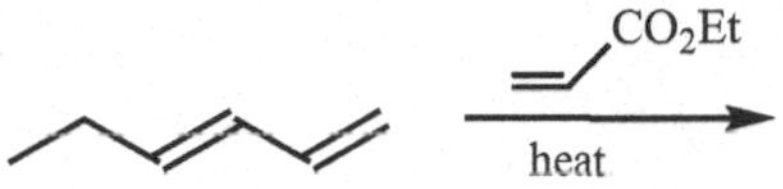 CO_2Et heat (b) 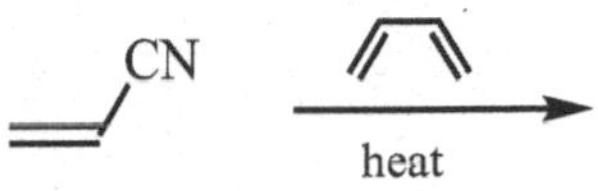 CN heat

(c) 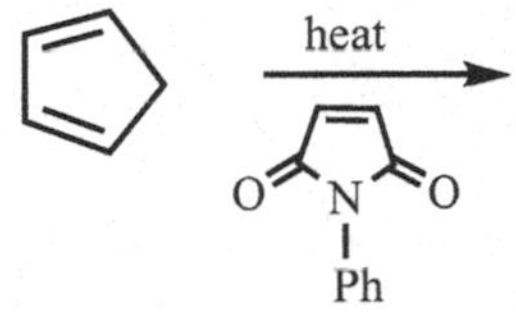 heat O N O Ph (d) 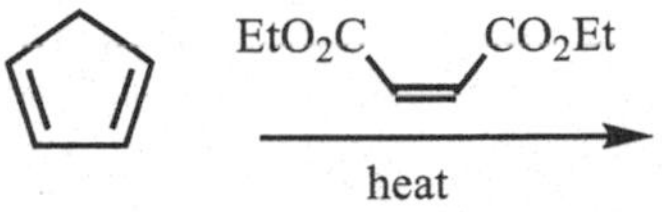 EtO_2C CO_2Et heat

14. Molecule **A** is known to require much lower reaction temperatures to undergo a Claisen rearrangement when compared with **B**. Explain.

(a) 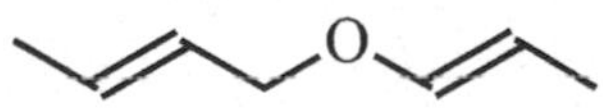 O (b)

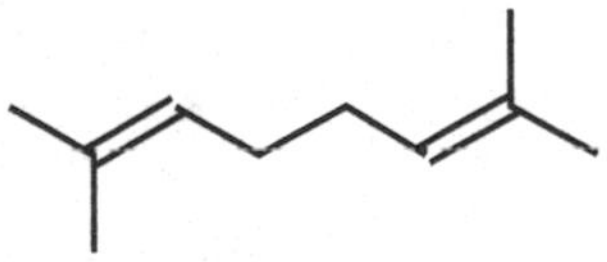

15. Give the major product for each of the following.

(a) 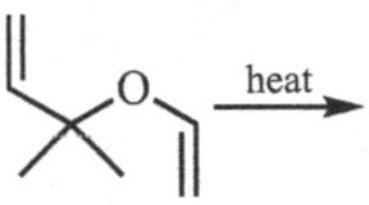 O heat (b) 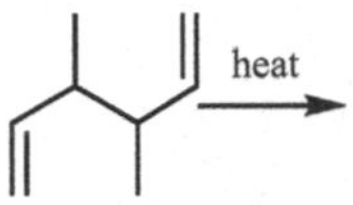 heat (c) 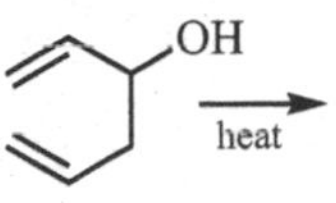 OH heat (d) 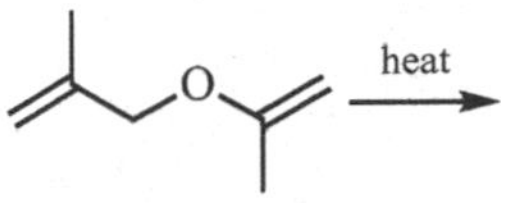 O heat

16. Draw the final product of the following reaction:

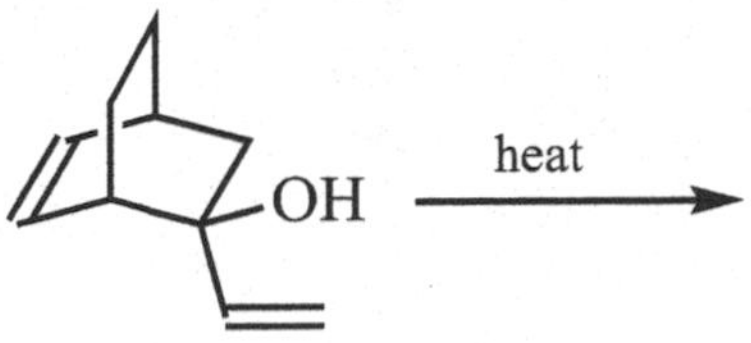

OH heat

17. Discuss the UV spectroscopic differences between hexa-1,3-diene and hexa-1,5-diene.

19

Amines

Amines are organic molecules with alkyl groups, aryl groups, or hydrogens attached to nitrogen (amines contain at least one alkyl or aryl group on nitrogen). Other nitrogen-containing molecules include nitriles, nitro compounds, and amides. Amines are a distinct class of compounds whose main characteristic is the basicity of the lone electron pair on nitrogen. Amines are useful as basic reagents in a variety of reactions. They also serve as intermediates in many reactions.

19.1 STRUCTURE AND PROPERTIES

What is an amine?

An amine is an organic molecule that contains a basic nitrogen atom with a lone electron pair that is attached to carbon atoms (alkyl groups). Using a simple analogy, amines can be considered to be derivatives of ammonia where one or more of the hydrogen atoms are replaced with alkyl or aryl groups: RNH_2, R_2NH, or R_3N.

What are generic examples of a primary amine, a secondary amine, and a tertiary amine?

A primary amine is characterized by two hydrogens on the nitrogen (RNH_2). A secondary amine is characterized by one hydrogen on the nitrogen (R_2NH), and a tertiary amine is characterized by no hydrogens on the nitrogen (R_3N).

What is the distinguishing feature of a tertiary amine?

A tertiary amine has three carbon groups on the nitrogen and no hydrogen atoms.

What is the IUPAC nomenclature system for alkyl amines?

Alkyl amines can be named as with an alkylamine or as an alkanamine, alkenamine, or alkynamine. The primary amine $CH_3CH_2CH_2CH_2NH_2$ is, therefore, butylamine or butanamine (note the -e of -ane is dropped).

What are the structures of 3-methylpentanamine, 2,2-diethylhexanamine and dodecaneamine?

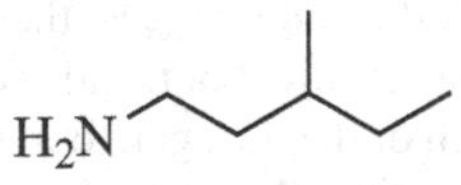

H_2N — 3-methylpentanamine

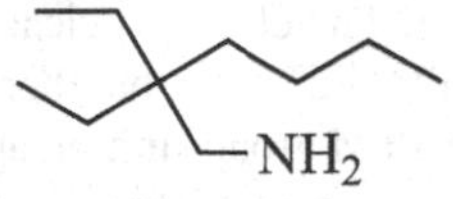

NH_2 — 2,2-diethylhexanamine

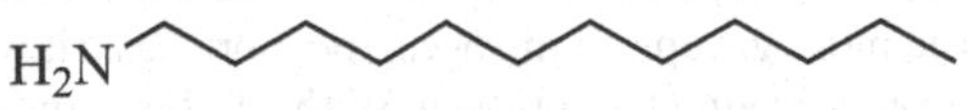

H_2N — dodecaneamine

What is the IUPAC nomenclature system for amine benzene derivatives?

Aryl amines are generally named as the parent aromatic amine. Aniline is the name of the amine formed when NH_2 is attached directly to a benzene ring. Aniline, 2-bromoaniline, and 3-nitro-aniline are typical examples. If a methyl group is also attached to the benzene ring, the common name is *ortho*-toluidine, *meta*-toluidine, and *para*-toluidine.

NH_2 NH_2 Br O_2N NH_2

aniline 2-bromoaniline 3-nitroaniline

How are substituents on the nitrogen of amines treated in the IUPAC system?

When a group is attached to the nitrogen, it is placed in the name with a *N*- preceding it. An example is $CH_3CH_2CH_2NHCH_2CH_3$, which is named *N*-ethylpropanamine. If there are two groups on nitrogen, each uses the *N*- designation. The amine $CH_3CH_2CH_2N(CH_3)_2$ is named *N,N*-dimethylpropanamine and $PhN(CH_3)Et$ is *N*-ethyl-*N*-methylaniline.

What are the structures of *N*-ethylbutanamine, *N*-butyl-*N*-methyloctanamine, 3,4,*N*-trimethylheptanamine, and 3-methoxy-*N*-ethylaniline?

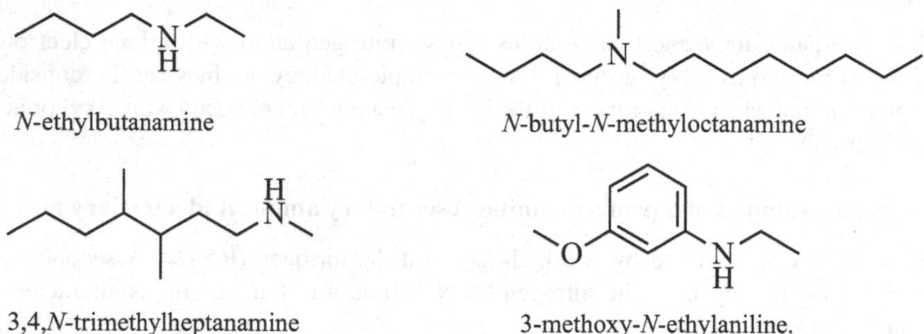

N-ethylbutanamine *N*-butyl-*N*-methyloctanamine

3,4,*N*-trimethylheptanamine 3-methoxy-*N*-ethylaniline.

How is an amine classified as a reagent?

An amine is both a nucleophile (if it reacts with carbon) and a base (if it reacts with a proton or a Lewis acid).

What is the product when an amine reacts with HCl?

The product is an ammonium chloride. For a secondary amine, the reaction is:

$$R_2NH + HCl \rightarrow R_2N^+H_2Cl^-$$

Which is more basic, a primary amine, a secondary amine, or a tertiary amine? Explain.

A secondary amine is the most basic when in a solvent. The electron-releasing alkyl groups suggest that the more groups on nitrogen, the more basic it will be (3° > 2° > 1°), but there is a steric effect of the alkyl groups around the nitrogen. With a tertiary amine, the alkyl groups inhibit approach of the nitrogen to the acid, decreasing the basicity. Another important factor is the presence of N—H groups in the ammonium salt product (the product after the amine reacts with the acid). These N—H groups are capable of hydrogen bonding with the solvent ($N—H—OH_2$), further stabilizing the product. This parameter suggests 1° > 2° > 3°. When in solution, the electronic effects, the solvent effects, and the steric effects are balanced to make secondary amines the most basic. *The usual order of basicity in solution is, therefore, 2° > 1° > 3°.*

What is the product when an amine reacts with $AlCl_3$?

The product is the usual Lewis acid–Lewis base "ate" complex (Section 3.1). For a secondary amine, the complex is: $R_2HN^+ : {}^-AlCl_3$.

Which is more basic, R_2NH or R_2N^-? Explain!

In R_2N^-, an amide anion, the charge is concentrated on the nitrogen with a formal charge of −1. The amide anion is clearly a stronger base (a better electron donor) relative to the neutral amine, which has only a δ^- charge on nitrogen due to the unshared electron pair.

Which is the strongest nucleophile, a primary amine, secondary amine, or a tertiary amine? Explain!

For essentially the same reasons described for basicity in the preceding question, secondary amines are usually the more nucleophilic in solution.

What is the product of the reaction between trimethylamine (a tertiary amine) and iodomethane?

The product is tetramethylammonium iodide: $Me_4N^+ I^-$.

What is a distinguishing feature of amines that can be correlated with their solubility characteristics?

Amines have a polarized C—N bond and also a polarized N—H bond for primary and secondary amines. The strong dipole of the C—N bond in small molecular weight amines promotes solubility in polar solvents. For primary and secondary amines, the ability of polarized molecules to hydrogen bond to the N—H moiety makes solubility in water and other protic solvents very high, if the molecular weight of the amine is not too great.

If an amine contains three different groups (RR^1R^2N), is the nitrogen chiral? Why or why not?

Such amines are considered to be chiral, racemic molecules, but the nitrogen is *not* considered to be stereogenic. Although there are three different alkyl groups and the lone electron pair can be considered a fourth "group," there is rapid inversion of configuration around nitrogen (*called fluxional inversion*) that generates a racemic mixture of the possible enantiomers. Fluxional inversion occurs faster than virtually any reaction that is possible for an amine. For this reason, the nitrogen of such amines is not considered to be a stereogenic center when determining the absolute configuration of chiral centers (they are chiral but exist as a racemic mixture). Note that if the amine is configurationally immobilized then nitrogen is a stereogenic center (see the following question).

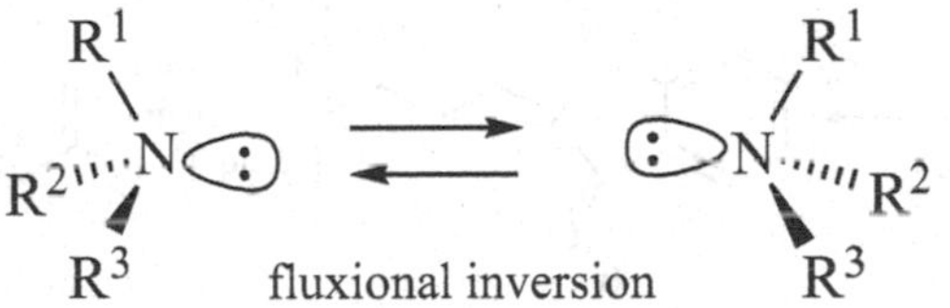

R^1, R^2, R^3 — N — R^1, R^2, R^3

fluxional inversion

How can the rapid fluxional inversion characteristic of an amine be prevented by structural modification of the amine?

If the alkyl groups are "tied back," as in 1-azabicyclo[2.2.2]octane (3,3,5-trimethylquinuclidine), inversion around nitrogen is not possible, the nitrogen is a stereogenic center, and 3,3,5-trimethylquinuclidine is a chiral, non-racemic molecule.

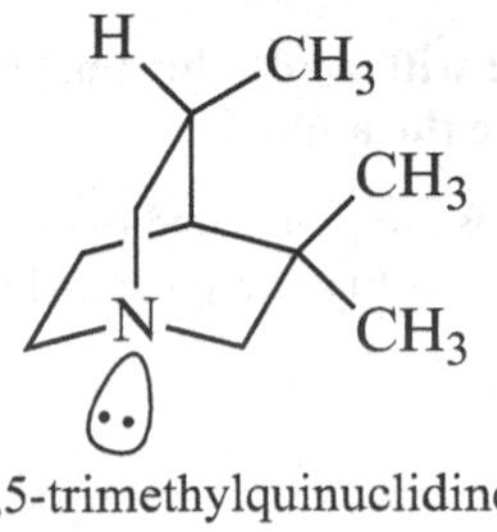

H CH_3 CH_3 N CH_3

3,3,5-trimethylquinuclidine

Do amines have a distinguishing nmr signal and an ir absorption?

Yes! The nmr signals for a CH-NR_2 signal is 2–3 ppm. The proton nmr signal for the hydrogen atoms of the N—H unit of an amine appears at 1–5 ppm.

Primary amines show two peaks at 3500 and 3300 cm^{-1} due to the two N—H units whereas secondary amines show one peak in this region due to one N—H unit. Tertiary amines have no N—H units and do not show a peak in this region. The C—N peak usually occurs in the 1200–1350 cm^{-1} region and is often difficult to detect, or if detectable it is difficult to correlate with an amine.

19.2 PREPARATION OF AMINES

What is the structure of phthalimide?

Phthalimide has the structure shown in the figure and it is the imide of phthalic acid.

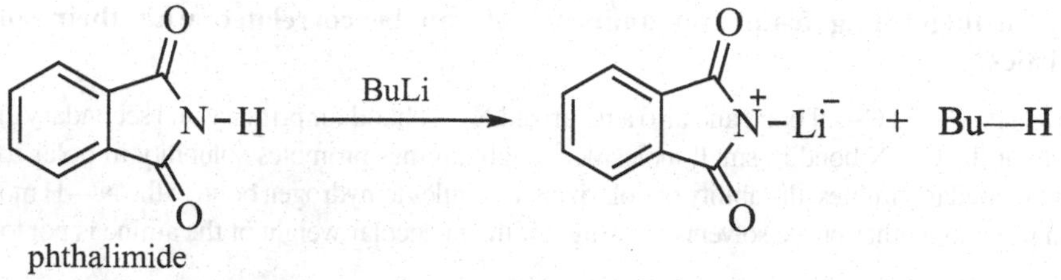

BuLi

phthalimide

What is the product when phthalimide reacts with n-butyllithium?

The imide N—H is relatively acidic (pK_a of about 17) and treatment with a strong base such as butyllithium will give the imide anion, as shown in the preceding question.

What is the product when the sodium salt of phthalimide reacts with 1-bromopentane?

The phthalimide anion (*A*) is a good nucleophile and it reacts with 1-bromopentane via a S_N2 reaction to give *N*-pentylphthalimide, *B*.

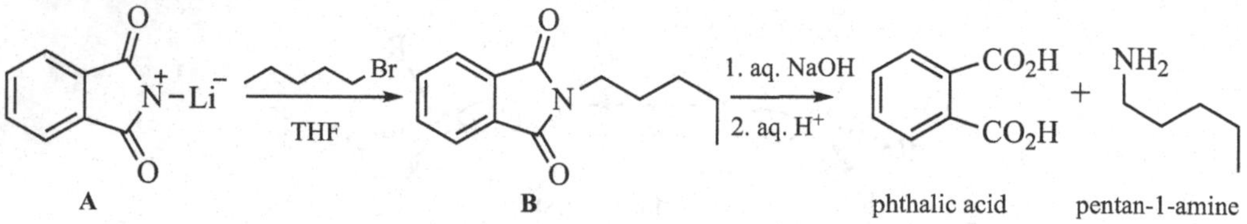

THF

1. aq. NaOH
2. aq. H^+

A B phthalic acid pentan-1-amine

What reaction conditions can be used to convert *B* in the preceding question to pentan-1-amine and phthalic acid?

As shown in the preceding question, saponification conditions (treatment with aqueous hydroxide followed by reaction with aqueous acid) converts the phthalimide unit to phthalic acid and the amine, pentan-1-amine.

If *N*-butyl phthalimide is hydrolyzed with acid, why must the pH of that solution be adjusted to about 8–9 prior to attempts to isolate the amine?

Under slightly acidic conditions, amines are protonated to give the ammonium salt. Adjusting the pH to about 8–9, which is slightly basic, removes that proton and "liberates" the free amine.

Is there another reagent to generate the primary amine from a *N*-alkylphthalimide?

Yes! The reaction of ***B*** in the preceding question with hydrazine gives pentan-1-amine and the phthalazine shown in what is called the *Ing–Manske procedure.*

$$\mathbf{B} \xrightarrow{NH_2NH_2} \text{2,3-dihydrophthalazine-1,4-dione} + \text{pentan-1-amine}$$

What is the name of the reaction sequence that uses phthalimide as an amine surrogate in reactions with alkyl halides followed by conversion to the amine?

This reaction sequence is called the *Gabriel synthesis.*

Why is polyalkylation not a problem in reactions of an alkyl halide with phthalimide?

The product of the alkylation is a *N*-alkyl phthalimide, which does not react as a base since the electron density of the nitrogen is diminished by the proximal carbonyls of the imide and cannot react further with the alkyl halide.

What is reductive amination of carbonyls?

Amines react with aldehydes and ketones to form imines (see Section 12.2). These imines can be reduced *in situ* or in a second step without isolation of the imine to form a new amine.

What is the product of the reaction between pentan-1-amine and formaldehyde?

In general, aldehydes react with primary amines to form an imine. In this example, the initial reaction of pentan-1-amine and formaldehyde will generate an iminium salt (*A*), which can be deprotonated to give the imine, *N*-pentylmethanimine. Imines formed from reaction of a primary amine and simple aldehydes such as formaldehyde are very reactive and difficult to isolate. Note that simple imines such as *N*-pentylmethanimine are highly reactive (not very stable) and tend to give secondary product. In other words, it is very difficult to isolate simple imines such as this one.

$$\text{pentan-1-amine } (NH_2) \xrightarrow{HCHO} [\,\text{A}: N^{+}(H){=}CH_2\,] \xrightarrow{-H^{+}} \text{N-pentylmethanimine } (N{=}CH_2)$$

If formaldehyde were to react with pentan-1-amine and the imine product was not isolated but rather exposed to hydrogen and a palladium catalyst, what would the product be?

The initial reaction of pentan-1-amine and formaldehyde generates an imine, as shown in the preceding question. Rather than try to isolate the imine, addition of hydrogen gas and a palladium catalyst leads to reduction to the corresponding amine (see Section 15.6). In this case the product is *N*-methylpentanamine.

$$\text{pentan-1-amine } (NH_2) \xrightarrow{HCHO} \text{N-pentylmethanimine } (N{=}CH_2) \xrightarrow[\text{ethanol}]{Pd^{\circ},\ H_2} N\text{-methylpentan-1-amine } (NH{-}CH_3)$$

If 3-methylpentanal were to react with pentan-1-amine and the imine product was not isolated but rather exposed to hydrogen and a palladium catalyst, what would the product be?

The initial reaction of pentan-1-amine and 3-methylpentanal generates an imine, (*E*)-3-methyl-*N*-pentylpentan-1-imine. After the addition of a palladium catalyst and hydrogen gas, reduction occurs to give the corresponding amine (see Section 15.6). In this case the product is 3-methyl-*N*-pentylpentan-1-amine.

NH_2 NH_2 N Pd°, H_2 ethanol H N

pentan-1-amine (*E*)-3-methyl-*N*-pentylpentan-1-imine 3-methyl-*N*-pentylpentan-1-amine

What is a Schiff base?

A Schiff base is the imine derived from reaction of a primary amine and an aromatic aldehyde. Reaction of benzaldehyde and ethanal, for example, leads to $PhN{=}CHCH_3$.

What is the product of the reaction between the Schiff base $PhN{=}CHCH_3$ and $LiAlH_4$?

The powerful reducing agent $LiAlH_4$ is capable of reducing the C=N bond to the amine, via delivery of hydride to the δ^+ carbon of the C=N bond (see Section 14.3). In this case, $Ph{-}N{=}CH_3$ reacts with $LiAlH_4$ and is then hydrolyzed to give the amine product, $Ph{-}NHCH_3$.

What is the product between a Schiff base and hydrogen gas, in the presence of a catalyst?

The product will be the amine, via reductive amination (see the reaction with formaldehyde).

What is the product when the imine derived from aniline and butanal is treated with $NaBH_4$?

Aniline and butanal will form the Schiff base, $PhN{=}CHCH_2CH_2CH_3$. Subsequent reaction with sodium borohydride reduces this imine to the amine, $PhNHCH_2CH_2CH_2CH_3$, although the reaction can be slow in the absence of an acid catalyst (which generates the iminium salt).

What is the product when 1-bromobutane reacts with KCN in THF?

The product is pentanenitrile via a S_N2 reaction.

What is the product when hexanenitrile is reduced with $LiAlH_4$?

When hexanenitrile is reduced with $LiAlH_4$, the product is hexan-1-amine.

What is the product when benzonitrile (PhCN) is reduced with hydrogen and a palladium catalyst?

The product is benzylamine ($PhCH_2NH_2$).

What is the product of the $LiAlH_4$ reduction of 1,6-hexanedinitrile?

The hydride-reducing agent reacts with both nitrile units to give the diamine. The product is the diamine, 1,6-hexanediamine [$H_2N{-}(CH_2)_6{-}NH_2$].

What is the product when *N*-ethylpentanamide is treated with $LiAlH_4$?

As mentioned in Section 15.6, amides react with $LiAlH_4$ to remove only the carbonyl groups and so they are reduced to amines rather than an alcohol. In this case, the product is *N*-ethylpentanamine after mild hydrolysis.

What is the product when 2-pyrrolidinone is reacted with $LiAlH_4$ followed by mild hydrolysis?

Reduction of lactams gives cyclic amines. Reduction of 2-pyrrolidinone gives pyrrolidine.

What is the structure of sodium azide?

Sodium azide has the structure NaN_3. The azide anion is N_3^-.

How stable is the azide anion?

The azide anion is a resonance-stabilized structure, as shown.

$$N_3^- \equiv \left[{}^-N{=}\overset{+}{N}{=}N \longleftrightarrow {}^-N{-}\overset{+}{N}{\equiv}N \longleftrightarrow N{=}\overset{+}{N}{=}N^- \right]$$

What is the major product of the reaction between sodium azide and 1-iodohexane?

The product is 1-azidohexane, $CH_3CH_2CH_2CH_2CH_2CH_2N_3$.

What is the major product when 1-azidopentane reacts with $LiAlH_4$? With H_2 and a catalyst?

In both cases, the azide is reduced to the primary amine. In this case, 1-azidopentane is reduced to pentanamine with both reagents.

Can the reaction of azide and alkyl halides ever react to give a secondary or tertiary amine?

No! Reduction of the azide moiety always leads to $-NH_2$, the primary amine.

Aromatic amines are generally considered to be derivatives of what simple compound?

Aniline, $PhNH_2$.

How is nitrobenzene prepared from benzene?

Reaction of benzene with nitric and sulfuric acid gives nitrobenzene. This chemistry was discussed in Section 16.2.

What is the major product when nitrobenzene is reacted with hydrogen and a palladium catalyst?

Reduction with hydrogen and a transition metal catalyst leads to aniline as the product.

Why do these conditions not reduce the benzene ring?

The benzene ring is aromatic (resonance stabilized) and an excess of hydrogen and very vigorous conditions (heat and pressure) are required to reduce it. The nitro group is relatively easy to reduce relative to the benzene ring, and the conditions used will not affect the benzene ring.

What is the major product of the reaction between a catalyst, H_2 and nitrobenzene?

Reduction of the nitro group by catalytic hydrogenation leads to aniline. Note that lithium aluminum hydride reacts differently with aromatic amines such as aniline. The mechanism will not be discussed here, but the product is *not* the amine (aniline) but rather a diazo compound, 1,2-diphenyldiazene.

$$PhNH_2 \xleftarrow[\text{EtOH}]{H_2\text{, EtOH}} PhNO_2 \xrightarrow[\text{2. dilute aq. } H^+]{\text{1. LiAlH}_4} Ph{-}N{=}N{-}Ph$$

1,2-diphenyldiazene

What is the major product of the reaction between 1-nitrobutane and $LiAlH_4$?

Unlike aromatic nitro compounds, alkyl nitro derivatives are cleanly reduced to the amine. In this case, the product is butan-1-amine ($CH_3CH_2CH_2CH_2NH_2$).

Is reduction of aromatic nitro compounds with $LiAlH_4$ a viable synthetic route to aromatic amines?

No! In general, diazo compounds are produced rather than amines. This chemistry was discussed in Section 16.4.

19.3 REACTIONS OF AMINES

Are there a large number of new reactions of amines?

Several reactions of amines have been presented in preceding chapters. The questions in this section will review those important reactions, and the reader is referred to the appropriate chapter where each reaction was first introduced.

Can amines be prepared by S_N2 reactions?

Yes! Since amines are nucleophiles, they can react with alkyl halides via a S_N2 process (Section 8.2) to produce new amines. However, over-alkylation is a problem, which limits the utility of the reaction. Since amines are also basic, however, E2 reactions (Section 9.1) may be competitive with the substitution with secondary amines and will dominate with tertiary amines.

What is the initial product when butan-1-amine reacts with iodomethane?

The nitrogen of butan-1-amine is a nucleophile, and it will displace iodide in an S_N2 reaction to give the ammonium salt, $CH_3CH_2CH_2CH_2NH_2CH_3^+ I^-$,

If *N*-methylbutan-1-ammonium iodide is the initially formed product in the preceding reaction, why is *N*-methylbutan-1-amine the isolated product?

Pentan-1-amine is a base and the hydrogen atoms on nitrogen of the ammonium salt are acidic. Therefore, the ammonium salt is deprotonated *in situ* and the product is the amine, pentan-1-amine.

Which is the more nucleophilic, butan-1-amine or *N*-methylbutan-1-amine?

The secondary amine, *N*-methylbutan-1-amine, is more nucleophilic since there are two alkyl groups releasing electrons to nitrogen.

Why is monoalkylation of a primary amine with iodomethane very difficult?

If a primary amine such as ethanamine reacts with iodomethane, the initial product is *N*-methylethanamineammonium iodide ($EtNHMe^+I^-$). Since ethanamine is also a base, deprotonation of the ammonium salt is possible to give the secondary amine, EtNHMe. Secondary amines are more nucleophilic and will react faster than primary amines, so EtNHMe will likely react with unreacted MeI faster than $EtNH_2$ and will give a tertiary amine. Remember that after one half-life of the reaction (see Section 8.2), only half of the MeI has reacted. Since the products of the initial reaction with $EtNH_2$ are more reactive than the starting material, it is difficult to stop the reaction at the secondary amine stage.

How can polyalkylation be minimized in reactions of amines?

If a large excess of the primary amine is used relative to the alkyl halide, polyalkylation is minimized.

Why is elimination a problem when amines react with alkyl halides?

Amines are relatively good bases that can initiate the E2 reaction if the rate of the S_N2 reaction is relatively slow. With secondary and especially tertiary halides, elimination of the halide leaving group will lead to an alkene via an E2 reaction (see Section 9.1).

What is the product when 2-bromo-2-methylpentane reacts with triethylamine?

This reaction is an E2 reaction and the product is 2-methylpent-2-ene.

Is elimination a major problem when primary amines react with alkyl halides? Why or why not?

In general, elimination is slower than substitution for primary halides. In other words, reaction at the primary carbon atom is faster than the acid–base reaction to remove to weakly acidic β-hydrogen atom. The ammonium intermediate ($RCH_2NR_3^+$) is susceptible to both S_N2 and E2 reactions since $-NR_3^+$ is a good leaving group. For primary amines, substitution is faster than elimination and elimination is usually not a significant problem in alkylation reactions of primary amines.

What is a protic solvent?

A protic solvent has an acidic hydrogen atom due to polarized X—H bonds as found in water alcohols (methanol or ethanol), ammonia, or amines (methanamine or *N*-methylmethanamine).

What is an aprotic solvent?

An aprotic solvent does not contain an acidic proton and all hydrogen atoms are generally attached to carbon. Examples, are diethyl ether, pentane, tetrahydrofuran (THF), etc.

What is solvation?

Solvation is the process by which solvent molecules surround and interact with solute ions or molecules. Polar solutes such as alcohols, carboxylic acids, or alkoxide ions are solvated by polar solvents such as water or alcohols, but they are not solvated by non-polar solvents such as hexane.

Does solvent play a role in the S_N2 versus E2 reactions?

Yes! In general, protic solvents such as methanol, ethanol, or water favor E2 elimination when S_N2 and E2 reactions compete. Conversely, aprotic solvents such as diethyl ether of THF favor S_N2 reactions. A protic solvent will solvate a polar and often ionic nucleophile, which inhibits approach of the nucleophile to the electrophilic carbon that reacts to give a S_N2 reaction. Approach to a hydrogen atom is more facile and the E2 reaction is faster.

Why does the reaction of a tertiary alcohol with thionyl chloride and triethylamine lead directly to an alkene?

Thionyl chloride first converts the alcohol to the tertiary chloride *in situ* and the triethylamine present in the reaction medium reacts to induce an E2 elimination to give the alkene directly.

What is the product of reactions (a), (b), and (c)?

(a) 1-iodopentane —(Me_2NH, THF)→

(b) butan-1-amine (NH_2) —(excess CH_3I, THF)→

(c) 2,3-dimethylhexan-2-ol (OH) —($SOCl_2$, pyridine heat)→

In reaction (a) the nucleophilic secondary amine reacts with the primary alkyl iodide to give *N,N*-dimethylpentan-1-amine. In reaction (b), the amine reacts with an excess of iodomethane to give the ammonium salt, *N,N,N*-trimethylbutan-1-ammonium iodide. In reaction (c), thionyl chloride reacts with the tertiary alcohol to give the tertiary chloride, and in the presence of the basic amine, pyridine, an E2 reaction gives the product, 2,3-dimethylhex-2-ene.

(a) NMe_2 N,N-dimethylpentan-1-amine

(b) $\overset{+}{N}(CH_3)_3\ I^-$ N,N,N-trimethylbutan-1-aminium iodide

(c) 2,3-dimethylhex-2-ene

What is the product when 2-bromo-2-methylpentane is heated with triethylamine in ethanol?

The conditions described promote an E2 reaction, so the product is 2-methylpent-2-ene. Note that the E2 reaction will give the more-substituted alkene (see Section 9.1).

What is the product when 2-(trimethylammonium)butane bromide reacts with (1) Ag_2O/H_2O and is then (2) heated?

This reaction is the *Hofmann elimination* (see Section 9.4). The initial reaction will exchange the bromide ion for the hydroxide ion. Since the base is tethered to the molecule, heating will induce syn- elimination and the product is the less-substituted alkene, but-1-ene.

$NMe_3^+\ Br^-$ —(Ag_2O , H_2O)→ $NMe_3^+\ OH^-$ —(heat)→ but-1-ene

What is the product when *N,N*-dimethylbutan-2-amine is reacted with (1) H_2O_2 and then (2) heated?

This reaction is the *Cope elimination* (see Section 9.4). The initial reaction will convert the amine to the amine *N*-oxide, *A*. Since the base is the oxygen of the *N*-oxide, heating will induce syn- elimination and the product is the less-substituted alkene, but-1-ene.

Me–N–Me —(H_2O_2)→ $^+N(Me)_2$–O^- **A** —(heat)→ but-1-ene + Me_2NOH

What is the product when pentan-2-one reacts with propan-1-amine?

A primary amine such as propan-1-amine reacts with an aldehyde or a ketone to give an imine. Therefore, pentan-2-one reacts to give *N*-propylpentan-2-imine. In general, primary amines react with an aldehyde or a ketone to give the imine (see Section 12.2).

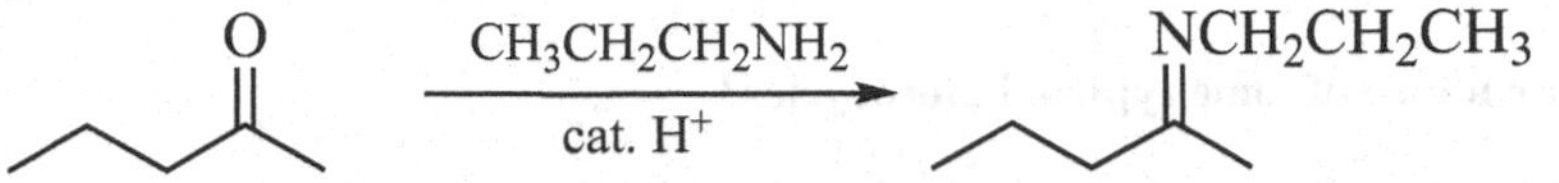

O $CH_3CH_2CH_2NH_2$ cat. H^+ $NCH_2CH_2CH_3$

N-propylpentan-2-imine

What is the product when butan-2-one reacts with pyrrolidine?

A secondary amine such as pyrrolidine reacts with a ketone to give an enamine. Therefore, butan-2-one reacts to give 1-(but-1-en-2-yl)pyrrolidine. In general, secondary amines react with a ketone to give the enamine. Although the reaction with an aldehyde also gives an enamine (see Section 9.2), the reaction of aldehydes is more complicated due to over-reaction with the amine. The secondary reactions of aldehydes will not be discussed further, however. Note that in the enamine, the 1- in the name refers to the group attached to nitrogen.

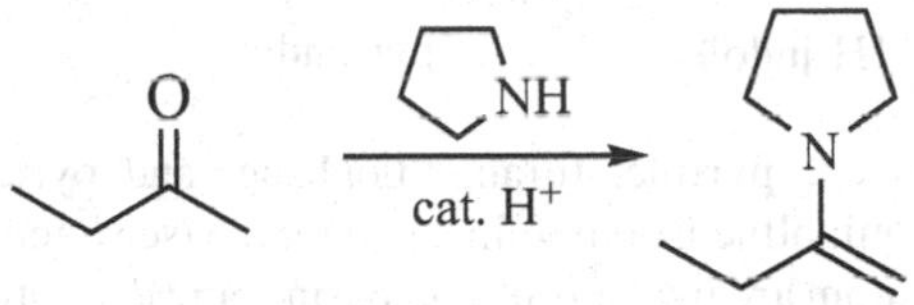

O NH cat. H^+ N

1-(but-1-en-2-yl)pyrrolidine

What is the product when aniline reacts with HONO and then CuBr?

Aniline reacts with nitrous acid (HONO) to give benzenediazonium chloride. The diazonium salt reacts with CuBr in what is called the *Sandmeyer reaction* to give bromobenzene. See Section 16.4.

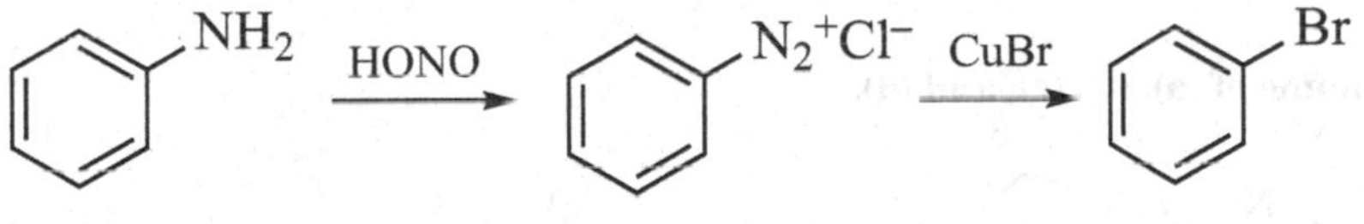

NH_2 HONO $N_2^+Cl^-$ CuBr Br

What is the product when aniline reacts with $NaNO_2$/HCl and then anisole?

The reaction of sodium nitrite and HCl generates HONO, which reacts with aniline to give benzenediazonium chloride. Diazonium salts react with activated aromatic rings to give an azo dye (see Section 16.4). In this case, reaction with anisole gives the azo dye, 1-(4-methoxyphenyl)-2-phenyldiazene.

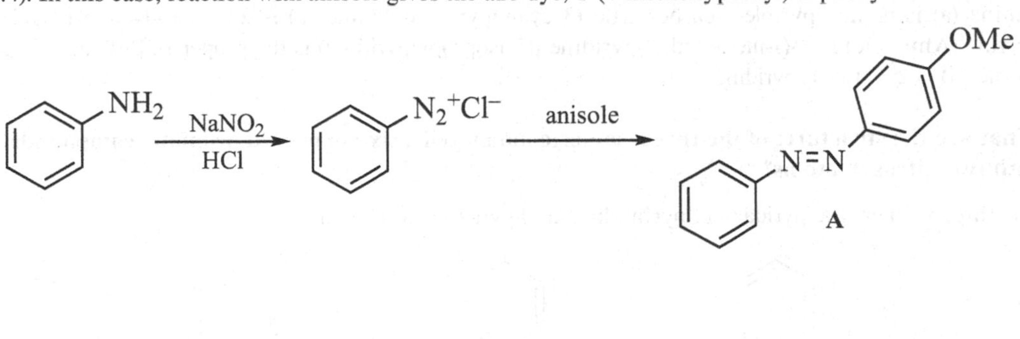

NH_2 $NaNO_2$ HCl $N_2^+Cl^-$ anisole OMe N=N

A

19.4 HETEROCYCLIC AMINES

What is a heterocyclic amine, sometimes just called a heterocycle?

A heterocyclic amine is defined as an aromatic compound that contains nitrogen in a ring.

What is the structure of some typical heterocycles?

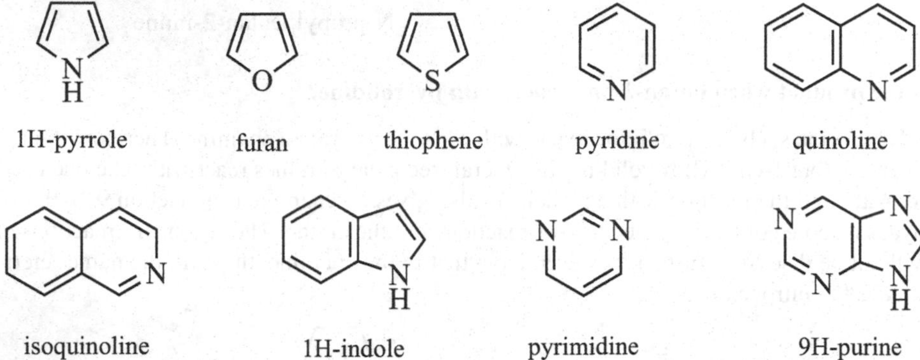

Common monocyclic heterocycles are pyrrole, furan, thiophene, and pyridine (see Section 16.6). Common bicyclic heterocycles are quinoline isoquinoline, and indole (see Section 16.6). Typical heterocycles with more than one nitrogen atom are pyrimidine and purine, and derivatives of these heterocycles are found in DNA and RNA.

What is the nomenclature system for substituted pyrroles and pyridines?

The name pyrrole and pyridine constitute the IUPAC base name of all derivatives of these compounds. The nitrogen always receives the lowest number (1). The ring is numbered to give the smallest combination of substituent numbers.

What is the name of (a), (b), (c), and (d).

(a) (b) (c) (d)

Amine (a) is named pyrrole-3-carbonitrile (3-cyanopyrrole). Amine (b) is 2-bromo-4-ethyl-1-methylpyrrole. Amine (c) is 3-(1-methylethyl)pyridine [(3-isopropylpyridine) is the proper IUPAC name], and amine (d) is 2,3-dinitropyridine.

What are the structures of the three isomeric monocyclic, six-membered aromatic compounds with two nitrogen atoms?

The three isomers are pyridazine, pyrimidine, and pyrazine, as shown.

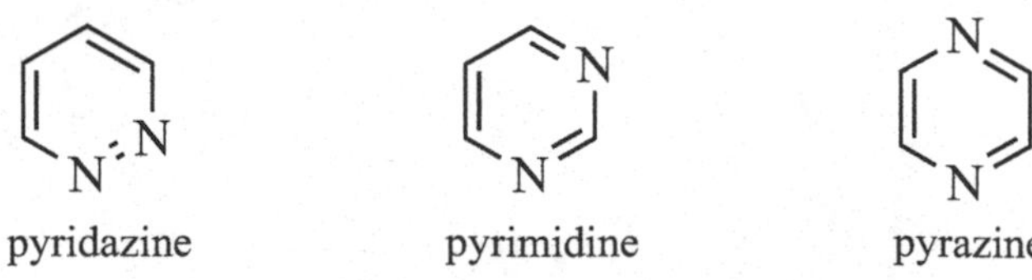

Which pyrimidine units are found in nucleic acid structures (see Section 21.5)?

The more important pyrimidine derivatives found in DNA and RNA are cytosine (4-aminopyrimidin-2(1*H*)-one), thymine (5-methylpyrimidine-2,4(1*H*,3*H*)-dione), and uracil (pyrimidine-2,4(1*H*,3*H*)-dione).

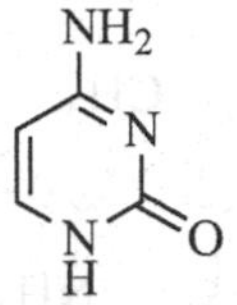

cytosine
(cytosine-4-aminopyrimidin-2(1H)-one)

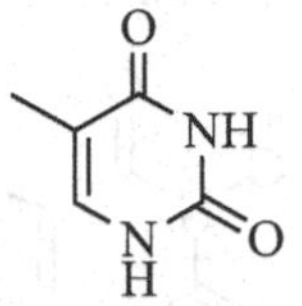

thymine
(5-methylpyrimidine-2,4(1H,3H)-dione)

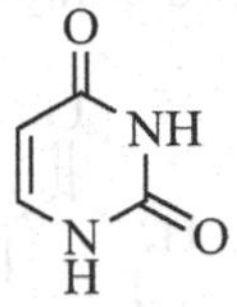

uracil
(pyrimidine-2,4(1H,3H)-dione)

What is the structure of purine?

The structure of 9H-purine is shown. Note that the position of the H atom on the atom that is not sp^2-hydrbiridzed in the molecule is indicated by "H" in the name, so this isomer is 9*H*-purine.

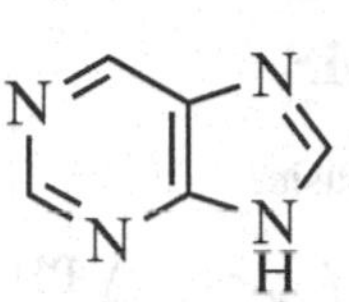

9*H*-purine

Are there isomers of 9*H*-purine?

Yes! There are several isomers based on the position of the NH or the CH_2 units, where the other atoms are part of a π-bond. The position of the NH or CH_2 units are indicated by 1*H*, 2*H*, etc. The isomers and the IUPAC names are shown in the figure.

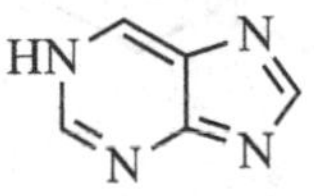

1*H*-purine 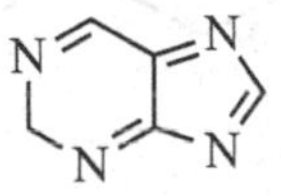 2*H*-purine 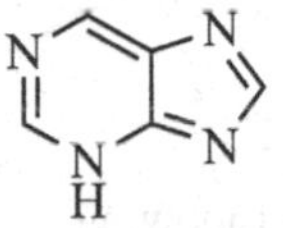 3*H*-purine 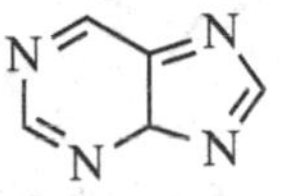 4*H*-purine 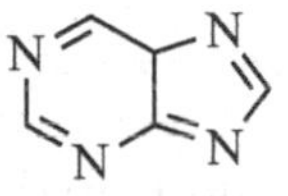 5*H*-purine

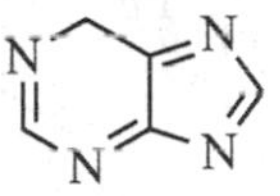

6*H*-purine 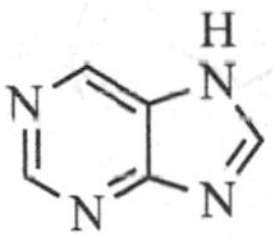 7*H*-purine 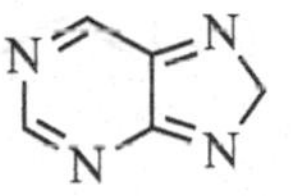 8*H*-purine 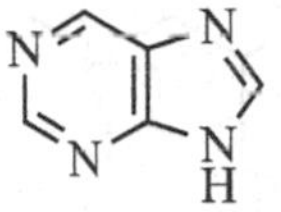 9*H*-purine

Which purine units are found in nucleic acid structures (see Section 21.5)?

Two important purine derivatives are found in DNA and RNA. They are adenine (9*H*-purin-6-amine) and guanine (2-amino-1,9-dihydro-6*H*-purin-6-one).

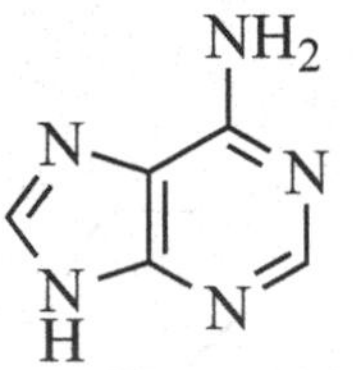

adenine
9H-p(urin-6-amine)

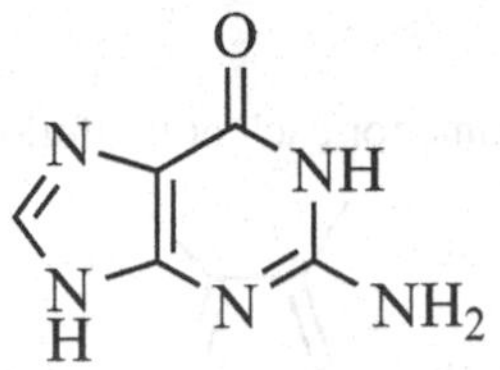

guanine
(2-amino-1,9-dihydro-6H-purin-6-one)

Are purine units found in other biologically important molecules?

Three common purine derivatives are uric acid (7,9-dihydro-1*H*-purine-2,6,8(3*H*)-trione), found in urine, caffeine (1,3,7-trimethyl-3,7-dihydro-1*H*-purine-2,6-dione), found in coffee and tea, and theobromine (3,7-dimethyl-3,7-dihydro-1*H*-purine-2,6-dione), found in chocolate.

uric acid (7,9-dihydro-1H-purine-2,6,8(3H)-trione)

caffeine (1,3,7-trimethyl-3,7-dihydro-1H-purine-2,6-dione)

theobromine (3,7-dimethyl-3,7-dihydro-1H-purine-2,6-dione)

END OF CHAPTER PROBLEMS

1. Which of the following is the more basic?

   PH_2 PH (2) P (3)

2. Choose the more basic molecule in each pair. Assume the basicity of the molecules are examined in solution. Explain your choice.

   (a) (b)

3. Give the IUPAC name for each of the following.

   (a) (b) (c)

   (d) (e) (f)

4. Give the correct name for each of the following.

   (a) (b) (c) (d)

5. Give the major product for each of the following reactions. If there is no reaction, indicate by N.R.

(a) 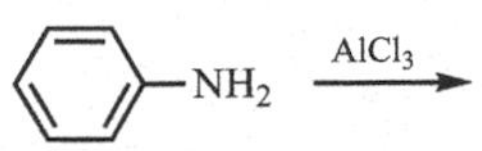 NH_2 — $AlCl_3$ →

(b) 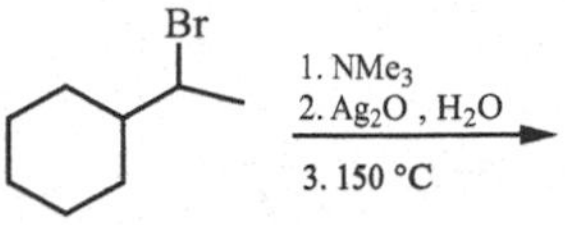 Br — 1. NMe_3 2. Ag_2O, H_2O 3. 150 °C →

(c) N 3 — Br →

(d) NMe_2 — 1. MeI 2. Ag_2O, H_2O 3. 150 °C →

(e) PPh_3 — iodopentane →

(f) OH — $POCl_3$, pyridine →

(g) NMe_2 — H_2O_2, 25 °C →

(h) Br — pyridine, heat →

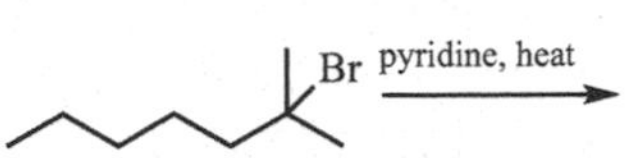

(i) 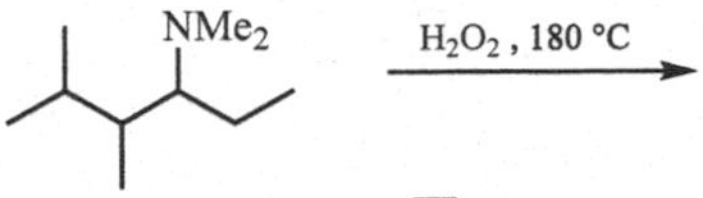 NMe_2 — H_2O_2, 180 °C →

(j) 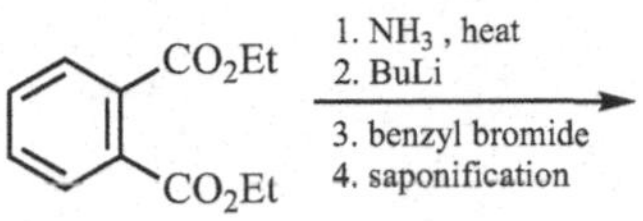 CO_2Et CO_2Et — 1. NH_3, heat 2. BuLi 3. benzyl bromide 4. saponification →

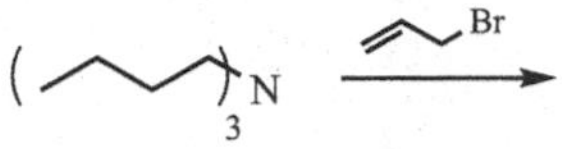

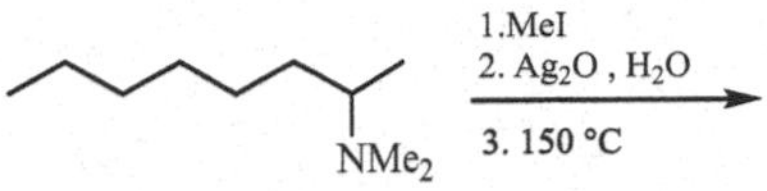

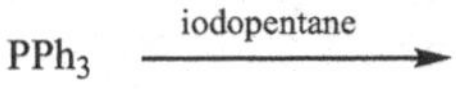

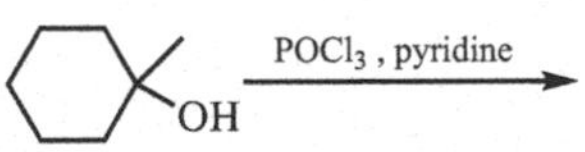

(k) 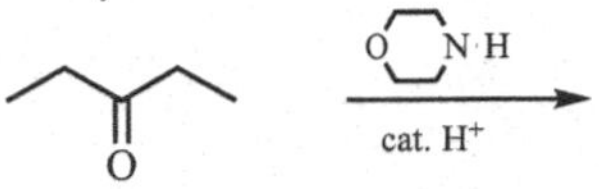 O — O N H, cat. H^+ →

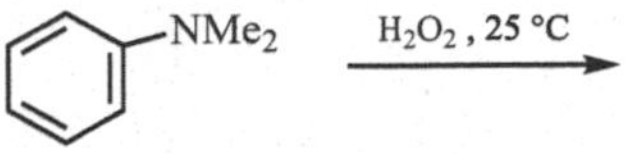

(l) 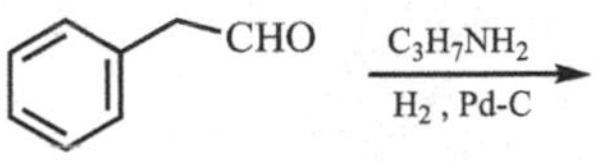 CHO — $C_3H_7NH_2$ H_2, Pd-C →

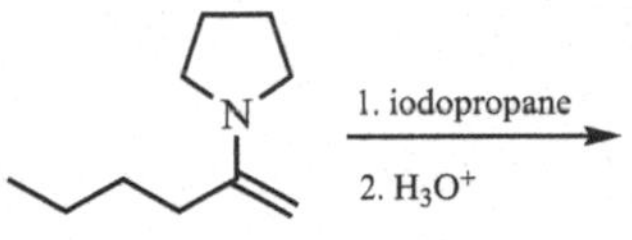

(m) N — 1. iodopropane 2. H_3O^+ →

(n) NH_2 — PhCHO, cat. H^+ →

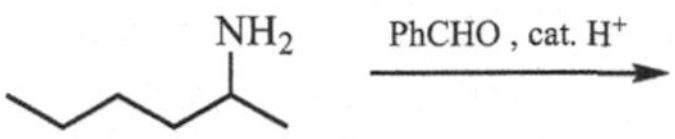

(o) 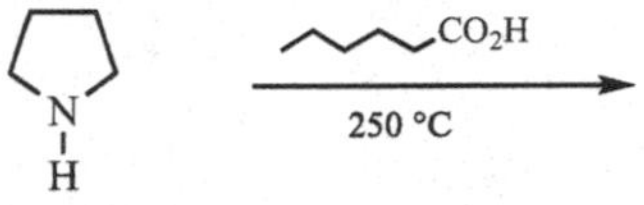 N H — CO_2H 250 °C →

(p) 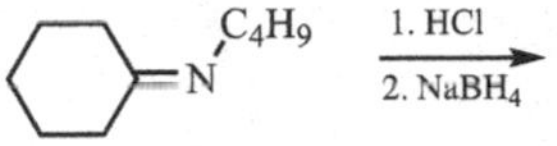 C_4H_9 N — 1. HCl 2. $NaBH_4$ →

(q) 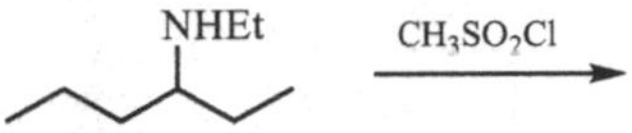 NHEt — CH_3SO_2Cl →

(r) 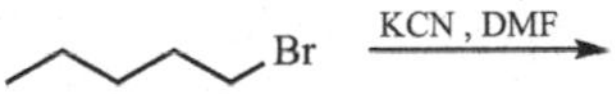 Br — KCN, DMF →

(s) 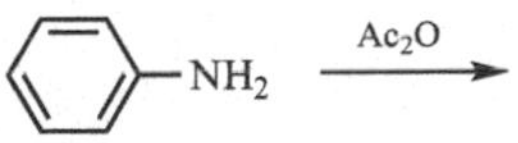 NH_2 — Ac_2O →

(t) 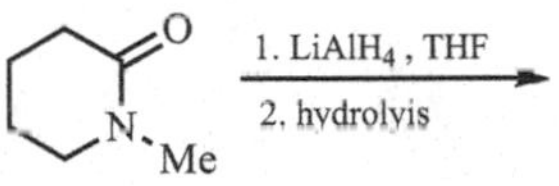 O N Me — 1. $LiAlH_4$, THF 2. hydrolyis →

(u) 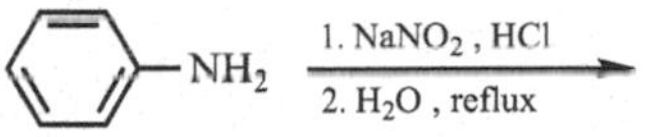 NH_2 — 1. $NaNO_2$, HCl 2. H_2O, reflux →

(v) 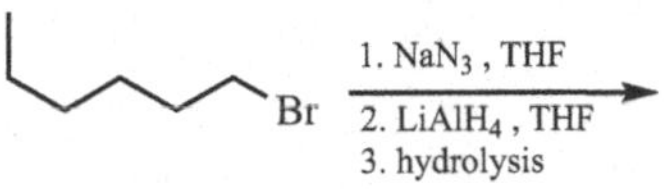 Br — 1. NaN_3, THF 2. $LiAlH_4$, THF 3. hydrolysis →

(w) 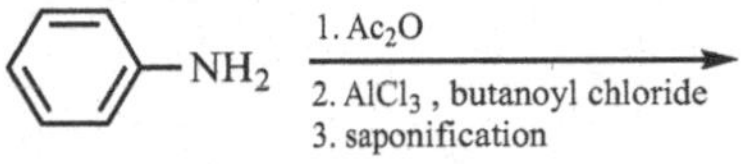 NH_2 — 1. Ac_2O 2. $AlCl_3$, butanoyl chloride 3. saponification →

6. Give the structure of: (a) 2-ethylpyrazine (b) 2,4-dibromopyrimidine (c) 9-ethylpurine (d) 3-cyclopentyl-9-methylguanine.

20

Amino Acids, Peptides, and Proteins

Organic molecules that contained two or more functional groups have been seen only sparingly in this book. This chapter discusses one of the most important classes of multi-functional organic molecules, amino acids. Amino acids are important biologically as constituents of peptides and proteins. They are important chemically since their properties and chemical reactions graphically illustrate the problems that arise when two different functional groups are in a single molecule and what happens when those groups interact with each other. Since amino acids are the important building blocks of proteins and peptides, a brief overview of that chemistry will be given as well.

20.1 AMINO ACIDS

What is an amino acid?

An amino acid is a difunctional molecule that contains an amino group (NH_2) and a carboxylic acid group (CO_2H).

What is the generic structure of an α-amino acid?

The general structure will be $HO_2CCH(R)NH_2$. An example is glycine, which is 2-aminoethanoic acid: $H_2NCH_2CO_2H$.

Why are these amino acids called α-amino acids?

The NH_2 group is attached to the carbon that is α- to the carboxyl group, C2 relative to the carboxyl group. Therefore α-amino acids are 2-amino-alkanoic acids. It is important to note that there are amino acids other than α-amino acids. In a long chain carboxylic acid, the NH_2 group can appear on any carbon of the chain to give a "non-α-amino acid."

What are β-amino acids, γ-amino acids, and δ-amino acids? What is an example of each?

A β-amino acid has the amino croup of C3 relative to the carbonyl, a γ-amino acid has the amino group of C4, and a δ-amino acid has the amino group on C5. A β-amino acid is $H_2NCH_2CH_2CO_2H$, (3-amino-propanoic acid), a γ-amino acid is $H_2NCH_2CH_2CH_2CO_2H$ (4-aminoobutanoic acid), and a δ-amino acid is $H_2NCH_2CH_2CH_2CH_2CO_2H$ (5-aminopentanoic acid).

Are α-amino acids chiral molecules?

Yes, all except glycine! The C2 of an α-amino acid is a stereogenic center in all amino acids except glycine, which has no substituent at C2.

Do α-amino acids exist with the NH_2 and the CO_2H structures at neutral pH?

No! An amine is a base and the CO_2H unit is an acid, so an internal acid–base reaction occurs at neutral pH so amino acids exist as the zwitterion, $^+NH_3CHRCO_2^-$. The formal charge of this molecule is zero (electrically neutral) since the + and – charges cancel.

What is a zwitterion?

A zwitterion is a dipolar ion that has a positive and a negative charge in the same molecule.

What is the zwitterionic structure of glycine (2-aminoethanoic acid)?

The zwitterion structure is H_3N^+-CH_2-CO_2^-.

Why does an amino acid exist as a zwitterion?

At neutral pH, the NH_2 group is a base and reacts with the acidic proton of the COOH group to form the zwitterion.

What is the absolute configuration of most biologically important amino acids?

These amino acids will have the (*S*)-configuration, as shown. The older nomenclature of amino acids with this absolute configurate is the L-configuration. This amino acid is also shown in its Fischer projection (see Section 6.1). The α-amino acids with the opposite absolute configuration are (*R*)-amino acids, and the older designation is D.

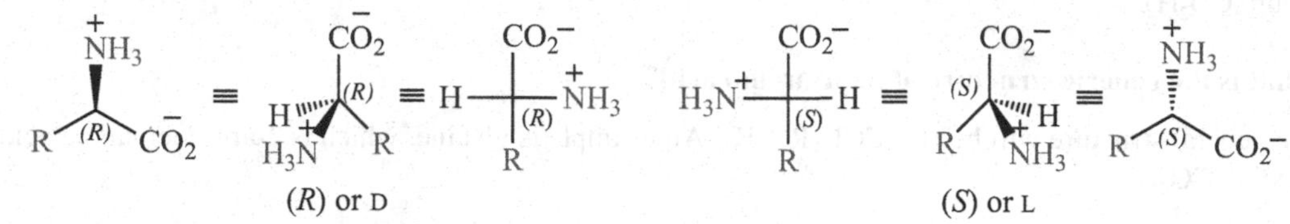

(*R*) or D

(*S*) or L

How is the D- and L-configuration of an α-amino acid determined?

The terms D and L designations are based on glyceraldehyde. When drawn in a Fischer projection with the CHO unit at the top and the CH_2OH unit at the bottom, as shown, (*R*)-glyceraldehyde has the OH unit on the right and is assigned a D-configuration. Similarly, (*S*)-glyceraldehyde will have the OH unit on the left and is assigned the L-configuration. When α-amino acids are drawn in Fischer projection with the CO_2^- group on the top and the α-substituent (*R*) on the bottom, as in the preceding question, the D-configuration has the NH_3 group on the right, and the L-configuration has the NH_3 unit on the left, as shown.

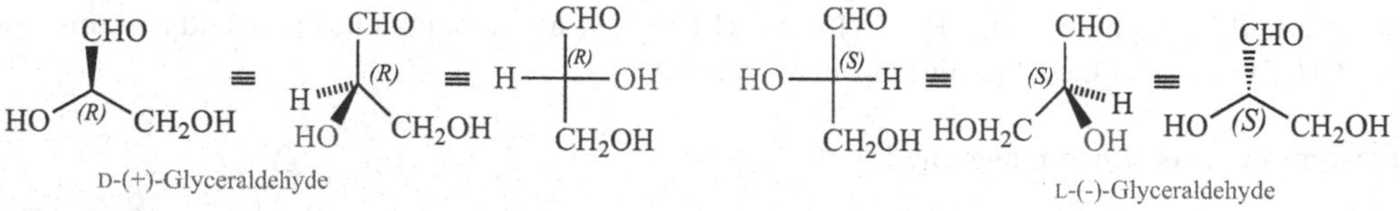

D-(+)-Glyceraldehyde

L-(-)-Glyceraldehyde

Draw D-(+)-glyceraldehyde in Fischer projection.

The structure of D-(+)-glyceraldehyde in Fischer projection is shown in the preceding question.

What are the common α-amino acids by name, three-letter code, and one-letter code, and give R group in $^{+}NH_3CHRCO_2^{-}$?

C2 Substituent	Name	Three-Letter Code	One-Letter Code
H	Glycine	gly	G
Me	Alanine	ala	A
$CHMe_2$	Valine	val	V
$CHMe_2$	Leucine	leu	L
CH(Me)Et	Isoleucine	ile	I
CH_2Ph	Phenylalanine	phe	F
CH_2OH	Serine	ser	S
CH(OH)Me	Threonine	thr	T
CH_2(4-hydroxy-C_6H_4)	Tyrosine	tyr	Y
CH_2SH	Cysteine	cys	C
CH_2CH_2SMe	Methionine	met	M
CH_2CONH_2	Asparagine	asn	N
$CH_2CH_2CONH_2$	Glutamine	gln	Q
CH_2COOH	Aspartic acid	asp	D
CH_2CH_2COOH	Glutamic acid	glu	E
$CH_2CH_2CH_2CH_2NH_2$	Lysine	lys	K
CH_2(2-indolyl)	Tryptophan	trp	W
CH_2(4-imidazolyl)	Histidine	his	H
$CH_2NHC(=NH)NH_2$	Arginine	arg	R
2-Pyrrolidinyl	Proline	pro	P

What are the actual structures of the α-amino acids shown in the preceding question?

The important amino acids are: glycine (Gly, G, ***A***), alanine (Ala, A, ***B***), leucine (Leu, , ***C***), isoleucine (Ile, I, ***D6***), valine (Val, V, ***E***), phenylalanine (Phe, F, ***F***), serine (Ser, S, ***G***), cysteine (Cys, C, ***H***), methionine (Met, M, ***I***), threonine (Thr, T, ***J***), asparagine (Asn, N, ***K***), glutamine (Gln, Q, ***L***), proline (Pro, P, ***M***), tyrosine (Tyr, Y, ***N***), tryptophan (Trp, W, ***O***), aspartic acid (Asp, D, ***P***), glutamic acid (Glu, E, ***Q***), arginine (Arg, R, ***R***), histidine (His, H, ***S***), and lysine (Lys,, K ***T***). Note that the indole nitrogen in tryptophan is not very basic.

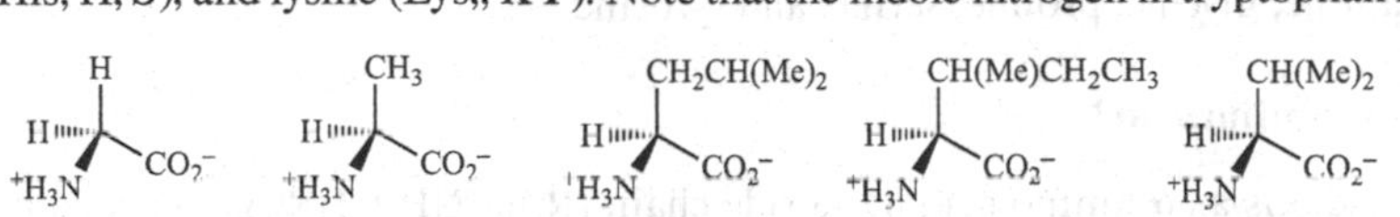

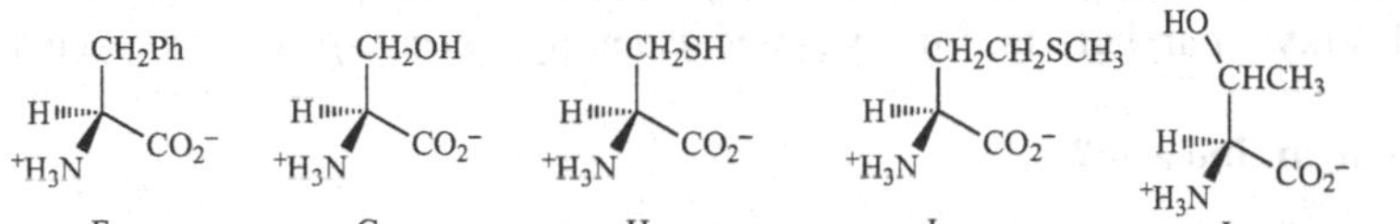

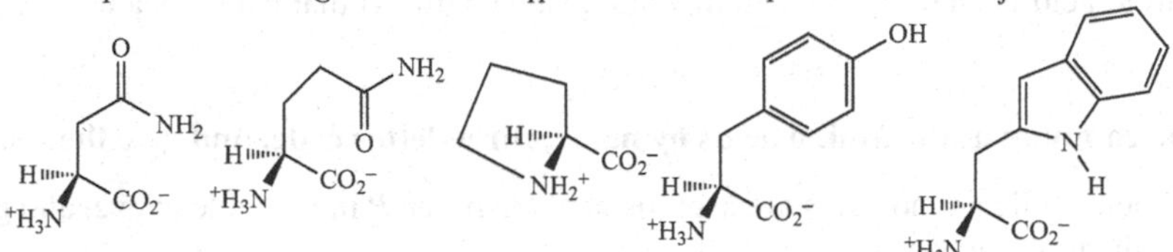

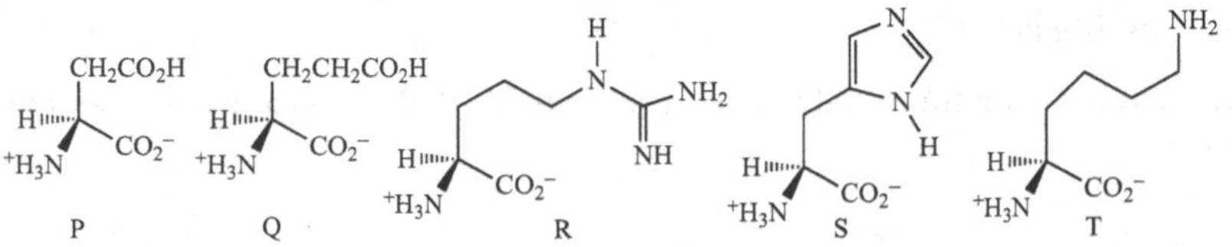

How is D-(+)-glyceraldehyde structurally related to D-alanine?

Analysis of the Fischer projections shows that the CHO of glyceraldehyde correlates with CO_2H of alanine and the NH_3 of alanine correlates with the OH of glyceraldehyde.

What is the Fischer projection of L-phenylalanine? Of D-leucine? Of L-serine? Of D-cysteine?

L-phenylalanine: CO_2H (top), NH_2 (left), H (right), CH_2Ph (bottom)

D-leucine: CO_2H (top), H (left), NH_2 (right), CH_2CHMe_2 (bottom)

L-serine: CO_2H (top), NH_2 (left), H (right), CH_2OH (bottom)

D-cysteine: CO_2H (top), H (left), NH_2 (right), CH_2SH (bottom)

What is the IUPAC nomenclature for glycine, alanine, phenylalanine, leucine, serine, aspartic acid, glutamic acid, and lysine.

The IUPAC name for glycine is 2-aminoethanoic acid. Alanine is 2-aminopropanoic acid. Phenylalanine is 2-amino-3-phenylpropanoic acid. Leucine is 2-amino-4-methylpentanoic acid. Serine is 2-amino-3-hydroxypropanoic acid. Aspartic acid is 2-amino-1,4-butanedioic acid. Glutamic acid is 2-amino-1,5-pentanedioic acid and lysine is 2,5-diaminohexanoic acid.

What are essential amino acids?

The essential amino acids must be taken in by food since they cannot be made by the human body. The nine essential amino acids are: histidine, isoleucine, leucine, lysine, methionine, phenylalanine, threonine, tryptophan, and valine.

What are non-essential amino acids?

The non-essential amino acids can be made by the human body and so are not essential to the human diet. There are 11 nonessential amino acids: alanine, arginine, asparagine, aspartic acid, cysteine, glutamic acid, glutamine, glycine, proline, serine, and tyrosine

What is a neutral amino acid?

A neutral amino acid is an α-amino acid has a side chain (R in $^+NH_3CHRCO_2^-$) and at neutral pH it is neither acidic nor basic (no amine or carboxylic acid substituents are present). In general, neutral amino acids are simple alkyl or aryl groups (methyl, ethyl, isopropyl, phenyl, *p*-methoxyphenyl, etc.).

What is an acidic amino acid?

An acidic amino acid is an α-amino acid that has a side chain (*R*) that contains a carboxylic acid unit, COOH.

What are the common acidic amino acids by name, three-letter code, and give their structure?

The two common acidic amino acids are aspartic acid (Asp, see ***P*** in the table above) and glutamic acid (Glu, see ***Q*** in the table above).

What is a basic amino acid?

A basic amino acid is an α-amino acid that has a side chain (*R*) that contains a free amino group ($-NH_2$ or NHR).

What are the common basic amino acids by name, 3-letter code, and give their structure?

The most common basic amino acids are arginine (Arg, see ***R*** in the table above), histidine (His, see ***S*** in the table above), and lysine (Lys, see ***T*** in the table above).

There are two pK_a values for neutral amino acids. What are the reactions in each acid–base process?

Glycine is used to illustrate these reactions. In acidic solution, the NH_2 group is converted to the ammonium salt and the carboxylate is protonated as the acid to give the ammonium acid (***A***). Neutralization with base removes the most acidic hydrogen (from the carboxyl) to generate the zwitterion, ***B***. Further reaction with base removes the proton from the ammonium ion, which is also acidic. This reaction liberates the free amine, amino carboxylate salt, ***C***. These reactions with acid or with base are general.

CO_2H / NH_3^+ **A** $\underset{H^+}{\overset{\text{base}}{\rightleftharpoons}}$ CO_2^- / NH_3^+ **B** $\underset{H^+}{\overset{\text{base}}{\rightleftharpoons}}$ CO_2^- / NH_2 **C**

Why is the first pK_a of glycine 2.34 and the second 9.6?

In general, the carboxyl proton is the more acidic and will be removed first. The presence of an amino group of the α-carbon allows internal hydrogen bonding which makes the carboxyl proton more acidic than acetic acid), with a relatively low pK_a of 2.34. Removal of the proton from the zwitterion is analogous to the acidity of most other ammonium salts, which have pK_a values around 9–10. The observed 9.6 pK_a is, therefore, typical.

Why is the pK_a of the carboxyl group of glycine lower than the pK_a of acetic acid?

The nitrogen on the α-carbon can hydrogen bond with the acidic proton (through-space inductive effect; Section 3.4), weakening the O—H bond, so glycine is a stronger acid.

In aspartic acid, the pK_a of the carboxyl of the α-amino acid is 2.09 and the pK_a of the "side chain" carboxyl is 3.86. Why is the side chain carboxyl less acidic?

The electron-withdrawing nitrogen group is close to the COOH of the "α-amino acid unit" and the inductive effect is rather large (see the preceding question). This nitrogen is much further away from the COOH on the side chain and the effects are minimal to the acidity, which is typical of most other aliphatic carboxylic acids.

What is the isoelectric point for an amino acid?

The isoelectric point is the pH at which the amino acid is completely neutral (no longer exhibits a charge). The structure at the isoelectric point is the zwitterion form (such as $^+NH_3CHRCO_2^-$). The point in the equilibrium when this neutral species is formed is the *isoelectric point, pI*, which is defined as the pH at which the material carries no net electrical charge. If p*I* is used to represent the isoelectric point, then p*I* is defined by the following equation:

$$pI = \frac{pK_{a_1} + pK_{a_2}}{2}$$

How is p*I* determined?

A pH curve for an amino acid is shown in the figure in which the isoelectric point and both K_{a_2} and K_{a_2} are marked. The value of K_{a_1} and the value of K_{a_2} varies with the substituents attached to the amino acid. The point of this figure is to show that K_{a_1} and K_{a_2} can be experimentally determined for any amino acid, and the isoelectric point can then be determined. A practical answer is that $pI = (pK_1 + pK_2)/2$.

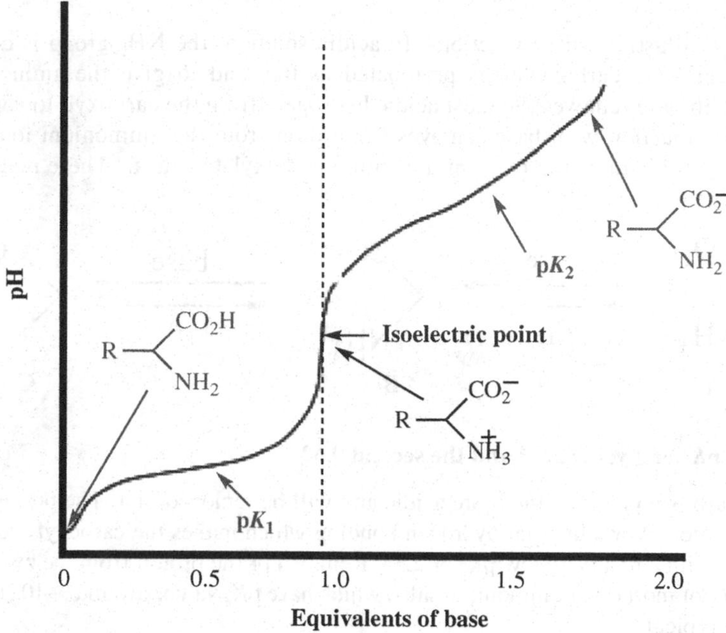

How can the isoelectric point be related to the acid/base equilibrium species present in glycine?

At the isoelectric point, the zwitterion of an amino acid represents the major species in solution.

How does the presence of an acidic side chain influence the isoelectric point of an amino acid?

The presence of the second carboxyl group will lower the pH of the isoelectric point (to pH 3.2–3.5, typically).

How does the presence of a basic side chain influence the isoelectric point of an amino acid?

The presence of the basic amino groups will raise the pH of the isoelectric point (to pH 7.6–10.8 in most cases).

What is the equilibrium for glutamic acid, which has an acidic side chain?

The presence of a third acidic proton on the acidic side chain leads to a more complex equilibrium. The initial reaction with base generates the zwitterion ***A***. Further reaction with base deprotonates the next more acidic proton on the COOH side chain to give ***B***. Finally, the least acidic proton on the ammonium salt is removed to give ***C***.

Glutamic acid $\overset{K_1}{\rightleftharpoons}$ **A** $\overset{K_3}{\rightleftharpoons}$ **B** $\overset{K_2}{\rightleftharpoons}$ **C**

What is the equilibrium for lysine, which has a basic side chain?

With the basic side chain there is a possibility of a third acidic site since the amino group can be converted to an ammonium ion. Treatment of lysine with base generates the zwitterion, ***A***. The zwitterion can be converted to the ammonium salt ***B*** and reaction with base generates the carboxylate anion, ***C***.

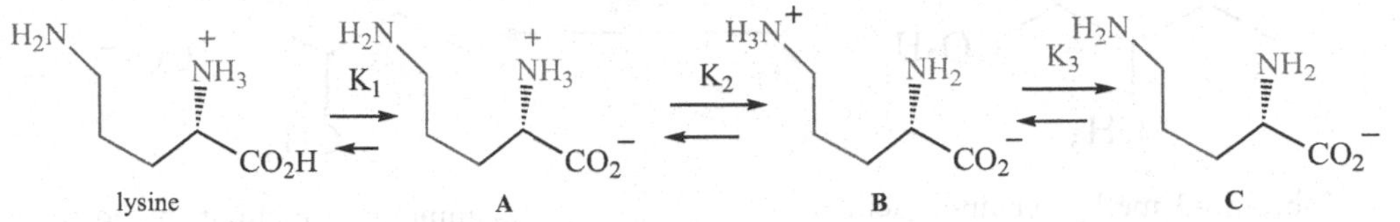

lysine A B C

What is allothreonine? What is alloisoleucine?

The term *allo* is used to denote the diastereomer of the amino acid. Two of the amino acids have a second chiral center in the side chain, threonine and isoleucine, and in Fischer projection show that L-threonine is (2*S*,3*R*) and L-isoleucine is (2*S*,3*S*). The diastereomer of L-threonine is called allothreonine with (2*S*,3*S*) stereocenters. The diastereomer of L-isoleucine is alloisoleucine with the (2*S*,3*S*) stereocenters.

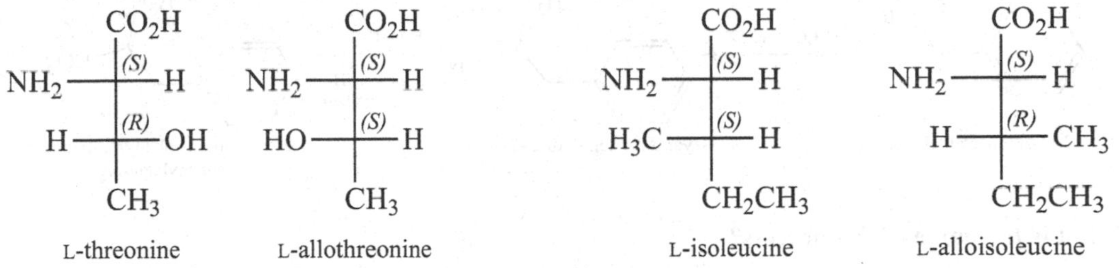

L-threonine L-allothreonine L-isoleucine L-alloisoleucine

Is there any correlation between the *d,l* designator and the D,L designators?

No! The (*d,l*) nomenclature refers to specific rotation (+,–) whereas the (D,L) refers to the name of the absolute configuration (analogous to *R,S*).

Is there any correlation between the D,L designator and the *R,S* designators?

Both refer to absolute configuration but (*R,S*) is based on the Cahn–Ingold–Prelog selection rules and (D,L) is based on a comparison with glyceraldehyde.

20.2 SYNTHESIS OF AMINO ACIDS

What is the product when 2-bromoethanoic acid is heated with an excess of ammonia?

The product is glycine

What is the product when 2-bromo-3-methylpentanoic acid is heated with excess ammonia?

The product is isoleucine

Does the reaction if an α-bromocarboxylic acid and ammonia produce a single enantiomer or a racemic mixture? A single diastereomer or a mixture? Explain!

If the starting bromide (2-bromo-3-methylpentanoic acid) is racemic, the final product 2-ammonio-3-methylpentanoate will also be racemic, so it will be a mixture of isoleucine and alloisoleucine. There may be some enantioselectivity if the bromide is chiral since displacement will be via a S_N2 reaction. There is no stereocontrol in this reaction; a mixture of diastereomers in 2-bromo-3-methylpentanoic acid (note the squiggle line) will result in a diastereomeric mixture of isoleucine and alloisoleucine (2-ammonio-3-methylpentanoate).

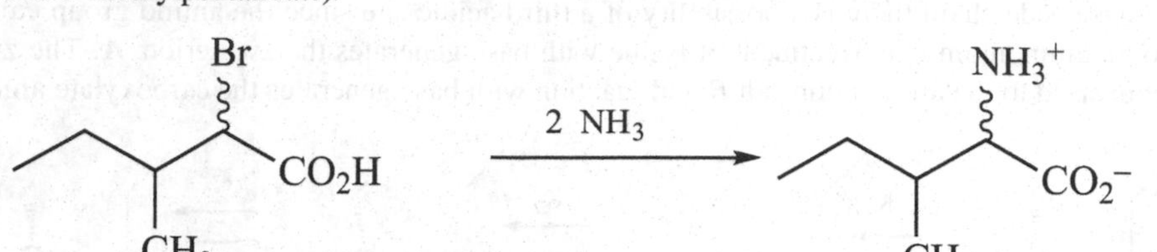

2-bromo-3-methylpentanoic acid $\xrightarrow{2\ NH_3}$ 2-ammonio-3-methylpentanoate

What is the product when phenylacetaldehyde is reacted with sodium cyanide and ammonium chloride?

The initial product of the reaction with phenylacetaldehyde is the aminonitrile, 1-cyano-2-phenylethan-1-aminium. Saponification of the nitrile leads to the amino acid, phenylalanine.

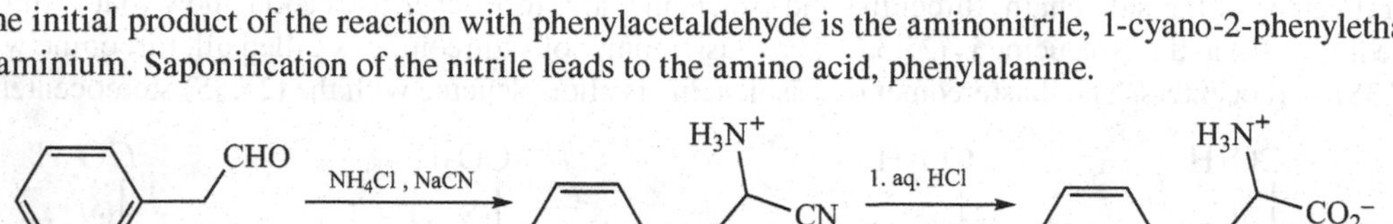

2-phenylacetaldehyde $\xrightarrow{NH_4Cl,\ NaCN}$ 1-cyano-2-phenylethan-1-aminium $\xrightarrow{1.\ aq.\ HCl;\ 2.\ aq.\ NaOH\ (neutralize)}$ 2-ammonio-3-phenylpropanoate (phenylalanine)

What is the name of this process?

This reaction sequence is called the *Strecker synthesis.*

What is the major product for the reactions of (a), (b), and (c)?

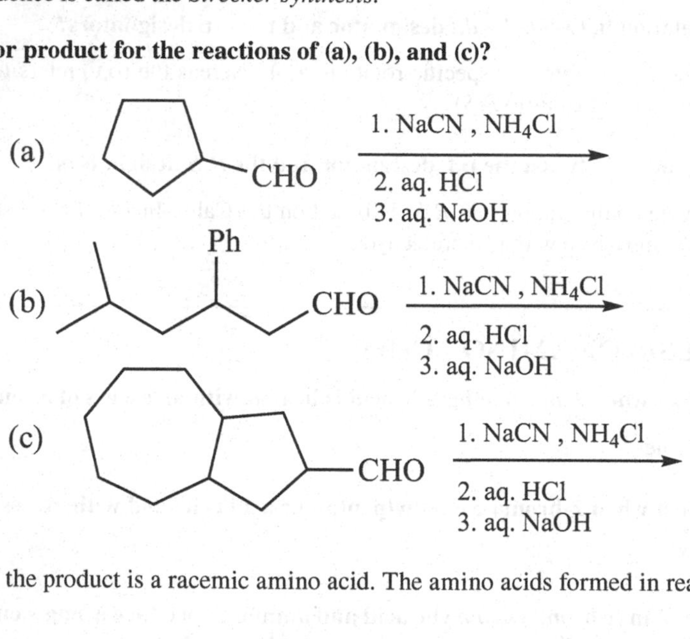

(a) cyclopentyl–CHO: 1. NaCN, NH_4Cl; 2. aq. HCl; 3. aq. NaOH

(b) aldehyde bearing Ph: 1. NaCN, NH_4Cl; 2. aq. HCl; 3. aq. NaOH

(c) bicyclic–CHO: 1. NaCN, NH_4Cl; 2. aq. HCl; 3. aq. NaOH

In all three cases, the product is a racemic amino acid. The amino acids formed in reaction (a), (b), and (c) are shown.

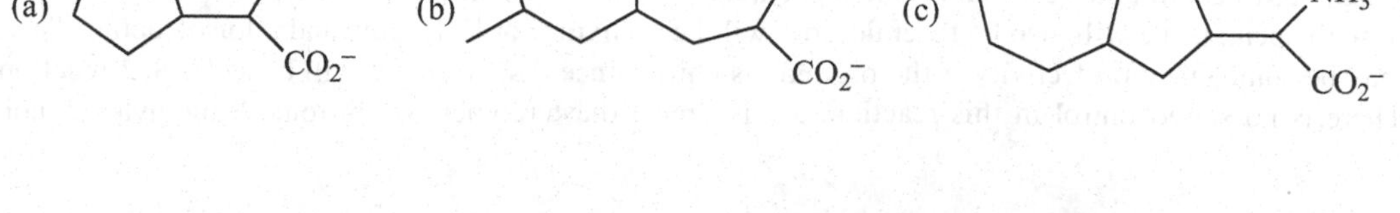

(a) NH_3^+, CO_2^- (b) Ph, NH_3^+, CO_2^- (c) NH_3^+, CO_2^-

What is the product when the sodium salt of phthalimide is reacted with diethyl 2-bromomalonate?

The nucleophilic phthalimide anion (*A*) displaces the bromide of diethyl 2-bromomalonate via a S_N2 reaction to give to give ***B***.

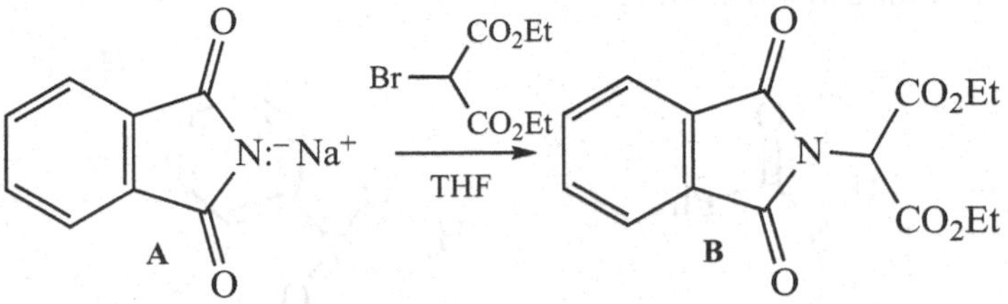

If *B* in the preceding question is reacted with Na/EtOH, what is the resulting product? If iodomethane is added in a subsequent step, what is the product? What is the final product after decarboxylation?

Treatment of ***A*** with diethyl 2-bromomalonate gives ***B***. The reaction of ***B*** with base deprotonates the acidic α-proton to form the enolate anion (***C***) and subsequent reaction with iodomethane gives the alkylated product, ***D***. Saponification of ***D*** (Section 15.5) generates the racemic amino acid, alanine.

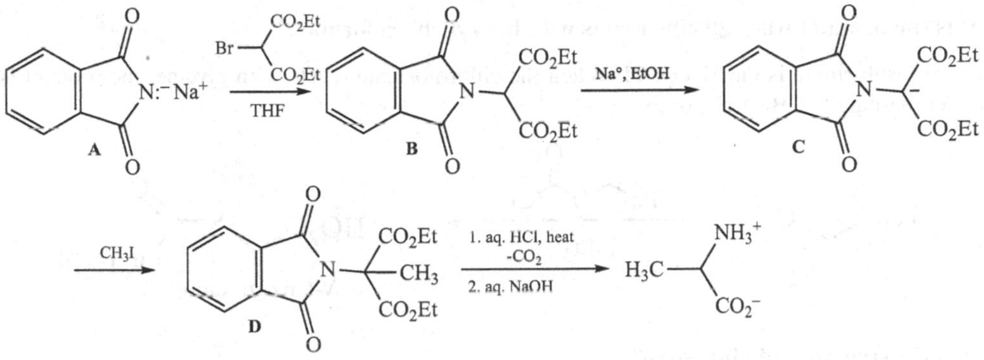

What is the name of this overall process?

The name of this synthetic sequence is the *Gabriel synthesis*.

20.3 REACTIONS OF AMINO ACIDS

What product is formed when alanine is treated with methanol and HCl?

Under these conditions, the amino acid is converted to the ammonium acid NH_3^+-CH(R)-COOH and in the presence of methanol, the methyl ester is formed. In this case the product is the methyl ester of alanine [H_3N^+-CH(Me)CO_2Me].

What is the product when isoleucine is treated with acetic anhydride?

Under these conditions, isoleucine is converted to the acetamide derivative, *N*-acetylisoleucine.

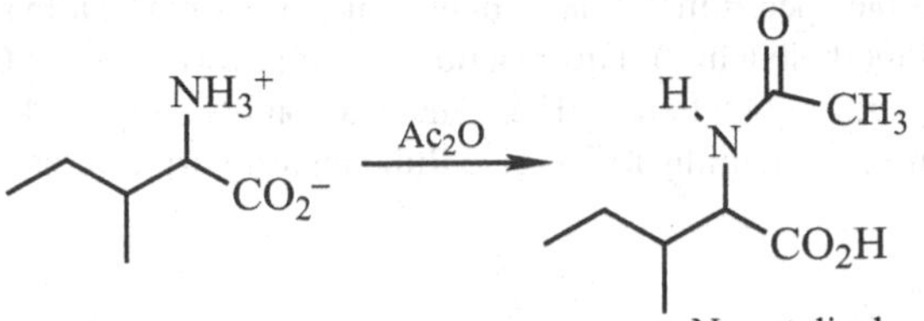

N-acetylisoleucine

What is the product when alanine treated with benzoyl chloride in the presence of an amine? With tosyl chloride in the presence of an amine?

In the first reaction, the benzamide derivative (*N*-benzoylalanine) is formed and in the second, the *N*-tosyl derivative is formed (*N*-tosylalanine).

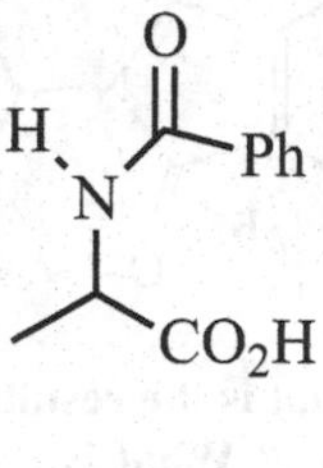

N-benzoylalanine 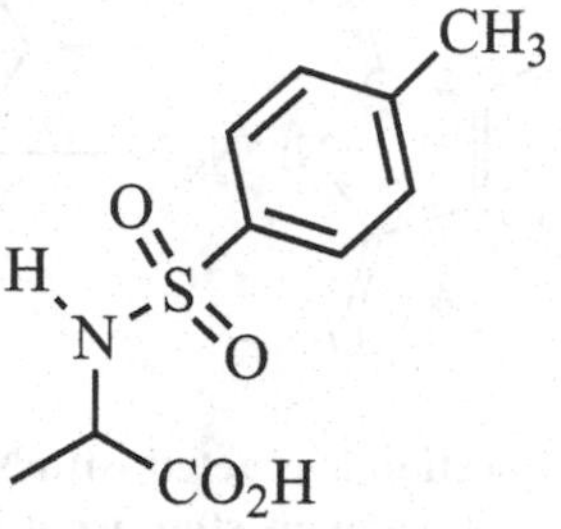 N-tosylalanine

What is a carbamate?

A carbamate has the basic functional group O–(C=O)–N = (O_2C—N).

What is the product when glycine reacts with benzyl chloroformate?

Benzyl chloroformate is $PhCH_2O_2CCl$. When the chloroformate reacts with glycine, the product is the benzyl carbamate (a CBz derivative).

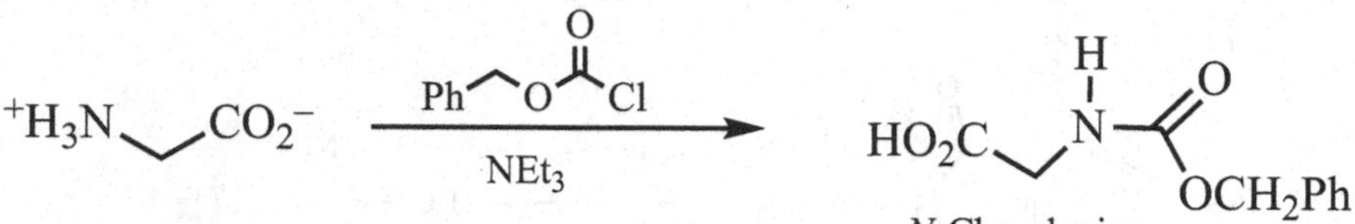

$$^{+}H_3NCH_2CO_2^{-} \xrightarrow[NEt_3]{PhCH_2OC(=O)Cl} HO_2CCH_2NHC(=O)OCH_2Ph$$

N-Cbz-glycine

What is the structure of ninhydrin?

The structure of ninhydrin is shown: the chemical name is 2,2-dihydroxy-1*H*-indene-1,3(2*H*)-dione.

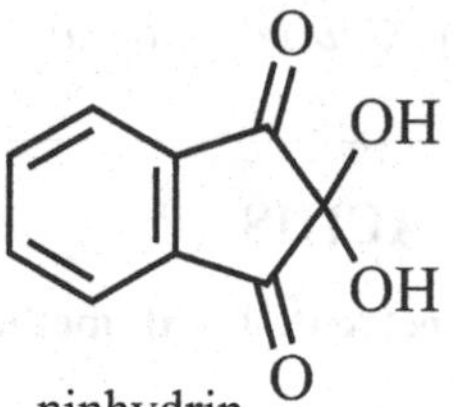

ninhydrin

What is the initial product when ninhydrin reacts with leucine?

In the initial reaction, ninhydrin reacts with the amine portion of the amino acid to produce an imine, ***A***. This initially formed imine decarboxylates under the reaction conditions to form a new imine, ***B***, that reacts with more ninhydrin to form the product imine (***C***), which is known as *Ruhemann's Purple* and it absorbs strongly at 570 nm in the visible spectrum – it has a bluish-purple color. The alkyl side chain of the amino acid is lost as an aldehyde (3-methylbutanal). This reaction with ninhydrin to form ***C*** is diagnostic for amino acids that contain a primary amino function (-NH_2). This reaction does *not* work with secondary amines. Proline, therefore, does not react with ninhydrin to give Ruhemann's Purple, although there is a reaction.

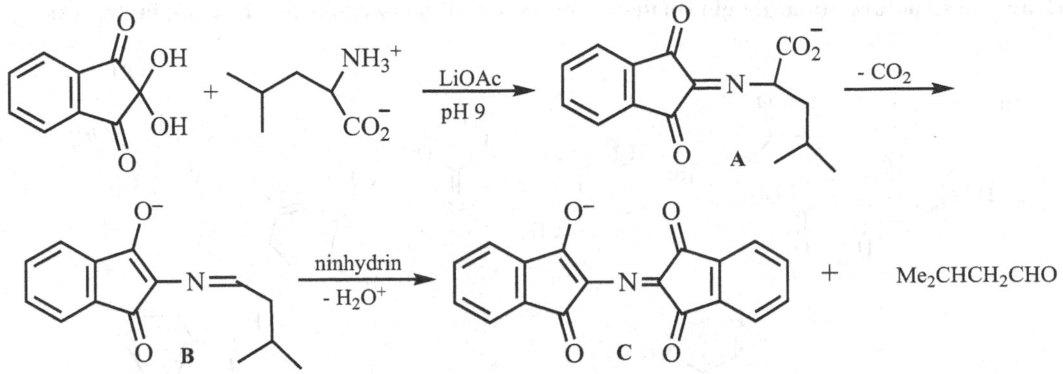

What is the final product of the reaction between ninhydrin and leucine? Of any amino acid?

The final product from the reaction of ninhydrin in an amino acid is Ruhemann's Purple (*C* from the preceding question) and an aldehyde, *if* the amino acid contained a primary amino functionality.

What is a peptide?

A peptide is a biologically important molecule composed of several amino acids, linked together by amide bonds (called peptide bonds). An example is the tetrapeptide ala-ser-val-met. A polypeptide can be composed of hundreds of amino acid residues.

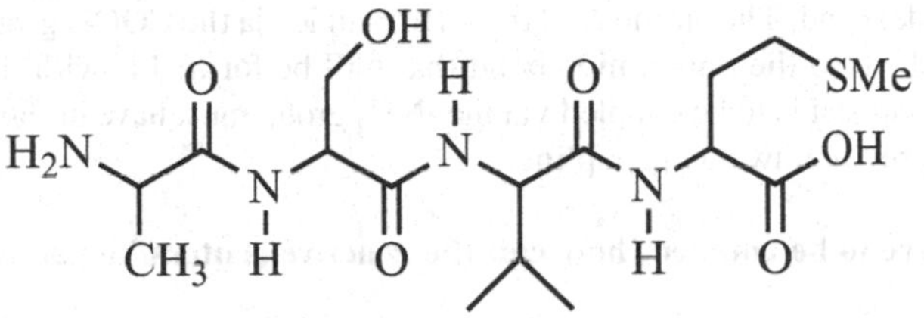

ala-ser-val-met

What is a dipeptide? A pentapeptide?

A dipeptide is a molecule composed of two amino acid residues. A pentapeptide is a molecule composed of five amino acid residues.

What is a residue?

Residue is the term used for each amino acid unit in a peptide.

What is the C-terminus?

The C-terminus of a peptide is the portion of the peptide that terminates in COOH (the methionine residue in ala-ser-val-met in the preceding question).

What is the N-terminus?

The N-terminus of a peptide is the portion of the peptide that terminates in $-NH_2$ (the alanine residue in ala-ser-val-met in the preceding question).

Draw the structure of: (a) gly-glu (b) ile-ala (c) tyr-ser (d) met-arg-gly (e) pro-pro-phe-trp-val

Why is it necessary to protect the amino group of an amino acid or peptide if coupling is to occur at the C–terminus?

When a peptide is formed, the amino group of one amino acid reacts with the carboxyl of a second to form the amide (peptide) bond. The amino acid that is to couple via the COOH group *must* have its amino group protected (blocked) so the only amide bond that will be formed is with the second amino acid. Similarly, the amino acid that is to be coupled via the -NH_2 group must have its carboxyl group protected (blocked) in order to prevent unwanted coupling.

If two amino acids are to be coupled, how can the reactive centers be protected? Use general terms in the answer!

The amine group of one amino acid is protected (usually as an amide or a carbamate) and the carboxyl group of the second amino acid is blocked (usually as an ester). The free carboxyl group on one amino acid is then coupled to the free amino group of the second amino acid to give the amide bond. There are several methods for doing this coupling. In one, the COOH is converted to an acid chloride and then coupled with the amine. Alternatively, the carbonyl can be "activated" (by DCC for example), allowing reaction with the amino group.

What are suitable N-protecting groups?

The most common amine protecting groups for this purpose are amide (NHAc, NHCOPh, etc.) and carbamates [$NHCO_2CH_2Ph$ (called Cbz) and $NHCO_2CMe_3$ (called *t*-BOC or just BOC)].

What are suitable C-protecting groups?

The acid group is usually protected as a methyl or ethyl ester.

What is DCC?

DCC is dicyclohexylcarbodiimide (see Section 15.4): c-C_6H_{11}-N=C=N-c-C_6H_{11}.

How can the formation of a dipeptide between glycine and serine using DCC as the coupling agent be described?

The amino group of glycine is protected as the benzyl carbamate and the carboxyl group of serine is protected as the ethyl ester. The acid moiety of CBZ-glycine reacts with DCC to form *A* and the carbonyl of this intermediate is attacked by the amino group of the serine ethyl ester. This reaction displaces dicyclohexylurea and produces the protected dipeptide, ***B***. Saponification removes the ester group and reaction with hydrogen (Pd catalyst) removes the CBz group to give the dipeptide, gly-ser.

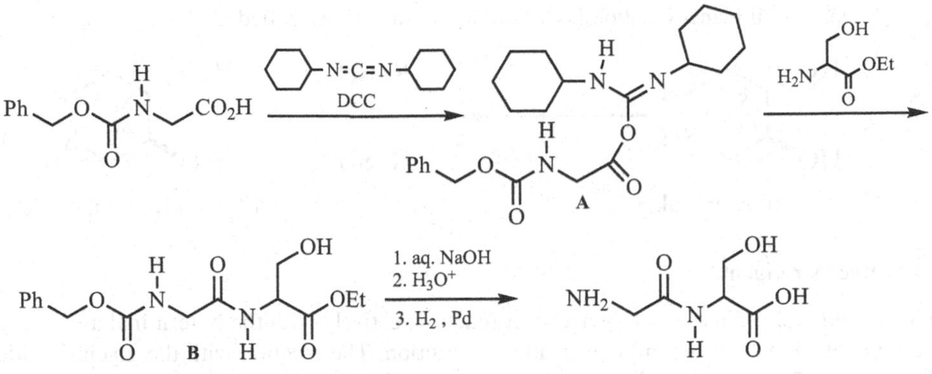

How are C-terminus ester protecting groups removed?

If the C-terminus (the COOH) is protected as an ester, saponification (1. aq. $^{-}$OH 2. aq. H^+) will convert the ester to the carboxylic acid.

How are N-terminus protecting groups removed?

If an amide group is used (acetamide, benzamide), basic hydrolysis followed by neutralization with acid usually removes the group. If the benzylic carbamate is used (CBz), catalytic hydrogenation with a palladium catalyst removes the protecting group.

20.4 PROTEINS

What is a protein?

A protein is a long chain biopolymer composed of amino acids joined together by amide bonds (usually called *peptide bonds*). There are two basic types of proteins: *simple proteins* that yield only amino acids and no other organic compounds upon hydrolysis and *conjugated proteins* that give other compounds along with amino acids upon hydrolysis.

What is a peptide bond?

A peptide bond is an amide bond that connects amino acid residues in a peptide or in a protein.

What is an enzyme?

Enzymes are proteins that are the biological catalysts required to initiate chemical reactions in biological systems.

What is the primary structure of a protein or peptide?

The primary structure of a peptide is the sequence of amino acids that comprise its fundamental structure.

What is the primary structure of ala-phe-ile-trp?

The amino acid sequence ala-phe-ile-trp *is* the primary structure.

What are disulfide bonds?

When two cysteine residues, each of which have a $-CH_2SH$ unit, are incorporated in a peptide or protein, conformational changes in the structure can bring two SH units together and they can react to form a disulfide bond (R–S—S–R).

What does dithiothreitol do when reacted with a disulfide bond?

Dithiothreitol reacts with a disulfide to "liberate" two thiol moieties and this reaction generates the cyclic disulfide, (4*S*,5*S*)-1,2-dithiane-4,5-diol. Dithiothreitol is sometimes called *Cleland's reagent.*

R–S–S–R + dithiothreitol → R–SH + R–SH + (4S,5S)-1,2-dithiane-4,5-diol

What is Sanger's reagent?

Sanger's reagent is 2,4-dinitrofluorobenzene. It reacts selectively with the N-terminal amino acid residue of a peptide (***A***) via nucleophilic aromatic substitution. The reaction with the glycine residue of a peptide generates ***B***. Aqueous acid hydrolysis with 6N HCl will "release" all amino acids, but only the N-terminal amino acid will be attached to the Sanger's reagent, forming ***C*** (2,4-dinitrophenyl)glycine. This N-aryl amino acid usually forms a derivative with a yellow color that is easily identified.

Sanger's reagent → (H_2N–CH_2–CO–NH-peptide-COOH, **A**) → **B**; aq. H_3O^+ → **C** + other amino acids

What is the structure of dansyl chloride?

Dansyl chloride is 5-dimethylamino-1-naphthalenesulfonyl chloride. The N-terminal amino acid of a peptide (***A***) will displace the fluorine to form an N-aryl derivative, sulfonamide ***B***. Hydrolysis leads to cleavage of the N-terminal amino acid residue from the peptide as a dansyl amino acid (***C***), (5-(dimethylamino)naphthalen-1-yl)sulfonyl)glycine. This compound is fluorescent and easily detected in the presence of the other amino acids liberated in the hydrolysis step.

dansyl chloride → (H_2N–CH_2–CO–NH-peptide-COOH, **A**) → **B**; 1. aq. HCl, heat 2. aq. NaOH → **C**

What is the Edmund degradation?

The *Edmund degradation* is the process for derivatizing and cleaving the N-terminal amino acid of a peptide by first treating the peptide with phenyl isothiocyanate (Ph–N=C=S) and then subjecting the peptide to acid hydrolysis. The N-terminal amino acid is converted to a *N*-phenyl-thiohydantoin by this procedure, cleaving only the terminal amino acid from the peptide and allowing easy identification of that amino acid.

What is the phenylthiocarbamoyl derivative resulting from the reaction of ala-phe and phenyl isothiocyanate?

The initial product of the reaction between dipeptide ala-phe and *N*-phenylisothiocyanate is an *N*-phenylthiourea derivative, ***A***, (phenylcarbamothioyl)phenylalanylalanine.

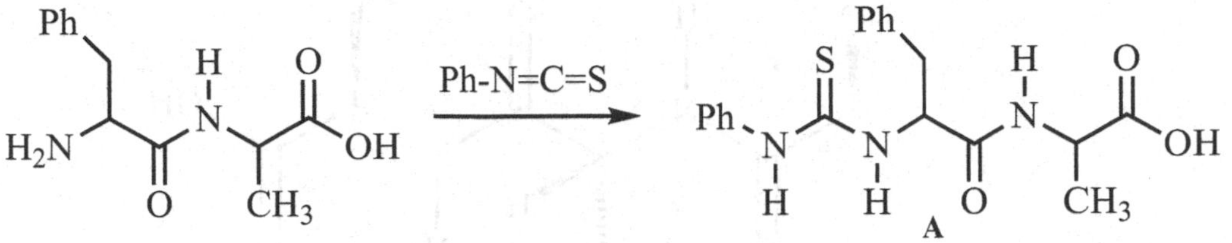

What is the final product of an Edman degradation of isoleucine?

An Edman degradation is the reaction of the C-terminus of a peptide with phenylisothiocyanate to give a phenylthiocarbamoyl derivative. Subsequent reaction with trifluoroacetic acid generates thiohydantoin. A *thiohydantoin* is actually a *thiazolone.* If isoleucine were the N-terminal amino acid, Ph-N=C=S would convert it into ***A*** and reaction with trifluoracetic acid would give hydantoin ***B*** (5*R*-*sec*-butyl)-3-phenyl-2-thioxoimidazolidin-4-one.

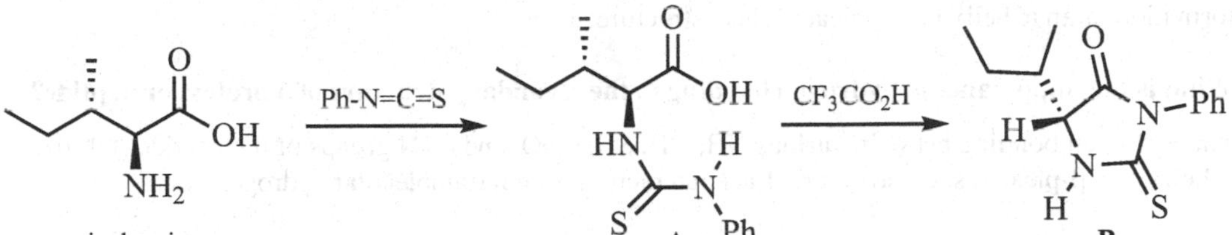

isoleucine

What is the structure of ala-phe, showing the relative positions of the carbonyl groups, amino groups, and side chains?

The fundamental structure of a protein involves amide bonds where the alkyl side chain of one amino acid residue is effectively "anti-" to the alkyl side chain of the adjacent amino acid residue, as shown. The amide carbonyls are also anti- in this low energy conformation of the peptide. This alternating pattern appears throughout most proteins or peptides.

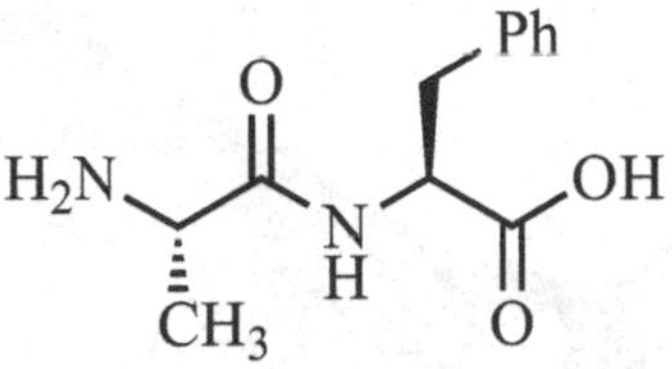

Why is there an anti- relationship of the R groups of adjacent amino acid residues in a peptide?

The amide unit is essentially planar since it exists as two resonance structures, one with the carbonyl unit and the other with an alkoxy-iminium salt unit. These resonance contributors lead to the C—N unit having "partial double-bond character." Rotation around the C—N bond in part depends on the amount of sp^2-hybridization leads to a geometry for the amide unit, so it is rather planar. The alkyl groups in each amino acid residue have a great influence on the magnitude of angles ψ and ϕ, and these angles of rotation define the conformation for that portion of the peptide. The groups attached to the carbonyl and the nitrogen may have different stereochemical relationships, and the relationship will vary with the nature of the R groups. As shown in the figure, the amide unit of one amino acid residue is anti- to the amide unit of the adjacent amino acid residue. And the carbonyl of one residue is anti- to the carbonyl of the adjacent residue. As a consequence, a peptide chain assumes an alternating or anti- pattern.

Rotational angle ψ, C—C=O

Rotational angle ϕ, C—NH

ala-val-ser

What is the secondary structure of a protein or peptide?

The secondary structure of a protein or peptide is the amount of structural regularity that results from intramolecular or intermolecular hydrogen bonding. The most common secondary structure features are formation of an α-helix or a β-pleated sheet structure.

What is the importance of hydrogen bonding in the secondary structure of a protein or peptide?

The hydrogen bonding between various NH, OH, SH, C=O, and C=N groups of the peptide stabilize an α-helix or a β-pleated sheet structure. Each interaction is an intramolecular hydrogen bond.

What is an α-helix?

An α-helix is the shape of peptide assumes due to the chirality of the individual L-amino acids, forming a spiral type structure, as shown in the figure for glucagon peptide hormone. The spiral structure is generated by intramolecular hydrogen bonding between NH, OH, C=O, and other heteroatom functional groups.

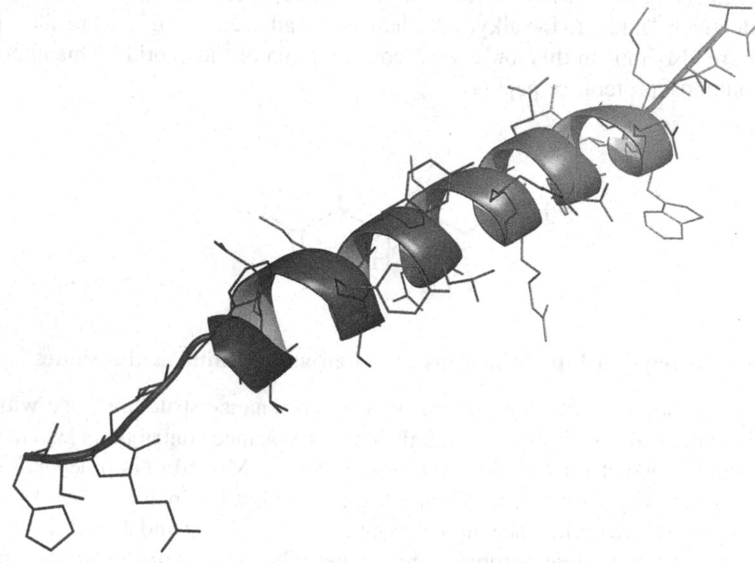

α-Helix of a protein. Glucagon peptide hormone, chemical structure. Glucagon is produced in the pancreas and has the opposite effect of insulin. Shutterstock image 117136321

What is the β-pleated sheet structure of a protein or peptide?

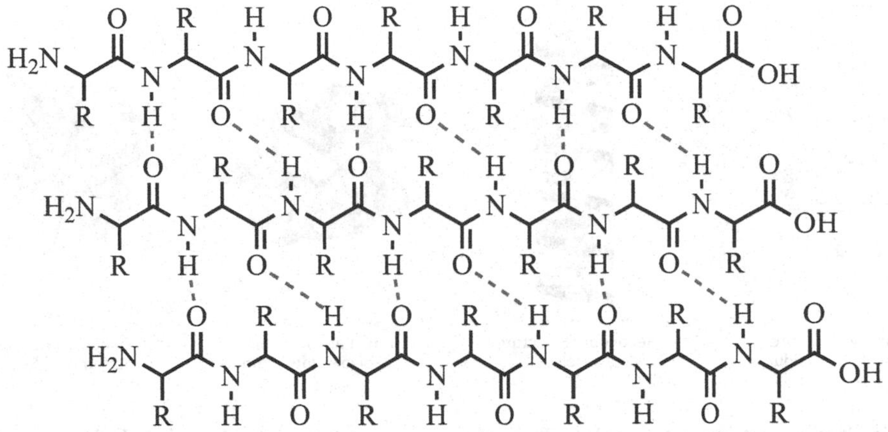

A

Two β-pleated sheet structures are shown. The antiparallel pleated sheet is shown in ***A***. In the pleated sheet the peptide chains align in a parallel manner, with all chain orientation N→C. In the antiparallel structure, ***B***, the chains alternate N→C, C→N, N→C, etc., as shown. In both cases, intermolecular hydrogen bonding allows "stacking" of the peptide chains.

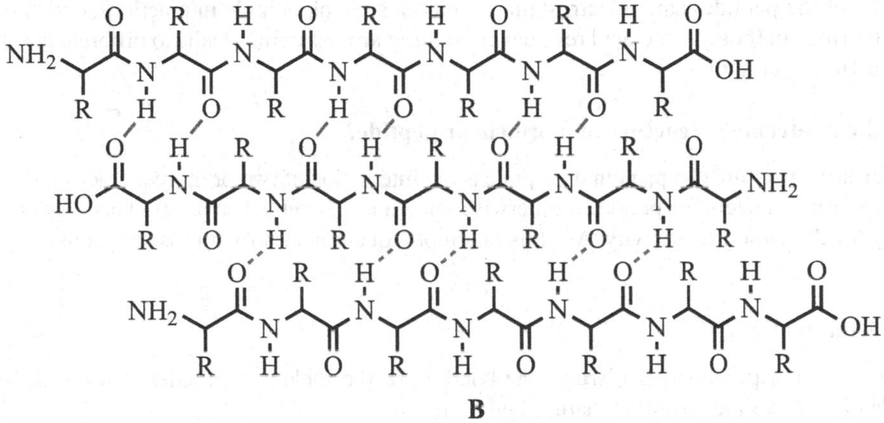

B

What is a random coil?

A random coil is a type of secondary structure that is "random" and does not conform to a distinct structure. The peptide chains arrange in a random manner, held together by hydrogen bonding.

Are most proteins composed of one of the above-mentioned secondary structures or mixtures of several?

Most proteins assume several different secondary structures and a typical protein is composed of various percentages of each of the structural types.

What is the tertiary structure of a protein or peptide?

The tertiary structure of a protein is its three-dimensional structure due to folding and coiling of the peptide chain. The tertiary structure will be the result of both the primary and secondary structure as well as "folding" of the peptide chains, loosely illustrated in the figure. Note that the general primary, secondary, tertiary and quaternary structures associated with a protein are illustrated in this figure.

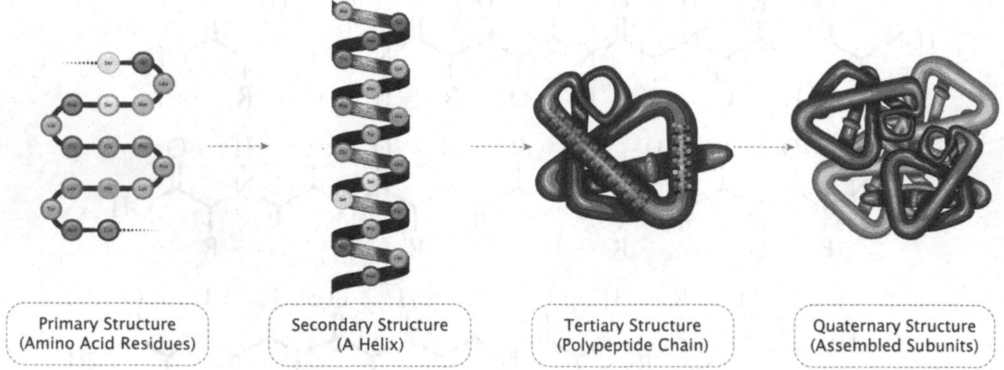

Protein Structure Primary Secondary Tertiary Quaternary Amino Acid residues Helix Polypeptide Chain Assembled Sub units Detailed Chemistry Education Color Full Vector Illustration. Shutterstock image 1474657079.

What physical properties are primarily responsible for the tertiary structure?

A combination of hydrogen bonding, disulfide linkages (R–S—S–R) between cysteine residues in different parts of the peptide chain, electrostatic interactions, dipole–dipole interactions, and "π-stacking" of aromatic rings in those amino acid residues containing aromatic rings leads to different tertiary structures for different proteins.

What is the quaternary structure of a protein or peptide?

The quaternary structure of a protein or peptide is the interaction of two or more peptide chains that join together to form "clusters" of peptides, otherwise known as assembled subunits. This cluster is usually necessary for the biological activity. An illustration of a quaternary structure is shown in the preceding question.

What is denaturation?

Denaturation is the process that disrupts the bonding of the folded or coiled tertiary structure of the protein, leading to a random coil (denatured protein).

What are some common denaturants?

Organic solvents, detergents, and concentrated urea solutions all act as denaturants. Heating a protein can also lead to denaturation.

Is a denatured protein biologically active?

The biological activity of a protein is often a function of its tertiary structure and denaturation usually deactivates the protein.

What are hydrophobic residues?

When two hydrocarbon fragments of different amino acids (such as the interaction of two isopropyl groups of two different valine residues) come in close proximity, the "like dissolves like" rule suggests these residues will interact with each other.

END OF CHAPTER PROBLEMS

1. Give the IUPAC name for each of the following:

(a) 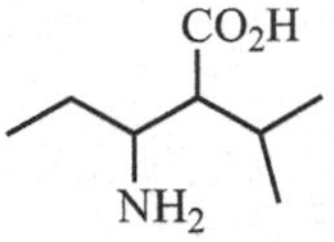 CO_2H NH_2 (b) 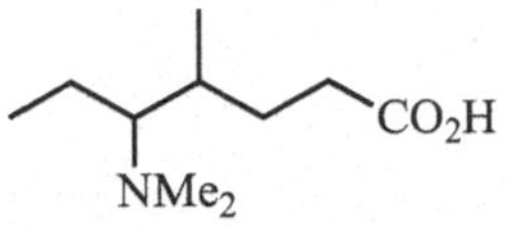 CO_2H NMe_2 (c) 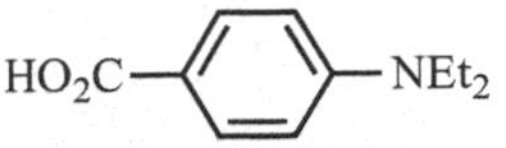 HO_2C–C_6H_4–NEt_2

2. Give the structure for each of the following, in Fischer projection:

(a) glu (b) val (c) ile (d) ser (e) pro (f) ala (g) asp (h) his (i) arg (j) met

3. In each case give the major product. If there is no reaction, indicate by N.R.

(a) 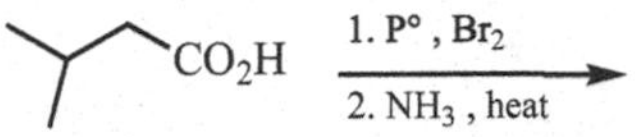 CO_2H — 1. P°, Br_2; 2. NH_3, heat →

(b) 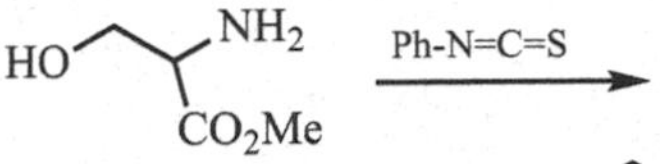 HO, NH_2, CO_2Me — Ph-N=C=S →

(c) OH — 1. PCC, CH_2Cl_2; 2. NaCN, NH_4Cl; 3. aq. HCl; 4. neutralize →

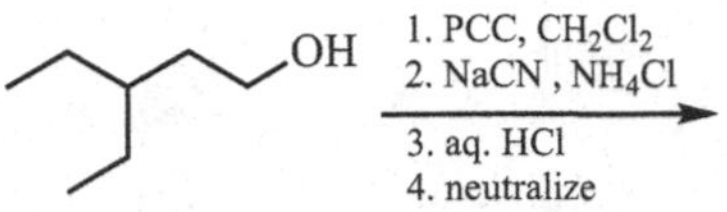

(d) 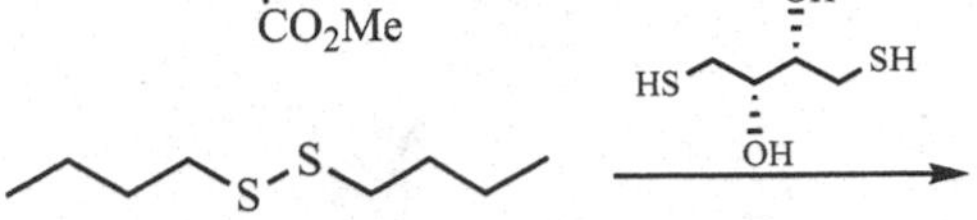 S–S — HS, OH, OH, SH →

(e) 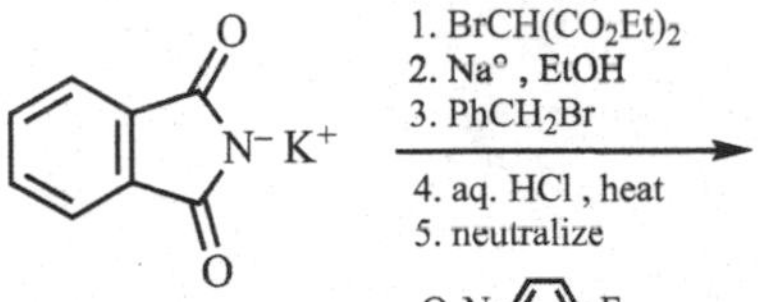 O, N^-K^+, O — 1. $BrCH(CO_2Et)_2$; 2. Na°, EtOH; 3. $PhCH_2Br$; 4. aq. HCl, heat; 5. neutralize →

(f) NH_3^+, CO_2^- — 1. Ac_2O, pyridine; 2. $SOCl_2$;, EtOH →

(g) NH_2, CO_2Et — O_2N–C₆H₃(F)(NO_2) →

(h) NH_2, CO_2Et — O, Cl, O →

(i) EtO_2C, O, Ph, N, O, H — H_2, Pd-C →

(j) NH_2, CO_2Et — NMe_2, SO_2Cl; LiOAc →

(k) H_3C–S, NH_3^+, CO_2^- + O, OH, OH, O →

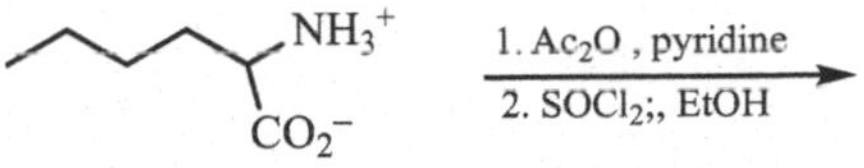

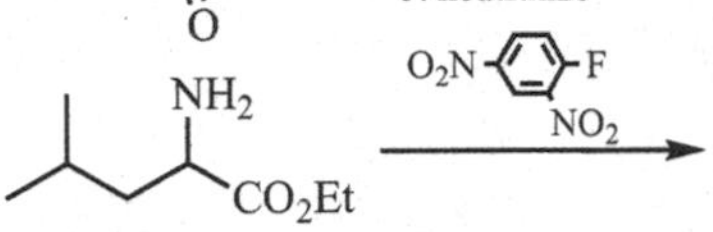

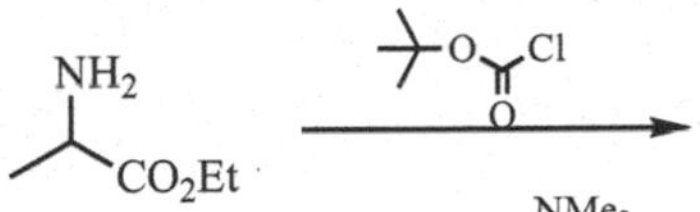

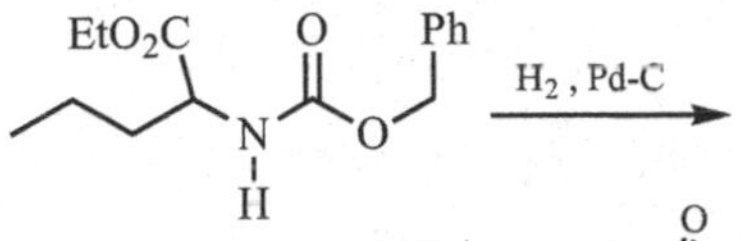

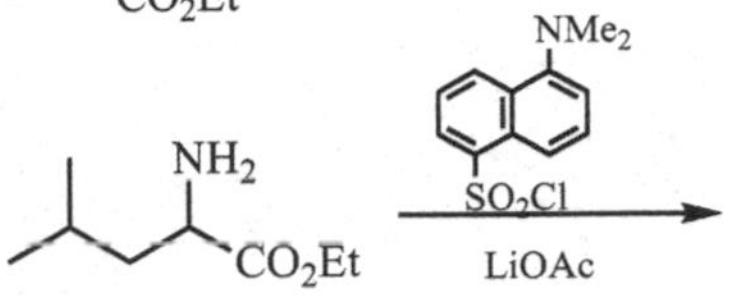

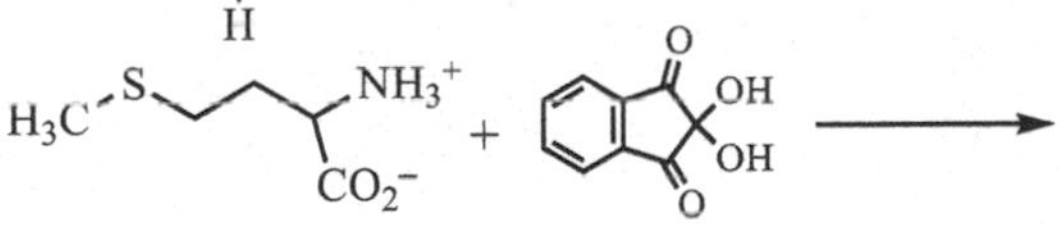

21

Carbohydrates and Nucleic Acids

Another important class of multifunctional molecules are carbohydrates, which have several hydroxyl groups in one molecule. Carbohydrates are very important components of naturally occurring molecules. There are many types of sugars, and one prominent feature is the unique chemistry and properties of these compounds. These properties are the result of the multifunctional nature of the molecules and the interaction of the functional groups with each other and with other chemical reagents. Nucleic acids have sugars as a key structural component. This section is not intended as an in-depth review of biological chemistry or biochemistry but simply as an illustration of the importance of carbohydrates.

21.1 CARBOHYDRATES

What is the definition of a carbohydrate?

A carbohydrate is literally a "hydrate of carbon." They are polyhydroxy aldehydes or ketones.

What is the general formula for a carbohydrate?

The general formula of a carbohydrate is $C_nH_{2n}O_n$, although the carbohydrate may have more or fewer hydrogens and more oxygens.

Why are carbohydrates also called sugars?

Many simple carbohydrates have a sweet taste. Sucrose is common table sugar, glucose is the common sugar used as an energy source in mammalian systems, lactose is milk sugar, and maltose is formed by the breakdown of starch. All of these compounds are carbohydrates and typical examples of this class of compounds. For these reasons, carbohydrates are often referred to as "sugars."

What is a saccharide?

Saccharide is another term for carbohydrates or sugars.

What is a monosaccharide?

Monosaccharides are sugars that *cannot* be hydrolyzed into simpler sugars.

What is the empirical formula for glucose? For fructose?

In both cases the formula is $C_6H_{12}O_6$.

What is the usual reaction of an aldehyde and an alcohol?

In general, aldehydes react with alcohols to form acetals [$RCH(OR')_2$] but the reaction proceeds by formation of an unstable hemiacetal [RCH(OH)OR′]. See Section 12.2.

What is the structure of a hemiacetal?

A hemiacetal has an OH and an OR on the same carbon [RCH(OH)OR′].

How can an aldohexose form a hemiacetal?

For acyclic aldehydes, a hemiacetal is rather unstable, especially in aqueous media. However, carbohydrates are polyhydroxy aldehydes and the cyclic hemiacetal is more stable than the acyclic aldehyde form. A carbohydrate such as D-glucose forms a hemiacetal by a hydroxy group reacting with the aldehyde carbonyl via acyl addition to form a stable six-membered ring, a so-called pyranose. The hemiacetal unit is marked in the box.

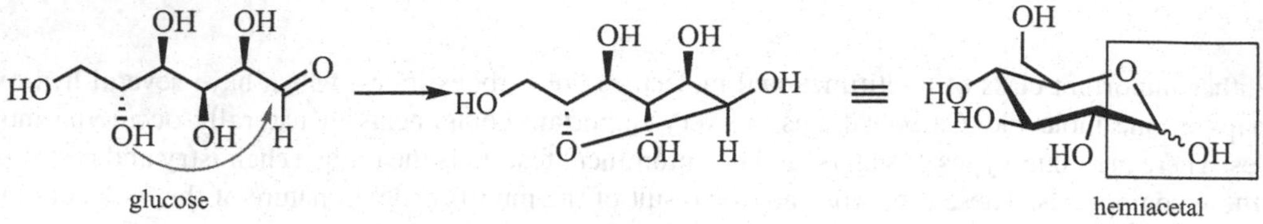

glucose

hemiacetal

What is the anomeric carbon?

The anomeric carbon is the carbon that bears on –OH(C–OH) that is attached to the ring oxygen of the pyranose. The hemiacetal (or hemiketal) carbon is the anomeric carbon.

What is an anomer?

The diastereomeric products of cyclized carbohydrates are referred to as anomers (α-D-glucose pyranose and β-D-glucopyranose are anomers). When the hemiacetal forms, the OH group of that carbon can be either (*R*) or (*S*).

What is a Haworth projection?

A Haworth projection takes the cyclic hemiacetal form of the sugar (glucose) and "flattens" it, making the H and OH groups appear either on the "top" or the "bottom," as in the Haworth projection shown in the figure. This method is a general way in which to present the structure and stereochemistry of sugars.

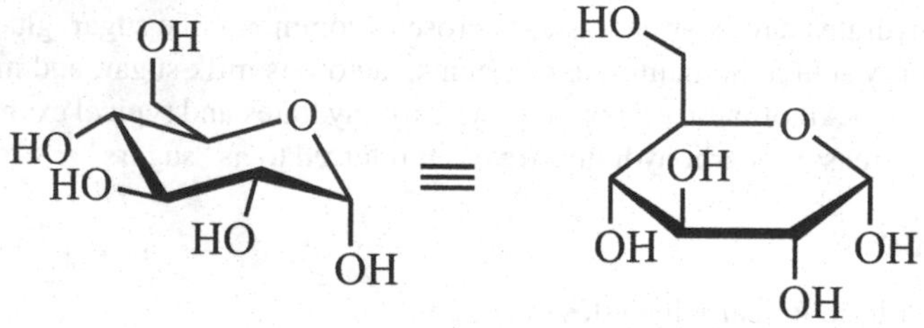

glucose

Haworth formula of glucose

What is a pyranose?

A *pyranose* is a saccharide in a six-membered ring that consists of five carbon atoms and one oxygen atom. Formally, a pyranose is a derivative of tetrahydropyran, a six-membered ring ether.

If the absolute configuration of all alcohol groups is fixed in glucose, why does the cyclic hemiacetal form two different cyclic structures? Draw both in Haworth projection.

When the hemiacetal forms, cyclization can occur from the top and also from the bottom faces of D-glucose, as written in the Haworth projection. Therefore, the OH on the anomeric carbon will be "up" or the OH "down" as the ring is drawn. Note that when D-glucose is draw as the six-membered pyranose form, it is named D-glucopyranose. The two isomers are α-D-glucose pyranose, where the anomeric OH is "up," and β-D-glucopyranose, where the anomeric OH is "down."

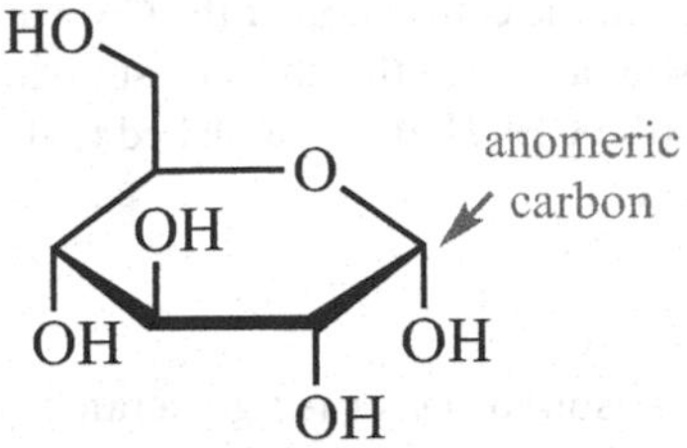

α-D-glucopyranose 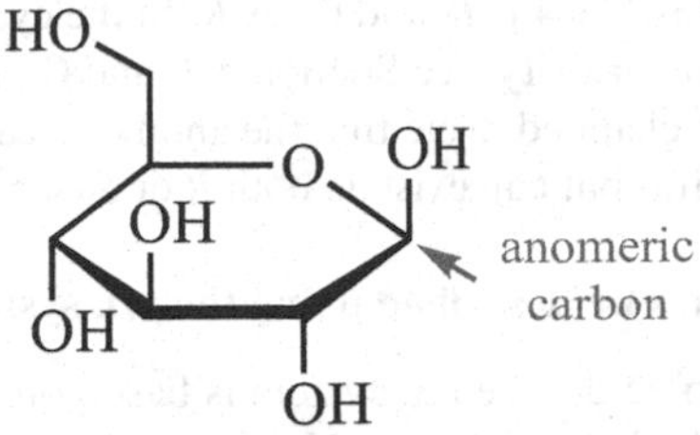 β-D-glucopyranose

What is a furanose?

A *furanose* is a saccharide in a five-membered ring that consists of four carbon atoms and one oxygen atom. Formally, a furanose is a derivative of tetrahydrofuran, a five-membered ring ether.

What is an aldohexose? A ketohexose? An aldopyranose? A ketofuranose?

An aldose is a polyhydroxy aldehyde and a ketose is a polyhydroxy ketone. A hexose is a six-carbon sugar and a pentose is a five-carbon sugar. A pyranose is the cyclic hemiacetal or hemiketal form of the sugar that exists in a six-membered pyran ring. Therefore, an aldopyranose is a polyhydroxy aldehyde in pyranose form. A furanose is the cyclic hemiacetal or hemiketal form of the sugar that exists in a five-membered tetrahydrofuran ring. Therefore, a ketofuranose is a polyhydroxy ketone in furanose form.

What is an example of an aldohexose, a ketohexose, an aldopyranose, and a ketofuranose?

An example of an aldohexose is D-glucose and an example of a ketohexose is D-fructose. An example of an aldopyranose is the pyranose form of D-glucose and an eample of a ketofuranose is the furanose form of D-fructose.

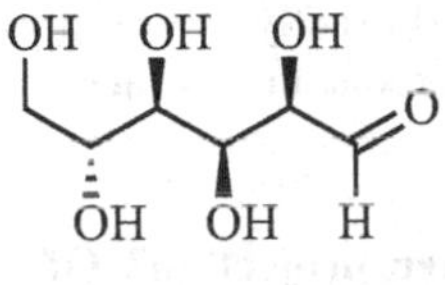

D-glucose 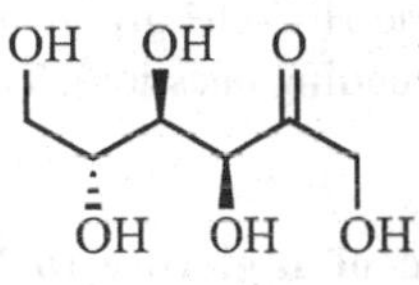 D-fructose 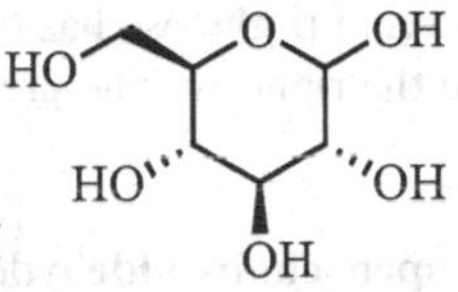 D-glucopyranose 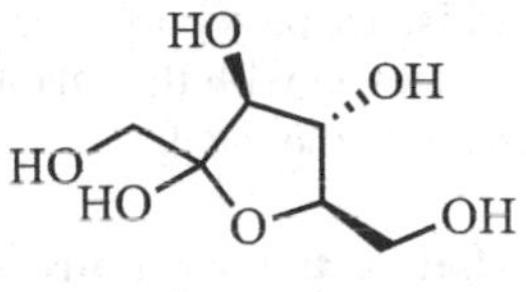 D-fructofuranose

Given the structure of D-glucose, how many stereogenic centers are present? Identify each using the R/S nomenclature.

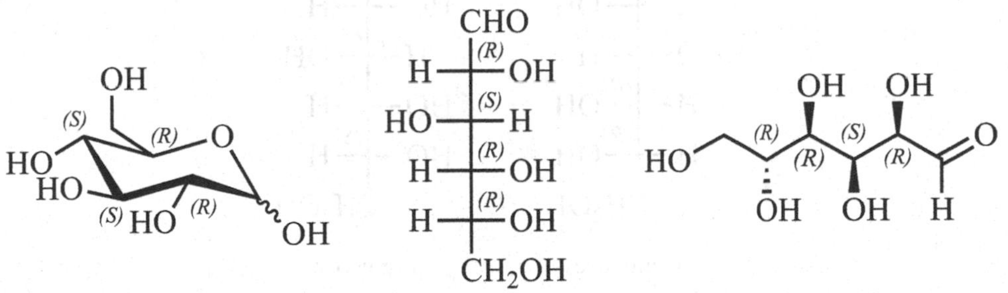

D-glucose

In the open-chain form, there are four stereogenic centers, although in the pyranose form there are five. The saccharide D-glucose is drawn in three forms, as the cyclic hemiacetal and as the open-chain aldehyde, and the Fischer projection of the open-chain aldehyde. In the open-chain forms, C2 (attached to

CHO) is *R*, C3 is *S*, C4 is *R*, and C5 is *R*. In the cyclic form, the conversion of the C=O unit to the acetal unit changes the priority (see Section 6.3) and C4 is now *S*, although the absolute sterochemistry of that carbon has not changed. Note that the anomeric carbon (the CHOH group) attached to the oxygen in the ring is also chiral but can exist as both *R* or *S* (see below).

How can sugars be described using the D/L system?

As with amino acids, the D,L system is based on comparison to (+)- or (−)-glyceraldehyde. Assigning (+)-glyceraldehyde as D-glyceraldehyde and (−)-glyceraldehyde as L-glyceraldehyde allows the comparison. When the OH of (+)-glyceraldehyde is "on the right" (in the box in D-glyceraldehyde) of the Fischer projection, it is given the label D-glyceraldehyde. If the OH on the next-to-last carbon in the open chain form of the carbohydrate (C5 in glucose) is on the right, it is a D-sugar. If the OH is on the left, it is an L sugar. In L-glucose, that OH (in the box) is on the left and this molecule is called L-glucose.

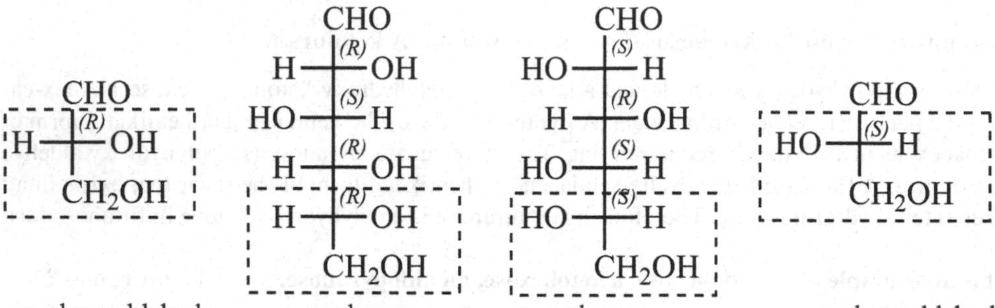

D-glyceraldehyde D-glucose L-glucose D-glyceraldehyde

How is D-glucose related to D-glyceraldehyde?

In Fischer projection, the C5 carbon in D-glucose has the H-C-OH group oriented exactly as in D-glyceraldehyde with the OH group on the right (see the preceding question). This stereoisomer is therefore assigned the label, D.

What is the structure of the open chain aldehyde of D-glucose in Fischer projection? Of L-glucose?

The Fischer projections of D-glucose and the enantiomer of D-glucose, L-glucose, are shown.

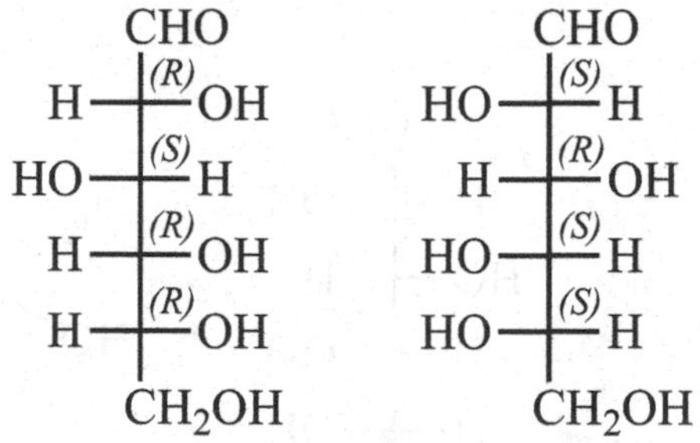

D-glucose L-glucose

What is the structure of the open chain aldehyde of D-fructose and L-fructose in Fischer projection?

The Fischer projections of D-fructose and the enantiomer of D-fructose, L-fructose, are shown.

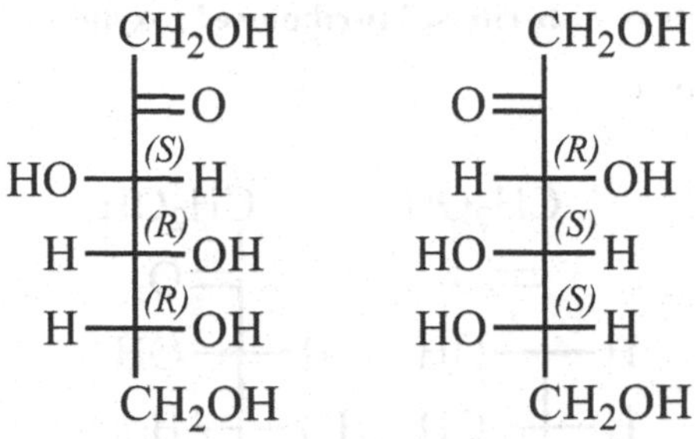

D-fructose L-fructose

What is the structure of the eight different α-D-isomers of glucose (including α-D-glucose) in their α-D-pyranose form? Give the name of each isomer!

The eight isomers are α-D-allose, α-D-altrose, α-D-glucose, α-D-mannose, α-D-gulose, α-D-idose, α-D-galactose, and α-D-talose.

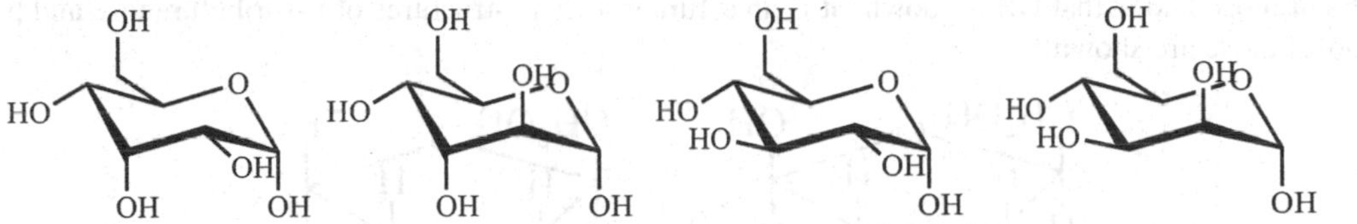

D-allose D-altrose D-glucose D-mannose

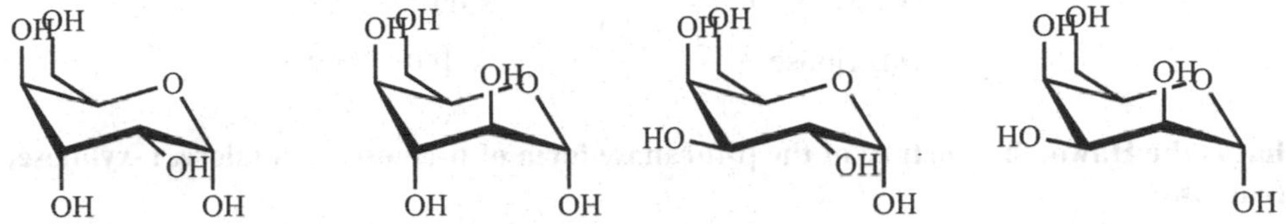

D-gulose D-idose D-galacatose D-talose

What is the structure of β-D-glucose, β-D-mannose, β-D-idose, and β-D-galactose in their α-D-pyranose form?

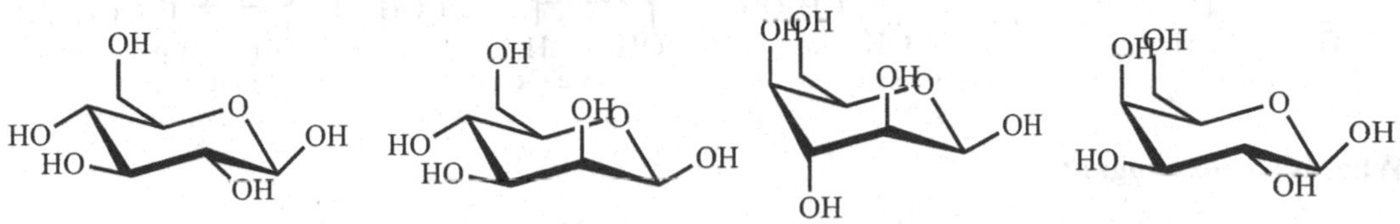

D-glucose D-mannose D-idose D-galacatose

What is a ketose?

A ketose is a polyhydroxy ketone.

What is a furanose?

A furanose is a five-membered ring hemiacetal or hemiketal in which the ring contains an oxygen. It is essentially a polyhydroxy tetrahydrofuran derivative.

What is the open chain structure of D-ribose? D-ribulose? L-xylulose? D-fructose?

The Fischer projections are shown.

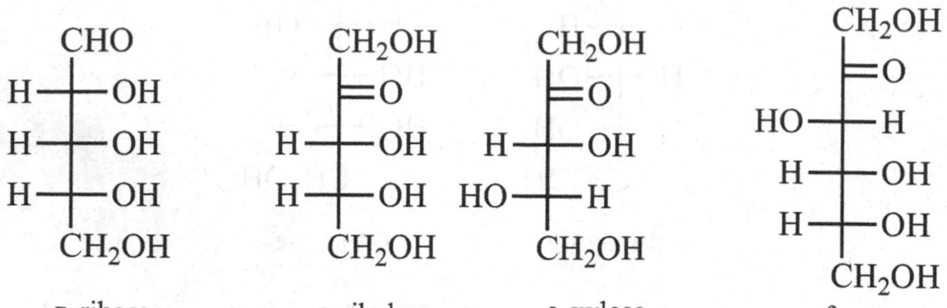

D-ribose D-ribulose L-xylose D-fructose

What are the α- and β-furanose forms of ribose as Haworth structures?

If the OH of the acetal moiety (the OH on the carbon atom connected to the ring oxygen) is "up," it is a β-furanose and if that OH is "down" it is an α-furanose. The structures of α-D-ribofuranose and β-D-ribofuranose are shown.

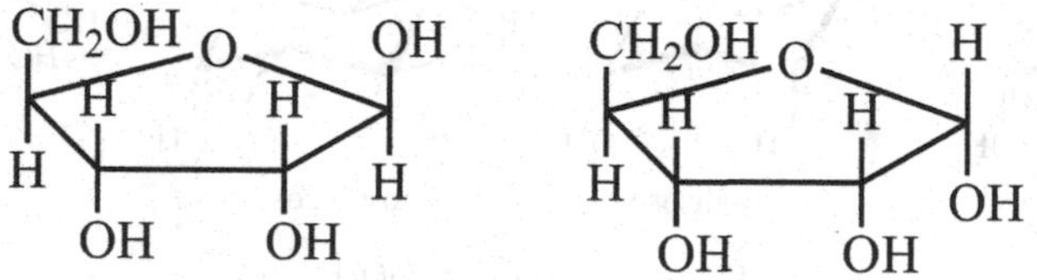

α-D-ribose β-D-ribose

What is the Haworth structure of the β-furanose form of D-ribose, D-ribulose, L-xylulose, and D-fructose?

In each case, the β-form of these sugars is shown. The Haworth formulas of β-D-ribose, β-D-ribulose, β-L-xylulose, and β-D-fructose are shown.

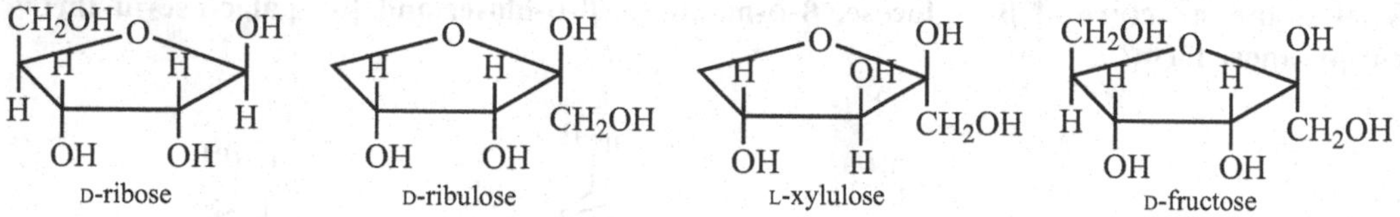

D-ribose D-ribulose L-xylulose D-fructose

What is a deoxy sugar?

A deoxy sugar is a carbohydrate in which at least one of the OH groups is missing. In other words, an OH unit has been removed so that one of the –CHOH units has been replaced with $-CH_2$.

What are the open-chain Fischer projections of 2-deoxy-D-glucose? Of 6-deoxy-L-mannose (L-rhamnose)?

The Fischer projections of 2-deoxy-D-glucose and the Fischer projection of 2-deoxy-L-mannose, otherwise known as L-rhamnose, are shown.

2-deoxy-D-glucose   6-deoxy-L-mannose (L-rhamnose)

What are the pyranose forms of α-D-2-deoxy-D-glucose? Of α-D-6-deoxy-L-mannose (α-L-rhamnose)?

The pyranose forms of α-2-deoxy-D-glucose is α-2-deoxy-D-glucpyranose and α-L-rhamnose is α-L-rhamnopyranose.

2-deoxy-D-glucopyranose   6-deoxy-L-mannopyranose (L-rhamnopyranose)

What is the structure of β-2-deoxy-D-ribofuranose?

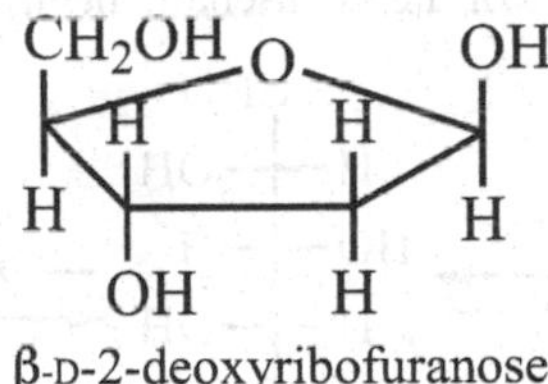

β-D-2-deoxyribofuranose

Does D-glucose exist primarily in the α-form or the β-form? Explain.

The pyranose D-glucose exists primarily as the β-anomer. However, there is actually an equilibrium mixture of 64% of β-D-glucose and 36% of the α-anomer, α-D-glucose.

Does D-glucose exist as the open-chain aldehyde? Explain.

Very little! There is a small percentage (usually less than 1%) of the open-chain aldehyde in equilibrium with the α- and β-D-glucose anomers.

If pure β-D-glucose is dissolved in water, why does the specific rotation of the solution change to a constant but different value over time?

Once dissolved in water, the β-anomer opens to the aldehyde and then can close again to either the β-form or the α-form. Similarly, if the pure α-anomer is dissolved in water, it will equilibrate to the same mixture of the two anomers. Note that the anomers are not enantiomers.

Which is more stable, α-D-glucopyranose or β-D-glucopyranose? Explain.

The most stable anomer is the β-anomer, where the OH group is in the axial position. The interaction of the lone electron pairs on the oxygen when it is in the equatorial position makes the axial orientation more stable. This orientation minimizes the electronic repulsion; also, the axial substituent is the more stable. This effect is called the *anomeric effect.*

Why does D-glucose have more than one value for specific rotation?

D-Glucose exists in two pyranose forms, α-D-glucopyranose and β-D-glucopyranose. Each anomer will have its own specific rotation when pure.

What is mutarotation?

Mutarotation is the equilibrium between the α- to the β-anomers of a carbohydrate. The equilibrium is established for a carbohydrate when dissolved in water that involves the α- and the β-anomers as well as the open-chain aldehyde form change, accompanied by a change in specific rotation. This equilibrium is established when the hemiacetal form of a carbohydrate changes the configuration of the O—CHOH group from C1-*R* to C1-*S* (or from C1-*S* to C1-*R*). The specific rotation will change to reflect the equilibrium mixture.

What properties of a sugar such as glucose lead to mutarotation?

Using glucose as an example, the open chain form (D-glucose) will close to the hemiacetal by attack of the C5 OH on the carbonyl of the aldehyde. In this hemiacetal, the carbon bearing the C1-OH can assume either the *R* (β-D-glucopyranose) or *S* (α-D-glucopyranose) configuration. The equilibrium established in water is, therefore, β-D-glucopyranose ⇄ D-glucose ⇄ α-D-glucopyranose. The position of this equilibrium can be monitored by examination of the specific rotation. The specific rotation of α-D-glucose is +112.2° and the specific rotation of pure β-D-glucose is +18.7°. When pure α-D-glucose is dissolved in water, the specific rotation changes to +52.6°, and if pure β-D-glucose is dissolved in water the specific rotation also changes to +52.6°. Each pure glucopyranose equilibrates to a mixture of 36% of α-D-glucose, 64% of β-D-glucose and <0.2% of the open-chain aldehyde.

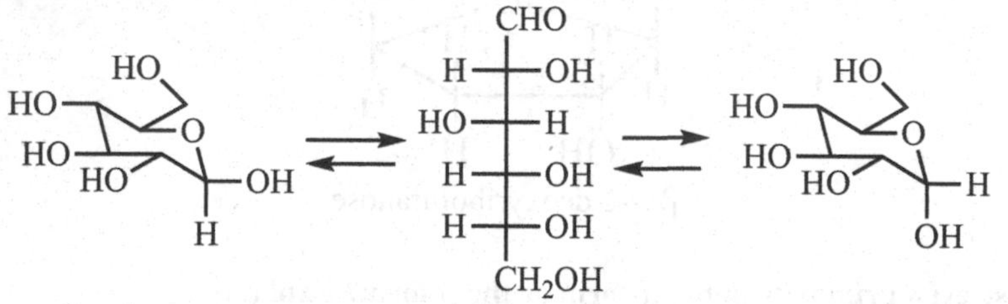

β-D-glucopyranose ⇄ D-glucose ⇄ α-D-glucopyranose

Does D-fructose undergo mutarotation?

Yes! At equilibrium there is about 4–9% of α-D-fructofuranose and 21–31% of β-D-fructofuranose. Complicating this picture is the fact that fructose also exists in the pyranose form. At equilibrium there is 0–3% of α-D-fructopyranose and the dominant isomer is 57–75% of β-D-fructopyranose.

What is the structure of β-D-fructopyranose?

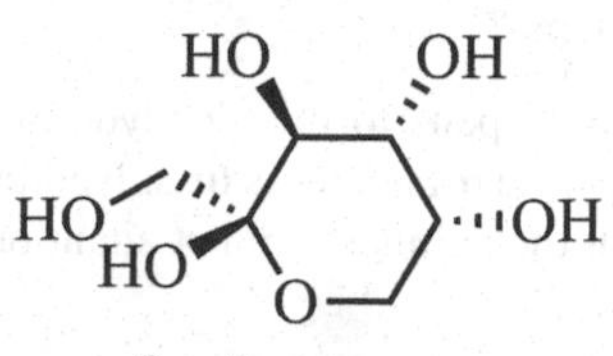

β-D-fructopyranose

21.2 DISACCHARIDES AND POLYSACCHARIDES

What is a disaccharide?

A *disaccharide* is a carbohydrate that is composed of two monosaccharides joined together and it gives two monosaccharides upon hydrolysis.

What is an oligosaccharide?

An *oligosaccharide* is a carbohydrate that is composed of a small number of monosaccharides, typically 3–10.

What is a polysaccharide?

A *polysaccharide* is a carbohydrate that is composed of a large number of monosaccharides, typically >10. Polysaccharides are also called *glycans* and are typically polymeric.

What is the structure of a disaccharide composed of two glucose molecules connected by an α-linkage between C1 and C1′? Of a β-linkage between C1 and C4′?

In the two disaccharides shown, the C1 and C4 carbon atoms of one glucose molecule in the disaccharide are marked, as well as the C1′ and C4′ carbons of the second glucose molecule. The "linkage" between the glucose molecules appears to be an ether-type linkage but it is, in fact, a linked acetal. The term "α-linkage" refers to the C1–C1′ connection (the anomeric carbons) being axial (α), as shown for the C2–C2′ disaccharides in the figure. The second disaccharide connects the anomeric OH (1) with the C_4 OH to give the C1–C4 disaccharide, which is a β-linkage with the anomeric C1 oxygen being equatorial. The name of the C1–C1′ disaccharide is maltose and the C1–C4′ disaccharide is cellobiose.

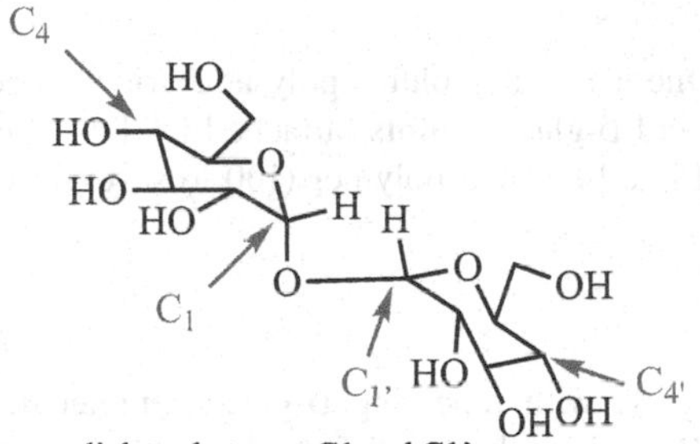

α-linkage between C1 and C1'.

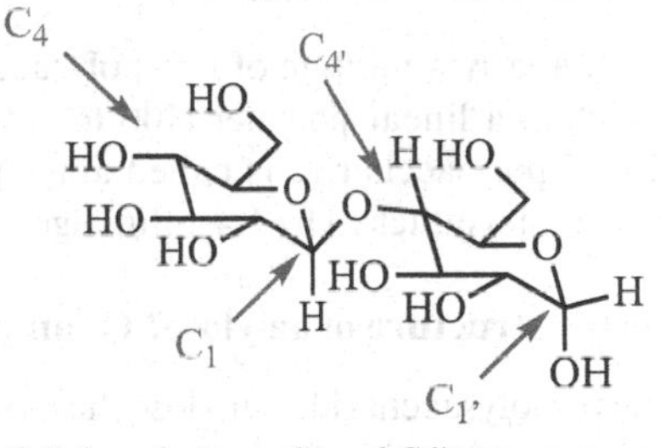

β-linkage between C1 and C4'

What is the structure of a D-glucose and a D-fructose disaccharide connected by a α-linkage between C1 and C21′?

This disaccharide has the structure shown. This molecule is called sucrose.

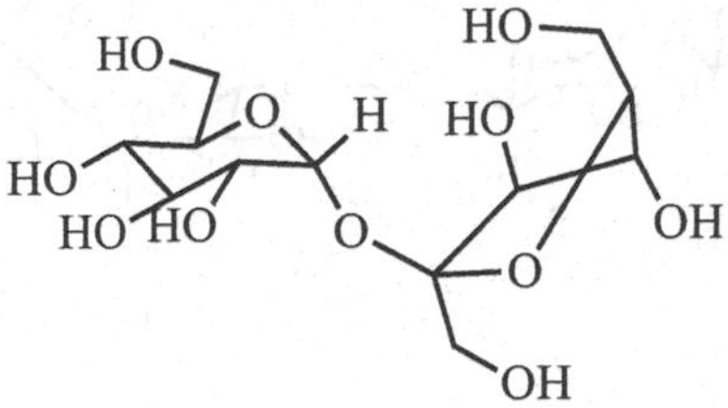

What is a head-to-head disaccharide?

A head-to-head disaccharide is a molecule composed of two monosaccharides linked by the C1–C1′ atoms.

What is a head-to-tail disaccharide?

A head-to-tail disaccharide is composed of two monosaccharides linked by the C1–C4′ atoms.

What is the structure of (a) maltose (b) cellobiose (c) lactose (d) sucrose?

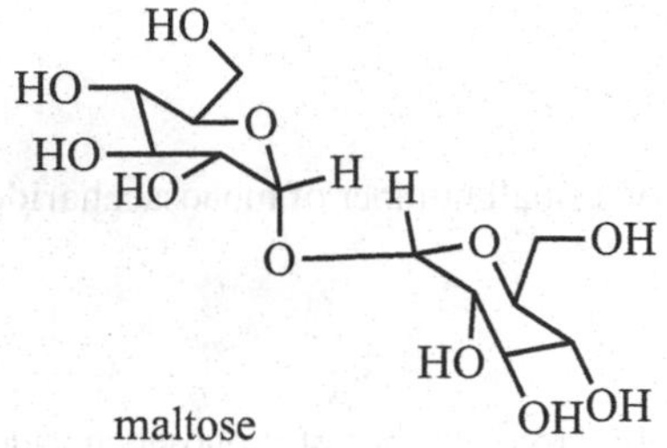

maltose 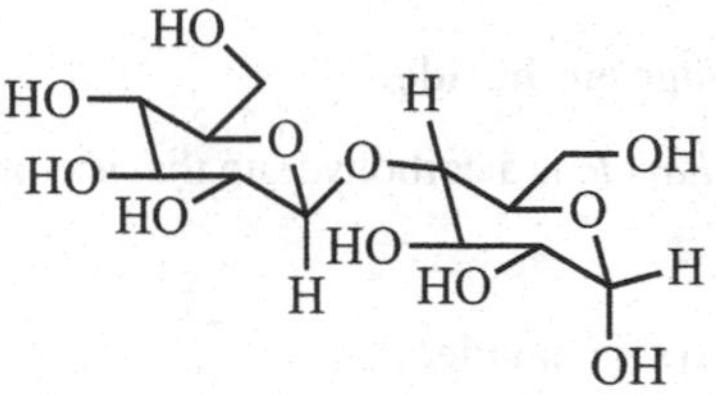 cellobiose

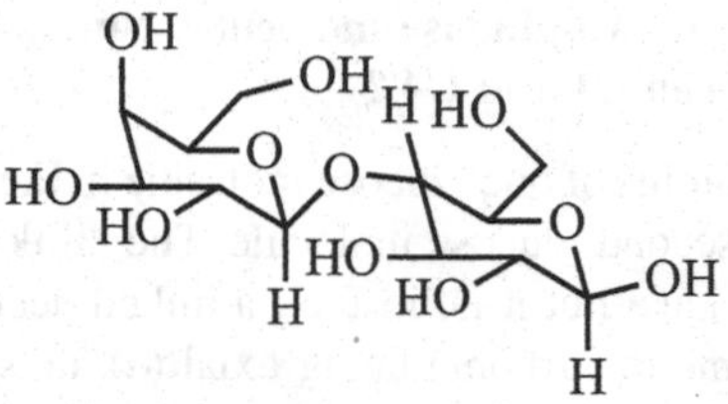

lactose 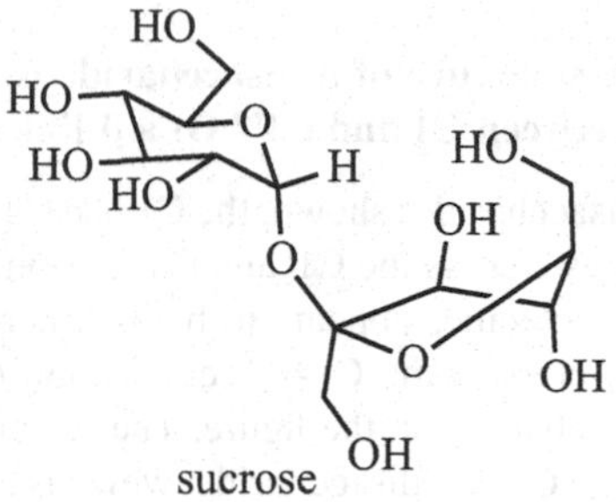 sucrose

What is the structure of starch?

Starch is actually a mixture of two polysaccharides. One is a water-soluble polysaccharide called amylose, which is a linear polymer (100 to several thousand D-glucose units) attached by 1,4-β-linkages. The second polysaccharide is called amylopectin and is a branched polymer (100 to several thousand D-glucose units) attached by 1,4-β-linkages.

What is the structure of amylose? Of amylopectin?

The linear polysaccharide amylose has the structure ***A***, with repeating D-glucose molecules. The branched polymer amylopectin can be represented as ***B***, again with repeating D-glucose units.

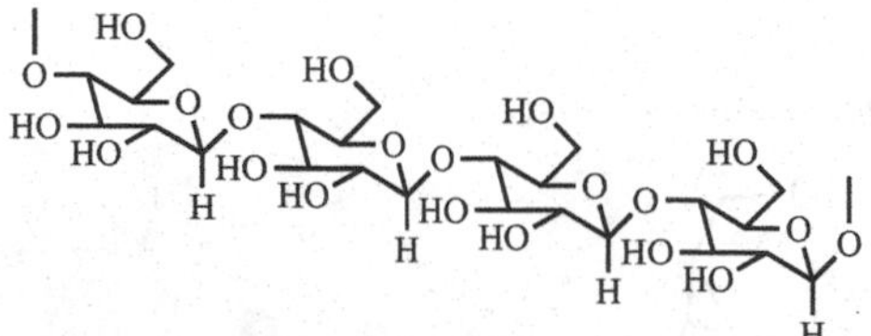

A (amylose)

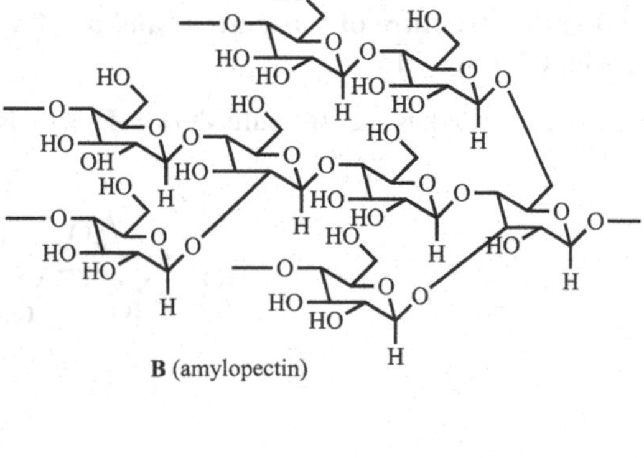

B (amylopectin)

What is the structure of cellulose?

Cellulose has a structure similar to amylose except that the linear D-glucose units are attached by an α-linkage as shown in the figure. Cellulose may be the most abundant organic material on earth and is the structural material that composes most plants.

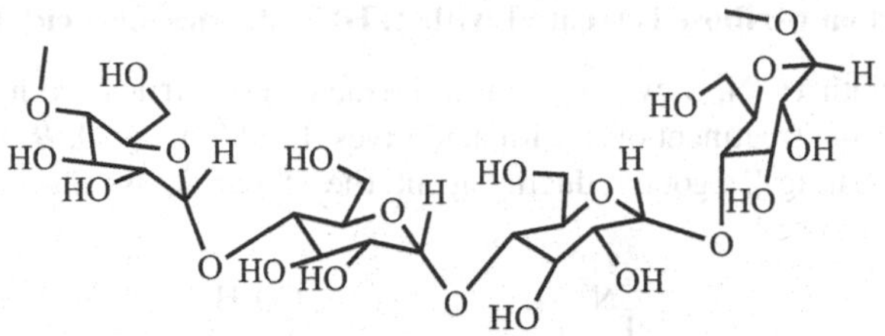

cellulose

What is the structure of *N*-acetylglucosamine?

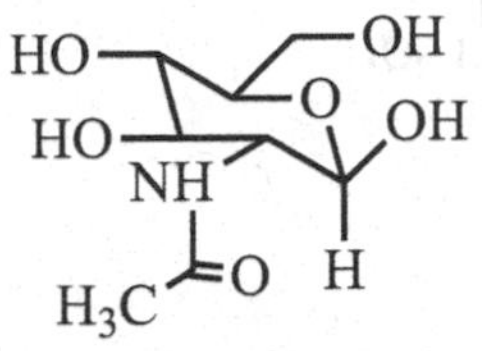

N-acetylglucosamine

What is the structure of chitin?

Chitin is a polysaccharide that comprises the exoskeleton of insects and is also found in crustaceans. It is a linear polymer of *N*-acetylglucosamine with β-linkages.

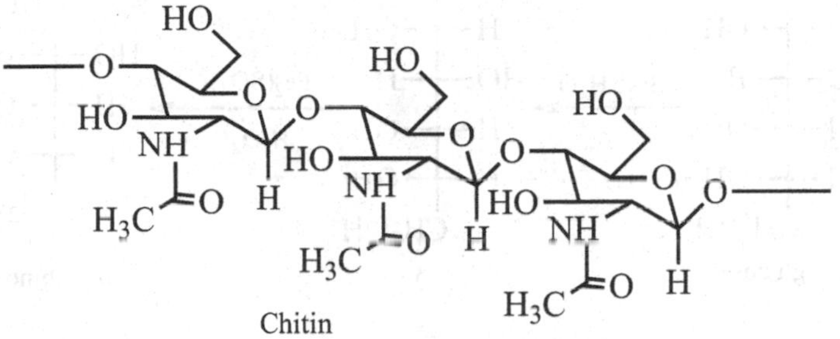

Chitin

What is a glycoprotein?

A glycoprotein is a protein bound to one or more carbohydrates. Glycoproteins play an important role in biological interactions.

21.3 SYNTHESIS OF CARBOHYDRATES

What is the Kiliani–Fischer synthesis?

The *Kiliani–Fischer synthesis* extends the chain length of a carbohydrate by reacting an aldose with HCN to form the cyanohydrin. Reduction of the nitrile then leads to a new aldose (with one additional carbon relative to the starting carbohydrate).

Does the Kiliani–Fischer synthesis provide pure D- or pure L-carbohydrates?

No! The initially formed cyanohydrin (see *A* in the following question) is a mixture of diastereomers. These diastereomers must be separated prior to conversion of the nitrile to the aldehyde in order to obtain pure D or pure L carbohydrates.

What is the product when D-ribose is treated with 1. HCN 2. aqueous acid 3. Na(Hg)?

When D-ribose reacts with HCN, a cyanohydrin is formed (***A***). Nitriles are hydrolyzed to carboxylic acids with aqueous acid and treatment of ***A*** with acid gives the aldonic acid, ***B***. When the acid is treated with sodium amalgam [Na(Hg)], a good reducing agent, the acid group is reduced to a racemic aldehyde, a mixture of allose and altrose.

CHO, H–OH, H–OH, H–OH, CH_2OH (D-ribose) —HCN→ CN, H~OH, H–OH, H–OH, H–OH, CH_2OH (**A**) —H_3O^+→ CO_2H, H~OH, H–OH, H–OH, H–OH, CH_2OH (**B**) —Na(Hg)→ CHO, H~OH, H–OH, H–OH, H–OH, CH_2OH (D-allose, D-altrose)

What is the Ruff degradation?

The *Ruff degradation* is the oxidation of an aldose to an aldonic acid with bromine in water, followed by oxidative cleavage to a new aldose with hydrogen peroxide (H_2O_2) and ferric sulfate [$Fe_2(SO_4)_3$]. This procedure gives a *carbohydrate with one fewer carbon* than the starting carbohydrate. An example is the oxidation of D-glucose to ***A*** with bromine, followed by cleavage to give D-arabinose with hydrogen peroxide and ferric sulfate.

CHO, H–OH, HO–H, H–OH, H–OH, CH_2OH (D-glucose) —Br_2, H_2O→ CO_2H, H–OH, HO–H, H–OH, H–OH, CH_2OH (**A**) —$Fe_2(SO_4)_3$, H_2O_2→ CHO, HO–H, H–OH, H–OH, CH_2OH (D-arabinose)

What is the Wohl degradation?

The *Wohl degradation* is virtually the opposite process to the Kiliani–Fischer synthesis. The aldehyde group in an aldose is converted to a nitrile (via conversion to the oxime and dehydration with acetic anhydride). The nitrile is then treated with base to give an aldehyde with loss of HCN (and one carbon from the carbohydrate chain).

What is the major product when D-xylose is treated with: 1. hydroxylamine 2. acetic anhydride and 3. sodium methoxide?

Hydroxylamine (NH_2OH) reacts with the aldehyde of the aldose (D-xylose) to give the oxime (***A***). Dehydration with acetic anhydride gives the nitrile, ***B***. When the α-hydroxy nitrile group is treated with base, HCN is lost to give the new aldose (D-threose). This overall process is called the *Wohl degradation.*

CHO, HO–H, HO–H, H–OH, CH_2OH (D-xylose) —H_2N-OH→ =N-OH, HO–H, HO–H, H–OH, CH_2OH (**A**) —Ac_2O, NaOAc→ CN, HO–H, HO–H, H–OH, CH_2OH (**B**) —NaOMe→ CHO, HO–H, H–OH, CH_2OH (D-threose)

21.4 REACTIONS OF CARBOHYDRATES

What is the product when β-D-glucopyranose reacts with excess acetic anhydride and pyridine?

As with any alcohol, treatment with acetic anhydride leads to an acetate ester. Since there are five OH groups in glucopyranose, this reaction gives 1,2,3,4,6-penta-*O*-acetyl-β-D-glucopyranose.

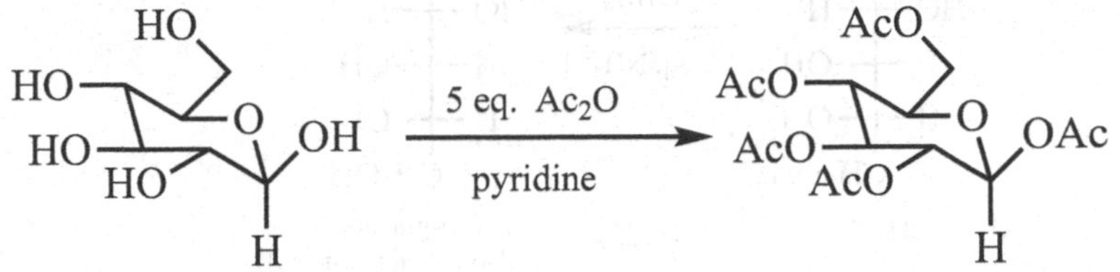

5 eq. Ac_2O, pyridine

What is the product when β-D-glucose is treated with dimethyl sulfate?

Dimethyl sulfate (Me_2SO_4) reacts with alcohols to give methyl ethers (R-O-Me). The reaction of β-D-glucopyranose with dimethyl sulfate forms 1,2,3,4,6-pentamethoxy-β-D-glucopyranose.

If pentamethoxy-D-glucopyranose from the preceding question is treated with aqueous HCl, what is the expected reaction product?

In general, methyl ethers are resistant to aqueous acid hydrolysis. The OMe at the anomeric carbon is not a simple ether, however, as it is part of an acetal structure. As such, the OMe hemiacetal is subject to acid hydrolysis. Treatment of 1,2,3,4,6-pentamethoxy-β-D-glucopyranose with aqueous HCl will, therefore, give the hemiacetal, 2,3,4,6-tetra-O-methyl-D-glucopyranose.

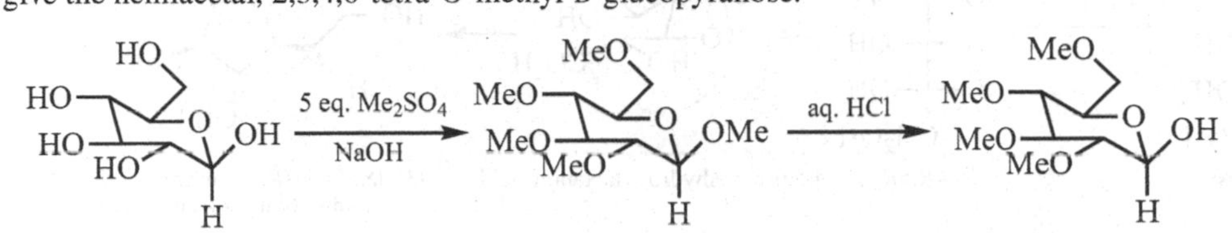

5 eq. Me_2SO_4, NaOH; aq. HCl

1,2,3,4,6-pentamethoxy-β-D-glucopyranose   2,3,4,6-tetramethoxy-β-D-glucopyranose

What is the product of the reaction between D-galactose and hydrogen with a nickel catalyst?

Catalytic hydrogenation will reduce the open-chain aldehyde form of the carbohydrate to the alcohol. In this case, D-galactose is reduced to D-dulcitol.

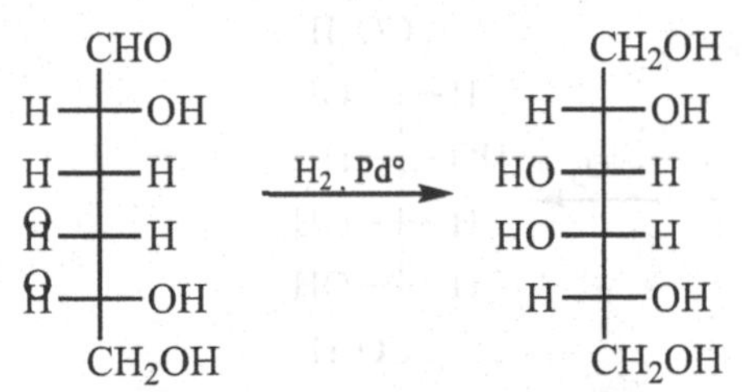

H_2, Pd°

D-galactose

D-dulcitol
(2*R*,3*S*,4*R*,5*S*)-hexane-1,2,3,4,5,6-hexaol

If D-glucose is treated with $NaBH_4$, what is the product?

If D-glucose is reduced with $NaBH_4$, the aldehyde group in the open-chain aldehyde is reduced to the alcohol, giving D-glucitol (also called D-sorbitol) as the major product.

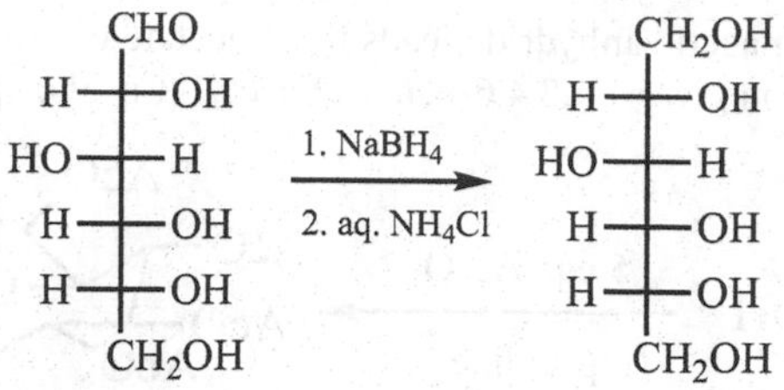

D-glucose → (1. $NaBH_4$; 2. aq. NH_4Cl) → D-glucitol (Also called D-sorbitol) (2*R*,3*R*,4*R*,5*S*)-hexane-1,2,3,4,5,6-hexaol

What is the product of D-glucose and aqueous bromine buffered with calcium carbonate?

When D-glucose is treated with bromine, the aldehyde group of the open-chain form is oxidized to a carboxylic acid (CHO → COOH), (2*R*,3*S*,4*R*,5*R*)-2,3,4,5,6-pentahydroxyhexanoic acid (called gluconic acid). In the presence of the various OH groups, one OH will react with the acid to form a five-membered ring. Therefore, this acid (drawn again in the figure) will cyclize to form a γ-lactone, (3*S*,4*S*,5*R*)-5-[(*R*)-1,2-dihydroxyethyl]-3,4-dihydroxydihydrofuran-2(3*H*)-one. There will also be a small amount of the six-membered ring lactone.

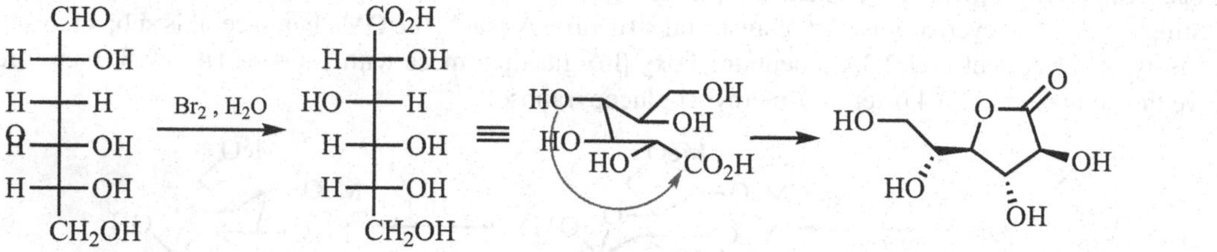

D-glucose → (Br_2, H_2O) → (2*R*,3*S*,4*R*,5*R*)-2,3,4,5,6-pentahydroxyhexanoic acid → (3*S*,4*S*,5*R*)-5-((*R*)-1,2-dihydroxyethyl)-3,4-dihydroxydihydrofuran-2(3*H*)-one

What is the product of D-altrose and dilute nitric acid when heated?

Under these conditions, nitric acid is a sufficiently strong oxidizing agent to oxidize not only the CHO group to a carboxylic acid but also to oxidize the terminal CH_2OH group to CO_2H. The final product is, therefore, the diacid, (2*R*,3*S*,4*S*,5*S*)-2,3,4,5-tetrahydroxyhexanedioic acid (glucaric acid).

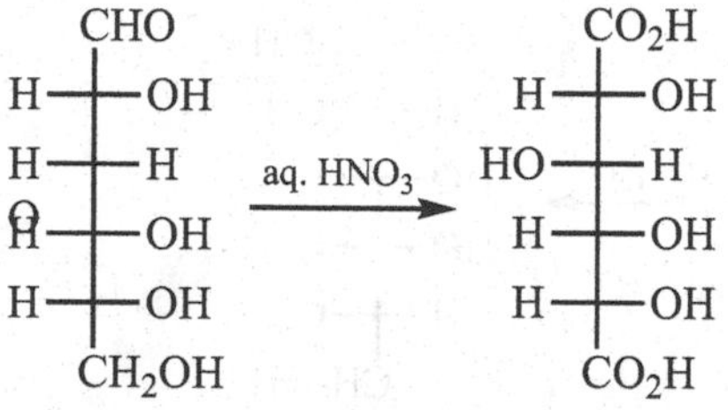

D-altrose → (aq. HNO_3) → (2*R*,3*S*,4*S*,5*S*)-2,3,4,5-tetrahydroxyhexanedioic acid

What is Fehling's solution?

Fehling's solution is an aqueous solution of copper (II) sulfate complexed with tartaric acid.

What is the product of the reaction between D-(–)-arabinose and Fehling's solution?

D-Arabinose is oxidized by this reagent to (2*S*,3*R*,4*R*)-2,3,4,5-tetrahydroxypentanoic acid (these mono acids are generically known as aldonic acids). Fehling's solution is, therefore, a mild and selective oxidizing agent.

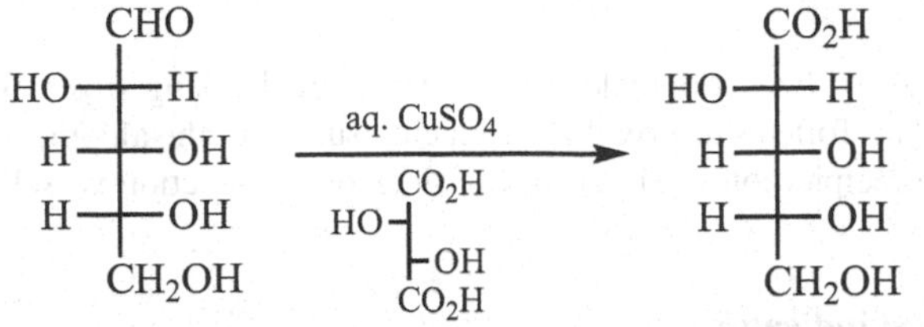

D-arabinose tartaric acid (2*S*,3*R*,4*R*)-2,3,4,5-tetrahydroxypentanoic acid

What is the Fehling's Test?

Both α-hydroxy aldehydes [CHOH-(C=O)H] and ketones as well as "normal" aldehydes react with Fehling's solution, When an aldose or ketose derivative with an α-hydroxy unit is treated with Fehling's solution, oxidation to the acid is accompanied by disappearance of the bluish color of the cupric solution and precipitation of a reddish-copper precipitate of cuprous oxide. This precipitation of a reddish-copper precipitate is taken as diagnostic of the presence of an aldehyde moiety (or an α-hydroxy aldehyde or ketone) in the carbohydrate. Sugars that react with Fehling's solution are called *reducing sugars.*

What is Benedict's reagent?

Benedict's reagent is a solution of cupric sulfate using citric acid as the complexing agent rather than tartaric acid.

What is the product when Benedict's reagent reacts with maltose?

Benedict's reagent also oxidizes an aldose to the aldonic acid (monocarboxylic acid) and is used to detect reducing sugars. In these examples, maltose (***A***) is oxidized to ***B***.

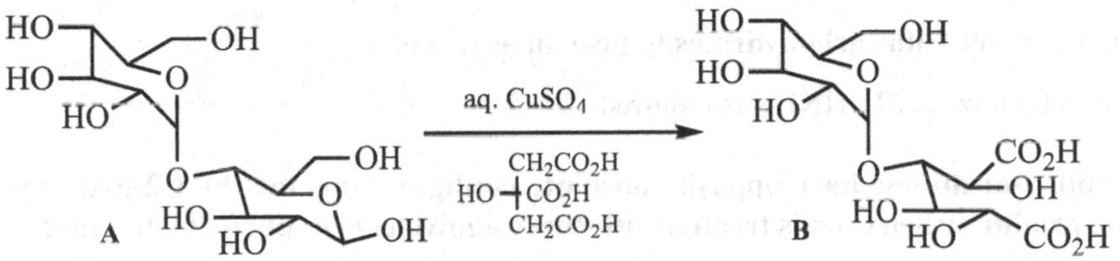

What is the product when Benedict's reagent reacts with D-fructose?

D-Fructose reacts by interconversion of the hydroxyketone to an enol which equilibrates to the aldehyde (D-glucose) and is then oxidized to the aldonic acid. Fehling's solution also oxidizes α-hydroxy ketones in this manner.

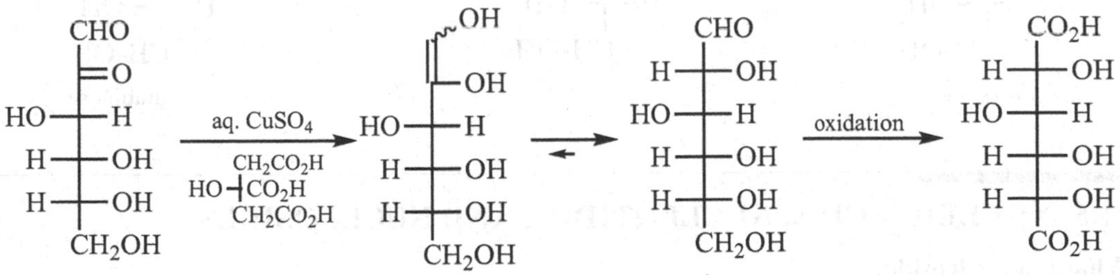

D-fructose D-glucose

What does a positive Benedict's test indicate?

A positive Benedict's test (loss of the blue color and precipitation of the red-copper cuprous oxide) indicates the presence of an aldehyde group or an α-hydroxy ketone or aldehyde moiety in the carbohydrate.

What is the Tollen's test?

The Tollen's test is a reaction that oxidizes aldehydes to carboxylic acids using silver oxide (Ag_2O) in aqueous ammonium hydroxide. The Tollen's test oxidizes reducing sugars to the aldonic acid. A positive Tollen's test is accompanied by precipitation of silver on the sides of the reaction vessel (usually a test tube), forming of a *silver mirror.*

What does a positive Tollen's test indicate?

As with other oxidizing tests, the Tollen's test indicates the presence of an aldehyde or an α-hydroxy ketone.

What is an osazone?

An osazone is a *bis*-hydrazone formed by reaction of carbohydrates with a hydrazine such as phenylhydrazine ($PhNHNH_2$). An example is the reaction of D-(+)-glucose with phenylhydrazine to give the osazone, ***A***.

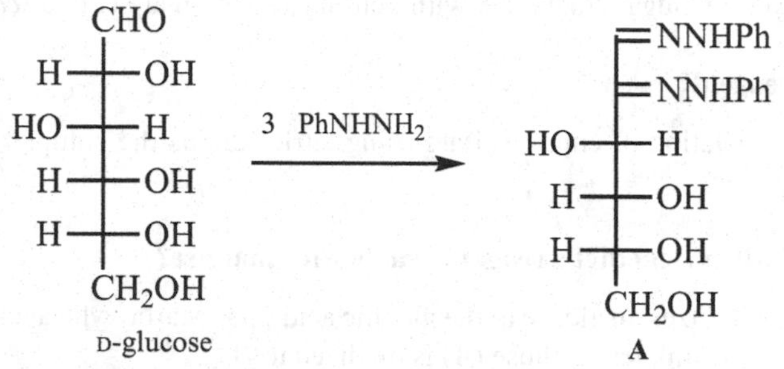

CHO
H—OH
HO—H
H—OH
H—OH
CH_2OH
D-glucose

3 $PhNHNH_2$ →

=NNHPh
=NNHPh
HO—H
H—OH
H—OH
CH_2OH
A

What reagents react with carbohydrates to give an osazone?

An excess of a hydrazine ($RNHNH_2$) is required.

D-Ribose and D-arabinose have opposite absolute configurations for the C2-hydroxyl group. What is the product when each is treated with three equivalents of phenylhydrazine?

The C2 hydroxyl is oxidized to a ketone group for both carbohydrates and in both cases the product is ***A***.

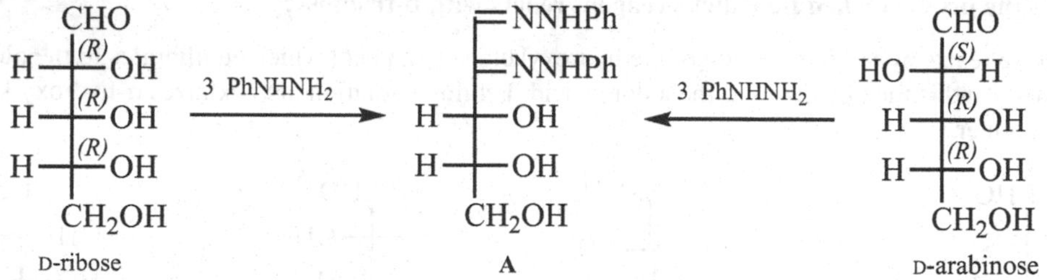

CHO
H—(R)—OH
H—(R)—OH
H—(R)—OH
CH_2OH
D-ribose

3 $PhNHNH_2$ →

=NNHPh
=NNHPh
H—OH
H—OH
CH_2OH
A

← 3 $PhNHNH_2$

CHO
HO—(S)—H
H—(R)—OH
H—(R)—OH
CH_2OH
D-arabinose

21.5 NUCLEIC ACIDS, NUCLEOTIDES, AND NUCLEOSIDES

What is a nucleoside?

A nucleoside is a carbohydrate, usually a cyclic furanose (ribofuranose), that is attached to a heterocyclic amine base at the anomeric carbon of a saccharide. The amine base is usually a purine or a pyrimidine derivative (see Section 16.6).

What sugars are usually involved in the structure of a nucleic acid?

The most common sugars are D-ribofuranose and D-2-deoxyribofuranose, although other sugars are sometimes seen. Both D-ribofuranose and D-2-deoxyribofuranose are shown.

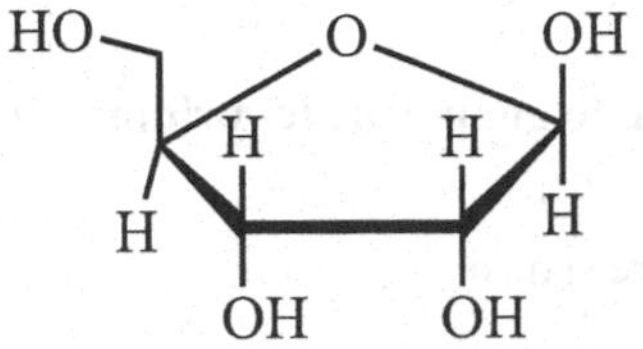

D-ribofuranose

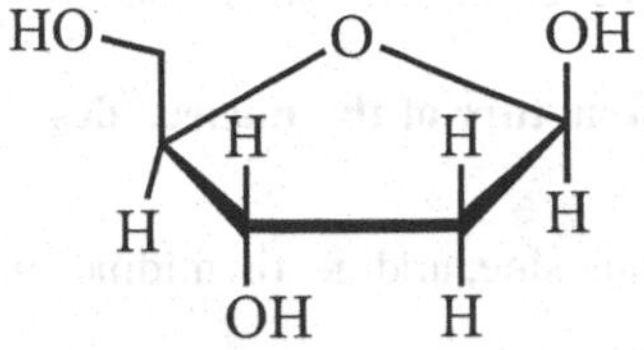

D-2-deoxyribofuranose

What is the base part of a nucleoside?

The amine base is usually a pyrimidine or a purine derivative, usually attached at the anomeric carbon of a D-ribofuranose and D-2-deoxyribofuranose.

What is the structure of pyrimidine? Of purine?

Pyrimidine is a six-membered aromatic ring containing two nitrogen atoms at the 1- and 3-position. Purine is a bicyclic amine, an imidazole unit fused to a purine unit, with four nitrogen atoms.

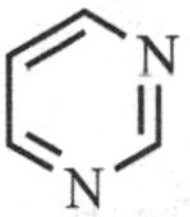

pyrimidine

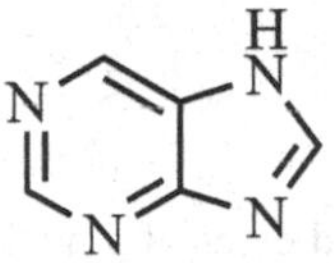

purine

What is the structure of: (a) cytosine (b) uracil (c) thymine?

Cytosine, uracil, and thymine are shown. All are pyrimidine bases.

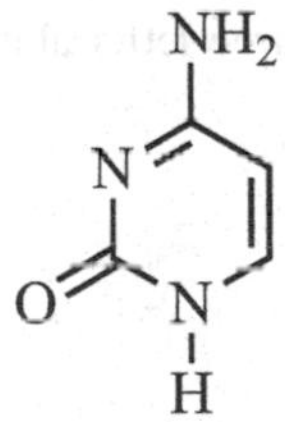

cytosine

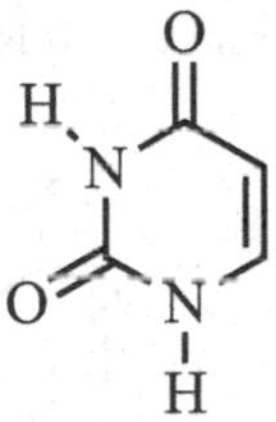

uracil

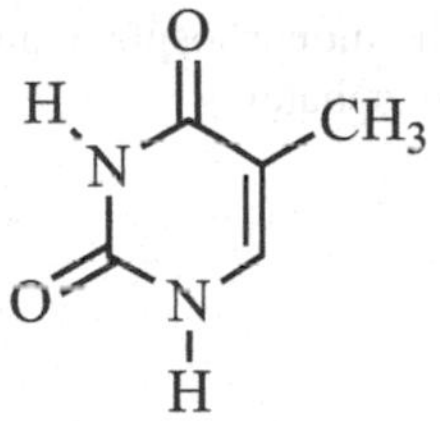

thymine

What is the structure of: (a) guanine (b) adenine?

Guanine and adenine are shown. Both are purine bases.

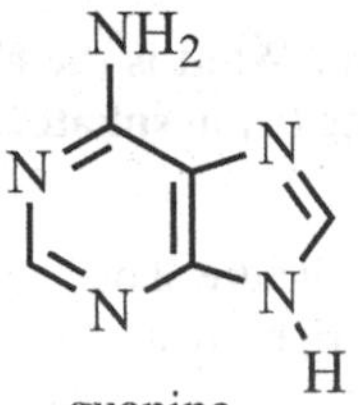

guanine

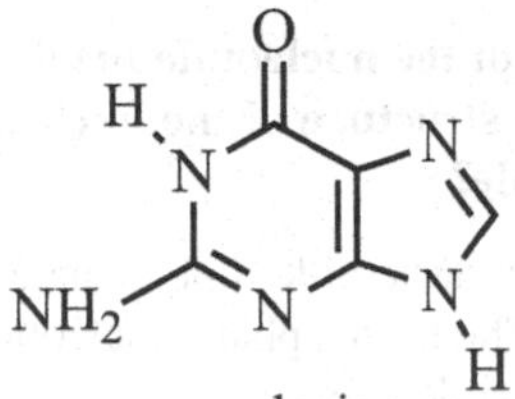

adenine

What are the two basic types of nucleosides?

The most common nucleosides are purine and pyrimidine nucleosides. When cytosine is attached to a ribose (a nucleoside) it is called cytidine, uracil gives uridine, thymine gives thymidine, guanine gives guanosine, and adenine gives adenosine.

What is the structure of the nucleosides: (a) adenosine b) guanosine (c) uridine (d) thymidine (e) cytidine?

Adenosine, guanosine, uridine, thymidine, and cytidine are shown.

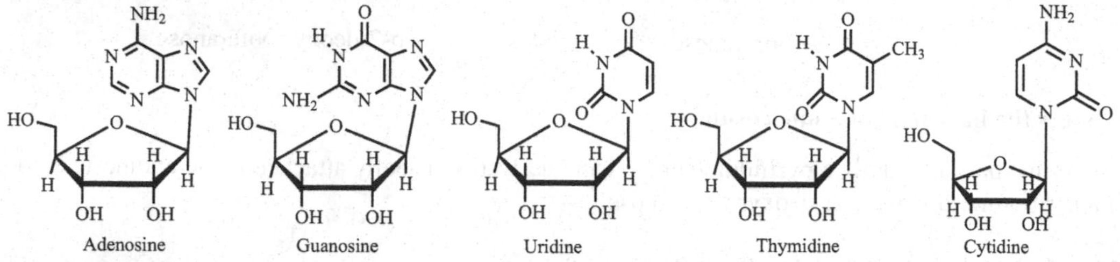

Adenosine Guanosine Uridine Thymidine Cytidine

What are the single-letter codes for the important nucleosides?

Each nucleoside has a single-letter code: **A** for adenosine, **G** for guanosine, **U** for uridine, **T** for thymidine, and **C** for cytidine.

What is a nucleotide?

A nucleotide is the phosphoric acid ester of a nucleoside. The $(HO)_2P(=O)$-O unit is attached at the C5 CH_2OH moiety of the sugar. If two phosphoric acids are attached, the molecule is called a diphosphate and if three phosphoric acids are attached it is a triphosphate.

What is the structure of the nucleotide adenosine monophosphate? What is the abbreviation for this molecule?

The structure of the monophosphate nucleotide is shown. It is given a three-letter abbreviation (AMP – adenosine monophosphate).

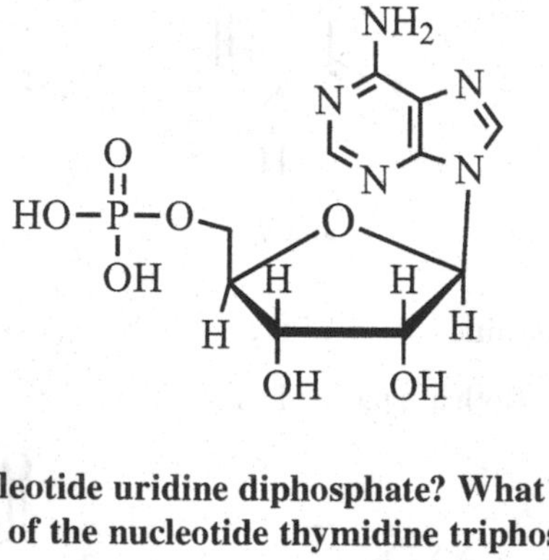

What is the structure of the nucleotide uridine diphosphate? What is the abbreviation for this molecule? What is the structure of the nucleotide thymidine triphosphate? What is the abbreviation for this molecule?

Uridine diphosphate is a nucleotide diphosphate and has the structure shown. The three-letter code for this molecule is UDP. The triphosphate nucleotide thymidine triphosphate has the structure shown and is given the three-letter code TTP.

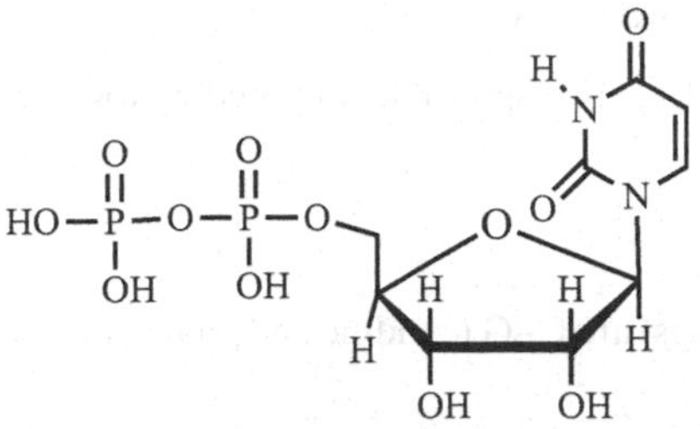

Uridine diphosphate

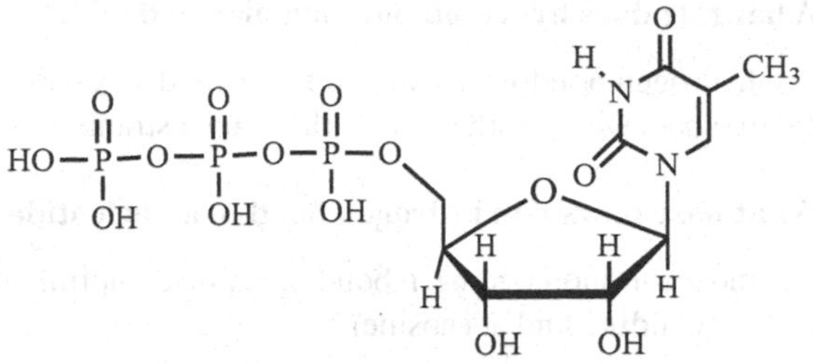

Thymidine triphosphate

What are the three-letter codes for all five important nucleotide triphosphates derived from the important purine and pyrimidine bases?

Adenosine triphosphate is ATP, uridine triphosphate is UTP, thymidine triphosphate is TTP, guanosine triphosphate is GTP, and cytidine triphosphate is CTP.

What is a polynucleotide?

A *polynucleotide* is a polymer of nucleosides linked together by phosphate linkages (usually monophosphate linkages). A polynucleotide of this type is called a *nucleic acid.*

What is a deoxyribonucleotide?

A *deoxyribonucleotide* is a nucleic acid that uses 2-deoxyribose as the carbohydrate portion of the nucleotide.

What is base pairing?

Purine bases in a nucleic acid will form strong hydrogen bonds using NH or amide carbonyl moieties when in close proximity to the NH or amide carbonyl moieties of pyrimidine bases in another nucleic acid or within the same nucleic acid. The two bases that form these hydrogen bonds are said to *base pair* and are referred to as *complementary bases.* The usual complementary bases are: C–G, T–A. These hydrogen bonds are shown for C–G and for T–A.

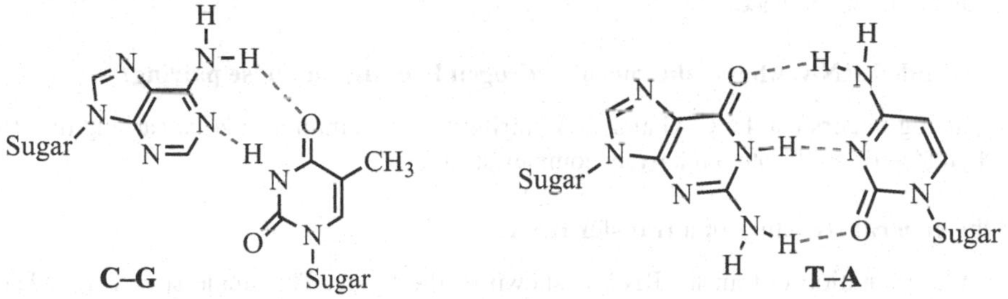

C–G **T–A**

What does the term "double stranded" mean?

Two nucleic acids are coordinated together in an antiparallel manner, as shown. Complimentary bases are usually important. In DNA the A–T and the C–G nucleotides are matched. Therefore, a T nucleotide in one nucleic acid will be matched with an A nucleotide in the second nucleic acid, and a C nucleotide is matched with a G nucleotide, as shown in the figure. In RNA, the C–G and the A–U nucleotides are paired.

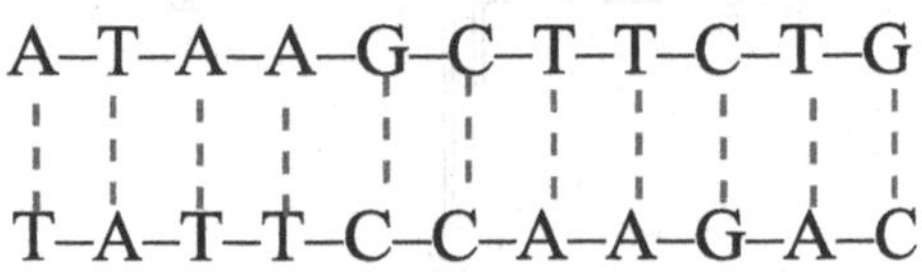

A–T–A–A–G–C–T–T–C–T–G

T–A–T–T–C–C–A–A–G–A–C

What role does hydrogen bonding play in double stranded nucleotides?

The hydrogen bonding between the C–G and T-A base pairs is largely responsible for "binding together" the two nucleic acid strands into the double strand.

What base pairs can hydrogen bond in a nucleotide?

The most common hydrogen bonding pairs (complimentary bases) are C–G (cytidine and guanosine) and T–A (thymidine and adenosine).

What is RNA?

RNA is a ribonucleic acid where the nucleotide backbone of the polymer is composed of ribose units.

What is the general structure of RNA?

The general structure of RNA is shown. Each nucleotide (linked by a monophosphate unit) is usually attached at the 3′-OH and the 5′-OH. The 5′-OH is the CH_2OH unit. Each sugar is a ribose unit and the "BASE" is one of the five bases described above. Therefore, RNA is a polymeric structure and may be relatively short with only a few nucleotides or can be composed of hundreds of nucleotides. Most RNA has thymidine rather than uridine in the structure.

RNA

Is RNA usually single stranded or double stranded?

RNA is usually single stranded.

In single stranded RNA, what is the role of hydrogen bonding and base pairing?

The base pairing occurs but the C–G and T–A pairing occurs intramolecularly, causing the RNA molecule to "bend" and "fold" into a relatively complex structure.

What is the general structure of a transfer RNA?

The usual representation of transfer RNA is shown in the figure. The single stranded nucleic acid is folded in a relatively specific pattern (a "cloverleaf"), allowing it to interact with messenger RNA (see below).

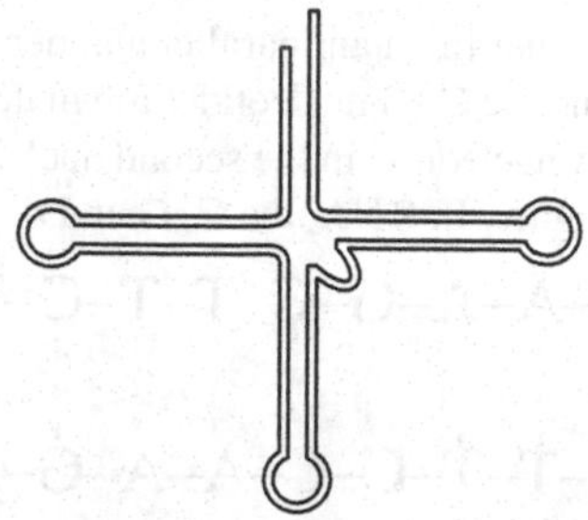

What is the role of transfer RNA?

Each molecule of transfer RNA (t-RNA) transports one specific amino acid, attached as an ester at the 3′-OH end. The transfer RNA contains a three-base-pair *anticodon*, the three highlighted nucleotides at the "bottom" of t-RNA in the figure, where the code corresponds to a single amino acid, and this allows the tRNA to bind to the messenger RNA (mRNA) at a specific site. This specificity allows transfer of only this particular amino acid in the biosynthesis of a growing peptide chain. As shown in the figure, the amino acid attached to the tRNA is transferred to the growing peptide chain and then the tRNA is released form the mRNA to obtain another specific amino acid. Ribosomes assemble protein molecules by using tRNA. The sequence is controlled by messenger RNA molecules (mRNA).

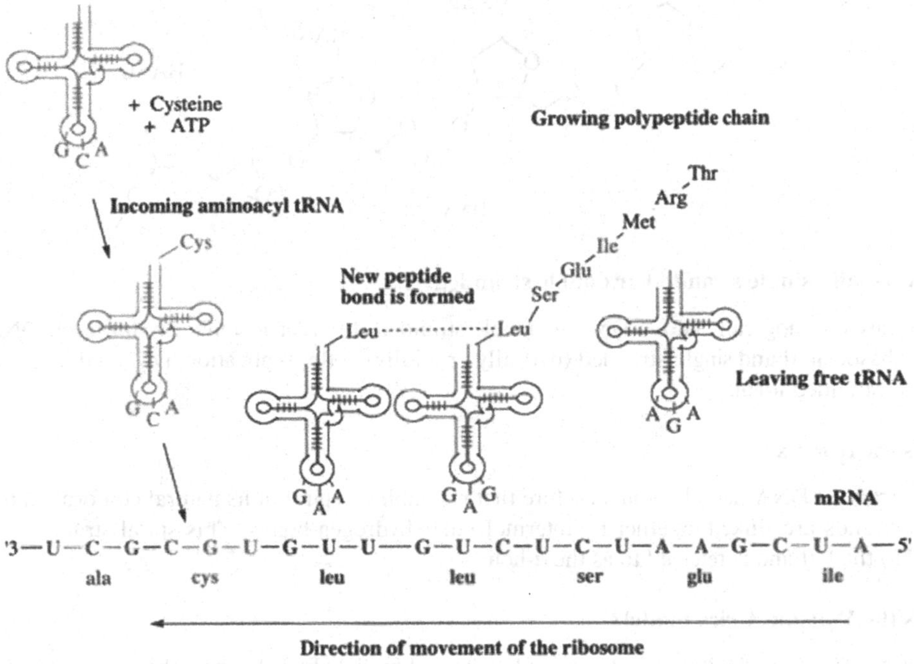

What is the general structure of a messenger RNA?

Messenger RNA (mRNA) is a nucleic acid that is generally single stranded and contains the three base-pair codons that correlate with the anticodons of the transfer RNA. The mRNA unit is found on a specific ribosome.

What is the role of messenger RNA?

Messenger RNA acts as a template, containing a series of three-base-pair codons, each of which correlates with a particular transfer RNA that carries a particular amino acid. The anti-codon of the transfer RNA binds to the codon of the messenger RNA and the amino acid is "unloaded" from the transfer RNA by formation of a peptide bond to the growing peptide chain. The transfer RNA is then "released" and the next transfer RNA (loaded with an amino acid) will attach itself to the appropriate codon. In this way, peptides, enzymes, etc. are synthesized so the chemical integrity and overall primary, secondary, tertiary, and quaternary structures are maintained.

What is the genetic code?

The genetic code is the three-letter (three base pair) codon on a messenger RNA that defines which amino acid is to be used in the biosynthesis of a peptide. Each amino acid usually has two or more codons (three letter code) that will allow the proper transfer RNA to interact with the messenger RNA.

What is DNA?

DNA is deoxyribonucleic acid and is a double stranded pair of nucleic acids composed of nucleotides using 2-deoxyribose as the sugar portion.

What is the general structure of DNA?

A fragmentary structure of DNA (single stranded) is represented by the structure shown in the figure. This single strand will be phase paired (complementary bases) in a double stranded array.

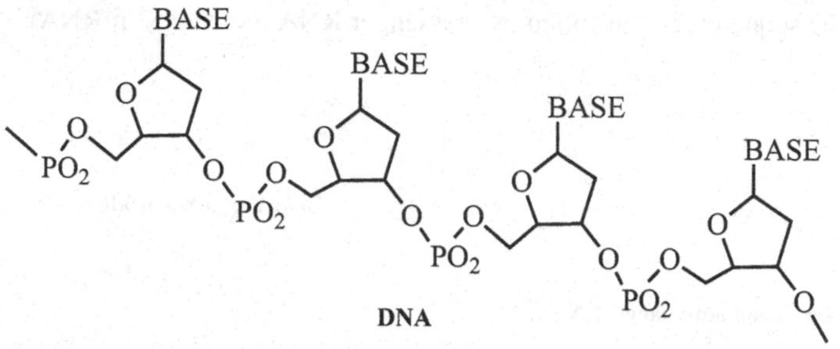

DNA

Is DNA usually single stranded or double stranded?

In most cases, biologically active DNA is double stranded. In order to replicate, however, DNA must become dissociated and single stranded (partially or totally). After replication, DNA will again resume its double stranded form.

What is the α-helix?

Double stranded DNA has a helical structure that resembles a spiral in its natural conformation, where the two strands are linked together by intermolecular hydrogen bonds. This spiral structure tends to "rotate" to the left and is referred to as the α-helix.

What is the Watson–Crick model?

The Watson–Crick model is the double-stranded, helical model of DNA where the structure is two anti-parallel stands of DNA held together by intermolecular hydrogen bonding. The figure shows an α-helix with connecting base pairs.

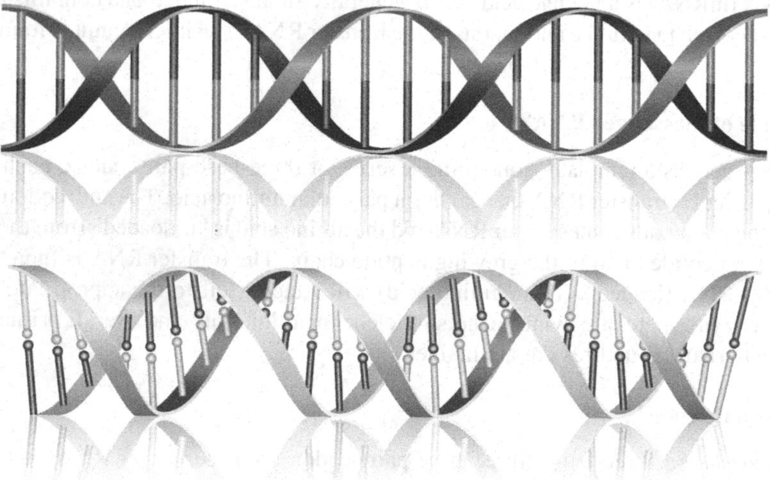

DNA. Shutterstock image 166096259

END OF CHAPTER PROBLEMS

1. Assign the absolute configuration to all stereogenic centers.

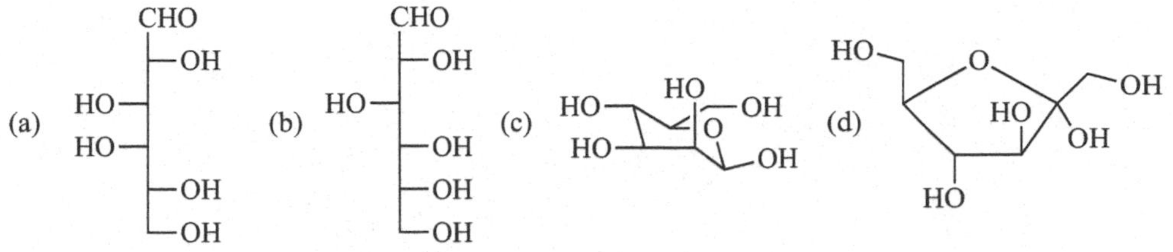

(a) (b) (c) (d)

2. Identify each of the following as a D- or an L- sugar.

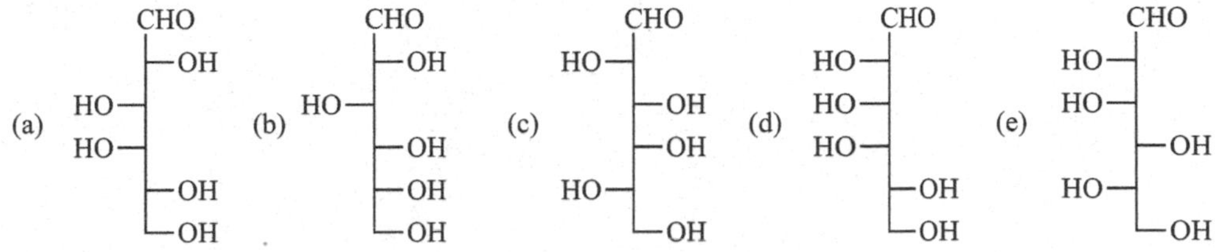

(a) (b) (c) (d) (e)

3. Draw each of the following in its Haworth formula:
   (a) α-D-glucose (b) α-L-mannose (c) β-D-gulose (d) β-L-altrose
4. Draw the Fischer projection of: (a) 3-deoxy-D-altrose (b) 2-deoxy-L-idose (c) 6-deoxy-D-galactose (d) 5-deoxy-D-talose
5. Draw: (a) α-D-fructofuranose (b) β-D-fructofuranose (c) α-D-fructopyranose (d) β-D-fructopyranose.
6. Draw the following disaccharides: (a) head-to-head α-D-gulose-L-altrose (b) head-to-tail-α-D-talose-D-galactose (c) head-to-tail-β-D-glucose-D-mannose.
7. Give the structures of: (a) dimethyl sulfate (b) diethyl sulfate (c) Ac_2O.
8. Draw the structures of: (a) CDP (b) ATP (c) GMP.
9. What is the complimentary strand for G-A-A-T-U-C-A-C-T-T-U-C?
10. In each case give the major product. Remember stereochemistry.

(a) α-L-mannose $\xrightarrow{5\ Ac_2O\text{, pyridine}}$

(b) L-altrose $\xrightarrow[2.\text{aq. } NH_4Cl]{1.\ NaBH_4}$

(c) β-D-gulose $\xrightarrow{5\ Me_2SO_4}$

(d) D-talose $\xrightarrow{\text{aq. } HNO_3}$

(e) D-ribulose $\xrightarrow{H_2\text{, Pd-C}}$

(f) β-D-fructose $\xrightarrow{3\ PhNHNH_2}$

11. In each case provide a suitable synthesis. Show all reagents and intermediate products.

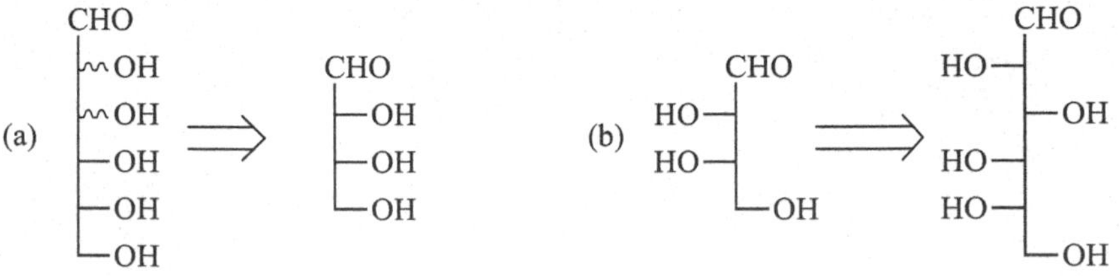

(a) (b)

Appendix: Answers to End of Chapter Problems

Chapter 1. Atomic Orbitals and Bonding

1. A 3s-orbital is spherically symmetrical, as are all s-orbitals. It is further from the nucleus than the 1s- or 2s-orbital and therefore electrons in the 3p-orbital are bound less tightly to the nucleus (they are more easily removed). A 3p-orbital is "dumbbell" shaped, as are all three degenerate p-orbitals. It is further from the nucleus than the 2p-orbitals and once again, any electrons in the 3p-orbital are bound less tightly to the nucleus (they are more easily removed)
2. The only difference is the direction of the orbital in three-dimensional space. Both are identical in energy. A p_x-orbital is directed along the *x*-axis of a three-coordinate system (*x*-*y*-*z*) and the p_y-orbital is directed along the y-axis.
3. Oxygen is $1s^2 2s^2 2p^4$. Fluorine is $1s^2 2s^2 2p^5$. Chlorine is $1s^2 2s^2 2p^6 3s^2 3p^5$.
   Sulfur is $1s^2 2s^2 2p^6 3s^2 3p^4$. Silicon is $1s^2 2s^2 2p^6 3s^2 3p^2$.
4. In (a), K—Cl is ionic and the N—Na bond in (e) is also ionic. In (b) the Na—C bond is ionic but the three bonds in the CN triple bond are covalent. In (c), the C—Br bond is covalent, as are all three C—H bonds. In (d), all three N—H bonds are covalent. In (f), the Na—O bond is ionic but the H—O bond is covalent. In (g) both O—H bonds are covalent.
5. (a) Carbon forms four bonds (b) Nitrogen forms three bonds with one electron pair remaining
   (c) Fluorine forms one bond, with three electron pairs remaining. (d) Boron forms three bonds
   (e) Oxygen forms two bonds with two electron pairs remaining.
6. Boron is in Group 13 and requires five electrons to complete the octet. It only has three valence electrons to form covalent bonds, however. When those three bonds are formed, boron remains electron deficient. It can react with a molecule that can donate an electron pair, a Lewis base, making BF_3 a Lewis acid.
7. Since fluorine is the most electronegative, the C—F bond is the most polarized.
8. In (a) the 2s- and 2p-electrons are valence electrons and this is N. Atom (b) is Na and the 3s-orbitals are the valence electrons. In (c) the 1s-electrons are valence and this is He. In (d) the 3s- and 3p-electrons are valence and this is P.
9. (a) C—O—H (H-bonding) (b) C—F (dipole–dipole)
   (c) C—C (van der Waals) (d) N—H (H-bonding)
10. 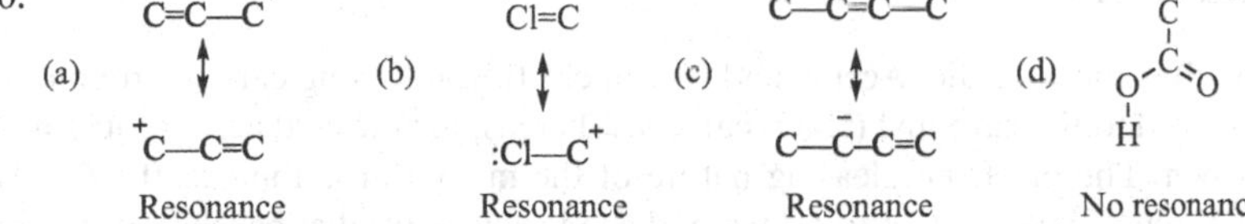

Chapter 2. Structure and Molecules

1. In (a), the third molecule (butan-1-ol) can hydrogen bond whereas the others cannot and has the highest boiling point. In (b) the first compound (butanoic acid) hydrogen bonds to a much greater extent than the other compound and has the higher boiling point. In (c) there is no hydrogen bonding or dipole–dipole interactions and the higher mass 7-carbon molecule (heptane) has the higher boiling point.

2. Molecular models of each molecule are shown. Molecule (a) is angular about the oxygen (bent), as is (c). Molecule (b) is tetrahedral about the central carbon. Molecule (d) is pyramidal with N at the apex of the pyramid and the H and two carbon groups at the other corners.

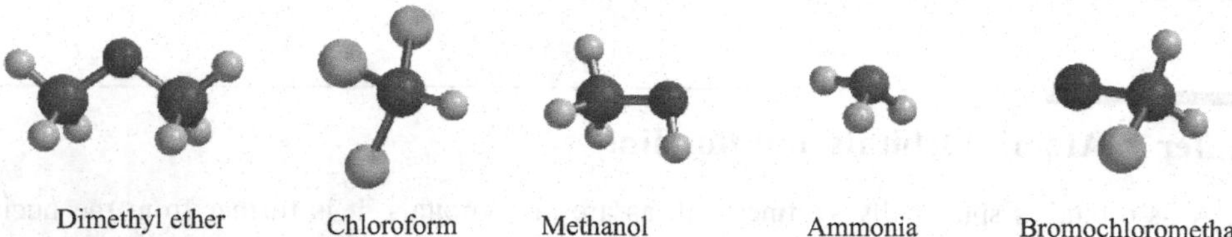

Dimethyl ether Chloroform Methanol Ammonia Bromochloromethane

3. Molecular models of the molecules are shown, with their dipole, which is shown by the yellow arrow. In (a), the dipole bisects the C—O—C bond, as it does in (c). In (b) the dipole is along the C—H bond (bisecting the three Cl atoms). In (d) the dipole is along the N-lone electron pair line and in (e) the dipole bisects the Br—C—Cl bond.

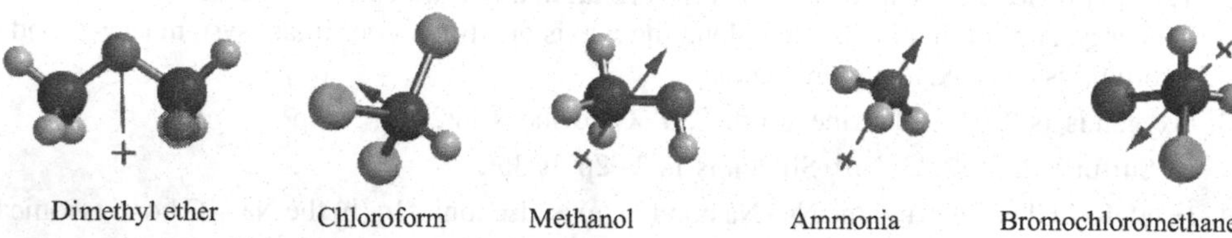

Dimethyl ether Chloroform Methanol Ammonia Bromochloromethane

4. The alcohol functional group is C—O—H. The ketone functional group is C=O where the carbonyl is flanked by two carbon groups (C—(C=O)—C). The alkyne functional group is C≡C and the aldehyde functional group is C=O, where at least one of the groups attached to the carbonyl carbon is a hydrogen (C—(C=O)—H). The thiol functional group is S—H and the nitrile functional group is C≡N.
5. For molecule (a); C^1, $C^2 = 0$; $N = +1$; H^1-$H^5 = 0$; $O^2 = 0$ and $O^1 = -1$. The formal charge for the molecule is 0 (+1−1). For (b) C^1, C^2 and $C^3 = 0$ but $C^4 = -1$. The $N = +1$ and H^1–$H^6 = 0$. The O = −1. For the molecule, the formal charge is −1 (−1+1−1 = −1).
6. In (a) the alcohol has the higher boiling point due to hydrogen bonding. In (b) the diol has the higher boiling point since two OH groups can hydrogen bond more extensively than one OH group. In (c) the carboxylic acid hydrogen bonds more than the alcohol and has the higher boiling point.
7. Of these three molecules, molecule (c) is more symmetrical and will "pack" into a crystal lattice more efficiently. For this reason, it will have the higher melting point.

Chapter 3. Acids and Bases

1. HCOOH (formic acid) is more acidic. Acetic acid has an electron-releasing carbon group (the methyl) directly attached to the carbonyl (C=O) carbon, whereas, formic acid has a H attached to the carbonyl carbon. The electron-releasing nature of the methyl group makes the O—H bond stronger via a through-bond inductive effect, and acetic acid is weaker because of it.
2. Since oxygen is more electronegative than nitrogen, oxygen retains electron density better than nitrogen. Therefore, nitrogen in CH_3NHCH_3 should be better able to donate electrons to a hydrogen atom than the oxygen in CH_3OCH_3. Therefore, the nitrogen compound is a better base.
3. (a) −4.53 (b) 8.63 (c) 1.24 (d) −7.9
4. (a) 4.68×10^{-3} (b) 2.82×10^{-24} (c) 8.91×10^{-18} (d) 1.66×10^{-4} (e) 7.08×10^{-11}
5. Although all three structures look identical, they represent delocalization of the charge on the carbon atom and all three oxygen atoms. A molecular model of the carbonate dianion is shown to give a better idea of the dispersion of electron density due to resonance.

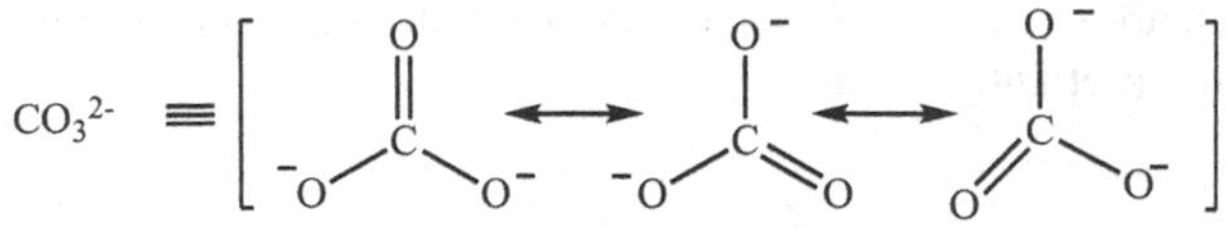

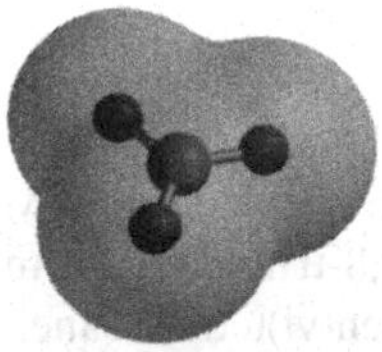

6. In this question, an aprotic solvent is assumed, where ***A*** is more acidic. In ***A***, the OH unit of the carboxyl group is held close in space to the electron withdrawing chorine, so there is a significant hydrogen bond (through-space effect) that makes the OH unit more polarized and more acidic. The COOH unit is held on the opposite side of the molecule from the chlorine atoms in ***B***, so the internal hydrogen bonding is ineffective or completely missing. Therefore, ***B*** does not have the enhancement in acidity and ***A*** is more acidic than ***B***.

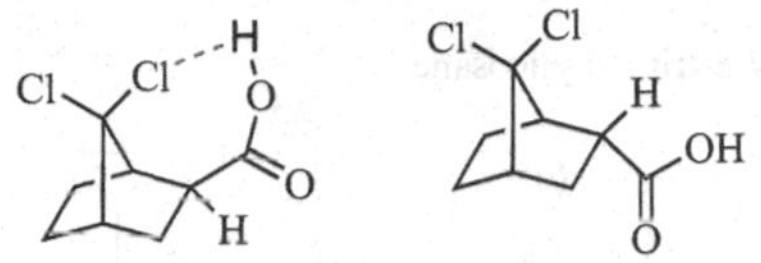

7. In this question, acid ***A*** is more acidic. In ***A***, there are two bromine atoms on C3, and the OH unit of the carboxyl group is close to the electron-withdrawing bromine, so there is a significant hydrogen bond (through-space effect), that makes the OH unit more polarized and more acidic. In ***B***, the bromine atoms are too far away from the COOH unit (on C6), so the internal hydrogen bonding is completely missing. Therefore, ***B*** does not have the enhancement in acidity and ***A*** is more acidic than ***B***.

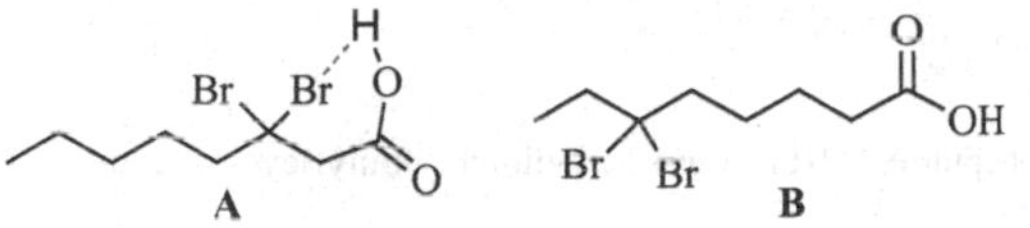

8.

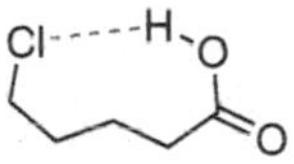

9. Water can solvate the two ions that are formed (H_3O^+ and acetate) much better than ethanol.
10. For many, if not most, organic chemical reactions, one starting material gives one product or two starting materials react to give one product, or two as in the case of a Brønsted–Lowry acid–base reaction. Because of this characteristic, the disorder of these reactions is small, which means that the changes in entropy ($\Delta S°$) is small. If the reaction generates multiples products, especially gases, then $\Delta S°$ is larger and cannot be ignored.
11. If ΔS is ignored, then $\Delta G°$ can be assumed to be equal to $\Delta H°$. If $\Delta H°$ is bonds formed – bonds broken, then $\Delta G°$ = 50.9 kcal – 72.9 kcal = –22.0 kcal. Since $\Delta G°$ is negative, the reaction is exothermic.

Chapter 4. Alkanes, Isomers, and Nomenclature

1. Formulae (b) and (f)
2. Formulae (a) and (e)

3. The longest continuous chain is 13, not 11, so this molecule is a tridecane. The correct name should be 5-ethyl-7-methyltridecane.

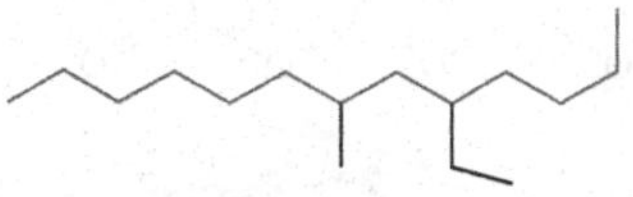

5-ethyl-7-methyltridecane

4. Molecule (a) is 3,3,6,6-tetramethylpentadecane. Molecule (b) is 8-(3-bromopropyl)-6-methylhexadecane. Molecule (c) is 5,7,8-trimethylisocane. Molecule (d) is 3,3,4,4-tetraethyloctane. Molecule (e) is 7-(3,3-dimethylpentyl)tetradecane.

(a) 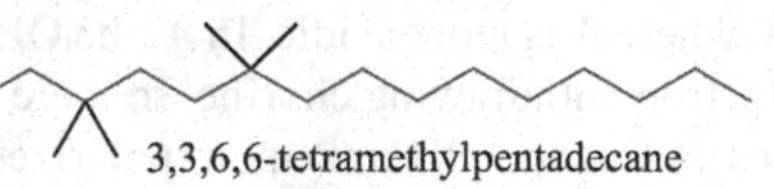 3,3,6,6-tetramethylpentadecane

(b) 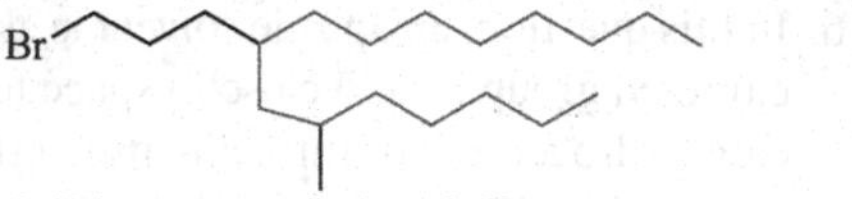 Br 8-(3-bromopropyl)-6-methylhexadecane

(c) 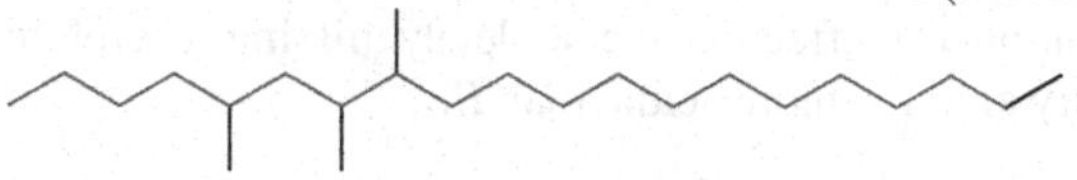 5,7,8-trimethylicosane

(d) 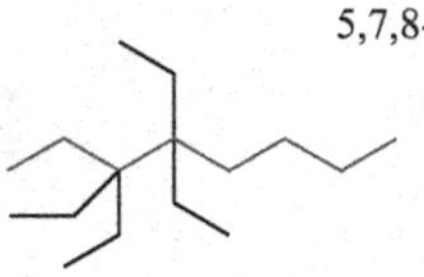 3,3,4,4-tetraethyloctane

(e) 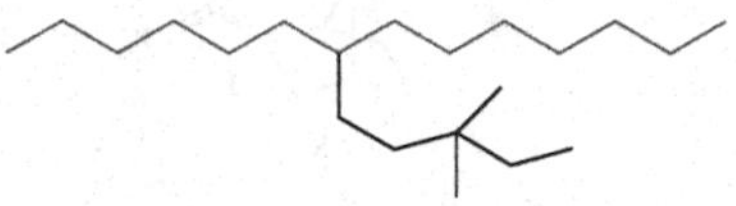 7-(3,3-dimethylpentyl)tetradecane

5.

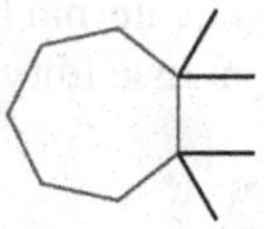

Br Br Br Br

3,3,4,4-tetramethylcycloheptane 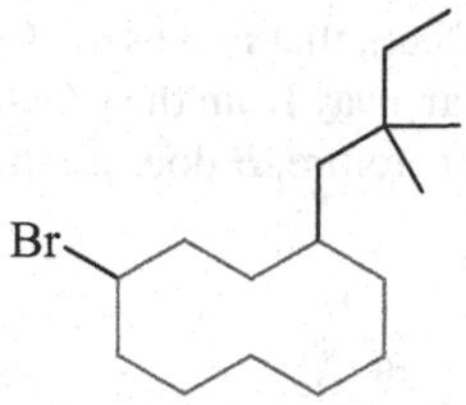 1-bromo-4-(2,2-dimethylbutyl)cyclodecane 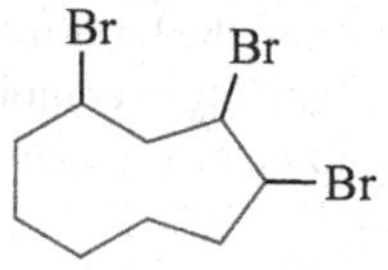 5,7,8-tribromocyclononane

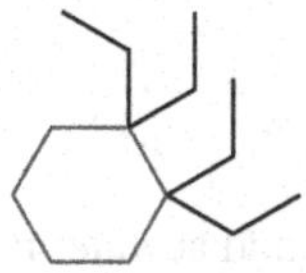

3,3,4,4-tetraethylcyclohexane 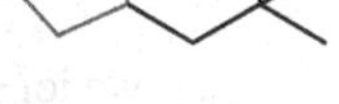 1-(2,2-dimethylpropyl)cyclopentane

6.
(a) 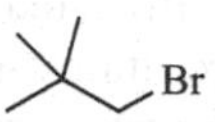 Br (b) 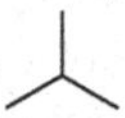 (c) 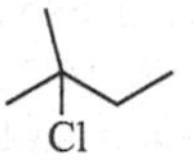 Cl (d) 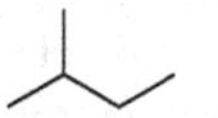 (e) 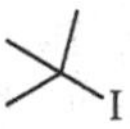 I

7. Eight isomers for (a) and (b) include:

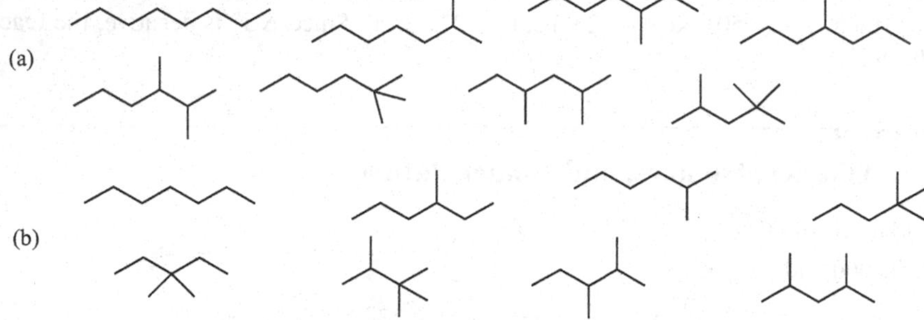

8. (a) 1,1-diethyl-3,3-dimethylcyclopentane (b) 1,2,2,4-tetramethyl-3-propylcylcohexane (c) 1,1,-dimethyl-4-(1-methylbutyl)cycloundecane.

Chapter 5. Conformations

1\.

Lowest Energy   Highest Energy

2\.

A   B

3. In the answer for question 2, conformation ***A*** has both chlorine atoms in the flagpole position whereas hydrogen atoms are in the flagpole positions of ***B***. The greater transannular strain in ***A*** (greater flagpole interactions) makes ***A*** higher in energy, and the equilibrium will shift to favor ***B***. Therefore, conformation ***B*** will be present in greater percentage because it is lower in energy relative to ***A***.

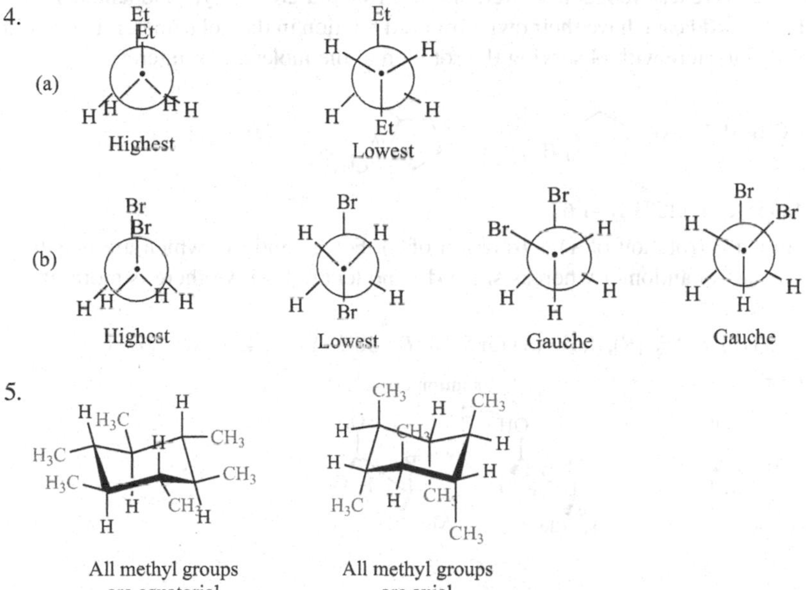

6. Cyclopropane has the greatest angle strain and also the greatest torsion strain.
7. Cyclopentane, in the envelope conformation, has more angle strain than the planar conformation, but the planar conformation has significantly more torsion strain than the envelope conformation. This observation indicates that relief of torsion strain is more important and cyclopentane exists primarily in the envelope conformation as the low energy form.

8. (a) Me, Me, Me ⇌ Me, Me, Me
lowest energy — highest energy

(b) Et, Et, Et ⇌ Et, Et, Et
lowest energy — highest energy

(c) Me, Me, Me, Me ⇌ Me, Me, Me, Me
lowest energy — highest energy

Chapter 6. Stereochemistry

1. (a) CH_2CH_3, (R), Br, CH_3, H, CH_3, CH_3 (b) H, Br, (S), (S), CH_3, Br, H (c) H, OH (d) HO, H, (S), CH_3

(e) CH_3, H, (S), HO, CH_2CH_3 (f) CH_3, (R), H, C≡C–CH_3, OH (g) Cl, (R), Br, CH_3, H (h) H, CH_3, $(CH_3)_3C$, (R), $CH(CH_3)_2$

2. The two alcohols that have a stereogenic center, butan-2*R*-ol and 2*R*-methylcyclopentan-1*R*-ol, are unsuitable. They would each have their own observed rotation in the polarimeter that would obscure or certainly interfere with observing the rotation of the molecule of interest.

CH_3OH H_2O (R), CH_3, HO, H (R), OH, (R), CH_3 CH_2Cl_2

3. (a) –5.23° (b) +10.95° (c) +0.12° (d) –1.67°

4. The observed rotation = (rotation of +) + (rotation of –). For (a) and (d), which are negative, there is more of the (*S*)-enantiomer whereas since (b) and (c) are positive there is more of the (*R*)-enantiomer.

(a) 44% (*R*), 56% (*S*) (b) 95.5% (*R*), 4.5% (*S*) (c) 52% (*R*), 48% (*S*) (d) 42% (*R*), 58% (*S*).

5.

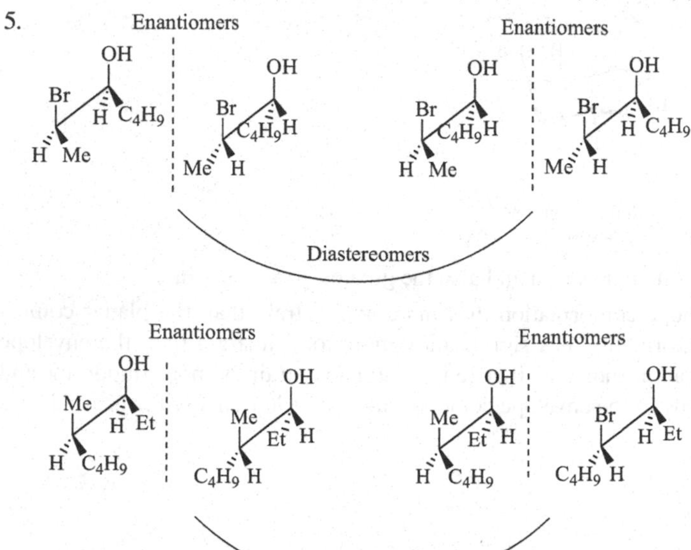

6. (2*R*,3*S*)-2-bromo-3-chloropentane (2*R*,3*R*)-2-bromo-3-chloroper

CH_3		CH_3		CH_3		CH_3
H—(S)—Br		Br—(R)—H		H—(S)—Br		Br—(R)—H
H—(R)—Cl		Cl—(S)—H		Cl—(S)—H		H—(R)—Cl
CH_2CH_3		CH_2CH_3		CH_2CH_3		CH_2CH_3

(2*S*,3*R*)-2-bromo-3-chloropentane (2*S*,3*S*)-2-bromo-3-chloropentane

7. In both cases, there are only three stereoisomers since both compounds can form a meso compound.

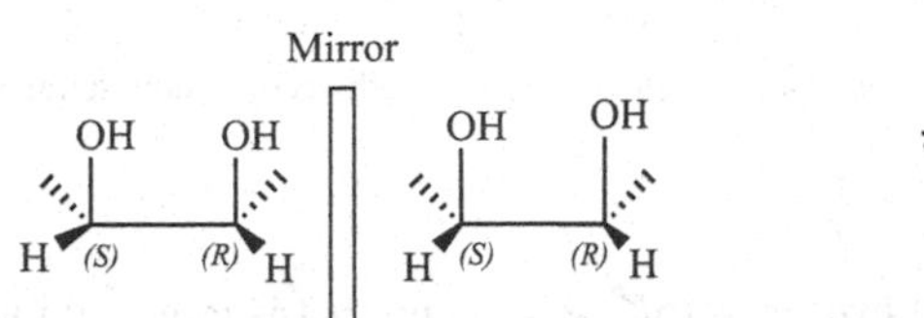

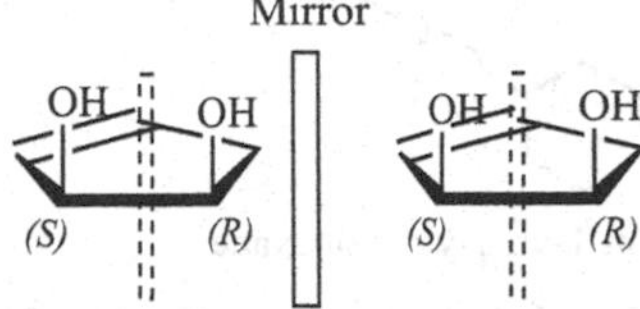

Chapter 7. Alkenes and Alkynes: Structure, Nomenclature, and Reactions

1. All of the carbon atoms are coplanar since each methyl-C=C unit is trigonal planar. Therefore, the C—C—C bond angles are about 120°.
2. The name is 1-bromo-1-chloropent-1-ene. The stereochemistry of the groups of C=C have not been established, so there are no cis-/trans- or E-/Z-isomers, so those terms are not included in the name.
3. The endocyclic (the C=C unit is within the ring) alkene (***A***) has three carbon groups attached to the C=C group whereas the exocyclic (the C=C unit is outside the ring) alkene (***B***) has only two. Since carbon groups release electrons into the π-bond and help to stabilize it, the more substituted alkene (***A***) is more stable.
4. (a) 4-chloromethyl-5-methyl-oct-3*Z*-ene. (b) 1,2-diethylcyclohexene.
   (c) 3-(2-methylbutyl)-2,4,4-trimethyldec-1-ene. (d) 3,4-dichlorohex-3*E*-ene.
   (e) 7-chloro-7-methyltridec-3*E*-ene. (f) 1,5,5-tribromo-3-butyl-3-ethylcycloheptene.

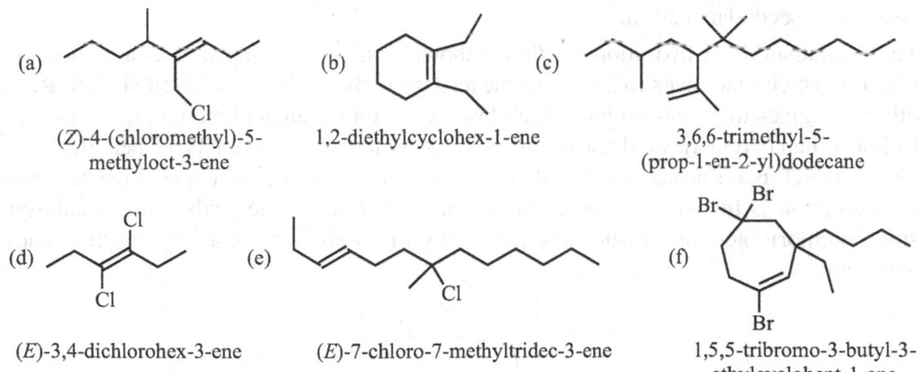

5. This is a Z alkene since the priority groups are Cl and ethyl. There are two identical groups (Et), however, on opposite sides of C=C, making it a trans- alkene.

6. (a) 5,9,9-trimethyldec-2-yne (b) 6-methylhept-1-yne (c) tridec-1-en-11-yne (d) 5-(1,1-dichloropropyl)-4-ethynyl-8-methyltetradecane (e) pent-1-yn-1-ylcyclohexane

(a) 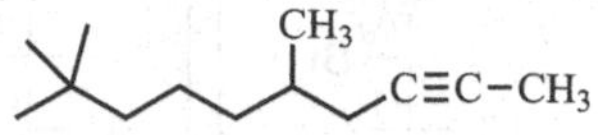 5,9,9-trimethyldec-2-yne

(b) 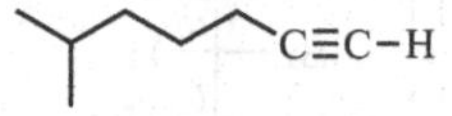 6-methylhept-1-yne

(c) 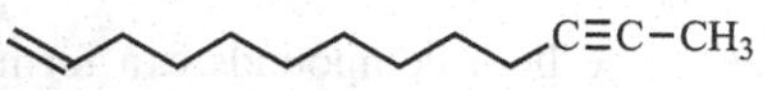 tridec-1-en-11-yne

(d) 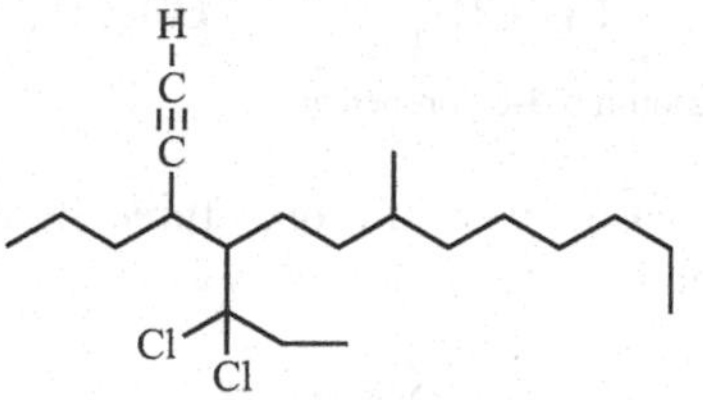 5-(1,1-dichloropropyl)-4-ethynyl-8-methyltetradecane

(e) 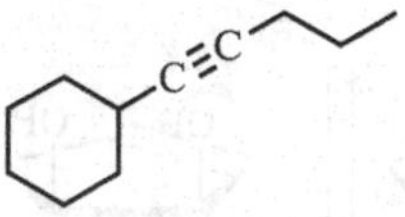 pent-1-yn-1-ylcyclohexane

7. The most acidic hydrogen is the O—H hydrogen (p$K_a \approx 4.5$) and that is removed much faster than the alkyne C—H (p$K_a \approx 25$).

8. (a) (b) 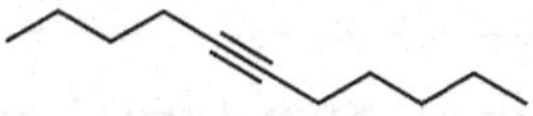 (c) No Reaction (d)

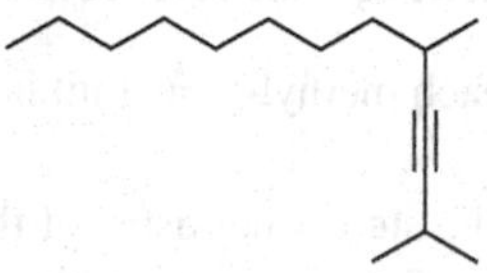

9. 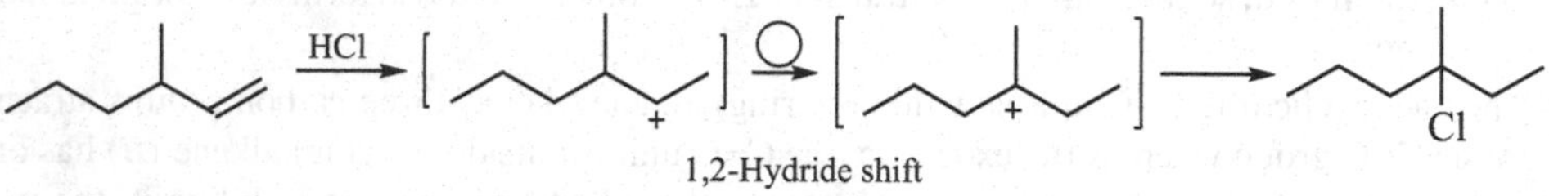 HCl

1,2-Hydride shift

10. When HCl reacts with 2-methylbut-2-ene, a tertiary cation is formed whereas reaction with but-1-ene gives a less stable secondary cation as the intermediate. The greater stability of the tertiary carbocation leads to a small energy of activation for formation of that carbocation, and therefore faster formation.

11. If a proton adds to C1, a tertiary cation is formed whereas addition of a proton to C2 generates a less stable secondary cation.

12. The mechanism of the hydration reaction is shown. Initial reaction generates a secondary carbocation, which rearranges to a more stable tertiary carbocation via a 1,2-ethyl shift. Reaction with water gives the oxonium ion, which loses a proton via an acid–base reaction to give the alcohol. When perchloric acid reacts with the C=C unit, the counterion is the perchlorate anion (ClO_4^-), which is resonance stabilized and not very nucleophilic. When HCl reacts similarly, the counterion is the nucleophilic chloride ion (Cl^-). Both of the acids act as a catalyst but using perchloric acid diminishes any possibility of by-products based on reaction with the counterion.

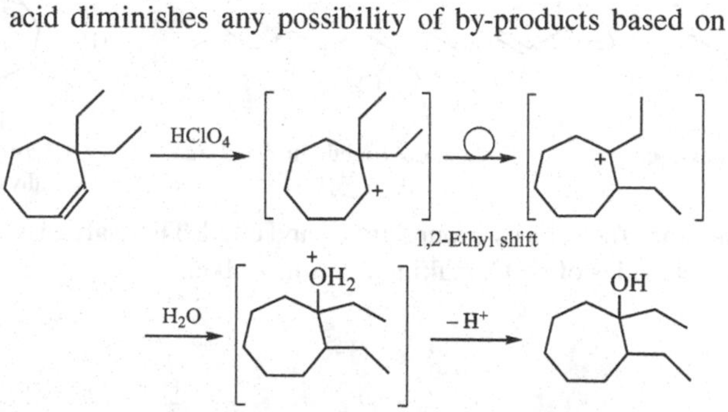

$HClO_4$

1,2-Ethyl shift

H_2O $-H^+$

13. When a molecule such as bromine (Br—Br) comes into close proximity to a polarized molecule, the negative pole will cause the electrons in the Br—Br bond to polarize. The Br closest to the negative pole will assume a δ^+ pole, making the other Br a δ^- pole. This phenomenon is known as an *induced dipole.*
14. When *trans*-but-2-ene reacts with I_2, the initially formed iodonium ion can be formed on the "top" or on the "bottom." Attack of the iodide counterion leads to a "trans-" diiodide. This molecule is a single diastereomer although it is racemic. *This diastereomer is the meso compound, not the* d,l *pair.* If *cis*-but-2-ene reacted with I_2, only the *d,l* diastereomer would be formed.
15. Initial reaction of the alkene with diatomic bromine gives a bromonium ion. Once the bromonium ion is formed, the nucleophile bromide ion will attack the less sterically hindered carbon in a substitution reaction.
16. (a) (b) (c) (d) (e) + (f) (g) (h)
17. (a) (b) (c) (d) (e) (f) (g) +
18. (a) (b) (c) (d) (e) (f)
19. $Hg(OAc)_2$ / EtOH → [$HgOAc$] → EtOH → [$HgOAc$] → $-H^+$ → $HgOAc$

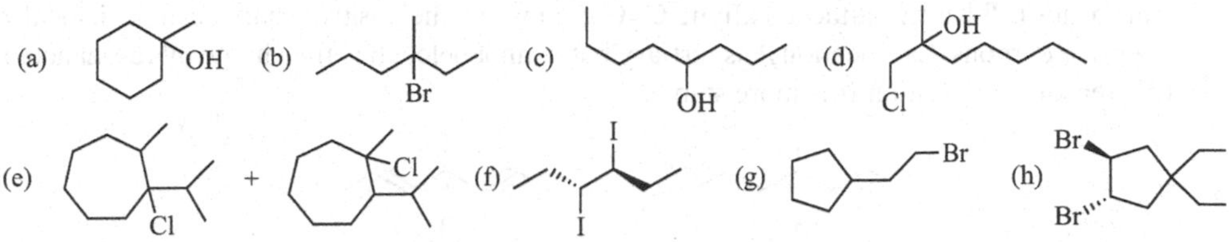

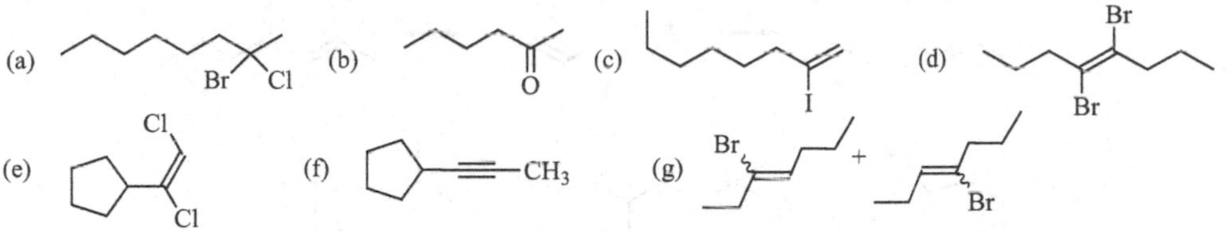

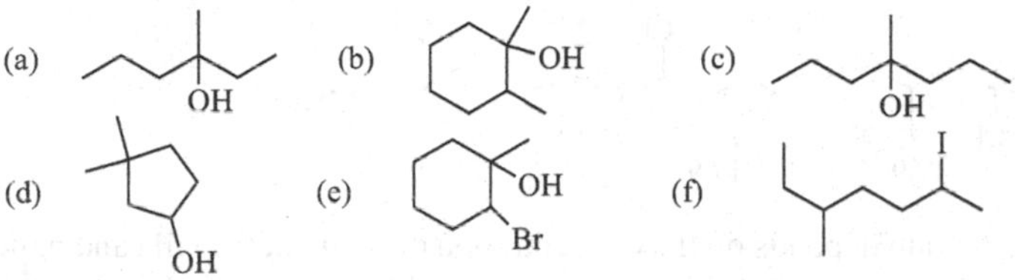

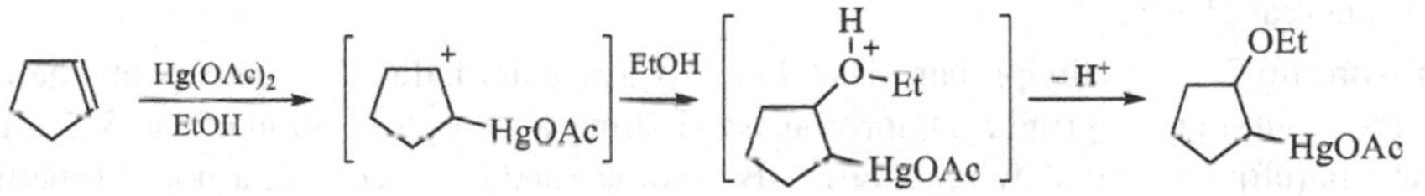

Chapter 8. Alkyl Halides and Substitution Reactions

1. (a) 1,1-dibromocyclopentane (b) 6-bromo-4-chloro-3,4-dimethyloctane (c) 9-cyclopentyl-8-(2-iodohexan-2-yl)-4,4-dimethylhexadecan-2-ol.

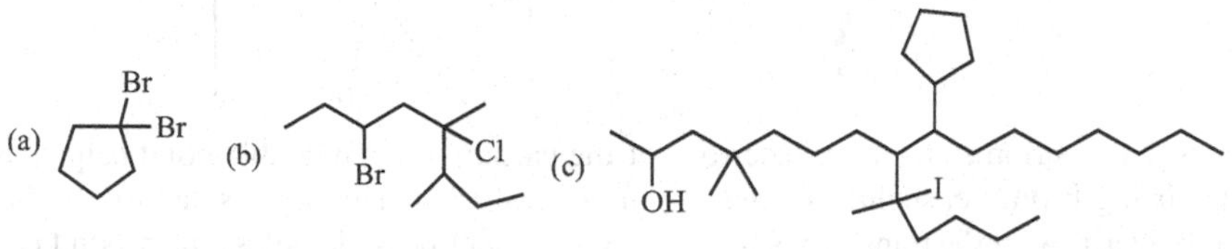

(a) 1,1-dibromo-cyclopentane

(b) 6-bromo-4-chloro-3,4-dimethyloctane

(c) 9-cyclopentyl-8-(2-iodohexan-2-yl)-4,4-dimethylhexadecan-2-ol

2.

(a)

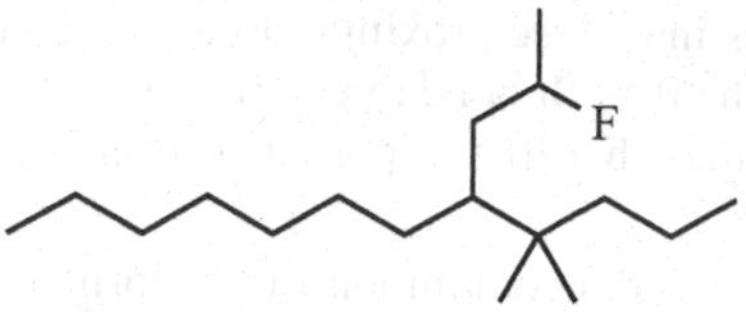

5-(2-fluoropropyl)-4,4-dimethyldodecane

(b)

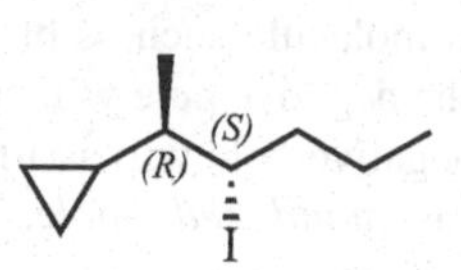

(2*R*)-cyclopropyl-(3*S*)-iodohexane

(c)

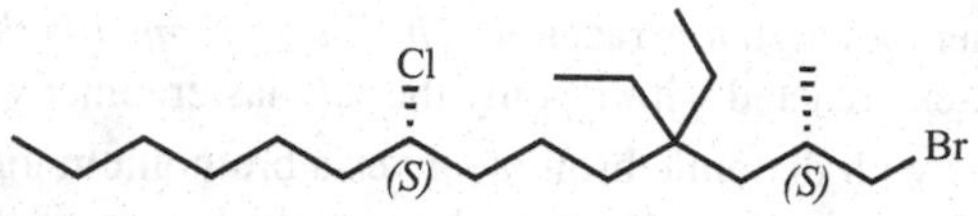

(2*S*,8*S*)-1-bromo-8-chloro-4,4-diethyl-2-methyltetradecane

3. Carbocation ***B*** has two attached allylic C=C groups and the positive charge can be delocalized over five carbons. Carbocation ***A*** is tertiary but cannot delocalize the charge by resonance. For this reason, carbocation ***B*** is more stable.

A **B**

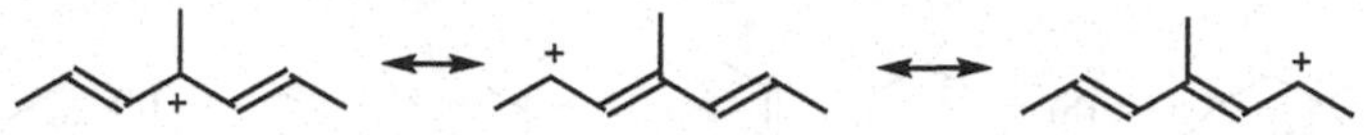

B

4.

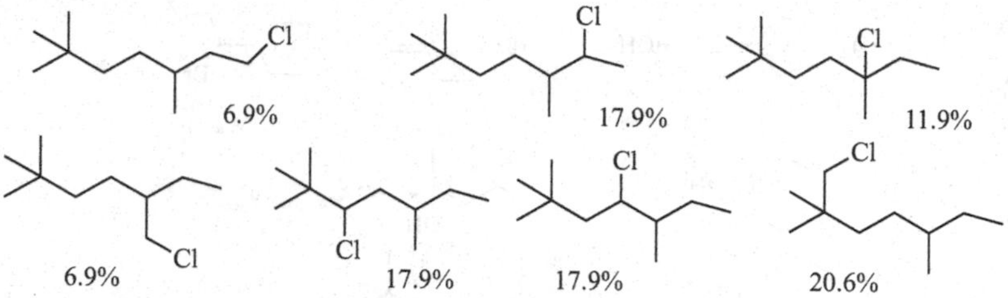

6.9% 17.9% 11.9%

6.9% 17.9% 17.9% 20.6%

5. This is a S_N2 reaction and the rate depends on the concentration of *both* nucleophile and halide. If the concentration of KI (the nucleophile) is increased 10-fold, the rate of the reaction is expected to increase by 10.
6. Although 1-bromo-2,2-dimethylpropane is technically a primary halide, it is a neopentyl halide and the large *t*-butyl group provides enormous steric hindrance to formation of the S_N2 transition state (therefore a very slow reaction). 1-Bromomethane is, of course, a normal methyl halide and reacts very fast.

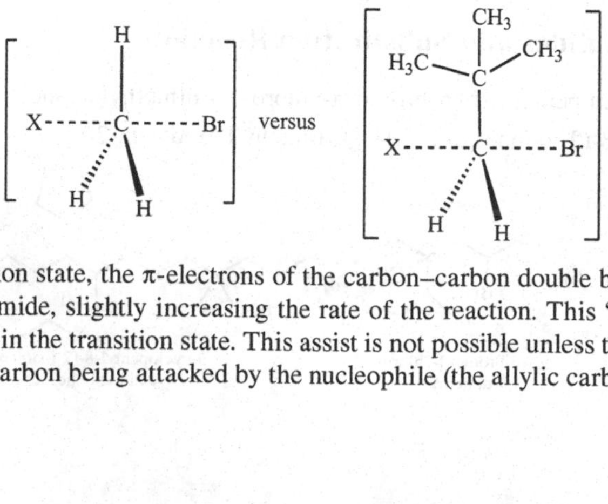

versus

7. In the S_N2 transition state, the π-electrons of the carbon–carbon double bond help "push out" the departing bromide, slightly increasing the rate of the reaction. This "assist" is illustrated by the blue arrow in the transition state. This assist is not possible unless the π-bond is in close proximity to the carbon being attacked by the nucleophile (the allylic carbon).

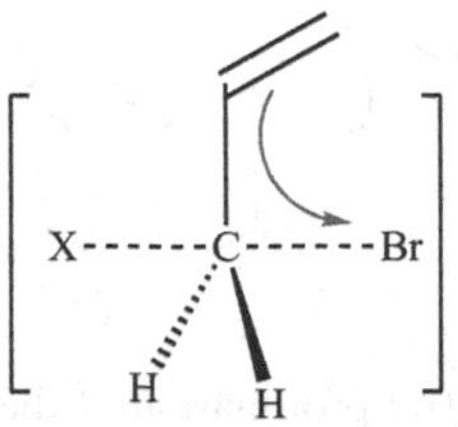

X------C------Br

H H

8. The S_N1 expression is: rate = k [RX]. Since the relative ratio of nucleophile to halide has no place in the rate expression (a first-order reaction), which means the reaction of the nucleophile with the carbocation is very fast relative to the initial ionization step, increasing the concentration has little or no effect. Increasing the concentration of the nucleophile will have no effect.
9. The energy required for the small hydrogen to migrate is less than for the larger methyl group. This energy difference is sufficient to make the H migrate is preference to the methyl.
10. The initially formed oxonium ion (by protonation of the OH) can either lose water to give the secondary cation (leading to a racemic mixture of chlorides) or have water displaced by chloride in an S_N2 reaction, giving the inverted chloride. The two are in competition but the cation reaction gives an equal mixture of inversion and retention and S_N2 gives only inversion. The inverted product must predominate if both processes are occurring. There may also be reaction of the nucleophile with the electrophilic carbon before the leaving group ($-OH_2^+$) has completely departed, which would favor more of the $S_N2$product.
11. (a) No Reaction (b) OH (c) N_3 (d) I (Racemic)

(e) Br (f) Cl Cl Cl Cl

(g) Br (h) CN (i) No Reaction (j) I

(k) C_5H_{11} (l) CN (m) CN (n) CN

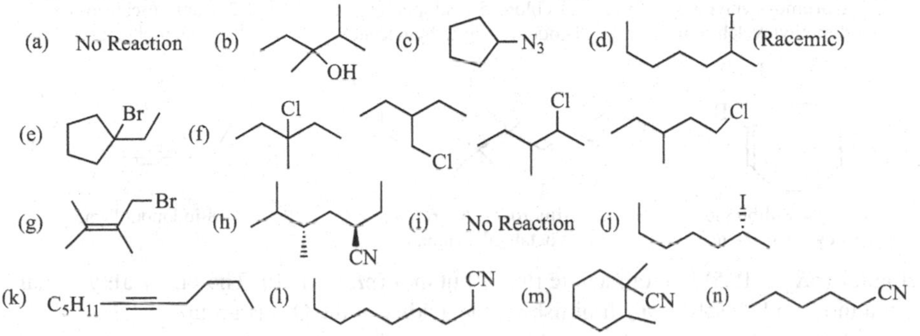

Reaction (f) shows four different chloride products (1-chloro-3-methylpentane, 2-chloro-3-methylpentane, 3-chloro-3-methylpentane and 1-chloro-2-ethylbutane), resulting from replacing each of the four different hydrogens. Reactions (a) and (i) give no reaction because they are tertiary halides under S_N^2 conditions.

12. (a) OH —HBr→ [$\overset{+}{O}H_2$] —$-H_2O$→ [+] —Br^-→ Br

(b) OH —HCl→ [$\overset{+}{O}H_2$] —$-H_2O$→ [+] —Cl^-→ Cl Racemic

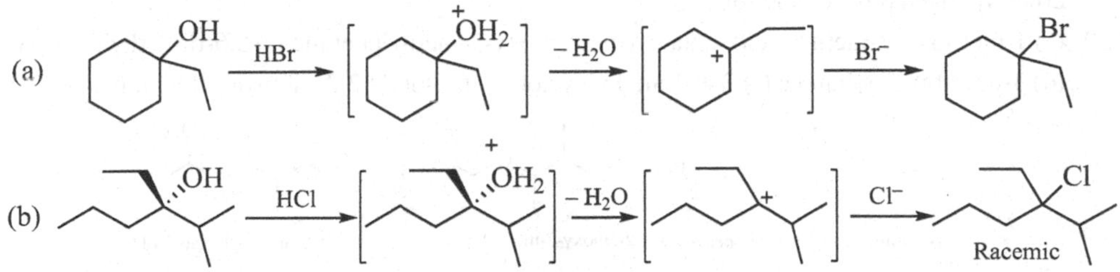

13. The basic oxygen of the alcohol reaction with the acidic hydrogen of HCl to form an *oxonium ion* (ROH_2^+). The energy required for this cation to ionize (by losing water) to form a primary cation is too high. The nucleophilic chloride displaces H_2O, which is a good leaving group, in a S_N2 reaction, giving 1-chloropentane as the product.

14. (a) (b) (c) (d) (e)

15. The initially formed oxonium ion (by protonation of the OH) can lose water to give the secondary carbocation leading to a racemic mixture of chlorides by a S_N1 reaction. Alternatively, once the oxonium ion is formed, water can be displaced by chloride in a S_N2 reaction giving the chloride with inversion of configuration. The two are in competition but the cation reaction gives an equal mixture of inversion and retention and S_N2 gives only inversion. The inverted product must predominate if both processes are in competition.

16. (a) 1-bromo-1-ethyl-3,3-dimethylcyclohexane (b) 3-chloro-5-cyclopentyl-7-iodo-4,9-dimethyldecane (c) 2-bromo-6-chloro-3,3-dimethylheptane (d) (*E*)-1,8-dibromocyclooct-1-ene (e) 1-fluoro-2,3,5,5,6,6,8,8-octamethylnonane (f) 8-iodonon-4-yne.

(a) 1-bromo-1-ethyl-3,3-dimethylcyclohexane (b) 3-chloro-5-cyclopentyl-7-iodo-4,9-dimethyldecane (c) 2-bromo-6-chloro-3,3-dimethylheptane

(d) (*E*)-1,8-dibromo-cyclooct-1-ene (e) 1-fluoro-2,3,5,5,6,6,8,8-octamethylnonane (f) 8-iodonon-4-yne

17. Methanol (pK_a = 15.5) is more acidic than *t*-butanol (pK_a = 19.0). The bulky alkyl groups in *tert*-butanol inhibits solvation, diminishing the acidity of the O—H group.

18. No! There is no possibility for overlap of the charge on oxygen with the π-bond of the alkene; the charge on oxygen is too far away from the C=C group (CH_2=$CHCH_2O^-$) for any delocalization of electron density from oxygen to the carbon atoms.

19. Since 2-methyl-2-iodopropane is a tertiary halide, a S_N2 reaction (required by the Williamson ether synthesis) is not possible.

20. (a) 1-methoxy-2-methylcyclopentane (b) 2-ethoxy-3-methylpentane (c) 5,6-dimethyloctan-3-ol (d) 1-(*tert*-butoxy)butane (e) 3,4-dimethylcyclohexan-1-ol (f) 2,2-diethylcyclobutan-1-ol.

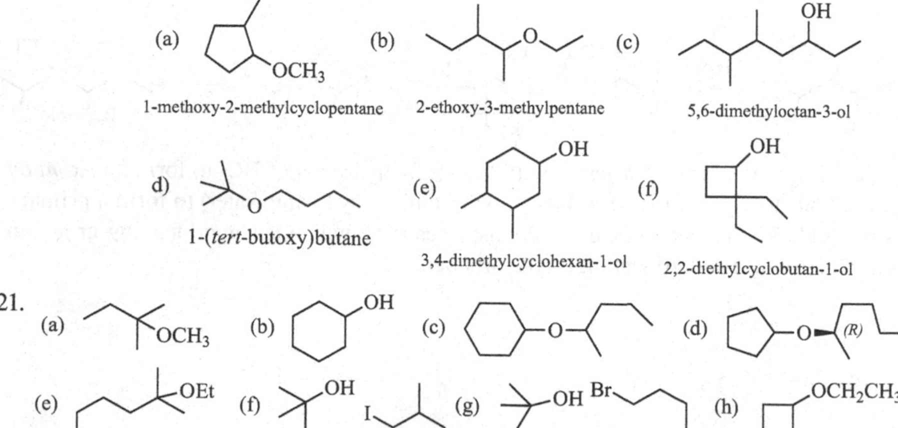

Chapter 9. Elimination Reactions

1. 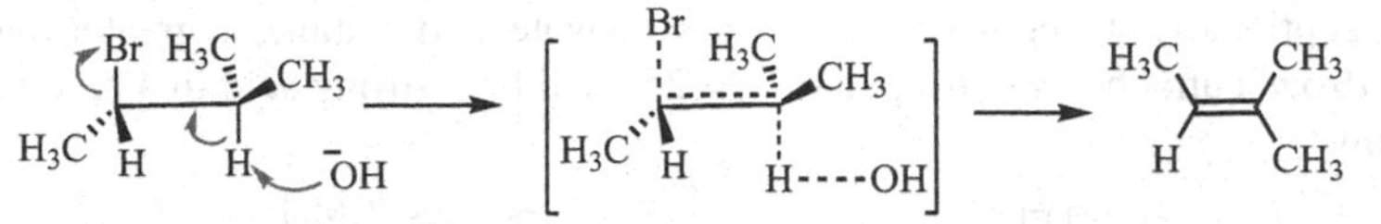 Br H_3C CH_3 H_3C H H $\bar{O}H$ → [Br H_3C CH_3 H_3C H H----OH] → H_3C CH_3 H CH_3

2. 3-Bromo-2,2,4,4-tetramethylpentane does not have a β-hydrogen atom relative to the bromine so there is no possibility of an E2. In addition, the bromine-bearing carbon is very sterically hindered, precluding any S_N2-type products.

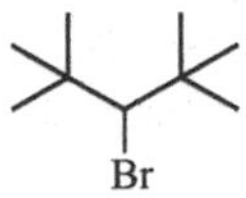

Br

3. (a) 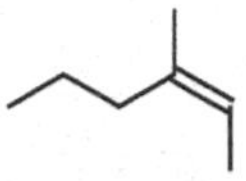 (b) (c) 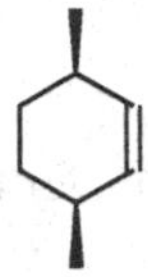 (d)

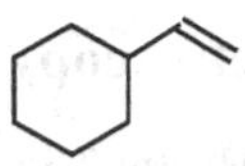

(e) 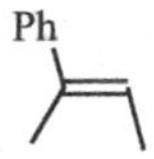 Ph (f) 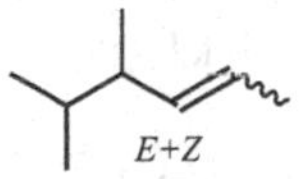 E+Z (g) 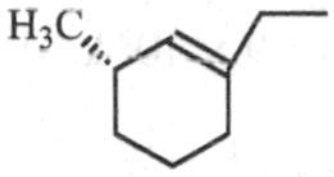 H_3C (h)

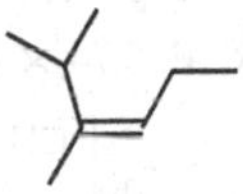

(i) 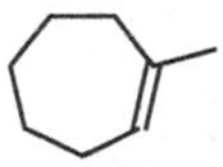 (j) 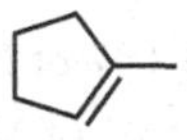 (k) 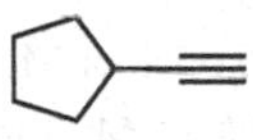 (l)

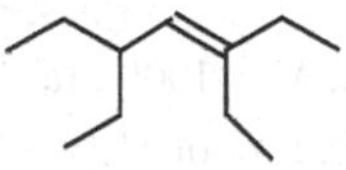

4. 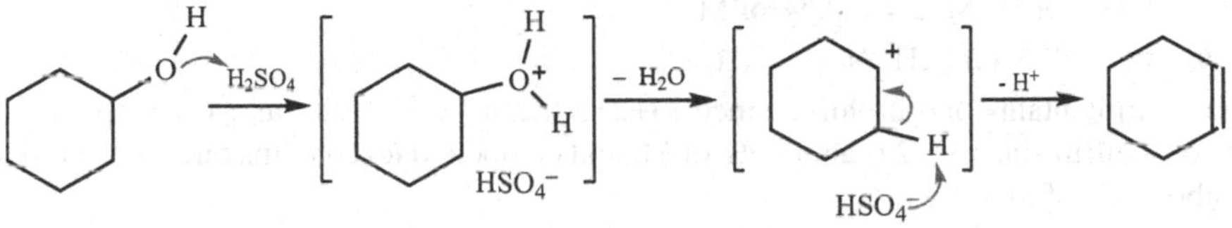 H O H_2SO_4 → [H O^+ H HSO_4^-] $- H_2O$ → [+ H HSO_4^-] $- H^+$ →

Chapter 10. Organometallic Compounds

1. Ethanol is a strong acid in the presence of the strongly basic Grignard reagent. Ethylmagnesium bromide will react with the ethanol solvent in an acid–base reaction to form ethane and the magnesium ethoxide faster than any other reaction.
2. Butyllithium is a powerful base, sufficiently strong to remove the weakly acidic hydrogen of an alkyne (pK_a of about 25). The conjugate acid of the reaction is the very weak conjugate acid, butane, which escapes from the medium and drives the reaction to the desired product. The butane does not interfere with isolation or further reactions of the alkyne anion product.

3. (a) 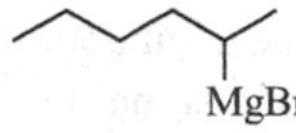 MgBr hexan-2-ylmagnesium bromide (b) 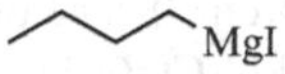 MgI butylmagnesium iodide (c) 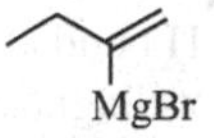 MgBr but-1-en-2-ylmagnesium bromide

(d) 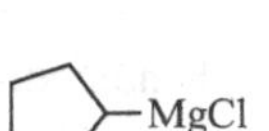 MgCl cyclopentylmagnesium chloride (e) 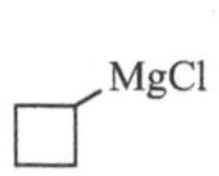 MgCl cyclobutylmagnesium chloride (f) 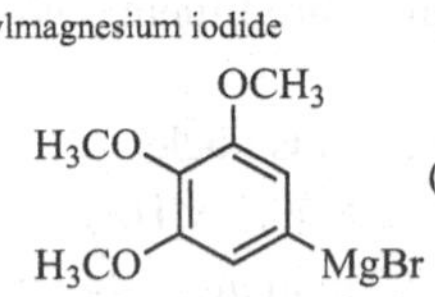 OCH_3 H_3CO H_3CO MgBr (3,4,5-trimethoxyphenyl)-magnesium bromide (g) 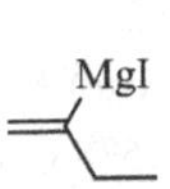 MgI but-1-en-2-yl-magnesium iodide

4. (a) $(\text{(CH}_3)_3\text{CCH}_2\text{CH}_2)_2\text{CuLi}$ (b) $(\text{pentyl})_2\text{CuLi}$ (c) $(\text{cyclohexyl})_2\text{CuLi}$ (d) $(\text{phenyl})_2\text{CuLi}$

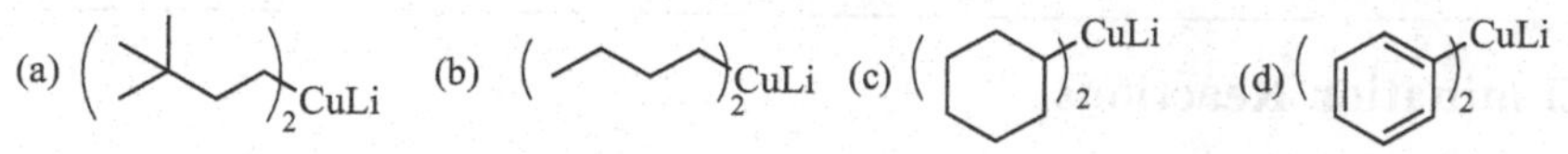

5. Butyllithium is an exceptionally strong base (pK_a of the conjugate acid, butane, is greater than 40) and an amine hydrogen attached to nitrogen (pK_a = 25) will be a strong acid in a reaction with an organolithium.

6. (a) [structure] (b) cyclohexyl–O^-Li^+ + pentane (c) naphthyl–MgI

(e) [structure]–Li (e) [structure] (f) [structure with Bu]

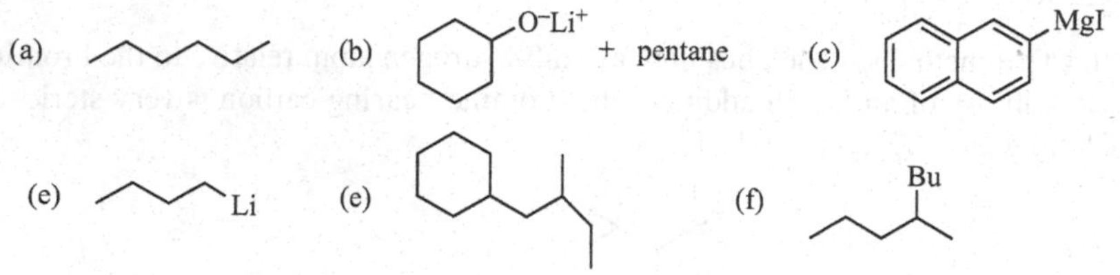

Chapter 11. Spectroscopy

1. (a) 6.16×10^{15} Hz. (b) 2.35×10^{-5} cm. (c) 4.34×10^{2} nm. (d) 3.8×10^{-4} μ. (e) 4.67×10^{7} Hz. (f) 6.09×10^{-2} m. (g) 1.14×10^{8}
2. (a) 1.61×10^{3} kcal, 6.74×10^{3} kJ. (b) 6.9×10^{2} kcal, 2.89×10^{3} kJ. (c) 52.2 eV. (d) 9.34 eV.
3. 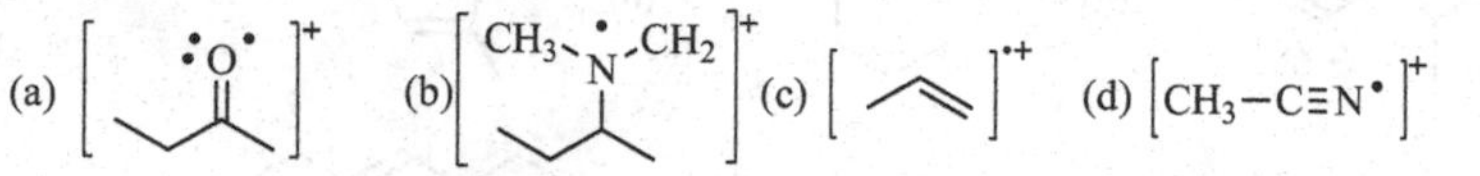 (a) [structure]$^{+}$ (b) $[CH_3\text{–}\dot{N}\text{–}CH_2 \ldots]^{+}$ (c) $[\text{[structure]}]^{\bullet+}$ (d) $[CH_3\text{–}C\equiv N^{\bullet}]^{+}$
4. In all cases, M = 100%. (a) M+1 = 5.55% of M, M+2 = 0.35% of M.
   (b) M+1 = 9.25% of M, M+2 = 0.39% of M. (c) M+1 = 5.55% of M, M+2 = 0.55% of M.
   (d) M+1 = 11.47% of M, M+2 = 0.82% of M.
5. (a) $C_8H_8O_2$ (b) $C_7H_{17}N$ (c) $C_5H_{12}N_2$ (d) $C_6H_{12}O$.
6. Compound (a) contains one bromine since M+2 is the same intensity as M. Compound (b) contains one sulfur since M+2 is about 5% of M, and compound (c) contains one chlorine since M+2 is about 1/3 of M.
7. (a) $-CH_3$ (b) $-H_2O$ (c) $-CH_2{=}CH_2$ (d) $-CH_2CH_3$ (e) $-C_3H_7$ (f) $-CO_2$.
8. Water can eventually dissolve pressed KBr. Brief exposure will "etch" or otherwise damage the surface of the plates, interfering with the transmission of light and the quality of the infrared absorption peaks. It also drastically reduces the lifetime of the plates.
9. A bending vibration describes a bond vibration in which the two atoms connected to the bond move "up and down" more or less in unison. A stretching vibration describes a bond vibration in which the two atoms connected to the bond move alternately away and toward each other, along the line between the two atoms (along the bond).
10. The strong but symmetrical C≡C bond gives a much less intense signal at higher energy. The C—O absorption band is also strong but appears at lower energy since it takes less energy to make that bond vibrate.
11. (a) The most prominent band is the carbonyl at 5.80 μ (1724 cm^{-1}). In (b) the most prominent band is the O-H band at about 2.8 μ (3571 cm^{-1}). The bromine in (c) appears at about 16 μ (625 cm^{-1}) but is not diagnostic. The OH band of COOH is a broad and strong signal between 3–4 μ (3333–2500 cm^{-1}) and is the most prominent, and the carbonyl band at 5.80 μ (1724 cm^{-1}) is also diagnostic.
12. (a) 3 (b) 1 (c) 1 (d) 1 (e) 1 (f) none – this nucleus does not lead to the NMR phenomenon.
13. (a) 122.5 MHz. (b) 538.6 MHz. (c) 1273.3 MHz.
14. (a) 5.21 ppm. (b) 16.39 ppm. (c) 7.2 ppm. (d) 4.24 ppm.

15. (a) HC-NR_2 (b) H-C-C=O (c) C=C-C-H (d) C≡C-H

16.

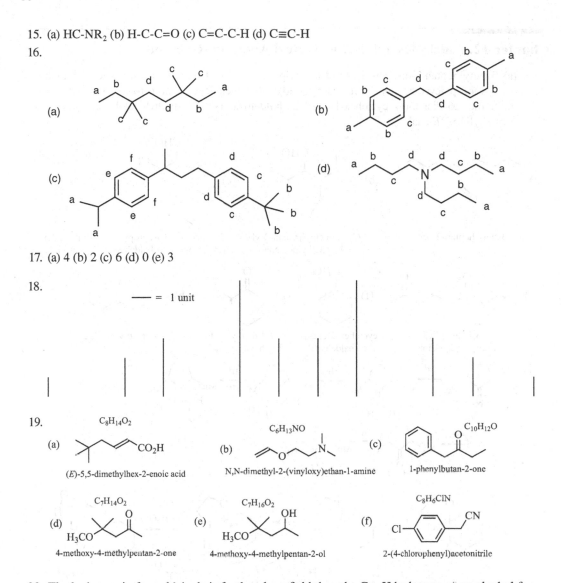

(a) 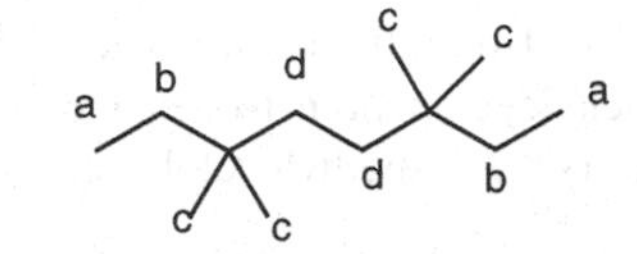 (b)

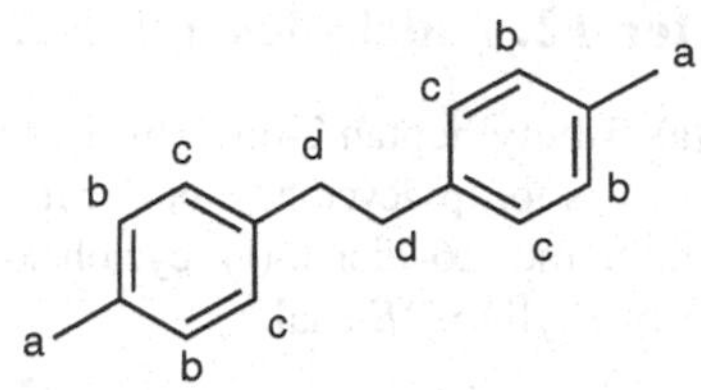

(c) 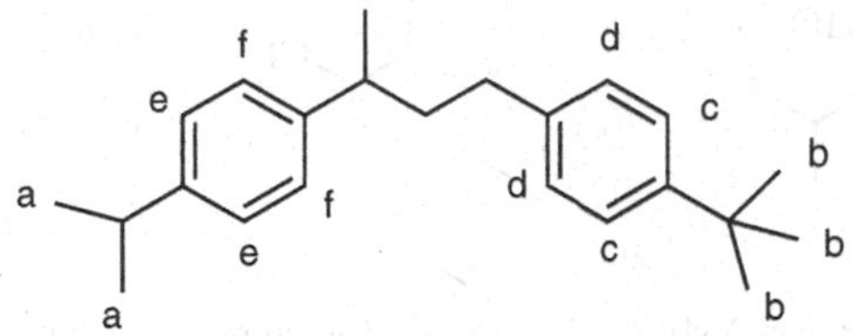 (d)

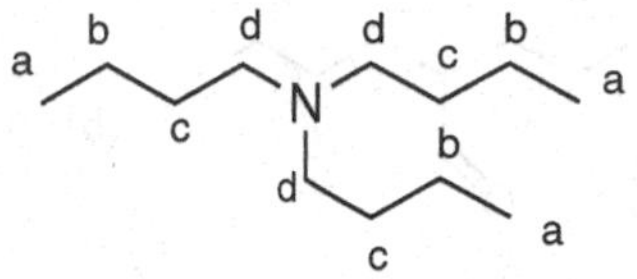

17. (a) 4 (b) 2 (c) 6 (d) 0 (e) 3

18.

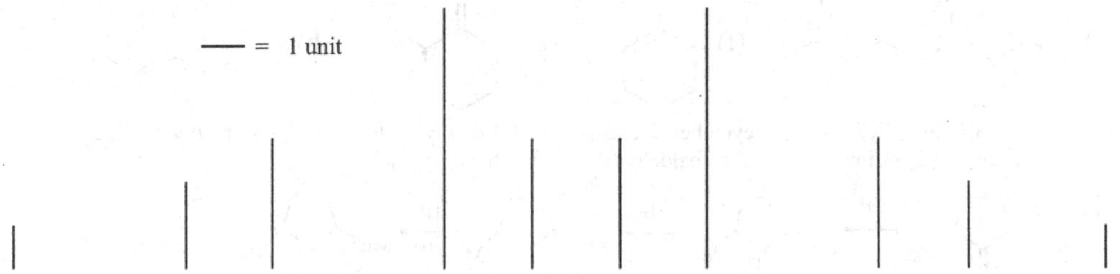

— = 1 unit

19.

(a) $C_8H_{14}O_2$

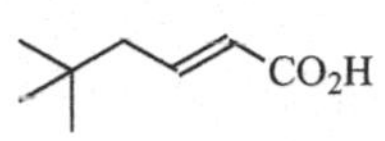

CO_2H

(*E*)-5,5-dimethylhex-2-enoic acid

(b) $C_6H_{13}NO$

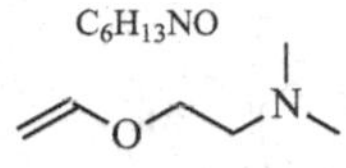

N,N-dimethyl-2-(vinyloxy)ethan-1-amine

(c) $C_{10}H_{12}O$

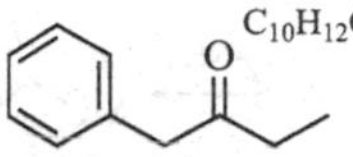

1-phenylbutan-2-one

(d) $C_7H_{14}O_2$

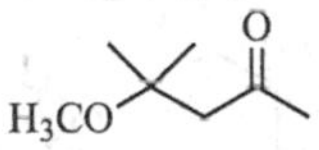

H_3CO

4-methoxy-4-methylpentan-2-one

(e) $C_7H_{16}O_2$

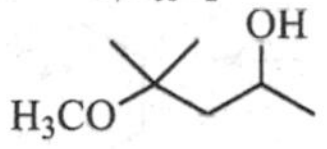

H_3CO OH

4-methoxy-4-methylpentan-2-ol

(f) C_8H_6ClN

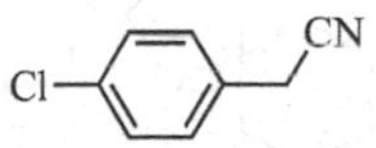

Cl CN

2-(4-chlorophenyl)acetonitrile

20. The hydrogen in formaldehyde is further downfield than the C—H hydrogen of an alcohol for two reasons. First, the proximity to the electron-withdrawing oxygen shifts the aldehyde hydrogen downfield. However, the π-bond of the carbonyl sets up a secondary field and the aldehyde hydrogen is shifted downfield due to magnetic anisotropy.

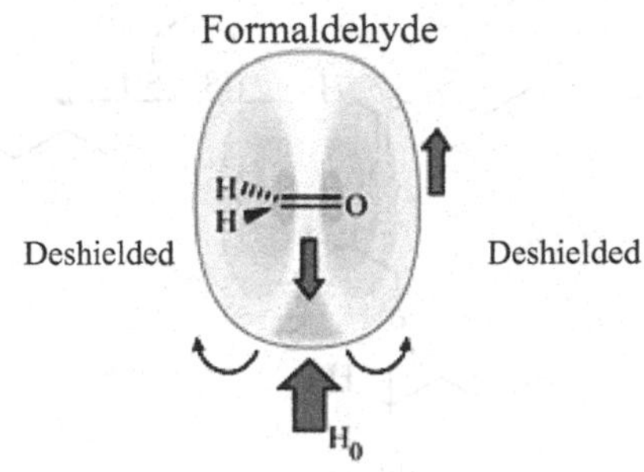

Chapter 12. Aldehydes and Ketones. Acyl Addition Reactions

1. (a) 3-butylheptan-2-one (b) 2-(2,4-dimethylpentan-3-yl)-3,4-dimethylpentanal (c) 2,5-dichloro-4-isopropylcyclohexane-1-carbaldehyde (d) 3,4-diphenylcyclopentan-1-one (e) 5,5-dimethylnonane-2,6-dione (f) cyclohex-1-ene-1-carbaldehyde (g) 2,2-diethylcyclohexan-1-one (h) 3-methylhex-2*E*-enal.

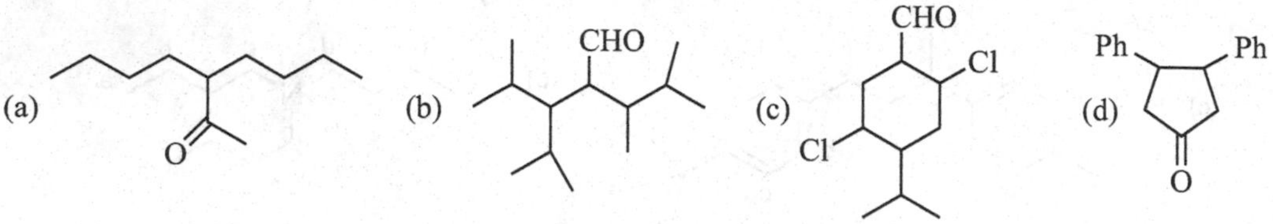

(a) 3-butylheptan-2-one (b) 2-(2,4-dimethylpentan-3-yl)-3,4-dimethylpentanal (c) 2,5-dichloro-4-isopropylcyclohexane-1-carbaldehyde (d) 3,4-diphenylcyclopentan-1-one

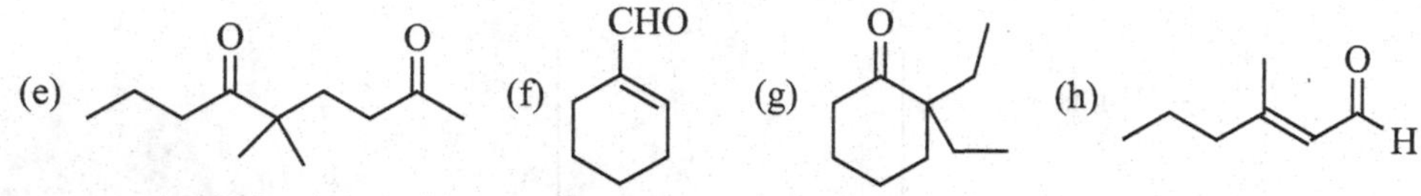

(e) 5,5-dimethylnonane-2,6-dione (f) cyclohex-1-ene-1-carbaldehyde (g) 2,2-diethylcyclohexan-1-one (h) (*E*)-3-methylhex-2-enal

2. H^+; $+ H_2O$; $-H^+$ / $+H^+$; $-NH_3$; $-H^+$

3.

(a) $+ H^+$; $+ H_2O$; $- H^+$; $+ H^+$; $- HOCH_2CH_2OH$; $- H^+$

(b) $+ H^+$; HS SH; $- H^+$; $+ H^+$; $- H_2O$; $- H^+$

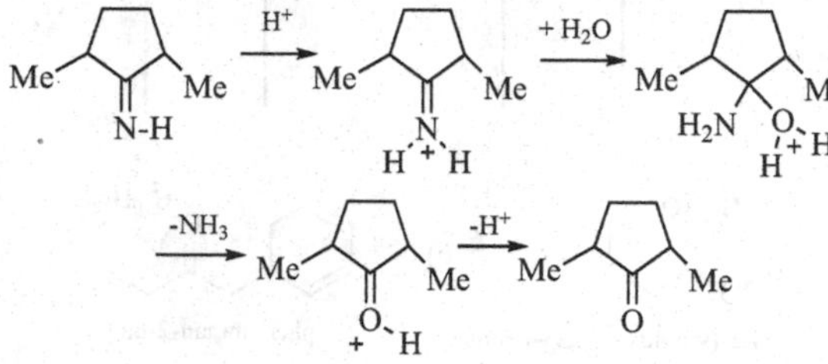

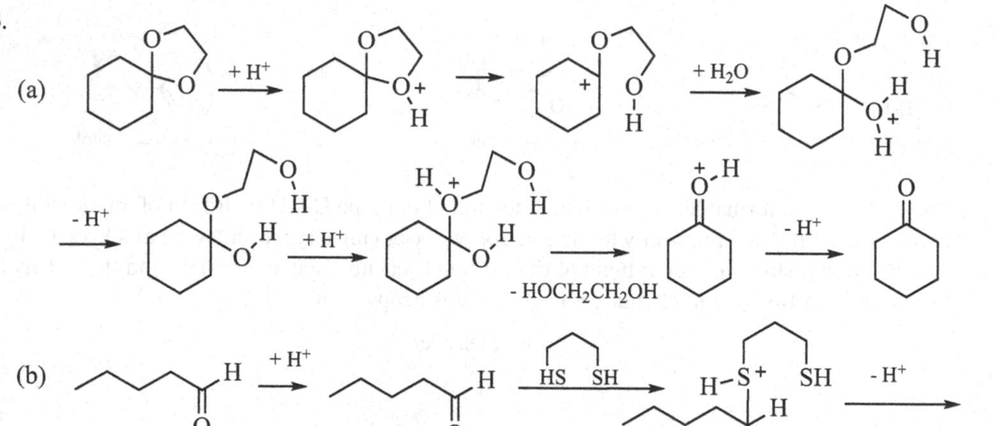

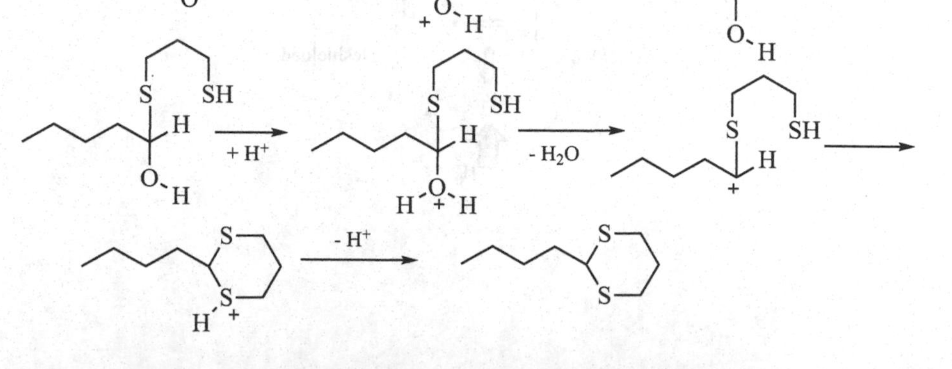

4. The initial product is an enol, which tautomerizes to the ketone, the isolated product.

5.

1,3-dioxane 1,3-dioxolane 1,3-dithiane 1,3-dithiolane

6.

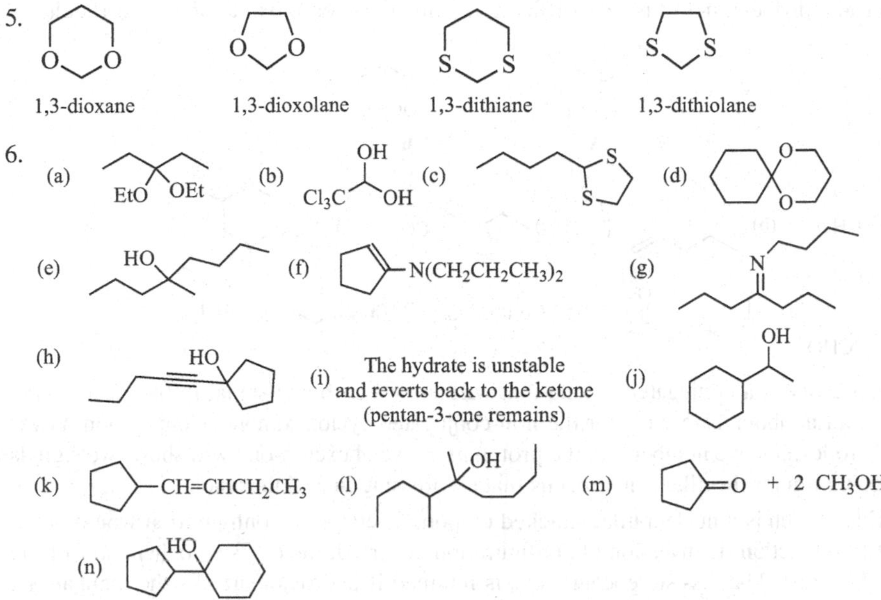

7. The reaction of triethylphosphine and 1-bromobutane will give phosphonium salt ***A***. When reacted with butyllithium to form the ylid, however, the most available, least hindered hydrogen will be removed, which is one of the hydrogen atoms on an ethyl group, which will give an ylid. If the goal is to transfer the butyl group, this ylid will not work since the ethyl group will be transferred instead. The reason why triphenylphosphine is used is because the hydrogen atoms on the alkyl halide group, here butyl, will be removed so the phosphonium salt will be converted to the ylid that will transfer the group of interest, here butyl.

BuLi **A** **B**

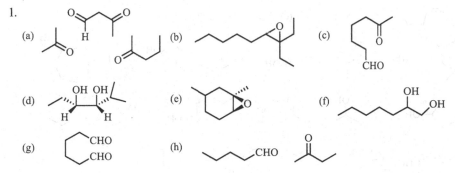

Chapter 13. Oxidation Reactions

1.

(a) (b) (c) CHO (d) OH OH H H (e) O (f) OH OH (g) CHO CHO (h) CHO O

2. Both alcohols form a chromate ester. A problem arises in the chromate ester of 2,2,4,4-tetramethylpentan-3-ol, ***A***, where the α-hydrogen atom to be removed by water (in light gray) is very sterically hindered. Therefore, generation of the ketone is much slower than removal of the α-hydrogen (in light gray) from the chromate ester formed by pentan-3-ol, ***B***. In other words,

approach of water to the sterically hindered hydrogen of the chromate ester derived from 2,2,4,4-tetramethylpentan-3-ol is very difficult, making the overall oxidation very difficult.

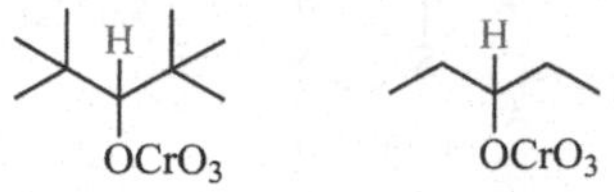

H H
$OCrO_3$ $OCrO_3$
A **B**

3.
(a) 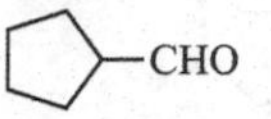 CHO (b) 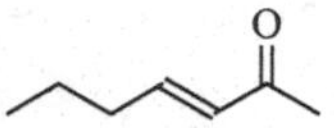 O (c) 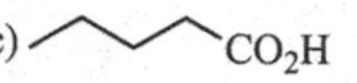 CO_2H (d) 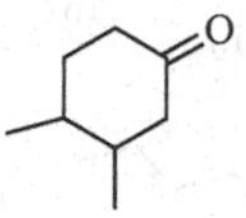 O
(e) 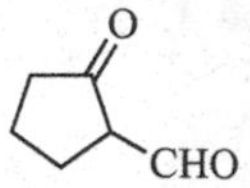 O CHO (f) 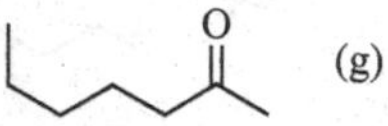 O (g) No Reaction (h) CHO

4. Cyclohexen-2-one is a conjugated ketone that will show a carbonyl signal in the IR at 1665–1685 cm^{-1} but at about 1715 cm^{-1} for the non-conjugated cyclohexanone. Conjugation moves the signals to lower wave numbers. In the proton nmr, cyclohexen-2-one will show two signals between 5–6 ppm for the alkene hydrogens that are missing in cyclohexanone.
5. If hydroxide, which is a nucleophile, attacked carbon, inversion of configuration would occur via a S_N2-like reaction. If inversion of configuration occurred, the cis- stereochemistry of the diol would be lost. The cis- stereochemistry is retained if hydroxide attacks the manganese, leaving the stereochemistry at carbon untouched.
6. The by-product of the epoxidation is a carboxylic acid which acidifies the reaction medium. Epoxides are reactive and in the presence of a Brønsted–Lowry acid in aqueous media will open to generate 1,2-diols. The sodium acetate acts as a buffer to prevent the reaction medium from becoming too acidic, and thereby preventing or minimizing deleterious reactions of the target product, which is the epoxide.
7. The disubstituted alkene is more electron rich and therefore a better electron donor than the monosubstituted alkene. Therefore, the reaction of the disubstituted alkene with peroxyacetic acid is faster. Remember that the alkene reacts with the electrophilic oxygen of the peroxy acid, so the more electron rich the alkene, the faster the reaction. A tetrasubstituted alkene is expected to react faster than a trisubstituted alkene, which reacts faster than a disubstituted alkene such as pent-2-ene, and a monosubstituted alkene such as pent-1-ene should be the least reactive of all.

Chapter 14. Reduction Reactions

1. (a) 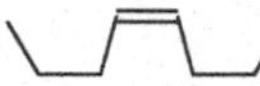 (b) N.R. (c) 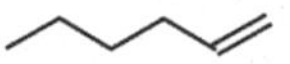
2.
(a) 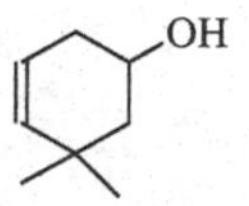 OH (b) 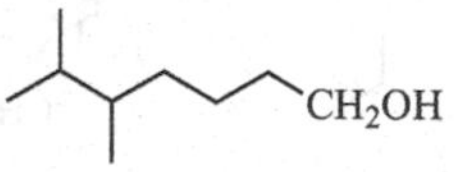 CH_2OH (c) 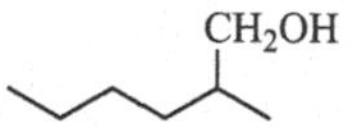 CH_2OH (d) 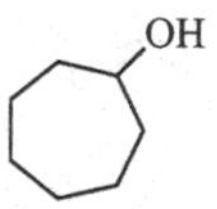 OH
(e) 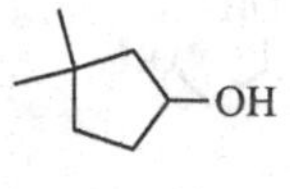 OH (f) 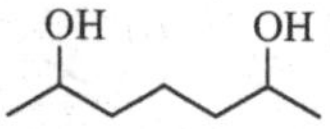 OH OH (g) 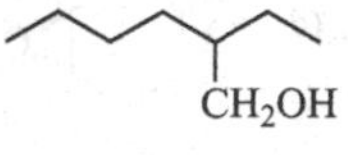 CH_2OH (h) 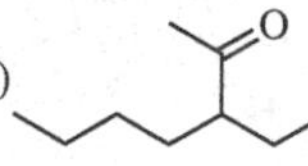 O

3. 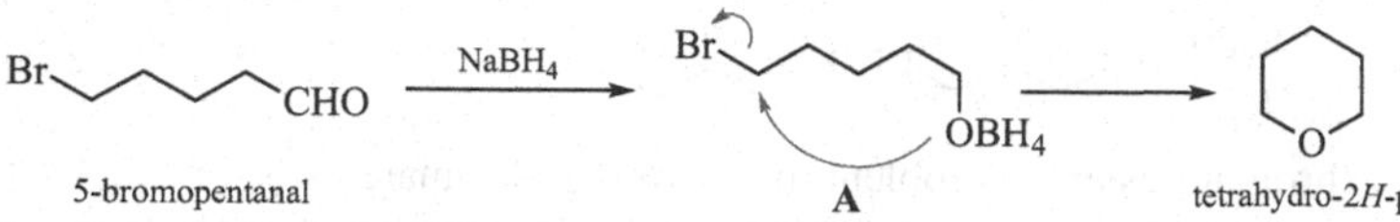
Br CHO → $NaBH_4$ → Br OBH_4 → O
5-bromopentanal **A** tetrahydro-2*H*-pyran

The initial reaction with $NaBH_4$ leads to the alkoxyborate *A*. Since the alkoxide is nucleophilic, an internal S_N2 reaction displaces the bromine to give the cyclic ether, tetrahydro-2*H*-pyran.

4.

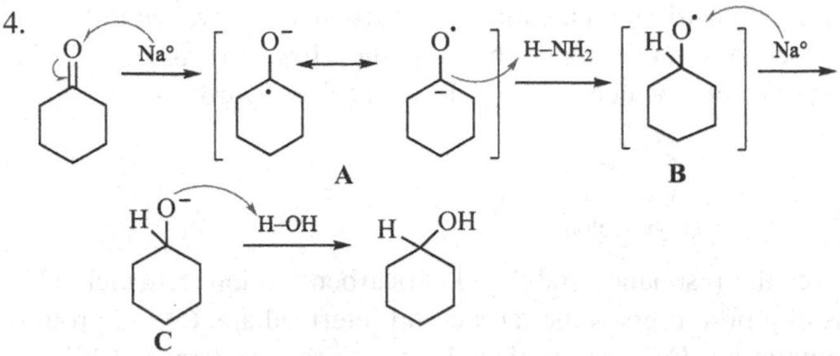

A B

C

The initial electron transfer from sodium to the ketone gives ketyl ***A***. In this medium, the ammonia reacts as an acid with the strong base (the carbanion resonance contributor of ***A***) to give radical ***B***. A second electron transfer from sodium gives alkoxide ***C***. In the second step, the alkoxide reacts with water to give cyclhexanol.

Chapter 15. Carboxylic Acids, Carboxylic Acid Derivatives, and Acyl Substitution Reactions

1. (a) 4-ethyl-2-(pentan-2-yl)heptanoic acid (b) 3,4,5-trimethylcyclohexane-l-carboxylic acid (c) 5,5-dichloro-2-methyl-7-phenylheptanoic acid (d) hex-2-ynoic acid (e) 4-methylhex-3*E*-enoic acid
   (f) 2-ethylhept-6-ynoic acid (g) 3-butyl-6-ethyl-2-pentyldecanoic acid.

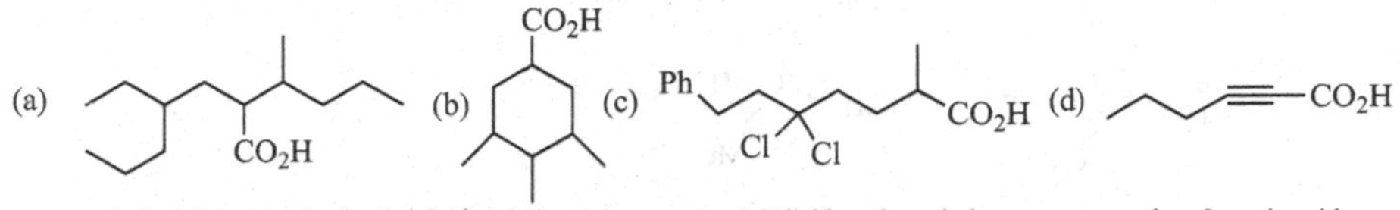

(a) 4-ethyl-2-(pentan-2-yl)-heptanoic acid (b) 3,4,5-trimethylcyclohexane-1-carboxylic acid (c) 5,5-dichloro-2-methyl-7-phenylheptanoic acid (d) hex-2-ynoic acid

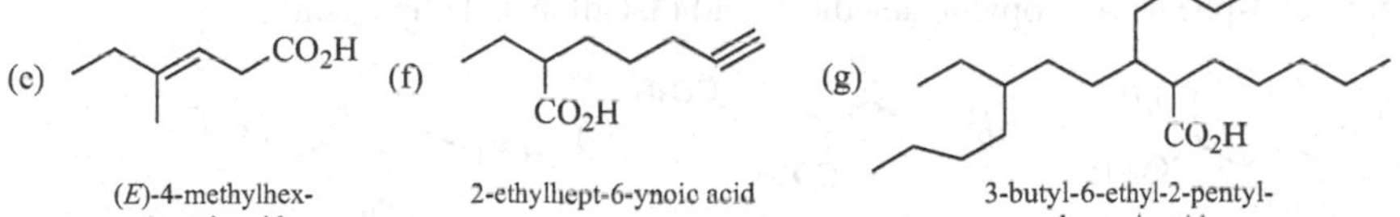

(e) (*E*)-4-methylhex-3-enoic acid (f) 2-ethylhept-6-ynoic acid (g) 3-butyl-6-ethyl-2-pentyl-decanoic acid

2. The strongest acid is 2-chlorohexanoic acid, where the Cl is closest to the carboxyl group. With this isomer, a pseudo five-membered ring through-space interaction is possible, which is more effective relative to the other chloroacids, as shown in the figure.

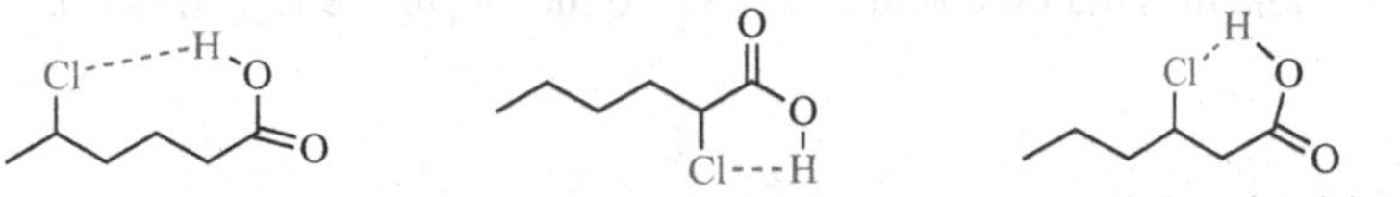

pseudo 8-membered ring pseudo 5-membered ring pseudo 6-membered ring

3.

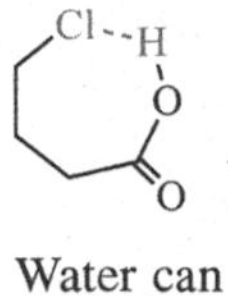

4. Water can solvate the two ions that are formed (H_3O^+ and acetate) much better than ethanol. Such solvation shifts the equilibrium toward the solvated ions, meaning there is greater ionization of the acid, which makes it stronger.

5. When the OH of an acid is in the C4 position, it can attack the carbonyl and cyclize to form a lactone. Indeed, the cyclized molecule is more stable than the uncyclized hydroxy acid. The product of this reaction is γ-butyrolactone, which does not have an acidic hydrogen.

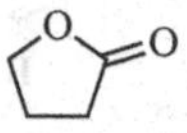

γ-butyrolactone

6. Protonation of the carbonyl gives the resonance stabilized oxocarbenium ion ***A***, which adds water to give oxonium ***B***. Loss of a proton gives the tetrahedral intermediate, ***C***, and protonation of the OEt unit gives oxonium ion ***D***. Loss of ethanol leads to the resonance-stabilized oxonium ion ***E***, and loss of a proton gives the product, 2-methylpentanoic acid.

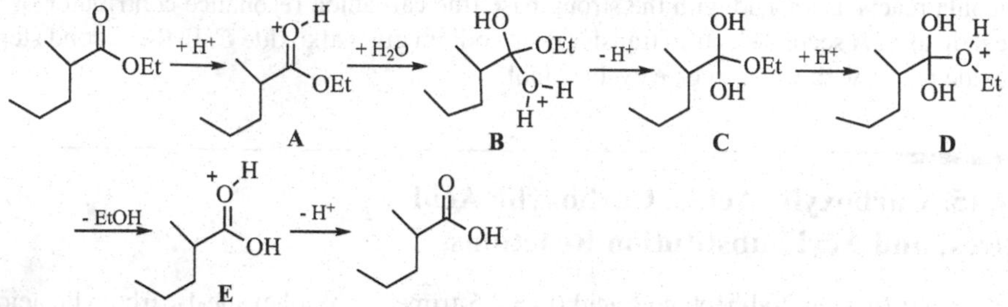

7.

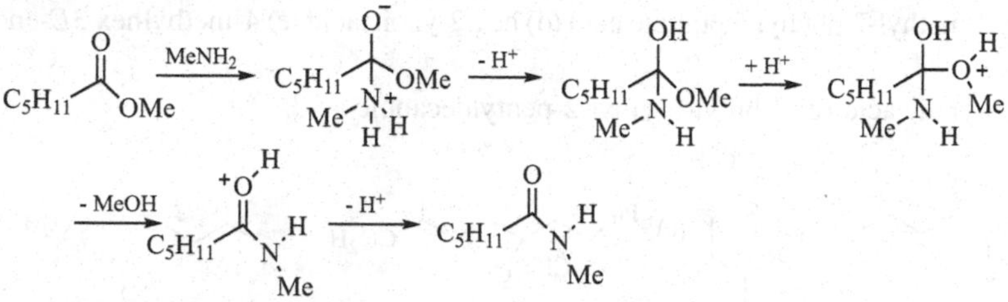

8. (a) 2-propylpropanedioc acid (2-propylmalonic acid) (b) 2-ethylpentanedioic acid (2-ethylsuccinic acid) (c) 3-phenyl-4-propylhexanedioic acid (3,4-diphenyladipic acid).

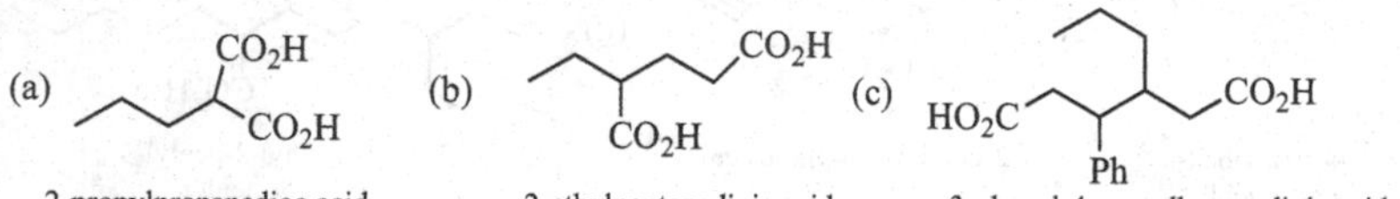

(a) 2-propylpropanedioc acid (2-propylmalonic acid)

(b) 2-ethylpentanedioic acid (2-ethylsucciic acid)

(c) 3-phenyl-4-propylhexanedioic acid (3-phenyl-4-propyladipic acid)

9. The first pK_a of malonic acid (2.83) is lower (stronger acid) because the electron-withdrawing carboxyl group is closer to the first carboxyl group. The first pK_a of glutaric acid (4.34) shows that it is less acidic than malonic acid and closer to the pK_a of acetic acid (4.75).

10.

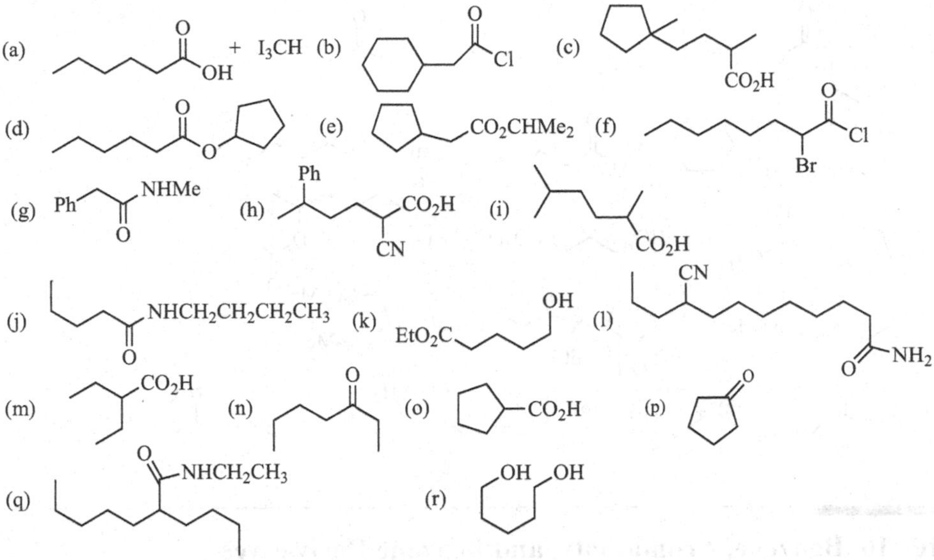

(a) + I_3CH (b) Cl (c) CO_2H

(d) (e) CO_2CHMe_2 (f) Cl Br

(g) Ph NHMe (h) Ph CO_2H CN (i) CO_2H

(j) $NHCH_2CH_2CH_2CH_3$ (k) EtO_2C OH (l) CN NH_2

(m) CO_2H (n) (o) CO_2H (p)

(q) $NHCH_2CH_3$ (r) OH OH

11.

$C_5H_{11}C(=O)OCH_3$ $\xrightarrow{+H^+}$ $C_5H_{11}C(=O^+H)OCH_3$ $\xrightarrow{+H_2O}$ $C_5H_{11}C(OH)(OCH_3)(O^+H_2)$ $\xrightarrow{-H^+}$ $C_5H_{11}C(OH)_2OCH_3$

$\xrightarrow{+H^+}$ $C_5H_{11}C(OH)_2O^+(H)CH_3$ $\xrightarrow{-MeOH}$ $C_5H_{11}C(=O^+H)OH$ $\xrightarrow{-H^+}$ $C_5H_{11}C(=O)OH$

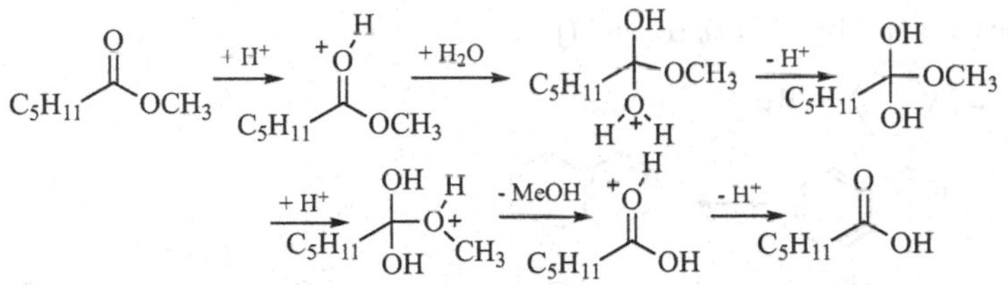

12. The OR unit of an ester is a better leaving group than a NR_2 unit of an amide, so a tetrahedral intermediate for an ester will lose OR faster than the tetrahedral intermediate for an amide will lose NR_2.

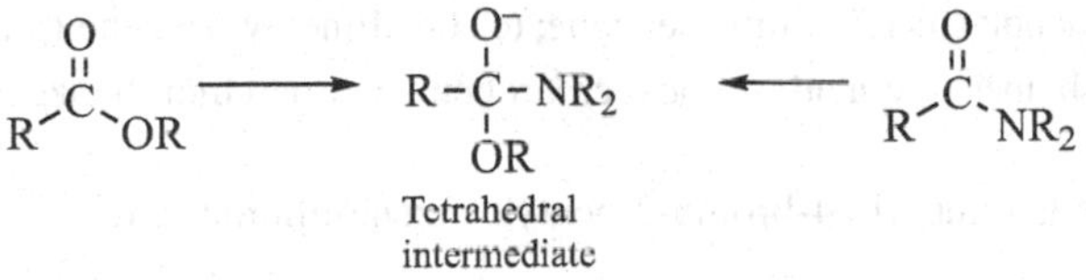

$R-C(=O)-OR$ $\longrightarrow$ $R-C(O^-)(OR)-NR_2$ $\longleftarrow$ $R-C(=O)-NR_2$

Tetrahedral intermediate

13.

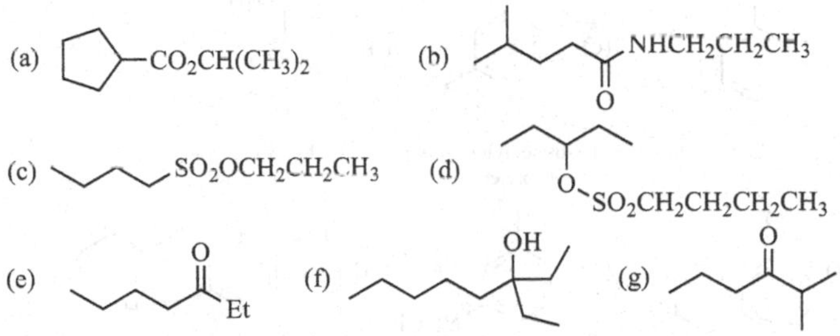

(a) $CO_2CH(CH_3)_2$ (b) $NHCH_2CH_2CH_3$

(c) $SO_2OCH_2CH_2CH_3$ (d) $O-SO_2CH_2CH_2CH_2CH_3$

(e) Et (f) OH (g)

14. The initial product is a ketone, which is more reactive than the ester starting material, and the ketone reacts further with the Grignard reagent to give the alcohol.

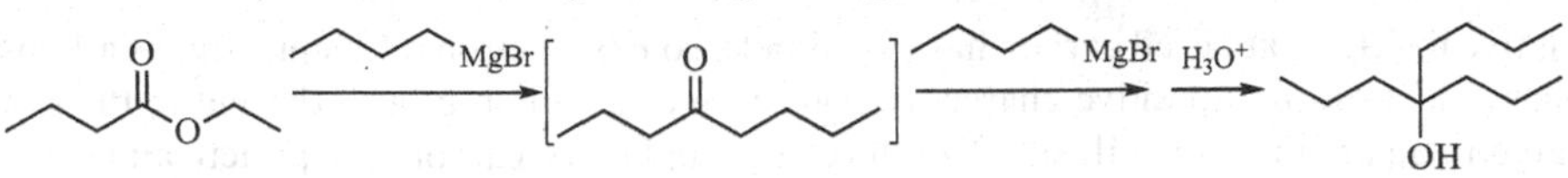

MgBr MgBr H_3O^+ OH

15. (a) (b) CN (c) (d) CO_2H CO_2H (e) (f) NH_2 (g) CH_3 (h) HO CO_2Et (i) (j) CO_2Me (k) N Et (l) CO_2Me CO_2Me (m) $NHCH_3$ (n) OH OH (o) CO_2NH_2 (p) NH_2

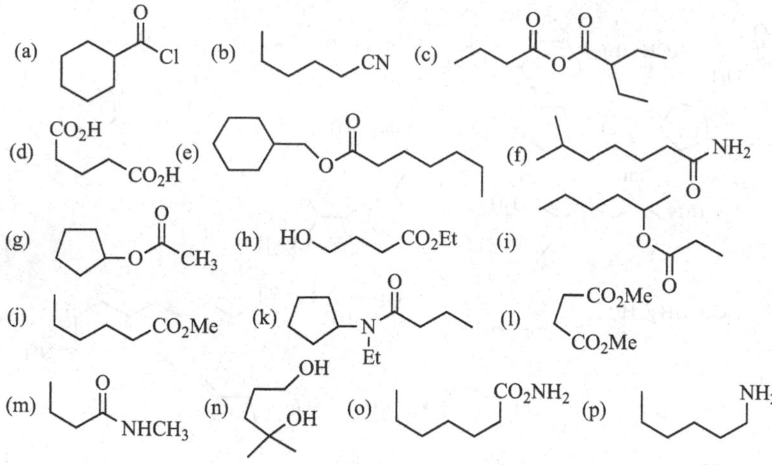

Chapter 16. Benzene, Aromaticity, and Benzene Derivatives

1. The aromatic molecules are (a), (b), (d), (h), (i), and (j).
2. (a) $-CH_3$ ⟷ $-CH_3$
(b)
(c)

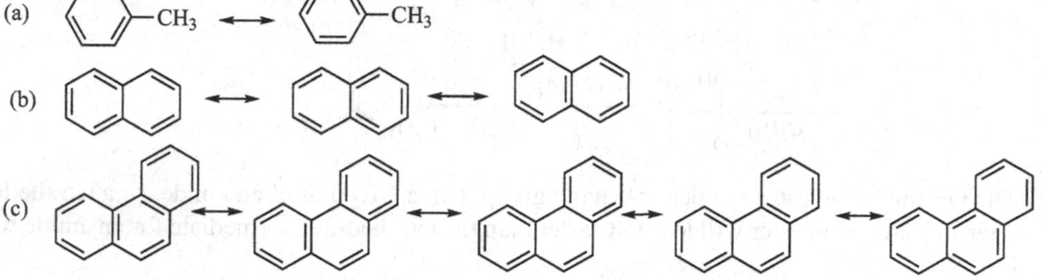

3. (a) 3,5-dichlorophenol; (b) 1,3-dinitrobenzene; (c) 1,4-dimethylbenzene (*para*-xylene); (d) 3-ethyl-5-methylbenzoic acid; (e) hexachlorobenzene (perchlorobenzene); (f) 3-(2-methylbutyl)phenol;
(g) *N*,3,5-trimethylaniline. (h) 4-bromo-2-pentylbenzenesulfonic acid.

(a) 3,5-dichlorophenol (b) 1,3-dinitrobenzene (c) 1,4-dimethylbenzene (*p*-xylene) (d) 3-ethyl-5-methylbenzoic acid

(e) hexachlorobenzene (perchlorobenzene) (f) 3-(2-methylbutyl)phenol (g) *N*,3,5-trimethylaniline (h) 4-bromo-2-pentylbenzenesulfonic acid

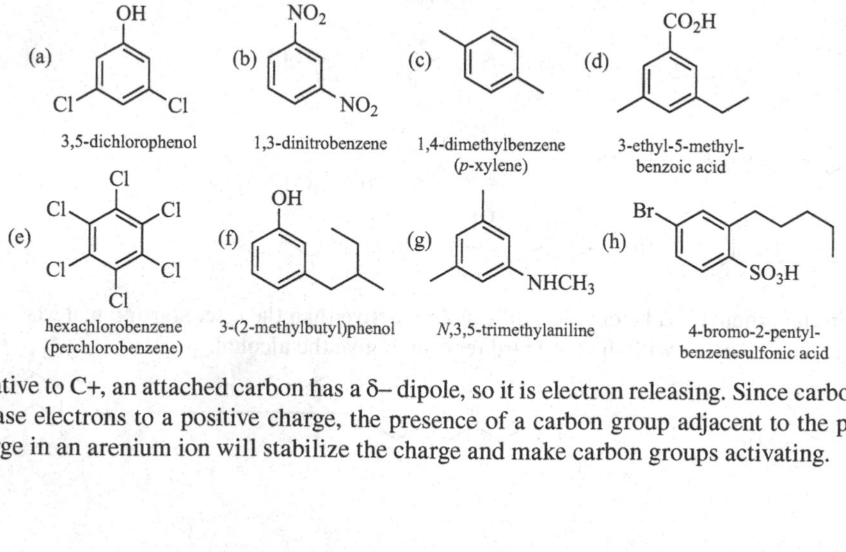

4. Relative to C+, an attached carbon has a δ– dipole, so it is electron releasing. Since carbons can release electrons to a positive charge, the presence of a carbon group adjacent to the positive charge in an arenium ion will stabilize the charge and make carbon groups activating.

5.

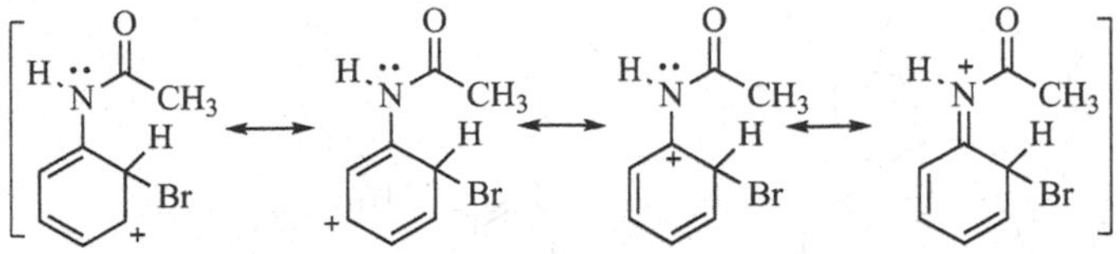

6. The reaction will produce a mixture of both the ortho- and the para- products. The only way to obtain a pure sample of the ortho- product is the separate the two products, usually via chromatography or, in some cases, fractional distillation (these products are liquids although the para- product is a low melting solid, mp 7.2 °C). Since the para- melts at 7.2°C and the ortho- at −72 °C, it is possible that fractional crystallization might separate them.

7. (a) 3,5-dibutylbenzoic acid; (b) methyl 4-phenylpentanoate; (c) 2-ethyl-3,5-diphenylheptanoyl chloride; (d) 3-bromo-4-methylbenzamide.

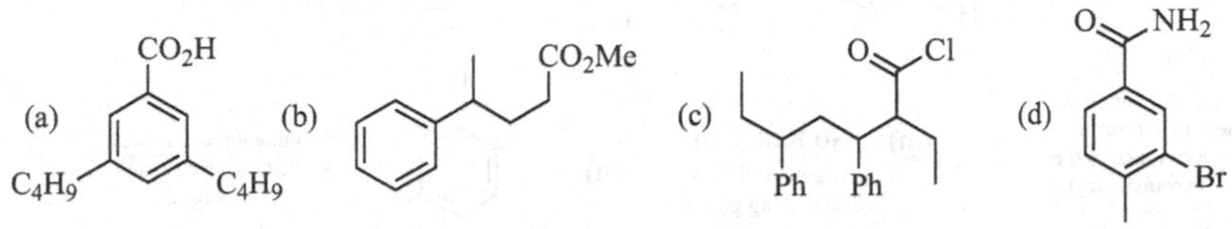

(a) 3,5-dibutylbenzoic acid (b) methyl 4-phenylpentanoate (c) 2-ethyl-3,5-diphenylheptanoyl chloride (d) 3-bromo-4-methylbenzamide

8. The polar nitro group will coordinate with the methoxy group via to dipole–dipole interactions, and this coordination will stabilize the ortho- attack arenium ion more than the para- attack arenium ion. This preference for the ortho- product due to interactions between the reagent and the substrate is called the ortho- effect.

9.

(a) separate the para product from the ortho product

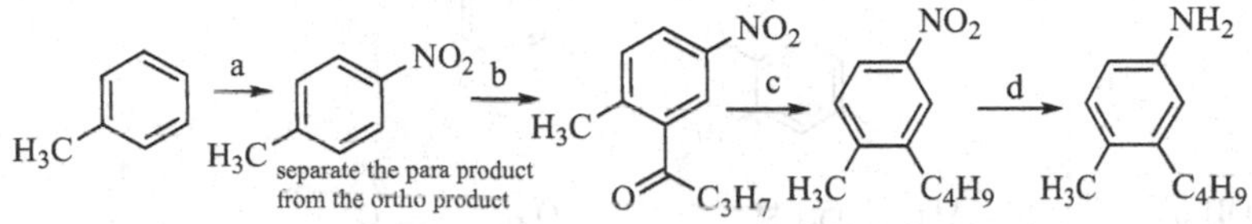

(a) HNO_3, H_2SO_4 (b) butanoyl chloride, $AlCl_3$ (c) NH_2NH_2, KOH (d) H_2, Ni

(b) (a) HNO_3, H_2SO_4 (b) H_2, Ni (c) $NaNO_2$, HCl (d) CuCN (e) HNO_3, H_2SO_4 (f) H_3O^+, heat (g) i. $SOCl_2$ ii. CH_3OH (h) H_2, Ni

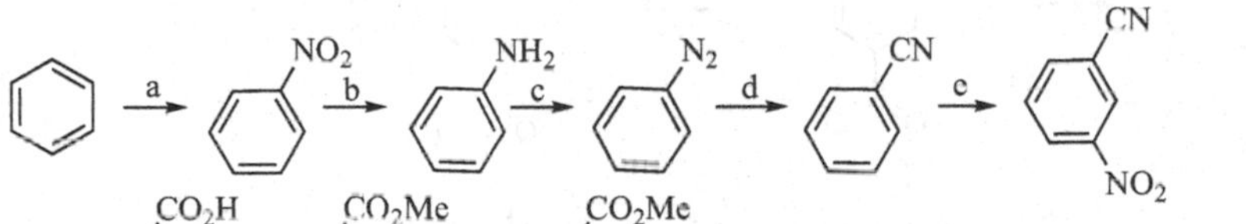

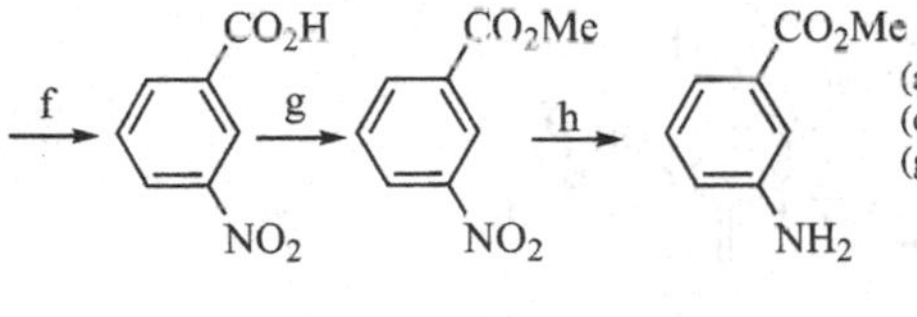

(c) separate the para product from the ortho product

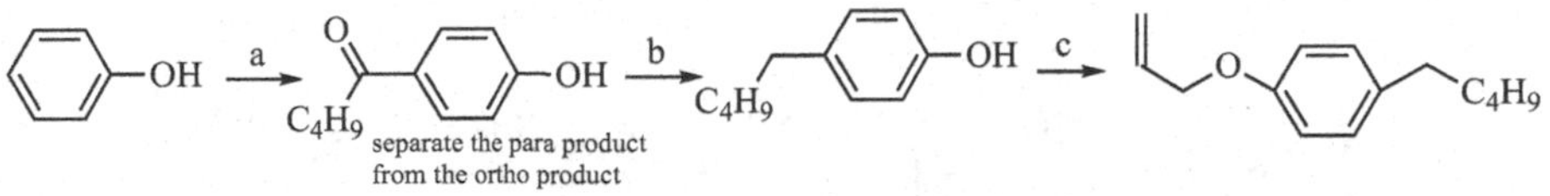

(a) pentanoyl chloride, $AlCl_3$ (b) NH_2NH_2, KOH (c) i. NaH ii. $CH_2{=}CHCH_2Br$

10. (a) NO_2 (b) Et_3C CEt_3 (c) Cl

(d) (e) O_2N OCH_3 OCH_3 NO_2 (f) C_3H_7 OCH_3 SO_3H

(g) NHAc Br NHAc Br (h) C_4H_9 O (i) O Br

(j) SO_3H OCH_3 H_3C CH_3 (k) Br C_4H_9 Br C_4H_9 (l) No Reaction

There is no Lewis acid catalyst

6-methoxy-2,3-dimethylbenzenesulfonic acid is not formed due to steric hindrance in the arenium ion transition state

(m) No Reaction

Friedel-Crafts with deactivating groups does not occur

(n) Br O_2N O

Bromination occurs next to the less deactivating groups

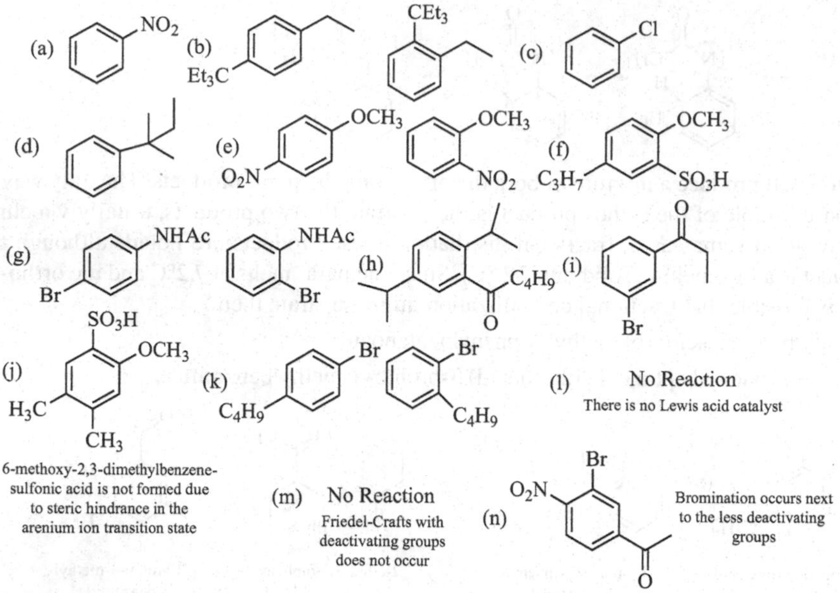

11. Bromination occurs exclusively in the more activated ring, with the OR and the methyl group, and since the para- position is blocked with methyl, bromination occurs ortho- to the OR group, as shown.

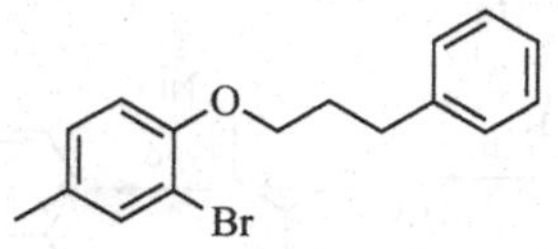

O Br

12.

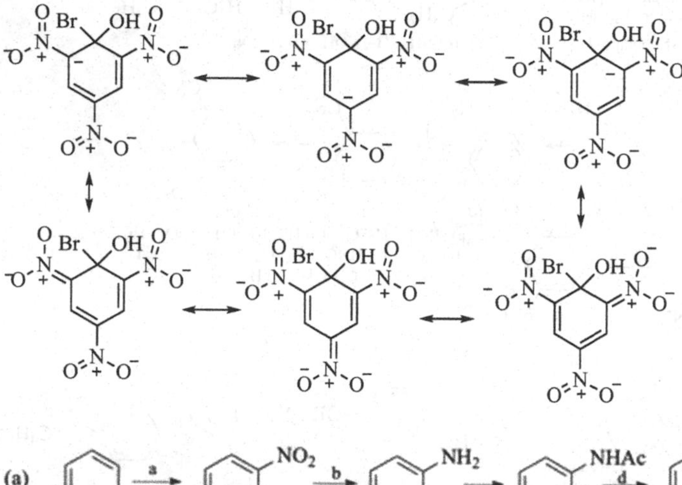

13. (a) a NO_2 b NH_2 c NHAc d O_2N NHAc

(a) HNO_3, H_2SO_4 (b) H_2, Pd (c) Ac_2O, NEt_3 (d) HNO_3, H_2SO_4

separate the para product from the ortho product

(b) Br a O b C_4H_9 c

C_4H_9 O d C_4H_9 C_4H_9

separate the para product from the ortho product

(a) 1. BuLi 2. 0.5 CuI 3. butanoyl chloride (b) NH_2NH_2, KOH
(c) butanoyl chloride, $AlCl_3$ (separate ortho) (d) NH_2NH_2, KOH

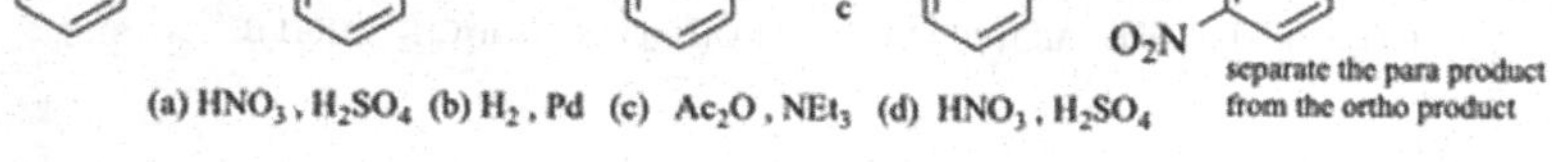

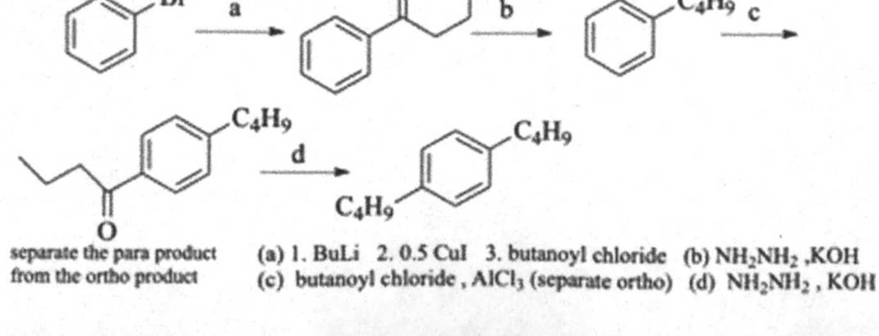

14. (a) 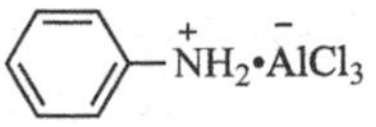 $C_6H_5-\overset{+}{N}H_2 \cdot \overset{-}{AlCl_3}$ (b) 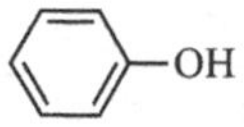 C_6H_5-OH (c) 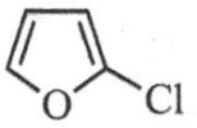 Cl (d) 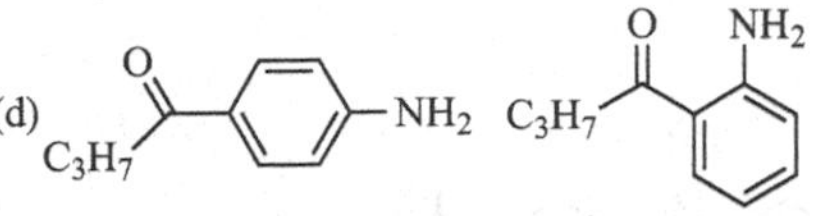 C_3H_7 NH_2 O NH_2 C_3H_7 (e) 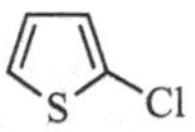 S Cl (f) 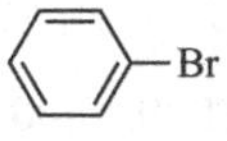 Br (g) 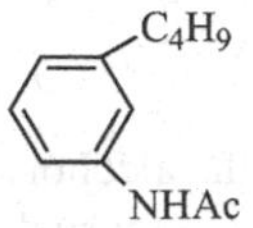 C_4H_9 NHAc (h) 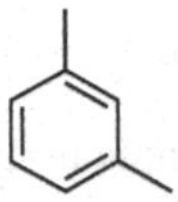 (i) 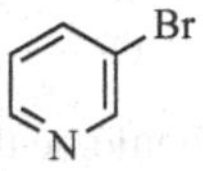 Br N

(j) No Reaction (k) 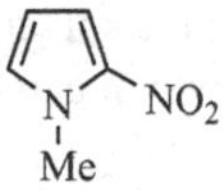 N Me NO_2 (l) 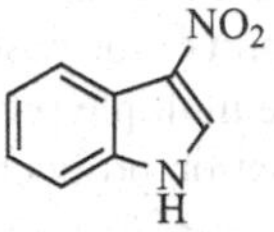 NO_2 N H

Chapter 17. Enolate Anions and Condensation Reactions

1. (a) H_b (b) H_a (c) H_b (d) H_a
2. The compound with the highest enol content is the 1,3-dicarbonyl compound, (c). The second carbonyl group increases the stability of the enol tautomer by increased internal hydrogen bonding.
3. Kinetic control is favored by the use of a dialkyl amide base such as lithium diisopropylamide (LDA), which has a conjugate base (diisopropylamine) that is less acidic than an aldehyde or ketone. An aprotic solvent such as diethyl ether or THF and a low reaction temperature is used (<0 °C), typically –78 °C. Short reaction times favor kinetic control to suppress the equilibrium reaction.
4. 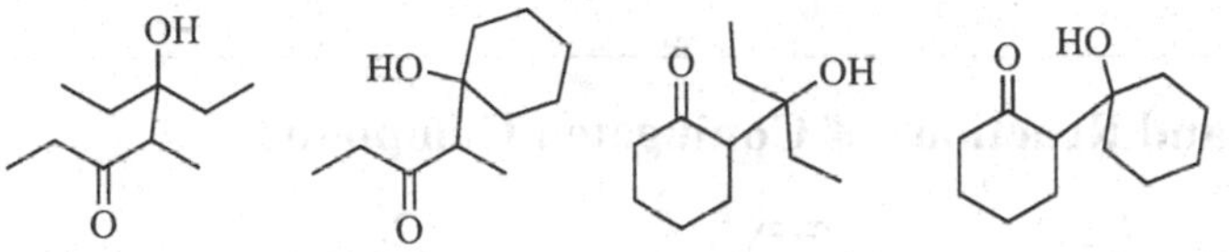 OH O HO O O OH O HO
5. The product is octan-2-one. O $\xrightarrow[\text{THF, -10 °C}]{Bu_2CuLi}$ Bu O octan-2-one
6. (a) 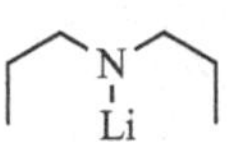 N Li (b) 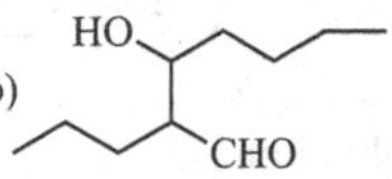 HO CHO (c) 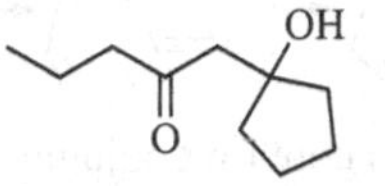 O OH (d) 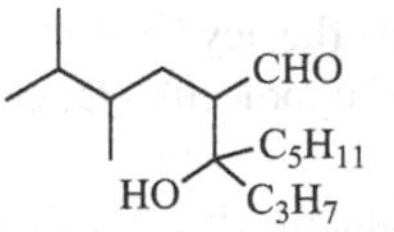 CHO C_5H_{11} HO C_3H_7 (e) 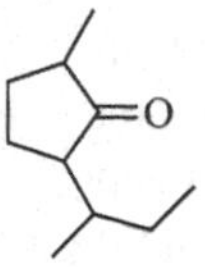 O (f) 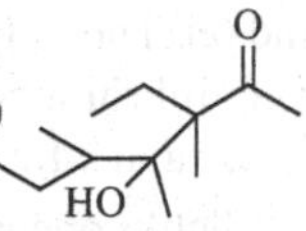 O HO (g) 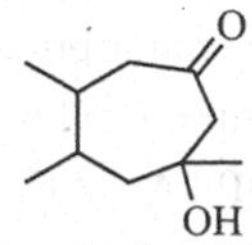 O OH (h) 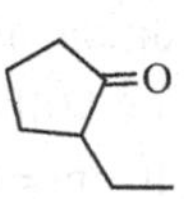 O (i) 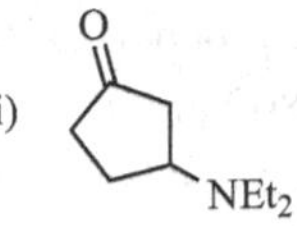 O NEt_2 (k) 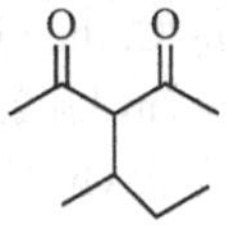 O O

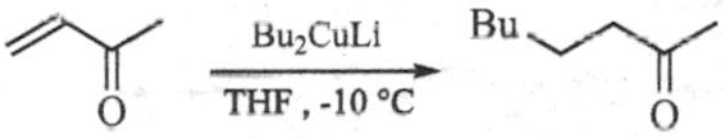

The 7-membered ring is formed preferentially to the other possible product, which is a difficult to form 8-membered ring

7. 1. $Hg(OAc)_2$, H_2O 2. $NaBH_4$, EtOH 3. aq. NH_4Cl → OH; CrO_3, H^+, acetone → O

1. NaOEt, EtOH reflux 2. EtBr → O; 1. LDA, THF -78 °C 2. PhCHO 3. H_3O^+ → Ph, O, OH

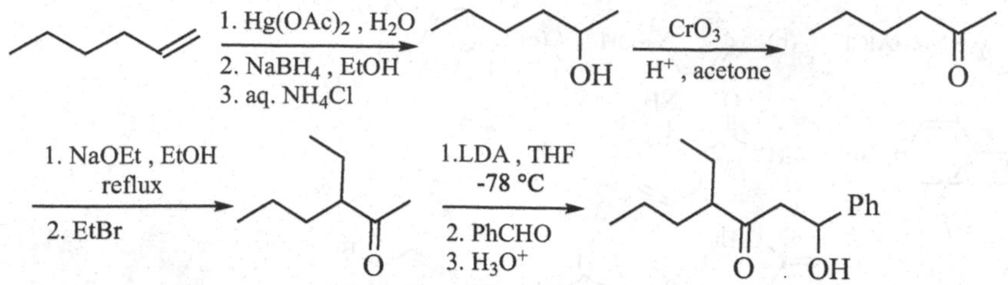

8. The alkoxide base (RO^-) should be the conjugate base of the alcohol solvent (ROH) and should match the OR unit of the ester ($R'CO_2R$). The primary reason for such correlation is transesterification, which can occur if the OR unit of the base and/or the solvent is used. Transesterification of $R'CO_2R$ to $R'CO_2R^2$ will produce multiple products, which can complicate the isolation and purification of any Claisen condensation products.
9. A weaker base can be used because of the enhanced acidity of malonic ester derivatives: pK_a of diethyl malonate is 12.9.

10. (a) CO_2Me (b) CO_2Et, O (c) O, CO_2Et

(d) CO_2H, =O (e) CO_2Me, OH (f) CO_2Et, =O (g) CO_2H

(g) CO_2Me, HO (h) O (i) OH, CO_2Me

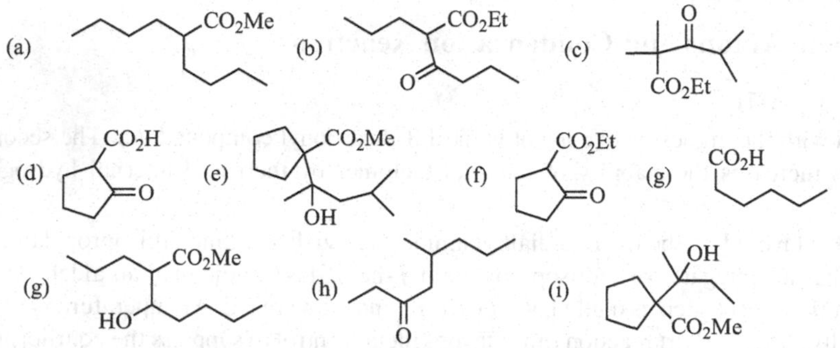

Chapter 18. Conjugation and Reactions of Conjugated Compounds

1. (a) $\overset{+}{C}H_2$ ↔ $=CH_2$ ↔ $=CH_2$ ↔ $=CH_2$

(b) + ↔ + ↔ +

(c) + ↔ + ↔ + ↔ + ↔ +

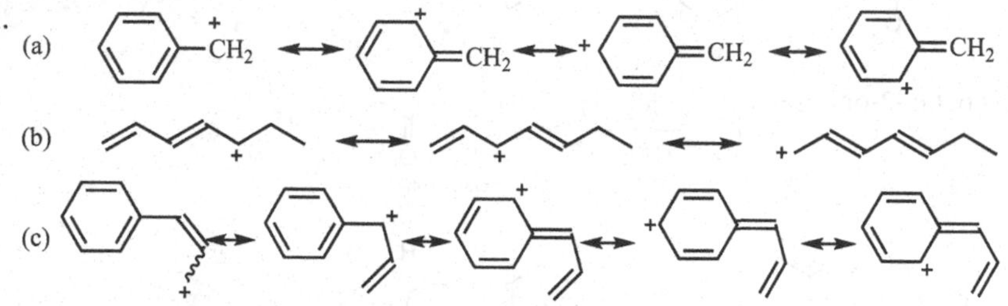

2. Molecules (a), (b), (d), and (e) contain conjugated double bonds.
3. The s-cis- dienes are (a), (b), and (e). The only s-trans diene is (d). Only the acyclic (a) has both s-cis- and s-trans- rotamers in equilibrium because it is the only acyclic molecule. Diene (c) is not conjugated and the terms s-cis- and s-trans- do not apply.
4. Both the 1,2-products (*E*+*Z* 1,2-dichloropent-3-ene) and the 1,4- products (*E*+*Z* 1,4-dichloropent-2-ene) are formed. At –78°C, the kinetic products (1,2-addition) are the major products.
5. (a) 83 kcal = 347.4 kJ = 2929.9 cm^{-1} = 2,373,800 nm. (b) 132 kJ = 901863 nm = 31.5 kcal. (c) 0.45 nm = $1.57x10^{-5}$ kcal = $5.55x10^{-3}$ cm^{-1} (d) 2.4 kcal = 68640 nm = 686400 Å = 847.2 cm^{-1}.
6. Only the conjugated double bonds will absorb strongly in the UV: (a), (c), (d), and (e).
7. If A = (ε) × (*l*) × (*c*), then A = 6457 × 0.3 × 5 = 9685.5 for but-3-en-2-one. Similarly, A = 17 × 0.3 × 5 = 25.5 for butan-2-one.

8. Since 1,4-diphenylbuta-1,3-diene is more conjugated than buta-1,3-diene, it will absorb light more efficiently, leading to a larger extinction coefficient.

9. (a) and (b) HO Ph Ph (c) Br Ph Ph (d) Br

(e) Cl (f) Br Br (g) Br Br

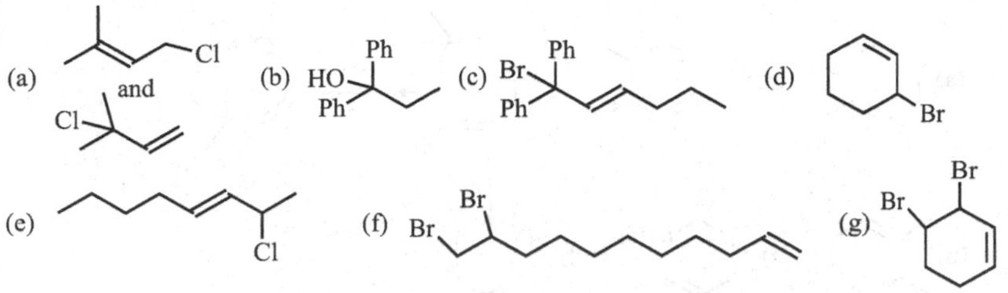

10.

(+1.0 eV) LUMO (+1.0 eV)

+1.5 eV, +2.0 eV, -0.57 eV

ΔE = 10.57 eV, ΔE = 11.07 eV, ΔE = 8.5 eV

(-9.07 eV) HOMO (-9.07 eV)

-9.05 eV, -10.52 eV, -11.95 eV

buta-1,3-diene; $H_2C{=}CH_2$ ethene; Furan-2,5-dione (maleic anhydride); ethoxyethene (OEt)

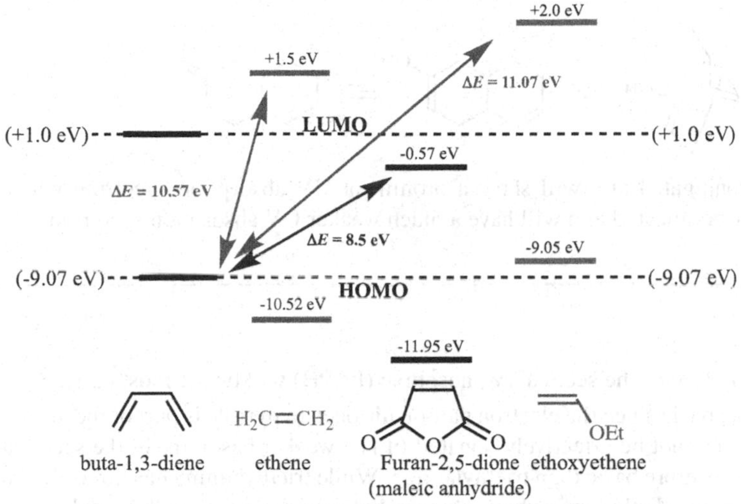

The ΔE for butadiene-ethene is 10.57 eV and is 8.5 eV for butadiene-maleic anhydride and 11.07 eV for butadiene-methyl vinyl ether. Maleic anhydride reacts faster since it has the smallest ΔE.

11. (a), (b), and (c). Triene (d) might react as an alkene with a diene in a Diels–Alder reaction but it cannot react as a diene with another alkene.

12. (a) Me, CO_2Et, Me (b) CO_2Et, CO_2Et (c) Ph, CN, CN, Ph (d) H, H, O, O, O

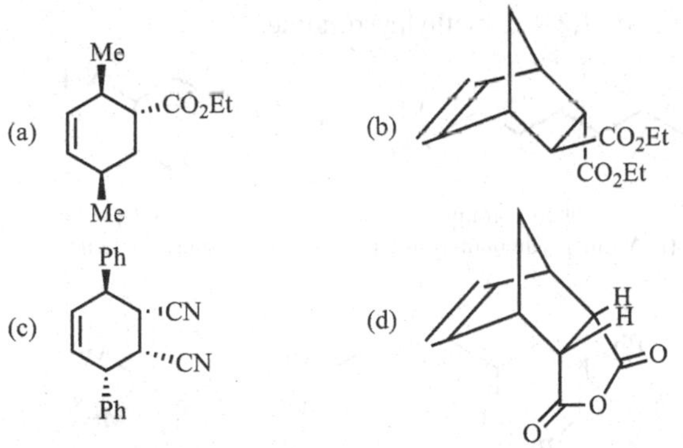

13. (a) CO_2Et, Et and CO_2Et, Et (b) CN (c) H, H, O, N, Ph, O (d) CO_2Et, CO_2Et

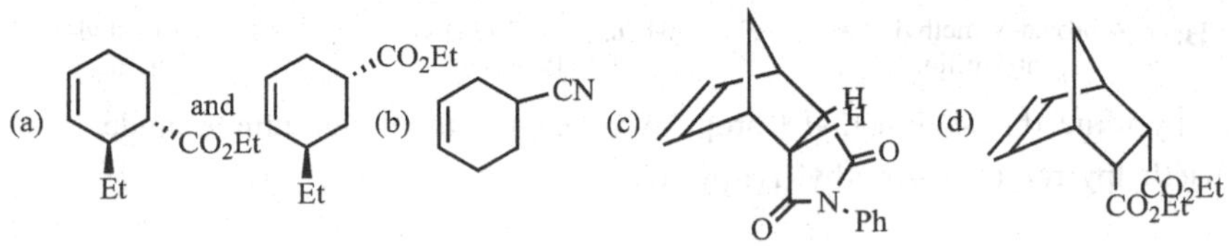

14. The Claisen rearrangement in reaction (a) gives a more stable product and has a lower activation energy to formation relative to the Cope rearrangement in reaction (b).

15.

16.

17. Hexa-1,3-diene is conjugated and will show a prominent UV absorption spectrum whereas hexa-1,5-diene is not conjugated and will have a much weaker UV absorption spectrum.

Chapter 19. Amines

1. Using the analogy of amines, the secondary phosphine (Pr_2PH) will be the most basic.
2. In (a) pyridine is more basic since the electron pair on nitrogen in pyrrole is part of the aromatic system and therefore cannot be effectively donated (it is a weaker base). In (b) the secondary amine (diethylamine) is more basic than triethylamine. While triethylamine has three electron-donating alkyl groups and diethylamine has only two, both amines exists as fluxional isomers. Therefore, the lone electron pair in triethylamine is more sterically hindered and any reaction with that lone electron pair is more difficult. In solvents, secondary amines are more basic and diethylamine is more basic than triethylamine.
3. (a) *N*-ethyl-2,3-dimethylbutan-1-amine (b) *N,N*-diheptylheptan-1-amine (triheptylamine) (c) 3-methyl-1-phenylbutan-2-amine (d) 4-bromo-*N*-methyl-*N*-pentylaniline (e) *N*-benzyl-*N*,2-diphenylhexan-1-amine (f) 1,2,2-trimethylpyrrolidine.

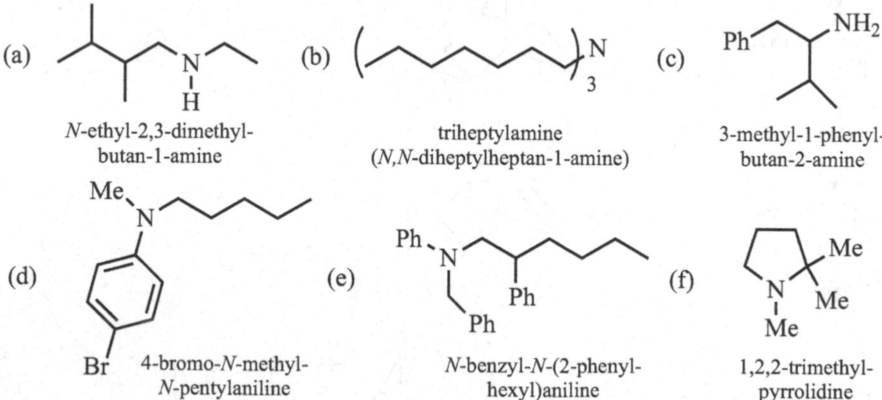

4. (a) 4-bromopyridine. (b) 3,4-dimethyl-1-propylpyrrole. (c) 1-ethylpyridinium bromide. (d) 2,3,4-triethylpyrrole (2,3,4-triethyl-1H-pyrrole.

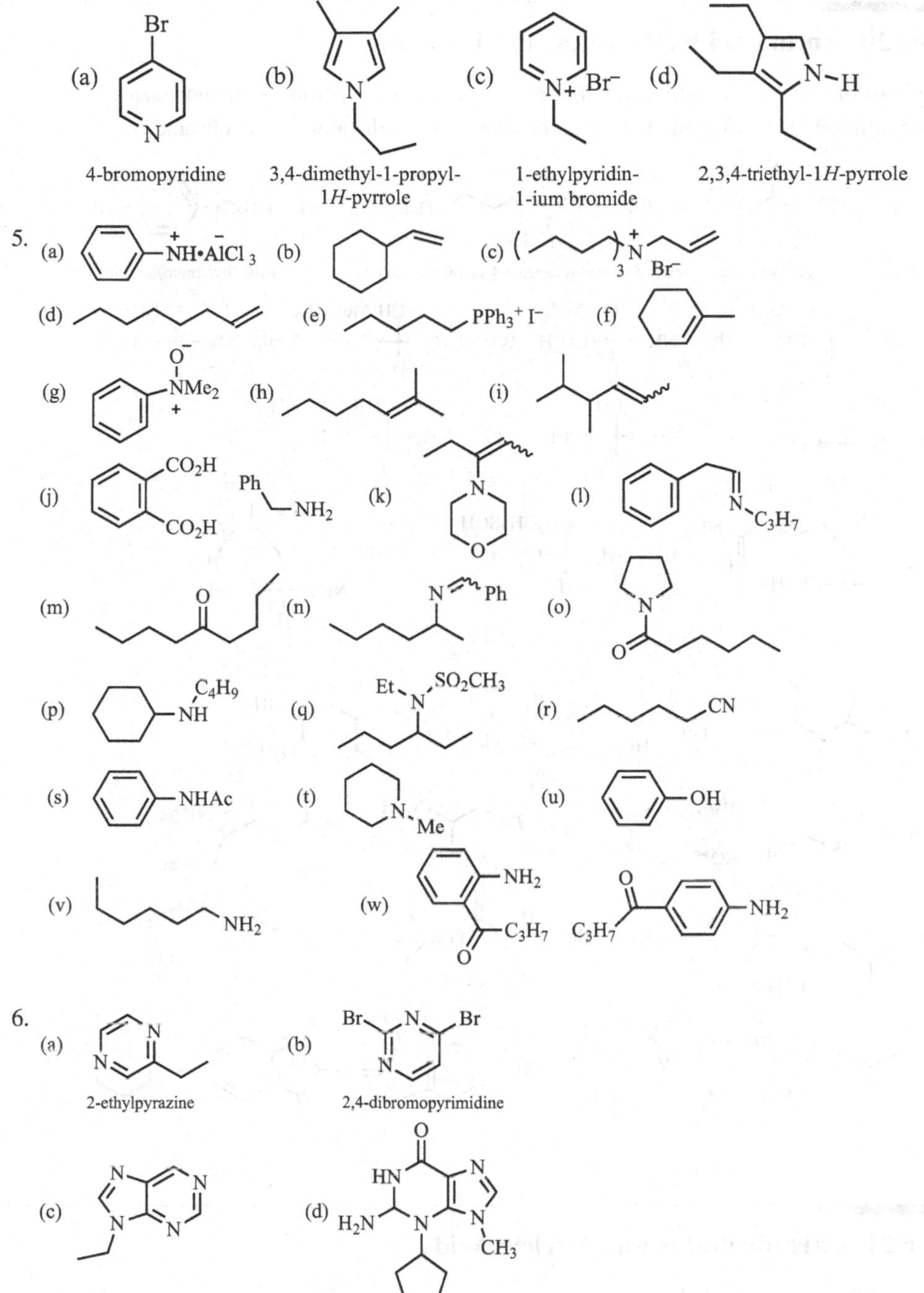
(a) Br N 4-bromopyridine
(b) N 3,4-dimethyl-1-propyl-1H-pyrrole
(c) N+ Br⁻ 1-ethylpyridin-1-ium bromide
(d) N-H 2,3,4-triethyl-1H-pyrrole
5.
(a) NH•AlCl3
(b)
(c) N Br⁻ 3
(d)
(e) PPh3+ I⁻
(f)
(g) O⁻ NMe2 +
(h)
(i)
(j) CO2H CO2H Ph NH2
(k) N O
(l) N C3H7
(m) O
(n) N Ph
(o) N O
(p) C4H9 NH
(q) Et N SO2CH3
(r) CN
(s) NHAc
(t) N Me
(u) OH
(v) NH2
(w) NH2 C3H7 O C3H7 O NH2
6.
(a) N N 2-ethylpyrazine
(b) Br N Br N 2,4-dibromopyrimidine
(c) N N N N 9-ethylpurine
(d) O HN N H2N N N CH3 3-cyclopentyl-9-methylguanine

Chapter 20. Amino Acids, Peptides, and Proteins

1. (a) 3-amino-2-(1-methylethyl)pentanoic acid or -amino-2-(isopropyl)pentanoic acid (b) 5-(dimethylamino)-4-methylheptanoic acid (c) 4-(diethylamino)benzoic acid.

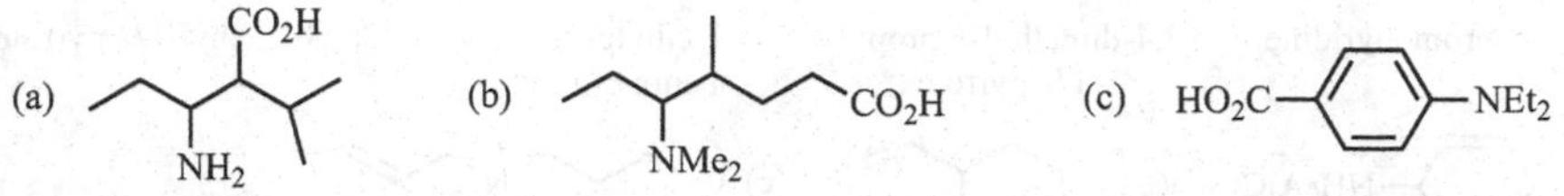

(a) 3-amino-2-isopropylpentanoic acid (b) 5-(dimethylamino)-4-methylheptanoic acid (c) HO_2C–C_6H_4–NEt_2 4-(diethylamino)benzoic acid

2. (a) NH_2–C(CH_2CO_2H)(H)–CO_2H (b) NH_2–C($CH(Me)_2$)(H)–CO_2H (c) NH_2–C($CH(Me)CH_2CH_3$)(H)–CO_2H (d) NH_2–C(CH_2OH)(H)–CO_2H (e) proline (f) NH_2–C(CH_3)(H)–CO_2H (g) NH_2–C($CH_2CH_2CO_2H$)(H)–CO_2H (i) arginine (j) NH_2–C($CH_2CH_2SCH_3$)(H)–CO_2H (h) histidine

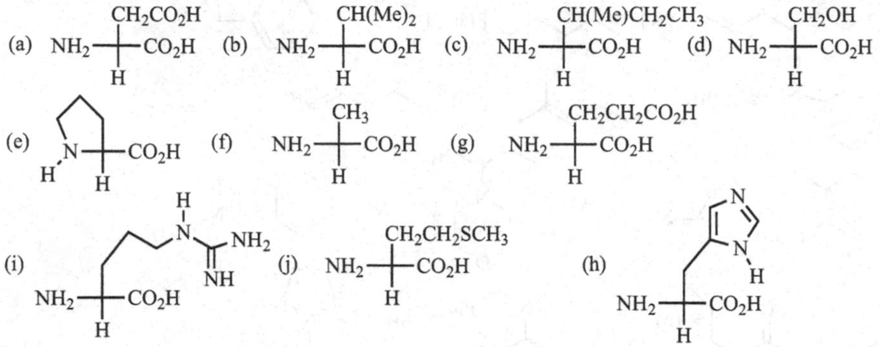

3. (a)–(k) structures

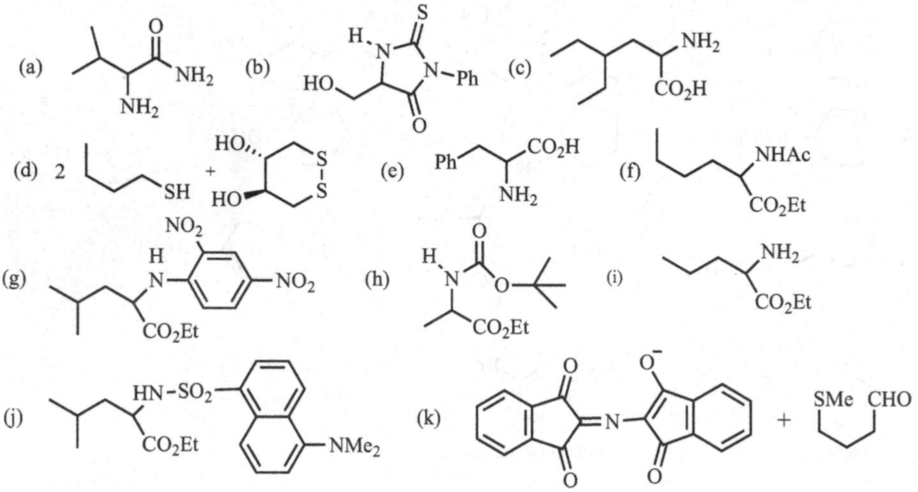

Chapter 21. Carbohydrates and Nucleic Acids.

1. (a) CHO, (R) OH, HO (S), HO (S), (R) OH, OH (b) CHO, (R) OH, HO (S), (R) OH, (R) OH, OH (c) (d)

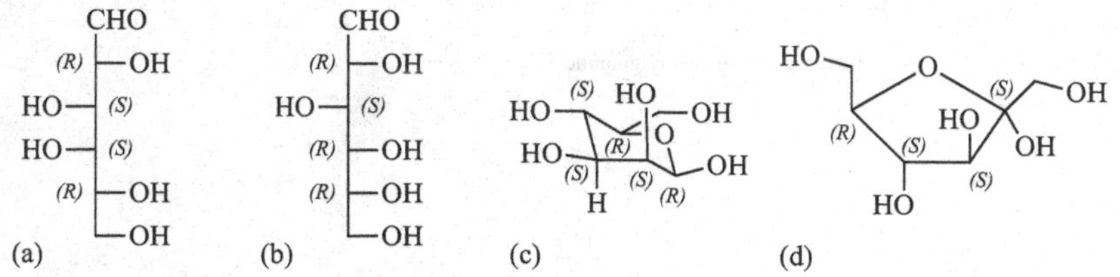

2. (a) D (b) D (c) L (d) D (e) L.

3. 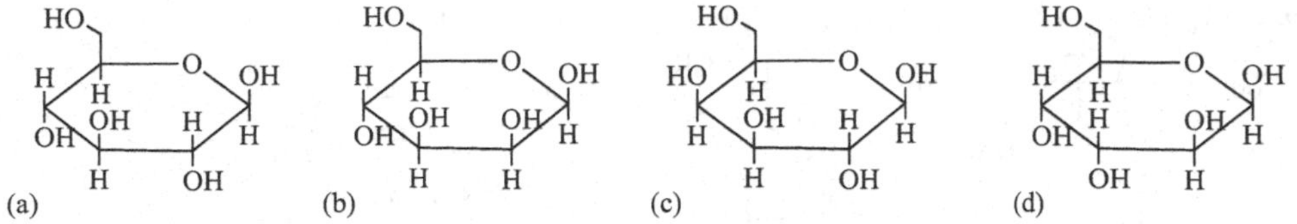 (a) (b) (c) (d)

4. 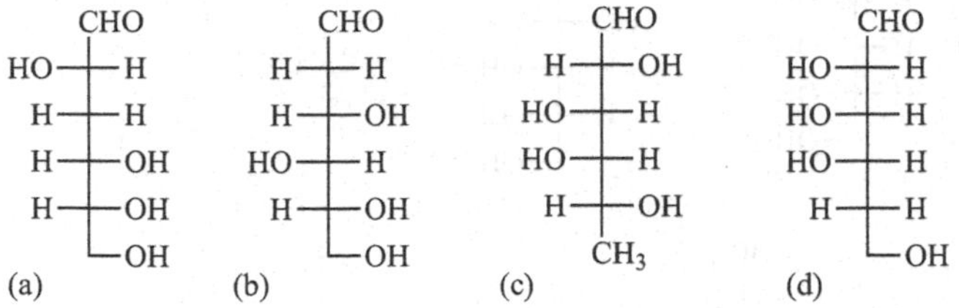 (a) (b) (c) (d)

5. 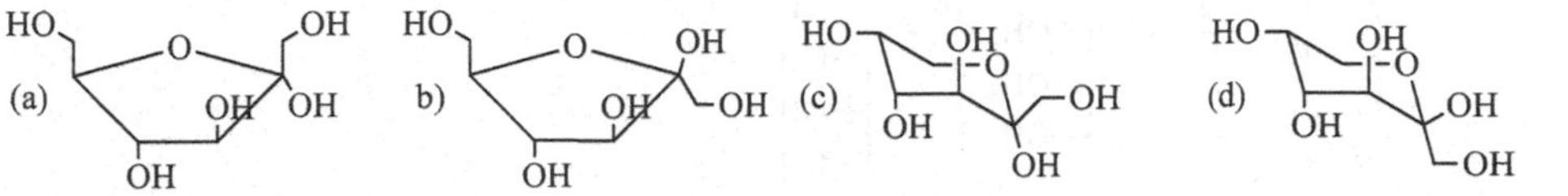 (a) b) (c) (d)

6. 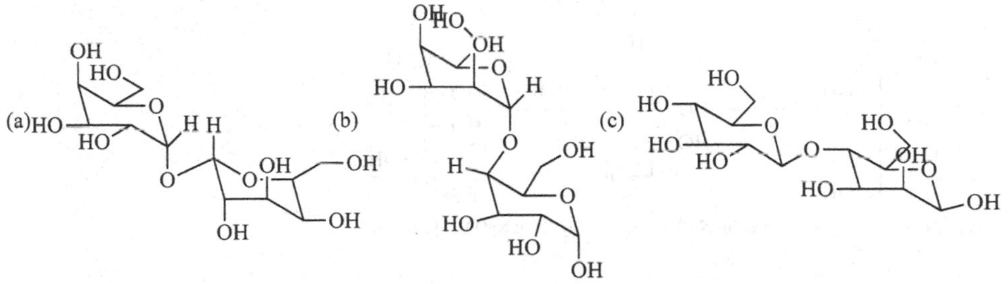 (a) (b) (c)

7. 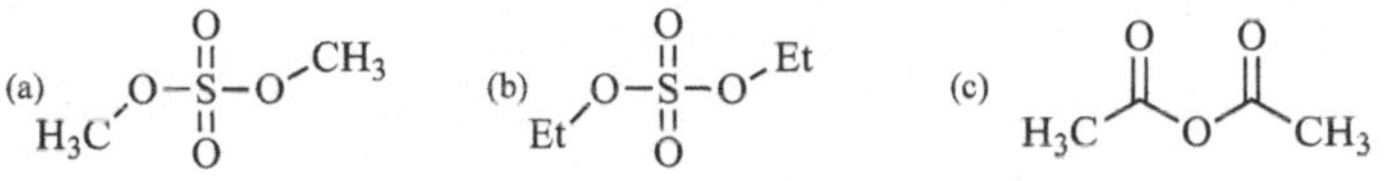 (a) (b) (c)

8. 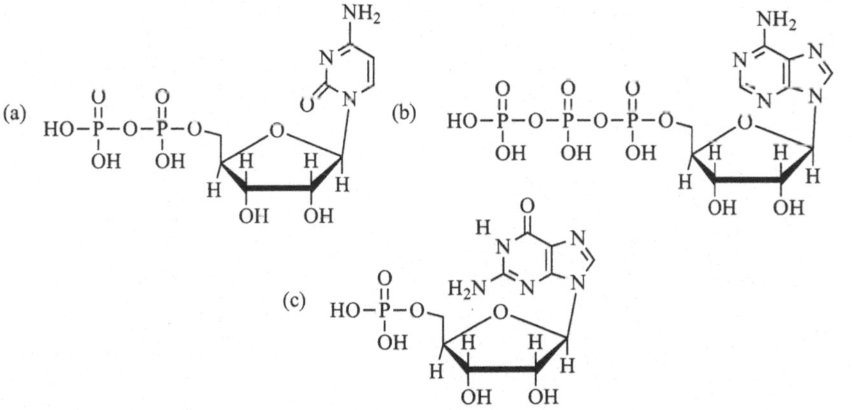 (a) (b) (c)

9. C-T-T-A-G-G-T-G-A-A-C-G

10.

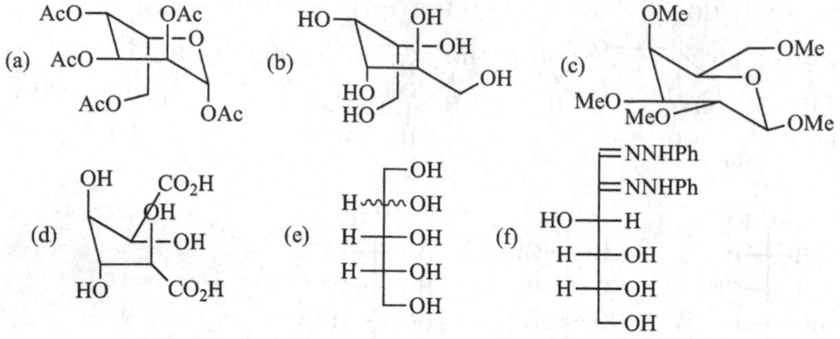

(a) AcO, AcO, OAc, O, AcO, OAc

(b) HO, OH, OH, HO, HO, OH

(c) OMe, OMe, O, MeO, MeO, OMe

(d) OH, CO_2H, OH, OH, HO, CO_2H

(e) OH, H, OH, H, OH, H, OH, OH

(f) NNHPh, NNHPh, HO, H, H, OH, H, OH, OH

11.

(a) CHO, OH, OH, OH → (a) CHO, OH, OH, OH, OH → (b) CHO, OH, OH, OH, OH, OH

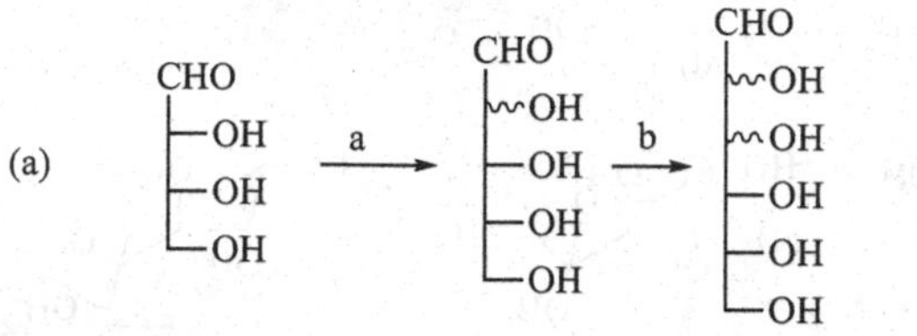

(a) i. HCN ii. H_3O^+ iii. Na(Hg) (b) i. HCN ii. H_3O^+ iii. Na(Hg)

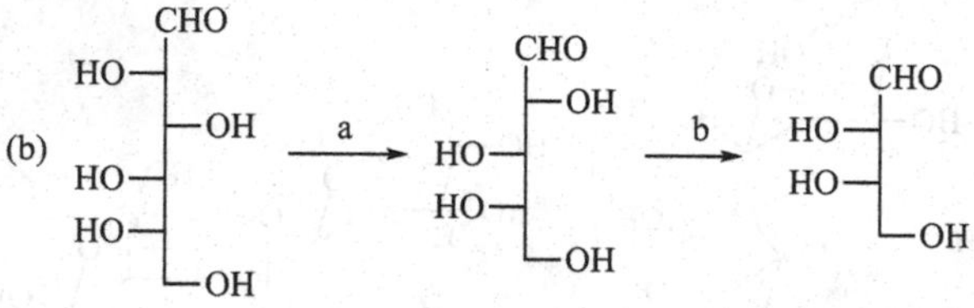

(b) CHO, HO, OH, HO, HO, OH → (a) CHO, OH, HO, HO, OH → (b) CHO, HO, HO, OH

(a) i. NH_2OH ii.NaOAc, Ac_2O iii. NaOMe (b) i. NH_2OH ii.NaOAc, Ac_2O iii. NaOMe

Index

A-strain, *see* $A^{1,3}$-strain
$A^{1,3}$-strain, 73, 74
AB quartet, nmr, 211
Absolute configuration, 83–88
  carbohydrates, 450, 451
Absorbance, and infrared spectrum, 198
Acetal formation, mechanism, 222
Acetals, 223–227, 449
Acetals, from aldehydes, 222–225
Acetate, 108
Acetic acid, 41–43, 108
Acetic anhydride, with carbohydrates, 461
  with oximes, 460
Acetoacetic acid, 376
Acetoacetic ester synthesis, 376, 377
Acetone, 11, 12, 222
  molecular ion, 193
  with HCl, 222
Acetylene, 122
Acetylides, 124, 230
Acid, aqueous, *see* Aqueous acid
Acid anhydrides, 284; *see also* Anhydrides
  with alcohols, 293
  with amines, 298
  cyclic, 285
  nomenclature, 284, 285
Acid–base reactions, 33, 38, 39, 98–106, 143, 165–176
Acid catalysts, 105
Acid chlorides, 284
  with alcohols, 293
  hydrolysis, 301, 302
  nomenclature, 284, 291
Acid chlorides, with amines, 298
  with amino acids, 438
  with carboxylic acids, 291
  with Grignard reagents, 305
  with Lewis acids, 332
  with lithium aluminum hydride, 306
  with organocuprates, 305
  with sodium borohydride, 306
Acid fluorides, 291
Acid halides, 284
Acidic amino acids, 432–434
Acid iodides, 291
Acidity, 170
Acidity constant, 38
Acids, 33
Activating groups, S_EAr reactions, 323–325
Activating groups, S_NAr reactions, 338
Activation energy, 36, 37, 136–138, 165, 167
  and the Diels-Alder reaction, 399
  and [4+2] reactions, 396–401
Acyl addition, 283, 372
  definition, 230
Acylium ions, 332
  and S_EAr reactions, 332
Acyl substitution, 294
1, 4-addtion, 369–371
Addition, conjugate, *see* Conjugate addition
Adenine, 425, 465
Adenosine, 466
Adenosine monophosphate, 466
Adenosine triphosphate, 467
Adsorption, and hydrogenation, 258
Alane, 265
Alanine, 45
β-alanine, 45
Alcohols, 23, 27, 31, 33, 40, 104, 106, 109–111, 121, 143, 147, 155, 172–175, 366–369
Alcohols, allylic, 385
  with HCl, 387
Alcohols, benzylic, 386, 387
  with HCl, 386, 387
Alcohols, from acid chlorides, 305, 306
  from aldehydes or ketones, 231, 232, 257, 266–272, 365–369
  from carboxylic acids, 306, 307
  from esters, 268, 305, 306
Alcohols, nomenclature, 143, 144
Alcohols, oxidation, 251–255
  mechanism, 252
Alcohols, with acid anhydrides, 293
  with acid chlorides, 293
  with aldehydes or ketones, 222–227, 449
  with amines and thionyl chloride, 421
  with amino acids, 437
  with base, 147
  with carboxylic acids, 294, 295
  with carboxylic acids and DCC, 295, 296
  with chromium trioxide, 280, 281
  with Grignard reagents, 187
  with HBr or HCl, 155
  with HX, 144, 155
  with Jones reagent, 252
  with organolithium reagents, 187
  with PDC or PCC, 254, 255
  with sulfonyl chlorides, 309
  with sulfur and phosphorus halides, 145
  with thionyl bromide, 145
  with thionyl chloride, 145
  with thionyl chloride + triethylamine, 145
Aldehydes, 27, 184, 219–235
Aldehydes, conjugated, 367
Aldehydes, from acetals, 225, 226
  from alcohols, 251–255
  from alkenes, 248–250
Aldehydes, hydride reduction, 265–269
  mechanism, 266, 267

Aldehydes, hydrogenation, 269–271
  dissolving metal reduction, mechanism, 272
  nomenclature, 220, 221
  pK_a, 357, 358
  reactivity, 220
  reductive amination, 417
  structure, 219
Aldehydes, with alcohols, 222–227, 449
  with alkyne anions, 231
  with amines, 228–230
  with diols, 226
  with enamines, 371, 372
  with enolate anions, 366–369
  with ester enolate anions, 381
  with Grignard reagents, 231, 232, 283
  with malonate anions, 382
  with NaCN and ammonium chloride, 436
  with sodium metal and ammonia, 271
  with thiols, 227, 228
  with ylids, 234
Alder endo rule, 401
Aldol condensation, 366–369
  intramolecular, 368, 369
  mixed, 366, 367
Aldols, 366
  dehydration, 367
Alkanes, 49, 50, 52, 62
  from alkenes or alkynes, 258–264
  cyclic, 57, 58, 67–75
  cyclic, nomenclature, 57, 58
  and radicals, 158–162
Alkenes, 14, 27, 28, 93–122, 382
  from aldehydes or ketones, 234
  from alkyl halides, 165–176
  from alkynes, 260–265
  from amine oxides, 180
  from ammonium salts, 178–180
  bromination, 392
  cyclic, 115
  dihydroxylation, 239–244
  exocyclic, 235
  halogenation, 114–117
  HOMO and LUMO, 395
  hydrogenation, 258–260
  nomenclature, 95–98
  oxidation, 239–250
  oxidative cleavage, 247–250
  stability, 170
Alkenes, with boranes, 117–121
  with bromine, kinetic control, 392, 393
  with bromine, thermodynamic control, 392, 393
  with bromine or chlorine, 114–117
  with hydroperoxides, 113
  with hypohalous acids, 117
  with Lewis acids, 107
  with mercuric acetate, 108
  with osmium tetroxide, 243, 244
  with ozone, 247–250
  with peroxyacids, 112, 245, 246
  with potassium permanganate, 240–242
  with radicals, 107
Alkoxides, 47, 138, 146, 188
  with alkyl halides, 147, 148
  with esters, 379
Alkoxyaluminates, 266, 267
Alkoxyborates, 267
Alkoxymercuration, 110, 111
Alkylation, Friedel–Crafts, 331
Alkylation, with enolate anions, 361–365, 373–375
Alkylboranes, 118–121
Alkyl groups, 53–56
Alkyl halides, *see* Halides
[3, 3]-alkyl shift, 404
Alkyne anions, 124, 230
  with aldehydes or ketones, 231
  with alkyl halides, 125
  with epoxides, 364
Alkynes, 14, 27, 28, 122–129
Alkynes, from vinyl halides, 176, 177
  hydrogenation, 258, 260–264
  nomenclature, 123, 124
  pK_a, 124, 187
  stereoselective reduction, 262, 265
  structure, 122, 123
Alkynes, with base, 230
  with HBr, 126
  with HCl, 126, 127
  with sodium and ammonia, 264, 265
  with sodium and ammonia, mechanism, 264, 265
Allo amino acids, 435
Allylic alcohols, *see* Alcohols
Allylic carbocations, *see* Carbocations
Allylic radicals, 161
Alumina, solid support, 259
Aluminum chloride, and amines, 414
  with alkyl halides, 331
  and aniline, 326
  with bromine, 319
Aluminum trichloride, 34
Amide bases, basicity, 415
Amides, 287, 288
Amides, from ammonium salts, 297, 298
  from aniline, 326
  from carboxylic acids, 297, 298, 299
  hydrolysis, 304
  with lithium aluminum hydride, 306, 418
  nomenclature, 287, 288
  with phosphorous pentoxide, 301
Amine N-oxides, 180, 422
Amines, 22, 23, 27, 28, 180, 413–426
Amines, and aluminum chloride, 414
  from amides, 306
  aromatic, 414
  basicity, 414, 415
  bicyclic, fluxional inversion, 415
  conjugate addition, 369, 370
  definition, 413
  and E2 reactions, 421, 422
  fluxional inversion, 415
  heterocyclic, 424–426
  from nitrobenzene, 419
  nomenclature, 413, 414

nucleophiles, 415
pK$_a$, 304
and S$_N$4 reactions, 420
and solvation, 421
spectroscopy, 416
Amines, with acid anhydrides, 298
with acid chlorides, 298
with alcohols and thionyl chloride, 421
with aldehyde or ketones, 228–230
with alkyl halides, 178, 420
with anhydrides, 300
with aryl halides, 341, 342
with carboxylic acids, 297
with carboxylic acids and DCC, 299
with formaldehyde, 417
with ketones, 423
with lactones, 299, 300
with sulfonyl chlorides, 309
Amino acids, 429–441
Amino acids, absolute configuration, 430
acidic, 432–434
allo, 435
α-amino acids, 429
β-amino acids, 429
γ-amino acids, 429
δ-amino acids, 429
basic, 432–434
and chirality, 429, 430
common, structures, 431
common, table, 431
d, l nomenclature, 435
definition, 429
essential, 432
neutral, 432–434
nomenclature, 431, 432
non-essential, 432
one letter code, 431
pK$_a$, 433–434
structure, 429
synthesis, 435–437
three letter code, 431
Amino acids, with acid chlorides, 438
with alcohols, 437
with anhydrides, 437
with chloroformates, 438
with ninhydrin, 438, 439
2-aminopropanoic acid, 45
3-aminopropanoic acid, 45
Ammonia, 19, 24, 34, 38, 45, 124, 264, 265
Ammonia, pK$_a$, 187
with anhydrides, 300
with aryl halides, 341
with halocarboxylic acids, 435, 436
with lactones, 299, 300
with organolithium reagents, 187
Ammonium chloride, 266–269
with NaCN and aldehydes, 436
Ammonium hydroxides, 422
Ammonium hydroxide/silver oxide, 464
Ammonium ions, 38
Ammonium salts, 178, 415, 416, 420, 433
and heat, 297
with silver oxide, 178
Amylopectin and amylose, 458
Angle, of rotation, 81
Angle strain, 67–69
Angular shape, 24
Anhydrides, cyclic, 292
with amines, 300
with amino acids, 437
with ammonia, 300
Aniline, and aluminum chloride, 326
protecting groups for, 326
with nitrous acid, 340
Aniline yellow, 341
Anions, 16
aromaticity, 317
Anomeric carbon, definition, 450
Anomers, 450
Antarafacial shift, 404
Anthracene, 347
Anti-Markovnikov orientation, 106
Antiparallel β-pleated sheet, 445
Anti-rotamers, 63, 64, 66, 67, 179
Aqueous acids, with dienes, kinetic control, 392
with dienes, thermodynamic control, 392
with epoxides, 246
Arenes, 330
from alkyl halides, 331
nomenclature, 330
Arenium ions, 320, 348
halogen substituents, S$_E$Ar reactions, 329, 330
and resonance, 324–329
stability, 324
Aromatic amines, 414
Aromatic compounds, 315–352
dissolving metal reduction, 345
functionalized, birch reduction, 345, 346
functionalized, hydrogenation, 344, 345
hydrogenation, 344, 345
reduction, 344–347
synthesis, 334–337
Aromaticity, 316
of anions and cations, 317
and functional groups, 317
and functional groups, nomenclature, 317, 322, 323
Aromatics, conjugate, structure, 390
Aryl halides, *see* Halides
Asymmetric center, 78
Asymmetry, 77
Ate complex, 34, 319, 414
Atomic number, 83–86
Atomic orbitals, 3, 5, 6
Atom transfer reaction, 159
Aufbau principle, 5
Axial–equatorial relationship, 74
Axial hydrogen atoms, 71, 72, 172
Azeotropes, 225
Azide ions, 138, 419
with oxiranes, 150
Azides, 150
Azides, alkyl, 419

Azides, with lithium aluminum hydride, 419
Azo dyes, 341, 423

Back donation, 108, 109, 110
Backside attack, 136, 139, 166
Baeyer strain, 67, 68, 69
Barium carbonate, 262
  as a solid support, 259
Base ion, mass spectrometry, 194
Base pairs, 467
Bases, 33
Bases, nonnucleophilic, 359
  Bases, with esters, 372, 373
  with carbonyls, 359
Basic amino acids, 432–434
Basicity, of amines, 414, 415
  of pyridine, 349
  of pyrrole, 349
9-BBN, 120
Beer–Lambert law, 407
Beer's law, 407
Benedict's reagent, 463
Benedict's test, 463
Bent shape, 24
Benzene, 315–319
  bromination, 319–321
  chlorination, 321
  nitration, 321
  resonance, 315
  secondary field effect, 208
  structure, 315
  substituents, 323
  sulfonation, 322
  with HCl, 316
Benzenediazonium chloride, 423
Benzenediazonium salts, 340, 341
Benzenesulfonic acid, 322
Benzyl chloroformate, 438
Benzylic alcohols, *see* Alcohols
Benzylic carbocations, 386
Benzyne formation, mechanism, 343
Benzyne reactions, and synthesis, 344
Benzynes, 342, 343
Betaines, 234
Bicyclic amines, fluxional inversion, 415
Bimolecular reactions, definition, 135
Biomolecular nucleophilic substitution, *see* S_N2 reactions
Birch reduction, 345, 346
  functionalized aromatic compounds, 345, 346
  mechanism, 346
Boat conformation, 70
Boiling point, 29, 30, 50, 276
Bond angles, 20, 24, 67–69, 220
Bond dipole moment, 10
Bond dissociation energy, 260
Bond dissociation enthalpy, 35
Bond distance, 25
Bonding, 93
Bond moments, 26
Bond polarity, 142, 275
Bond polarization, 42, 183, 184, 187, 266
Bond strength, and infrared spectroscopy, 197
9-borabicyclo[4.4.1]nonane, *see* 9-BBN
Boranes, 117–121, 265
  with alkenes, 117–121
  with carboxylic acids, 307
  structure, 117
Boric acid, 121
Boron, 8, 24
Boron trichloride, 34
  with chlorine, 321
Branched carbon, 20
Bromination, of benzene, 319–321
  of benzene, mechanism, 320
Bromine, and radicals, 159
  with alkenes, 114–117
    kinetic control, 392, 393
    thermodynamic control, 392, 393
  with aluminum chloride, 319
  with carbohydrates, 460, 461
  with ferric bromide, 320
Bromine radicals, 107
α-bromo acids, 383
Bromobenzene, with magnesium, 185
Bromoform, 281
Bromonium ions, 115, 128, 392, 393
Brønsted–Lowry acid–base reactions, 166
Brønsted–Lowry acids, 33, 34, 35, 38, 40, 45, 98, 99, 103, 107, 125, 126, 171, 275
  catalysts, 222
  definition, 33
  with oxiranes, 149
Brønsted–Lowry bases, 8, 34, 35, 38, 98, 99, 125, 126, 134, 319, 348
Buta-1, 3-diene, HOMO and LUMO, 394, 395
Butane, conformations, 65–67
Butanoic acid, 41
Butterfly conformation, 68, 69
Butyllithium, 124, 185, 186, 416
  with alcohols, 147
  with alkynes, 231
Butynes, 123

^{13}C, 203
Caffeine, 426
Cahn–Ingold–Prelog selection rules, 83–87, 97, 323
Calcium carbonate, 262
  solid support, 259
Calcium chloride, 225
Cannizzaro reaction, 371
  mechanism, 371
Carbamates, 438
Carbanions, 124, 135
Carbenium ions, 135
Carbocations, 98–106, 108, 110, 115, 126–128, 135, 142, 151–158, 172–176, 331
Carbocations, allylic, 16, 385–387, 391
  benzylic, 386
  definition, 98
  and S_EAr reactions, 331
  stability, 102, 154
  structure, 98

vinyl, 126–128
Carbohydrates, 449–465
absolute configuration, 450, 451
definition, 449
diastereomers, 450
D/L-nomenclature, 452, 453
furanose form, 454
hydrogenation, 461
nomenclature, 451, 452
open chain form, 452, 455
pyranose form, 453
sodium borohydride, 461, 462
synthesis, 459, 460
Carbohydrates, with acetic anhydride, 461
with bromine, 460
with dimethyl sulfate, 461
with Fehling's solution, 462, 463
with ferric sulfate, 460
with HCN, 460
with hydrazines, 464
with hydroxylamine, 460
with nitric acid, 462
with sodium amalgam, 460
Carbon, 8, 13
and hydrogenation, 259
Carbon dioxide, and decarboxylation, 307, 308
with Grignard reagents, 283
Carbon monoxide, 263
Carbon tetrachloride, 116
Carbonyl group, 219
Carbonyls, 27, 42, 43
conjugated, 369–371
Carboxylate anions, 40, 41, 280
Carboxyl groups, 275
Carboxylic acid derivatives, 284–304
enolate anions, 372–383
Carboxylic acids, 27, 40, 275–283
from alcohols, 280, 281
from aldehydes, 371
from alkenes, 281
from alkyl halides, 283
from dicarboxylic acids, 307
enols, 382
from epoxidation, 245
halo, with ammonia, 435, 436
halo, with phthalimide, 437
from nitriles, 282, 283, 304
nomenclature, 276, 277
pK_a, 277–280
structure, 275
Carboxylic acids, with acid chlorides, 291
with alcohols, 294, 295
with alcohols and DCC, 295, 296
with amines, 297
with amines and DCC, 299
with base, 280
with borane, 307
α-bromo, 383
with Grignard reagents, 305
lithium aluminum hydride, 306
with phosphorus and bromine, 382
with phosphorus and chlorine, 382
with phosphorus trichloride, 383
with sodium borohydride, 306
with thionyl halides, 290
Cartesian coordinates, 3
Catalysts, acid, 105
Brønsted–Lowry acids, 222
perchloric acid, 105, 175
sulfuric acid, 104, 105, 127, 174, 175
tetrafluoroboric acid, 175
transition metals, 258
Catalytic hydrogenation, *see* Hydrogenation
Cations, aromaticity, 317
Cellulose, 458, 459
Chain initiation step, 159
Chain propagation step, 159
Chain termination step, 159
Chair-chair equilibrium, 69, 72, 73
Chair conformation, 68–71
Chair cyclohexane, *see* Cyclohexanes
Chair-to-chair interconversion, 70
Charge cloud, 3, 4
Chemical shift, 206
Chichibabin reaction, 352
Chiral center, 78
Chirality, 77, 79
Chirality, peptides, 444
Chiral molecules, 79, 81
Chitin, 459
Chloral hydrate, 223
Chloride ion, 15
Chlorination, benzene, 321
Chlorine, with alkanes, 159, 160
with alkenes, 114–117
with boron trifluoride, 321
with radicals, 159
Chloroacetic acid, 43, 44
2-chlorobutanoic acid, 44
3-chlorobutanoic acid, 44
2-chloroethanoic acid, 43
Chloroform, 26
Chloroformates, with amino acids, 438
Chlorohydrins, 117
Chromate esters, 252
and steric hindrance, 252
Chromatography, 89
Chromic acid, 251, 252
Chromium trioxide, structure, 251
with alcohols, 280, 281
Circular dichroism, 83
Cisoid conformations, 390
Cis-stereoisomer, 96, 97
Citric acid/cupric sulfate, 463
Claisen condensation, 376–381
intramolecular, 380
mechanism, 376
Claisen rearrangement, 406
α-Cleavage, mass spectrometry, 196
Cleavage, of ethers, 148, 149
of peroxides, 107
Clemmensen reduction, 334

Cocoa butter, 303, 304
Codons, 469
Common amino acids, structures, 431
  table, 431
Common names, 56, 57, 144, 277, 286
Complementary bases, nucleotides, 467, 468
Concerted reactions, 136
Condensation reactions, 365
Condensed structure, 51
Conformational equilibrium, 69
Conformations, 61–66
  boat, 70
  butane, 65–67
  butterfly, 68, 69
  chair, 68–71
  cyclohexane, 75
  dienes, conjugate, 389
  envelope, 68
  gauche, 66, 68
  half-chair, 70
  peptides, 443
  s-cis, 390
  s-trans, 390
  twist boat, 70, 71
Conjugate acids, 38, 45, 46
Conjugate addition, 369–371
  of amines, 369, 370
Conjugate bases, 38–47
Conjugated aldehydes, 367
Conjugated aromatics, structure, 390
Conjugated carbonyls, 369–371
Conjugated compounds, 385–409
Conjugated dienes, conformations, 390
  isomers, 388
  sterochemistry, 388
  structure, 387–389
Conjugated ketones, 367
  structure, 389
Conjugated proteins, 441
Conjugation, and infrared spectroscopy, 201
Connectivity, 21, 22
Conrotatory motion, 400
Constitutional isomers, 22
Coordinate bonds, 34
Coordinate covalent bond, 34
Cope elimination, 180, 422
Cope rearrangement, 405
Copper (II) sulfate/tartaric acid, 462, 463
Core electrons, 12
Coupling constants, nmr, 209, 210, 212
Coupling reactions, 159
Covalent bonds, 7–9, 13, 14, 22, 50
C-protecting groups, peptides, 440, 441
C-terminus peptides, 439, 440
Cupric sulfate/citric acid, 463
Cuprous salts, with organolithium reagents, 189
Curtin–Hammett principle, 100
Curved arrows, 135
Cyanide ion, 138
  with alkyl halides, 282, 300
  with oxiranes, 150
Cyano, 27
Cyano group, 289
Cyanohydrins, 150
Cyclic alkanes, *see* Alkanes
Cyclic alkenes, *see* Alkenes
Cyclic ethers, *see* Ethers
[3+2]-cycloaddition reactions, 241, 243, 247, 401–404
  HOMO and LUMO, 402
[4+2]-cycloaddition reactions, 393–401
  activation energy, 396–401
  HOMO and LUMO, 396–401
  molecular orbital diagram, 396
Cycloalkanes, 57, 58
Cyclohexadiene, with HCl, 316
Cyclohexanes, chair, 71, 76, 171, 172
  conformations, 75
  planar, 71
Cyclohexanol, with acid, 174
Cyclohexenes, from dienes and alkenes, 393–401
  with HCl, 316
Cyclopentadiene, Diels-Alder reaction, 399
Cytidine, 466
Cytidine triphosphate, 467
Cytosine, 425, 465

Dansyl chloride, 442
Dative bond, 34
Daughter ions, 193
DCC, structure, 295
  with alcohols and carboxylic acids, 295, 296
  with alcohols and carboxylic acids, mechanism, 295
  with amines and carboxylic acids, 299
Deactivating groups, S_EAr reactions, 327–329
  S_EAr reactions, rate of reaction, 328, 329
Dean–Stark trap, 225
Debye, 10, 25, 26
Decarboxylation, 375, 380
  and enols, 308
  of dicarboxylic acids, 307
  and tautomerization, 308
  transition state, 307
Degenerate orbital, 4
Degenerate p-orbitals, 6, 12
Dehydrating agents, 300, 301
Dehydration, 385
  of aldols, 367
Dehydrohalogenation, 165–176
  definition, 169
  regioselectivity, 169, 170
Delocalization, 16
Delocalized charge, 15
Denaturants, 446
Denaturation, 446
Denatured proteins, 446
Deoxyribonucleotide, 467
Deoxy sugars, 454, 455
Deshielded protons, nmr, 207
Desulfurization, 228
Detergents, 446
Deuterium, and nmr, 209
Deuterium oxide, 363

Dialdehydes, from cyclic alkenes, 249
Diastereomer, definition, 87
Diastereomers, 87–90, 96, 97, 115, 116
  carbohydrate, 450
Diastereoselective reactions, 115
Diastereoselectivity, 241, 242
Diastereospecificity, 241, 242
Diastereospecific reactions, 115, 116
Diatomaceous earth, solid support, 259
Diazo compounds, 402, 403
Diazoethane, 403
Diazonium salts, 340, 341, 423
  and azo dyes, 341
  with CuCN, 340, 341
  with CuX, 340, 341
  with hypophosphorus acid, 340
Dibasic acid, nomenclature, 310, 311
Dibasic acids, 310–312
Dibasic carboxylic acids, *see* Dibasic acids
Diborane, *see* Borane
Dibromides, 392, 393
Dibromomethane, 26
Dicarboxylic acids, and decarboxylation, 307
  with phosphorus pentoxide, 292, 293
Dichloroacetic acid, 44
1, 4-dichlorocyclohexane, 70
Dichloromethane, 24
Dichromates, 252
Dicyclohexyl carbodiimide, *see* DCC
Dieckmann condensation, 379, 380
Diels–Alder reaction, 393–401
  activation energy, 399
  with cyclopentadiene, 399
  endo and exo products, 401
  isomeric products, 399, 400
  regioisomers, 399, 400
  stereoisomers, 399
Dienes, 404–406
  conjugate, conformations, 390
  conjugate, isomers, 388
  conjugate, sterochemistry, 388
  conjugate, structure, 387, 388
  conjugate, structure, nomenclature, 387, 388
  conjugated, and UV, 408
  s-cis and s-trans, 398
Dienes, with aqueous acid, kinetic control, 392
  with aqueous acid, thermodynamic control, 392
  with HCl, 391
  with HCl, kinetic control, 391
  with HCl, thermodynamic control, 391
  with HCl isomeric products, 391
Dienophiles, 397–399
Dihalides, alkyl, with base, 176, 177
  geminal, 176
  vicinal, 176
Dihydropyrazoles, 403
Dihydroxylation, 239–244
  and sodium hydroxide, 240
Diketones, from cyclic alkenes, 249
  pK_a, 358
5-dimethylamino-1-naphthalenesulfonyl chloride, 442
Dimethyl ether, 23, 29
Dimethyl sulfate, with carbohydrates, 461
Dimethyl sulfide, with ozonides, 249
2, 4-dinitrofluorobenzene, 442
Diols, 89, 113, 114, 239–244
  with aldehydes or ketones, 226
  with aldehydes or ketones, mechanism, 226
  from alkenes, 239–244
  from epoxides, 246
  from lactones, 306
  oxidative cleavage, 250, 251
  with periodic acid, 250, 251
  with periodic acid, mechanism, 250, 251
  vicinal, 240
Dioxolanes, 227
Dipolar compounds, 401, 402
Dipolar cycloaddition, 401–404
1, 3-dipolar cycloadditions, 241
Dipolar ions, 430
Dipolarophile, 402
Dipole–dipole interactions, 11, 29
Dipole interactions, 29, 31
Dipole moment, 10, 25, 26
  and infrared spectroscopy, 197
1, 3-dipoles, 402
Dipoles, 10, 25, 31, 41
Disaccharides, 457, 458
  definition, 457
  head-to-tail, 458
Disiamylborane, 120
Disproportionation, 189, 371
Disrotatory motion, 400
Dissolving metal reductions, 264, 265
  of aromatic compounds, 345
  and ethanol, 272
Disulfide bonds, 441, 442
Disulfide linkages, 446
Dithianes, 228
Dithioketals, 227, 228
Dithiols, 228
Dithiothreitol, 442
Diynes, conjugate, structure, 389
D, l nomenclature, amino acids, 435
D/L nomenclature, amino acids, 430
  carbohydrates, 452, 453
DMF, 125, 140
DMSO, 125, 140
DNA, 424, 425, 467, 470
  double stranded, 470
  α-helix, 470
  structure, 470
  Watson–Crick model, 470
Double-headed arrow, 15, 16
Double stranded, nucleotides, 467
Downfield signal, NMR, 206
Dulcitol, 461

E1 reactions, 172–176
  and S_EAr reactions, 320
E2 reactions, 165–172
  and amines, 421

transition state, 166
Eclipsed rotamers, 62, 63, 66, 179
Edmund degradation, 442, 443
Electric field, and the mass spectrometer, 192
Electromagnetic spectrum, 191, 406–409
Electron affinity, 7, 271, 394
Electron bombardment, 192
Electron configuration, 5
Electron density potential map, benzene, 315
Electronegativity, 9, 10, 26, 46, 133
Electronic configuration, 7, 12
Electronic potential map, 9
Electronic structure, 3
Electron-pair acceptor, 8
Electron-pair donor, 8
Electron releasing groups, 43
Electron-releasing substituents, 278
Electron transfer, 264, 265
Electron volt, 192
Electron withdrawing effects, 42
Electron-withdrawing substituents, 278
Electrophilic aromatic substitution, *see* S_EAr reactions
Electrophilic carbon, 134
Electrostatic interaction, 11
Elimination, syn, 178–180
Elimination reactions, 165–180
Elimination *vs.* substitution, 171
Empirical formula, 21, 31, 78
and nmr, 213
Enamines, 229, 364, 365
with aldehydes or ketones, 371, 372
with alkyl halides, 364, 365
from amines, 423
formation, mechanism, 229
from ketones, 423
Enantiomers, 79–87, 89, 116
IUPAC nomenclature, 83
Endo product, Diels–Alder reaction, 401
Endothermic, 35, 37
Energy barrier, 65, 67, 70, 73, 137
Energy curves, 36, 167, 168
Energy diagram, 64, 65
Energy levels, 3
Enolate alkylation, 361–365, 373–375
Enolate anions, carboxylic acid derivatives, 372–383
with aldehydes, 366–369
with alkyl halides, 361, 362, 373, 374
with epoxides, 363
ester, 372–383
formation, 359
with ketones, 366–369
kinetic control, 373, 381
malonate, stability, 374
reformatsky reaction, 381
regioisomers, 359
stability, 359
thermodynamic control, 373, 381
zinc, 381
Enols, 127, 128, 357–359, 376
carboxylic acids, 382
and decarboxylation, 308
Enophiles, 397–399
Entgegen, 98
Enthalpy, 35
Entropy, 35
Envelope conformation, 68
Enzymes, definition, 441
Epoxidation, 111, 112, 244–246
transition state, 112
Epoxides, 111, 112, 149
from alkenes, 244–246
with alkyne anions, 364
with enolate anions, 363
with Grignard reagents, 188, 246
with sodium hydroxide, 364
Equatorial hydrogen atoms, 71, 72
Equilibrium, chair-chair, 69, 72, 73
Equilibrium, conformation, 68
Equilibrium constant, 38, 39
chair-chair, 73, 74
conformations, 74
Equilibrium reactions, 17, 29, 38, 46, 47, 224, 297, 364, 404, 405
amino acids, 434, 435
Essential amino acids, 432
E-stereoisomer, 97
Ester formation, acid catalyzed, mechanism, 294
Esters, 246, 285, 286
Esters, enolate anions, 372–383
with aldehydes or ketones, 381
with esters, 376–381
Esters, from carboxylic acids, 293
from esters, 372
α-halo, 382
hydrogenation, 270
hydrolysis, 302
hydrolysis, mechanism, 302
nomenclature, 285, 286
pK_a, 373
saponification, 303
Esters, with alkoxides, 379
with bases, 372, 373
with ester enolate anions, 376–381
with Grignard reagents, 305
with LDA, 373, 378
with lithium aluminum hydride, 268, 306
with sodium borohydride, 268, 306
zinc enolate, 381
Ethane, 61–67
Ethanol, 109, 166
and dissolving metal reduction, 272
pK_a, 360
Ethene, 93, 94
secondary field effect, 208
Ethers, 23, 27, 28, 110, 111, 117, 118, 124, 146–148, 184, 231, 363, 461
Ethers, and Williamson ether synthesis, 147, 148
cleavage, 148, 149
cyclic, 106, 146
with HI, 148, 149
nomenclature, 146
vinyl, 405, 406

Ethylene, 93, 179
Ethylene glycol, 227
Ethyne, 122, 230
Ethyne, secondary field effect, 208, 209
Exocyclic alkenes, 235
Exo product, Diels–Alder reaction, 401
Exothermic reactions, 35, 36, 38, 150, 154, 167, 168, 234, 320
External magnets, and nmr, 201
Extinction coefficient, 407

Fatty acids, 303
Fehling's solution, 462, 463
  with carbohydrates, 462, 463
Fehling's test, 463
Ferric bromide, with bromine, 320
Ferric sulfate, with carbohydrates, 460
Field effect, 43
Fingerprint region, infrared spectrum, 199, 200
First-order kinetics, 151, 152, 173
First-order reaction, 141
Fischer projection, 88, 430–432, 452–454
  definition, 80
Flagpole steric interaction, 70
Fluorescence, 442
Fluorine, 7, 9, 10
Fluxional inversion, amines, 415
  bicyclic amines, 415
Formal charge, 7, 28
Formaldehyde, 219, 220
  with amines, 417
Formate anion, 17, 41, 47, 280
Formic acid, 17, 41, 42, 47, 48, 280
Four-centered transition state, 118, 119
Fragmentation, of radical cations, 193
Free energy, 167
Free radicals, *see* Radicals
Frequency, 191
  and infrared spectroscopy, 197
Friedel–Crafts acylation, and deactivated aromatic rings, 333
  S_EAr reactions, 331, 332
Friedel–Crafts alkylation, 331
  polyalkylation, 332
Frontier molecular orbitals, 393
Frontier molecular orbital theory, 393
Fumaric acid, 293
  pK_a, 312
Functional groups, 26, 27, 40, 196
  aromaticity, 317
  chemical shift, nmr, 206, 208
  and infrared spectroscopy, 198–201
  and oxidation, 239
  and UV, 407–409
Furan, 318, 348, 424
  S_EAr reactions, 350
Furanose, definition, 451, 453
Furanose form, carbohydrates, 454

Gabriel synthesis, 416, 417, 437
Gauche conformations, 66, 68
Gem-dimethyl, 52
Geminal dihalides, 176
Geminal dimethyl, 52
General formula, alkanes, 49
Genetic code, 469
Geometry, 20
Gibbs free energy, 35–37
Gibbs free energy equation, 35, 36
Gilman reagents, 189
Glucagon peptide hormone, 444
Glutaric acid, 292
Glutaric anhydride, 292
Glyceraldehyde, 430, 452, 453
Glycerol, 303
Glycoproteins, 459
Grignard reactions, 231, 232
Grignard reagents, 184, 185, 231, 232
  with acid chlorides, 305
  alcohols, 187
  with aldehydes or ketones, 231, 232, 283
  with aldehydes or ketones, mechanism, 232
  with alkyl halides, 232, 233
  basicity, 187
  with carbon dioxide, 283
  with carboxylic acids, 305
  with epoxides, 188, 246
  with esters, 305
  nomenclature, 184
  with oxiranes, 188
Group number, 8
Guanine, 425, 465
Guanosine, 466
Guanosine triphosphate, 467

^1H, 203
Half esters, 297
Half-chair conformation, 70
Half-life, 142
Halides, alkyl, 133–162
  from alcohols, 145
  nomenclature, 133, 134
  and S_N3 reactions, 151 158
  and S_N4 reactions, 134–151
  solvolysis, 153–156
  structure, 133
Halides, alkyl, with alkoxides, 147, 148
  with alkyne anions, 125
  with aluminum chloride, 331
  with amines, 178, 420
  with base, 165–176
  with cyanide ion, 282, 300
  with enamines, 364, 365
  with enolate anions, 361, 362, 373–375
  with Grignard reagents, 232, 233
  with lithium, 185
  with magnesium, 184, 185
  with organocuprates, 189
  with phosphines, 233, 234
  with phthalimide, 416
Halides, allylic, 391
Halides, aryl, 337

with amines, 341, 342
with ammonia, 341
with lithium, 186
with magnesium, 184
nomenclature, 321
with sodium amide, 342
with sodium hydroxide, 338, 339
Halides, phosphorous, 145
Halides, sulfur, 145
Halides, vinyl, 126, 176, 177, 184
with lithium, 186
α-Halo esters, 382
Haloforms, 281
Halogenation, of alkenes, 114–117
radical, 158–162
radical, rate of reaction, 159
regioselectivity, 160, 161
Halogens, 115–117
Halogen substituents, 55
S_EAr reactions, 329, 330
Halonium ions, 115–117
Hammond postulate, 169
Handedness, 84
Haworth formulas, 454
Haworth projections, 450, 451
HBr, 107
with alcohols, 155
with alkynes, 126
with ethers, 148, 149
HCl, 33, 38, 100, 101, 103
with acetone, 222
with alcohols, 155
with alkynes, 126, 127
with allylic alcohols, 387
with benzene, 316
with benzylic alcohols, 386, 387
with dienes, 391
with dienes, isomeric products, 391
with dienes, kinetic control, 391
with dienes, thermodynamic control, 391
with oxiranes, 149
with pyridine, 253, 254
with sodium nitrite, 339
HCN, with carbohydrates, 460
Head-to-tail disaccharides, 458
Heat of hydrogenation, 260
Heisenberg uncertainty principle, 3
Helium, 5
α-helix, DNA, 470
α-helix, peptides, 444
Hell–Volhard–Zelinsky reaction, 382, 383
Hemiacetals, 224, 449, 450
Heteroaromatic compounds, 318, 348–352
Heteroatoms, 10, 26, 31, 35, 43, 61–64
Heterocycles, 318, 424–426
nomenclature, 424
Heterocyclic amines, 424–426
Heterogeneous catalysis, hydrogenation, 259
Hexadecane, 30
HF, 10
HI, with ethers, 148, 149
Highest occupied molecular orbital, *see* HOMO
High field in nmr, 204
Hofmann elimination, 178, 179, 422
HOMO, 393, 394
buta-3, 55-diene, 394, 395
[3+2]-cycloaddition reactions, 402
HOMO, alkenes, 395
and ionization potential, 394
and [4+2] reactions, 396–401
Homogeneous catalysis, hydrogenation, 263
Homolytic cleavage, 158, 259
Hormones, 444
Hückel's rule, 316
Hybridization, 14, 94, 122, 124
Hybrid orbitals, 13
1, 2-hydide shifts, 102, 154
Hydrate formation, mechanism, 222
Hydrates, 222
Hydrates, stability, 222, 223
Hydration, mechanism, 103–105
Hydration reaction, 103
Hydrazines, with carbohydrates, 464
Hydrazones, 333, 334, 464
Hydride-bridged dimer, 117
Hydrides, with aldehydes or ketones, 265–269
Hydroboration, 106, 117–121
mechanism, 121
regioselectivity, 119, 120
sterochemistry, 118–120
transition state, 118–120
Hydrobromic acid, *see* HBr
Hydrocarbons, 31, 49, 140
Hydrochloric acid, *see* HCl
Hydrofluoric acid, *see* HF
Hydrogen, 6–10, 228, 258
Hydrogen, adsorption of metals, 258
Hydrogenation, 258–264
and adsorption, 258
and aromatic compounds, 344, 345
carbohydrates, 461
catalytic, 258
heterogeneous catalysis, 259
homogeneous catalysis, 263
and mechanism, 259
and nitrobenzene, 419
and solvents, 259
Hydrogenation, of aldehydes or ketones, 269–271
of alkenes, 258–260
of alkynes, 260–264
of aromatic compounds, 344, 345
of esters, 270
of imines, 417, 418
of nitriles, 418
Hydrogenation, solid supports, 259
stereoselectivity, 262
Hydrogen atoms, and nmr, 202, 203
Hydrogen bonding, 11, 29, 31, 275, 276, 446, 467, 468
internal, 279
peptides, 444
Hydrogenolysis, 109–111, 340
Hydrogen peroxide, 121, 281, 460

with ozonides, 249
[1, 3]-hydrogen shifts, 404
[1, 7]-hydrogen shifts, 404
Hydrogen sulfate anion, 103, 174
Hydroiodic acid, *see* HI
Hydrolysis, 150, 266, 416, 441, 442, 460, 461
of acid chlorides, 301, 302
of amides, 304
of esters, 302
of iminium salts, 365
of nitriles, 290, 304
Hydroperoxide anion, 121
Hydroperoxides, with alkenes, 113
Hydrophobic residues, 446
Hydroxy-esters, 381
Hydroxylamine, with carbohydrates, 460, 461
Hydroxylation, 107, 108
Hydroxyl unit, 27
Hypobromous acid (HOBr), 117
Hypochlorous acid (HOCl), 117
Hypohalous acids, with alkenes, 117
Hypophosphorus acid, and diazonium salts, 340

Imides, 288, 289
from anhydrides, 300
nomenclature, 288, 289
with organolithium reagents, 416
pK_a, 416
Imine–enamine tautomerism, 365
Imine formation, mechanism, 228
Imines, 228, 334, 417, 418
from amines, 423
hydrogenation, 417, 418
from ketones, 423
with lithium aluminum hydride, 418
Iminium salts, 228, 229, 364, 365, 417, 418
hydrolysis, 365
hydrolysis, mechanism, 365
Indole, 352, 424
S_EAr reactions, 351
Induced polarization, 114
Inductive effects, 42, 43, 278, 374
through-bond, 278
through-space, 279
Infrared light, 191, 192
Infrared radiation, 196
Infrared spectrometry, 196–201
Infrared spectrophotometers, 197
Infrared spectroscopy, and bond strength, 197
and conjugation, 201
and dipole moment, 197
and frequency, 197
and functional groups, 198–201
and wavelength, 197
Infrared spectrum, 198
and fingerprint region, 199, 200
Ing–Manske procedure, 417
Insertion reactions, 184, 185
Intact benzene rings, 348
Integration, nmr, 213
Intermediates, 98–102, 104, 106, 110, 115, 135, 342
Internal hydrogen bonding, 43
Internal standard, nmr, 205
International Union of Pure and Applied Chemistry, *see* IUPAC
Intramolecular aldol condensation, 368, 369
Intramolecular Claisen condensation, 380
Inversion of configuration, 137, 139, 145, 147
Iodoform, 281
Iodoform reaction, 281, 282
mechanism, 282
Iodoform test, 282
Ionic bonds, 7
Ionization, 117, 151, 154, 172–176
Ionization potential, 7, 394
Ipso carbon, 325
Isoelectric point, 433, 434
Isomerism, 50, 52
Isomers, 22, 51–55, 78, 96, 123, 318, 322, 382
and the Diels–Alder reaction, 399, 400
dienes, conjugate, 388
from dienes, with HCl, 391
S_EAr reactions, 323, 324
Isoquinoline, 352, 424
Isothiocyanates, 442, 443
Isotopic ratios, mass spectrometry, 194, 195
IUPAC nomenclature, 49, 52–57; *see also* Nomenclature

Jones reagent, 252, 280

K, *see* Equilibrium constant
K_a, 39, 41–44, 46, 47
K_a and pK_a, 278
Kekulé structures, 316, 348
Ketals, 224
Ketals, from ketones, 222–225
β-keto acids, 376
β-keto acids, pK_a, 376
Keto-enol tautomerism, 127, 128, 308, 357–359, 376
Ketones, 27, 29, 127, 184, 219–235
from acid chlorides, 305, 333
from alcohols, 251–255
from alkenes, 248–250
conjugated, 367
conjugated, structure, 389
dissolving metal reduction, mechanism, 272
from esters, 305
hydride reduction, 265–269
hydrogenation, 269–271
from ketals, 225, 226
from ketoacids, 308
ketones, oxidative cleavage, 281
nomenclature, 220, 221
pK_a, 357, 358
reactivity, 220
reduction, 333, 334
reductive amination, 417
structure, 219
Ketones, with alcohols, 222–227
with alkyne anions, 231
with amines, 228–230
with base, 359

with diols, 226
with enamines, 371, 372
with enolate anions, 365–369
with ester enolate anions, 381
with Grignard reagents, 231, 232
with iodine and sodium hydroxide, 281
with malonate anions, 382
with sodium metal and ammonia, 271
with thiols, 227, 228
with ylids, 234
Ketose, definition, 453
Ketyls, 271
Kieselguhr, solid support, 259
Kiliani–Fischer synthesis, 459
Kinetic control, alkenes, with bromine, 392, 393
dienes with aqueous acid, 392
dienes with HCl, 391
enolate anions, 373, 381
Kinetic enolates, 360, 361, 362, 366, 367
Kinetics, 100, 166
first order, 173
Knoevenagel condensation, 382

Lactams, 288
from lactones, 298, 299
with lithium aluminum hydride, 419
nomenclature, 288
Lactones, 286, 287
with amines, 299, 300
lactones, with ammonia, 299, 300
with lithium aluminum hydride, 306
nomenclature, 286, 287
λ_{max}, 407
LCAO method, 12, 13
LCAO model, 5, 6, 14
LDA, 359
with esters, 373, 378
Lead tetraacetate, 262
Leaving groups, 153, 337, 338
Le Chatelier's principle, 224
Lewis acid–Lewis base reaction, 108
Lewis acids, 8, 33, 34, 184, 331
with acid chlorides, 332
with alkenes, 107
Lewis bases, 8, 34, 134
Lewis dot structure, 8, 9
Lewis electron dot formula, 6
Lindlar catalyst, 262
Linear chain, 20
Linear Combination of Atomic Orbitals model, *see* LCAO model
Line notation, 21, 22
Lipids, 303
Lithium aluminum hydride, and amides, 418
and azides, 419
and imines, 418
and lactams, 419
and nitriles, 418
and nitrobenzene, 419, 420
structure, 265
Lithium aluminum hydride, with acid chlorides, 306
with aldehydes or ketones, 266–269
with amides, 306
with carboxylic acids, 306
with esters, 268, 306
with lactones, 306
Lithium diisopropyl amide, *see* LDA
Lithium fluoride, 6
Lithium metal, 143, 183, 185
London dispersion force, 29
London forces, 10, 29
Longest continuous chain, 51, 134
Louis Pasteur, 89
Low field, in nmr, 204
Lowest unoccupied molecular orbital, *see* LUMO
LUMO, 393, 394
alkenes, 395
buta-1, 3-diene, 394, 395
[3+2]-cycloaddition reactions, 402
and electron affinity, 394
and [4+2] reactions, 396–401

M+1 ions, 194, 195, 196
M+2 ions, 194, 195, 196
Magnesium metal, 183
Magnesium sulfate, 225
Magnet strength, 202
Magnetic anisotropy, nmr, 208
Magnetic field strength, and nmr, 202, 203
and the mass spectrometer, 192
Magnetic moment, 206
Magnets, and nmr, 202
Maleic acid, 311
Maleic acid, pK_a, 312
Maleic anhydride, 292
Malonate anions, with aldehydes, 382
with ketones, 382
Malonate esters, enolate anions, stability, 374
pK_a, 374
Malonic acids, and decarboxylation, 307, 375
pK_a, 311
Malonic ester synthesis, 375
Manganate esters, 113, 114, 240, 403
Markovnikov addition, 102
Mass spectrometer, 192
Mass spectrometry, 192–196
isotopic ratios, 194, 195
Mass spectrum, 193, 194
Maximum absorbance wavelength, 407
Mechanism, 112
acetal formation, 222
acid catalyzed ester formation, 294
alcohols + HX, 144, 155
aldehydes, hydride reduction, 266, 267
alkynes, with sodium and ammonia, 264, 265
alkenes + HX, 102–104
benzyne formation, 343
birch reduction, 346
bromination of benzene, 320
Cannizzaro reaction, 371
Claisen condensation, 376
DCC, with alcohols and carboxylic acids, 295

definition, 101
diols, with aldehydes or ketones, 226
diols with periodic acid, 250, 251
dissolving metal reduction of aldehydes, 272
dissolving metal reduction of ketones, 272
enamine formation, 229
epoxidation, 112
and hydrogenation, 259
Mechanism, esters, hydrolysis, 302
Grignard reagents, with aldehydes or ketones, 232
halogenation of alkenes, 115
hydrate formation, 222
hydration, 103–105
hydroboration, 121
hydrolysis iminium salts, 365
imine formation, 228
iodoform reaction, 282
nitration, benzene, 321
oxidation of alcohols, 252
ozonolysis, 248
peroxyacids, with alkenes, 246
pyridine, S_EAr reactions, 352
pyrrole, S_EAr reactions, 350
S_N1 reactions, 152, 174
S_NAr reactions, 338
solvolysis, 155
transesterification, 296, 297
Wittig reaction, 234
Wolff–Kishner reduction, 334
Melting point, 30, 31, 50
Mercaptans, 27
Mercuric acetate, 108, 128
Mercuric chloride, 108
Mercuric sulfate, 128
Mercury, 334
Meso compounds, 88, 89, 116
Messenger RNA, 469
Meta, ortho, para isomers, 318, 322
Metals, adsorption of hydrogen, 258
transition, catalysts, 258
Meta-periodic acid, *see* Periodic acid
Methane, 13, 20, 24, 26, 77
pK_a, 187
Methanesulfonic acid, 105
Methanoic acid, 41
Methanol, 11, 23, 29
Methoxyethanoic acid, 44
Methylcyclohexane, 72, 73
Methyl group, 53
Methyllithium, 187
1, 2-methyl shifts, 106
Michael addition, 369–371
Mineral acids, 33
with alkenes or alkynes, 135
Mirror images, 77–81, 88
Mixed aldol condensation, 366, 367
Mixed anhydrides, 284, 285
Mixed Claisen condensation, 378
Molecular ion, 192, 193
Molecular ions, even mass, 195, 196
fragmentation, 196
odd mass, 195, 196
Molecular models, 9, 10
Molecular orbital diagrams, 12, 122
[4+2] reactions, 396
Molecular orbitals, 5, 6, 12, 393–401
Molecular sieves, 225
Molecular vibration, 61
Monosaccharide, 449
mRNA, *see* Messenger RNA
Multiplet, nmr, 212
Multiplicity, nmr, 209–211
Mutarotation, 456

4n+2 π-electrons, 316
n→σ* transitions, 407
n⟶π* transitions, 407
N-acetylglucosamine, 459
N-bromosuccinimide, *see* NBS
N-chlorosuccinimide, *see* NCS
N-methylmorpholine-N-oxide, 244
N-protecting groups, peptides, 440, 441
N-terminus peptides, 439, 440
n+1 rule, nmr, 210, 211
Naphthalene, 347, 348
Naphthalene, S_EAr reactions, 347, 348
NBS, 161, 162, 289
NCS, 161, 162, 289
Neutral amino acids, 432–434
Newman projections, 63–65, 68, 179
Nickel, catalyst, 258, 259, 261, 270
Nickel, Raney, 228
Ninhydrin, structure, 438
with amino acids, 438, 439
Nitrate anion, 17
Nitration, benzene, 321
benzene, mechanism, 321
Nitric acid, 15, 33
nitric acid, carbohydrates, 462
nitric acid, with sulfuric acid, 321
Nitriles, 27, 28, 138, 289, 290
Nitriles, from alkyl halides, 300
from amides, 301
hydrogenation, 418
hydrolysis, 282, 283, 290, 304
with lithium aluminum hydride, 418
nomenclature, 289, 290
partial hydrolysis, 304
Nitrobenzene, 321, 419
with hydrogenation, 419
with lithium aluminum hydride, 419, 420
Nitro compounds, 419
Nitronium ion, 321
Nitrous acid, 339, 423
with aniline, 340
nmr, AB quartet, 211
coupling constants, 210, 212
deshielded protons, 207
deuterium, 209
downfield signal, 206
empirical formula, 212
and external magnets, 201

functional group chemical shift, 207, 208
high field and low field, 204
and hydrogen atoms, 202, 203
integration, 213
internal standard, 205
magnetic anisotropy, 208
and magnetic field strength, 202, 203
and magnets, 202
multiplet, 212
and radio wave frequencies, 202, 203
and spin quantum number, 201
nmr, multiplicity, 209–211
n+1 rule, 210, 211
Pascal's triangle, 212
ppm scale, 204
secondary field effect, 208
shielded protons, 207
shielding effect, 207
solvents, 203, 204
spectrum, 203–205, 214
spin-spin splitting, 209, 212
upfield signal, 206
zero point, 205
nmr spectrometer, 203
nmr spectroscopy, 201–214
Nodes, 3, 4
definition, 395
Nomenclature, 376
acid anhydrides, 284, 285
acid chlorides, 284, 291
alcohols, 143, 144
aldehydes, 220, 221
alkenes, 95–98
alkyl halides, 133, 134
alkynes, 123, 124
amides, 287, 288
amines, 413, 414
amino acids, 431, 432
arenes, 330
aryl halides, 321
carbohydrates, 451, 452
carboxylic acids, 276, 277
cis/trans, 96, 97
common names, 56, 57
cyclic alkanes, 57, 58
D/L, for amino acids, 430
dibasic acids, 310, 311
dienes, conjugate, structure, 387, 388
E/Z for alkenes, 97
Nomenclature, enantiomers, 83–87
esters, 285, 286
ethers, 146
functional groups, aromaticity, 317, 322, 323
Grignard reagents, 184
halogen substituents, 55
heterocycles, 424
imides, 288, 289
IUPAC, 49, 50
ketones, 220, 221
lactams, 288
lactones, 286, 287
nitriles, 289, 290
organocuprates, 189
organolithium reagents, 186
oxiranes, 149
prefix, 49, 50
suffix, 49, 50, 52
Non-essential amino acids, 432
Nonnucleophilic bass, 359
Nonsuperimposable, 79, 87
Nuclear magnetic resonance spectroscopy, *see* NMR
Nuclei, for nmr, 203
Nucleic acids, 465–470
Nucleic acid, definition, 467
Nucleophile, definition, 134
Nucleophiles, 100, 103, 124, 133, 134, 143–151, 221–233
amines, 415
backside attack, 136
with oxiranes, 150
strong, 230
Nucleophilic acyl addition, 221–233
Nucleophilic aromatic substitution, *see* S_NAr reactions
Nucleophilic substitution, *see* Substitution
with allylic rearrangement (*see* S_N2' reactions)
intramolecular (*see* S_Ni reactions)
Nucleoside, definition, 464, 465
Nucleosides, 465–470
one letter code, 466
Nucleotide, definition, 466
Nucleotide diphosphate, 466, 467
Nucleotide monophosphate, 466, 467
Nucleotides, 465–470
complementary bases, 467, 468
double stranded, 467
Nucleotide triphosphate, 466, 467

Observed rotation, 82
Octet rule, 8
Oleic acid, 303, 304
Oligosaccharide, definition, 457
One letter code, amino acids, 431
nucleosides, 466
Open chain carbohydrates, 452, 455
Optical resolution, 90
Orbitals, 4
Organoboranes, 118–121
Organocuprates, 188, 189
with acid chlorides, 305
with alkyl halides, 189
nomenclature, 189
structure, 189
Organolithium reagents, 185, 186, 304
with alcohols, 187
with ammonia, 187
basicity, 187
with cuprous salts, 189
and imides, 416
nomenclature, 186
reactivity, 186
Organomagnesium compounds, 184
Organometallic compounds, 183–189
Organometallics, 263

Ortho, meta, para isomers, 318, 322
Osazones, 464
Osmate esters, 113, 114, 243, 403
Osmium tetroxide, 113, 114, 402, 403
  with alkenes, 243, 244
  structure, 243
  toxicity, 244
Oxalic acid, 310
  pKa, 311
Oxaphosphetanes, 234
Oxaspiro compounds, 227
Oxidation, and steric hindrance, 252
  of alcohols, 251–255, 280, 281
  of alkenes, 239–250
  definition, 239
Oxidation reactions, 239–255
Oxidation state, 257
Oxidative cleavage, of alkenes, 247–250
  of diols, 250, 251
Oximes, with acetic anhydride, 460
Oxiranes, 111, 112, 149
  from alkenes, 244–246
  with azide ion, 150
  with Brønsted–Lowry acids, 149
  with cyanide ion, 150
  with Grignard reagents, 188
  with HCl, 149
  with nucleophiles, 150
  nomenclature, 149
  with sodium hydroxide, 150
Oxocarbenium ions, 16, 221–227, 294
Oxonium ions, 104, 106, 127, 155, 156, 173, 174, 294
Oxonium ions, structure, 103
Oxymercuration, 109
Oxymercuration-demercuration, 109
Ozone, 402
  with alkenes, 247–250
  structure, 247
Ozonides, 247, 248, 402
  with dimethyl sulfide, 249
  with hydrogen peroxide, 249
  with zinc and acetic acid, 249
Ozonolysis, 247–250, 281
  mechanism, 248

p-atomic orbitals, 13
p-orbitals, 4, 94, 124, 153, 241, 315
p-orbitals, adjacent to π-bonds, 385
Palladium, catalyst, 258, 259, 261, 270, 417, 418
Palladium chloride, 262
Palmitic acid, 303, 304
Para, ortho, meta isomers, 318, 322
Parallel β-pleated sheet, 445
Parent ion, 192, 193
Partial hydrolysis, 304
Pascal's triangle, nmr, 212
PCC, *see* Pyridinium chlorochromate
PDC, *see* Pyridinium dichromate
Pentacoordinate transition state, 136, 137, 139, 140
Pentane, 30
Peptide bonds, 441
Peptides, 441–446
  C-protecting groups, 440, 441
  C-terminus, 439, 440
  chirality, 444
  conformation, 443
  definition, 439
  and DCC, 440, 441
  α-helix, 444
  hydrogen bonding, 444
  β-pleated sheet, 445
  primary structure, 441, 446
  N-protecting groups, 440, 441
  quaternary structure, 446
  random coil, 445
  rotational angles, 444
  secondary structure, 444, 446
  sterochemistry, 443
  N-terminus, 439, 440
  tertiary structure, 445, 446
Percent transmittance, and infrared spectrum, 198
Perchlorate anion, 17
Perchloric acid, 33
  as a catalyst, 105, 175
Pericyclic reactions, 393–403
[2+2] Pericyclic reactions, 393
[4+2] Pericyclic reactions, 393–401
Periodic acid, structure, 250
Periodic table, 23, 34, 271
Permanganate, potassium, *see* Potassium
Peroxides, 107
Peroxyacids, 245
  with alkenes, 112, 245, 246
  with alkenes, mechanism, 246
  structure, 111–112, 245
Peroxycarboxylic acids, *see* Peroxy acids
Phenanthrene, 347
Phenols, from aryl halides, 338, 339
Phenylhydrazine, 464
Phenyl isothiocyanate, 442, 443
phosphines, 233
  with alkyl halides, 233, 234
Phosphonium salts, 233, 234
  pKa, 233
Phosphorus halides, with alcohols, 145
Phosphorus pentachloride, 145
Phosphorus pentoxide, 291–293, 301
Phosphorus tribromide, 145
Phosphorus trichloride, 145
  with carboxylic acids, 383
Phthalazines, 417
Phthalimides, 416
  with alkyl halides, 416
  with halocarboxylic acids, 437
Physical properties, 26, 28, 29, 50, 81–83, 89, 90, 133, 446
pI, 433, 434
π-back bonding, 108; *see also* Back bonding
π-bonds, 14, 15, 16, 27, 66, 93–129, 232, 260, 264, 383
π-bonds, adjacent to p-orbitals, 385
π-electrons, 16, 316
π-electrons, 4n+2, 316

$\pi \rightarrow \pi^*$ transitions, 407
2π systems, 393
4π systems, 393
π-type bonding, 14
Pitzer strain, 68
pKa, 39, 41–46
  alcohols, 143
  aldehydes and ketones, 357, 358
  alkynes, 124, 187
  amines, 304
  amino acids, 433
  ammonia, 187
  carboxylic acids, 277–280
  diisopropylamine, 360
  diketones, 358
  esters, 373
  ethanol, 360
  fumaric acid, 312
  imides, 416
  b-keto acids, 376
  maleic acid, 312
  malonate esters, 374, 382
  malonic acid, 311
  methane, 187
  oxalic acid, 311
  phosphonium salts, 233
  pyrrole, 349
  thiols, 143
Planar cyclohexane, *see* Cyclohexane
Plane-polarized light, 81, 83
Platinum, as a catalyst, 258, 259, 261, 270
Platinum oxide, as a catalyst, 258, 269
β-Pleated sheet, antiparallel, 445
β-Pleated sheet, parallel, 445
β-Pleated sheet, peptides, 445
Point charge, 15
Point of difference, 84
Polar covalent bond, 9, 10
Polarimeters, 81, 82
Polarity, 10
Polarizability, 114, 319
Polarizable atoms, 319
Polarization, 10, 81, 133, 134, 183
Polarized bonds, 246
Polarized covalent bond, 25
Polarized light waves, 81
Polyalkylation, 420
  Friedel–Crafts alkylation, 332
Polycyclic aromatic compounds, 347–348
Polynucleotide, 467
Polysaccharide, definition, 457
Potassium acetate, 41
Potassium bromide, pressed plates, 197
Potassium cyanide, 138
Potassium dichromate, 252
Potassium metal, 143
Potassium permanganate, 113, 114, 402, 403
Potassium permanganate, structure, 240
Potassium permanganate, with alkenes, 240–242
Ppm scale, nmr, 204
Primary structure, peptide, 441, 446
Product ions, mass spectrometry, 193
Propane, 29
Propanoic acid, 41, 42
Protecting groups, 326
Proteins, 441–446
  conjugated, 441
  definition, 441
  denatured, 446
  simple, 441
Pseudorotation, 61, 67–70
Purine, 424, 425, 465
Pyramidal shape, 24
Pyranose, definition, 450
Pyranose form, carbohydrates, 453
pyrazine, 424
Pyrazolines, 403
Pyridazine, 424
Pyridine, 349, 424
  with HCl, 253, 254
  S_EAr reactions, 351
  S_NAr reactions, 352
  structure, 253
Pyridinium chloride, 253, 254
Pyridinium chlorochromate (pcc), 254
  with alcohols, 254, 255
Pyridinium dichromate (PDC), 254
  with alcohols, 254, 255
Pyrimidine, 424, 425, 465
Pyrrole, 318, 348, 349, 424
  pKa, 349
  S_EAr reactions, 350
Pyrrolidine, 423

Quaternary structure, peptides, 446
Quinoline, 262, 352, 424

Racemates, 82, 116
Racemic mixture, 82
Racemic modification, 82
Racemization, in S_N1 reactions, 153, 156
Radical anions, 271
Radical cations, 192, 193
  fragmentation, 193
Radical chain reaction, 107
Radical halogenation, *see* Halogenation
Radical intermediates, 106
Radicals, 16, 18, 106, 107, 135, 158–162
  and alkanes, 158–162
  with alkenes, 107
  allylic, 161
  and bromine, 107, 159
  and chlorine, 159
  from peroxides, 107
  with radicals, 159, 160
  reaction with radicals, 107
  resonance stabilized, 161
  stability, 106
Radio wave frequencies, and nmr, 202, 203
Random coil, peptides, 445
Raney nickel, *see* Nickel
Rate constants, 137, 141, 142

S_N1 reactions, 152
S_N2 reaction, 137
Rate of reaction, 103, 140, 141
deactivating groups, S_EAr reactions, 328, 329
hydrogenation, 259
radical halogenation, 159
S_EAr reactions, 323, 324
S_N1 reactions, 152, 153
S_N2 reaction, 137
Reaction curves, 138
transition state, 138
Rearrangements, 102, 103, 107, 109, 121, 153, 154, 155, 331, 332, 386
sigmatropic, 404–406
S_N1 reactions, 153–155
transition state, 103
Reduction reactions, 257–272
aromatic compounds, 344–347
definition, 257
dissolving metal, 264, 265
ketones, 333, 334
Reductive amination, 417
Reference cells, infrared, 197
Reformatsky reaction, 381
Regioisomers, and the Diels-Alder reaction, 399, 400
enolate anions, 359
Regioselectivity, 150
alkynes with HX, 126
dehydrohalogenation, 169, 170
hydroboration, 119, 120
radical halogenation, 160, 161
Residue, definition, 439
Resonance, 15, 16, 40, 46, 174, 222, 280, 385, 386, 388, 402, 403
Resonance, and arenium ions, 324–329
azide ion, 419
benzene, 315
and radicals, 161
Resonance contributors, 16, 17, 47
Resonance delocalization, 40
Resonance energy, 319
Resonance stability, 16
Resonance stabilization, 40, 41
reversible reactions, 404, 405
Ribosome, 469
RNA, 424, 425, 467, 468
RNA, transfer, 468, 469
Robinson annulation, 370, 371
Rosenmund catalyst, 262
Rotamers, 61–65
Rotation, 61–65, 67
plane-polarized light, 81
Rotational angles, 81
of peptides, 444
Ruff degradation, 460

s-character, 124
s-cis-conformations, 390
s-cis dienes, 398
s-orbitals, 4, 13, 14, 124
s-trans dienes, 398
s-trans-conformations, 390
Saccharide, definition, 449
Sandmeyer reaction, 340, 423
Sanger's reagent, 442
Saponification, 303, 378
Sawhorse diagram, 62, 63
Schiff bases, 418
Schlenk equilibrium, 232
Schrödinger equation, 3, 4
S_EAr reactions, 319–337
activating groups, 323, 324, 325
acylium ions, 332
carbocations, 331
deactivating groups, 327–329
deactivating groups, rate of reaction, 328, 329
and E1 reactions, 320
Friedel–Crafts acylation, 331, 332
halogen substituents, 329, 330
halogen substituents, arenium ions, 329, 330
indole, 351
and isomers, 323, 324
mechanism, 320–322
naphthalene, 347, 348
pyridine, 352
pyridine, mechanism, 351
pyrrole, 350
pyrrole, mechanism, 350
and rate of reactions, 323, 324
thiophene, 350
Secondary field effect, benzene, 208
ethene, 208
ethyne, 208, 209
nmr, 208
Secondary orbital interactions, 401
Secondary structure, peptides, 444, 446
Second-order nucleophilic substitution, *see* S_n2 reactions
Second-order reactions, 141, 166
2^n rule, 87, 88
Self-condensation, 366, 377, 378
Sequence rules, 83
Shielded protons, nmr, 207
Shielding effect, nmr, 207
Sidedness, 94, 97
Sigma (σ) bond, 13–15, 94, 260
$\sigma \longrightarrow \pi^*$ transitions, 407
Sigmatropic rearrangements, 404–406
[1, 5]-Sigmatropic rearrangements, 404
[3, 3]-Sigmatropic rearrangement, 405, 406
Silver oxide, with ammonium salts, 178
Silver oxide/ammonium hydroxide, 464
Simple proteins, 441
Six-centered transition state, 405
S_N1 reactions, 151–158
mechanism, 152, 174
racemization, 153, 156
rate constants, 152
rate of reaction, 152, 153
and rearrangement, 153–155
S_N2 and S_N1 reaction competition, 156–158
S_N2 reactions, 124, 134–151, 165, 172, 282, 300, 361, 418
and amines, 420

definition, 135
rate constant, 137
reaction rate, 137
transition state, 136, 137
S_N4' reactions, 393
S_NAr reactions, 337–344
and activating groups, 338
mechanism, 338
pyridine, 352
S_Ni reactions, 145
Sodium amalgam, with carbohydrates, 460
Sodium amide, 124, 177
with alcohols, 147
with aryl halides, 342
Sodium azide, 138, 419
Sodium borohydride, 109–111
with acid chlorides, 306
with aldehydes or ketones, 266–269
with carbohydrates, 461, 462
with carboxylic acids, 306
with esters, 268, 306
structure, 266
Sodium chloride, 7
pressed plates, 197
Sodium cyanide, 138
with aldehydes and ammonium chloride, 436
Sodium dichromate, 252
Sodium ethoxide, 147
Sodium hydride, 124
Sodium hydroxide, 38, 47, 121, 166
with aryl halides, 338, 339
and dihydroxylation, 240
with epoxides, 364
with oxiranes, 150
Sodium metal, 143, 183, 264, 265
with ammonia, 271, 272
and ammonia with aldehydes or ketones, 271
Sodium methoxide, 146, 147
Sodium nitrite, with acid, 339
Sodium tetrahydridoborate, 109
Sodium thiosulfate, 243
Solid support, and hydrogenation, 259
Solubility, 31
Solute, 31
Solution, 81
Solvation, 153
and amines, 421
Solvent effects, 140
Solvents, 31, 45, 48, 81, 82, 116–118, 124, 125, 151, 180, 184, 186, 225, 231
aprotic, 140, 156–158, 171, 373, 421
hydride reduction, 267
and hydrogenation, 259
for nmr, 203, 204
nonpolar, 140, 171
polar, 140, 171
protic, 140, 153, 156–158, 171, 373, 421
Solvolysis, 155
of alkyl halides, 153–156
mechanism, 155
Sorbitol, 461
sp hybridized, 122
sp-hybrid orbital, 14
sp^2 hybridized carbons, 315
sp^2-hybrid orbitals, 94
sp^2-hybridization, 14, 94, 316
sp^3-hybrid orbitals, 13, 14
Space-filling models, 64, 70, 73
Specific rotation, 81–83, 89
carbohydrates, 455, 456
definition, 82
Spectroscopy, amines, 416
Speed of light, 191
Spin quantum numbers, 5
and nmr, 201
Spin-allowed, 408
Spin-forbidden, 408
Spin-spin splitting, nmr, 209, 212
Stability, arenium ions, 324
of alkenes, 170
carbocations, 102, 154
hydrates, 222, 223
malonate enolate anions, 374
of radicals, 106
transition states, 100, 101
Staggered rotamers, 62, 63, 66
Standard free energy, 167
Standard state, 167
Starch, 458
Stearic acid, 303, 304
Steering wheel model, 84–87
Stereochemistry, 147
dienes, conjugate, 388
hydroboration, 118–120
Stereogenic carbon, 83
Stereogenic centers, 78, 85–87, 139, 429
Stereogenic molecules, 79, 81
Stereoisomers, 78, 87–90, 96, 97, 116, 170, 240, 241
and the Diels–Alder reaction, 399
2^n rule, 87, 88
Stereoselectivity, 145, 241, 242
hydrogenation, 262
Stereospecific reactions, 170, 171
Steric hindrance, 11, 63–67, 118, 137, 174, 179
and chromate esters, 252
and oxidation, 252
Steric interactions, 63–68
flagpole, 70
transannular, 70, 73
Steric repulsion, 136
Sterochemistry, 261, 262
peptides, 443
Strecker synthesis, 436
Structural isomerism, 51
Structural isomers, 50
Structure, aromatics, conjugate, 390
carbohydrates, 451, 452
common amino acids, 431
dienes, conjugate, 387, 388
diynes, conjugate, 389
ketones, conjugate, 389
Styrene, 390

Substituents, 53–58, 133
 on benzene, 323
Substitution reactions, 134–162
 nucleophilic, definition, 134
Substitution *vs.* elimination reaction, 171
Succinic acid, 292
Sugars, 449–465
Sulfides, 27
Sulfonamides, 309
Sulfonate esters, 309
Sulfonation, benzene, 322
Sulfonic acids, 40, 105, 309
Sulfonyl chlorides, with alcohols, 309
 with amines, 309
Sulfonyl halides, 309
Sulfoxides, 78
Sulfur dioxide, 145
Sulfur halides, with alcohols, 145
Sulfuric acid, 15, 33, 103, 104
 as a catalyst, 104, 105, 127, 174, 175
 with nitric acid, 321
Sulfur trioxide, and benzene, 322
Sunlamp, 161
Superimposability, 79
Superimposable, 77, 78, 88
Suprafacial shift, 404
Symmetry, 116
Synchronous reactions, 135, 136, 241
Syn eliminations, 422; *see also* Elimination
Syn rotamers, 63, 64, 67, 179
Synthesis, benzyne reactions, 344
 of amino acids, 435–437
 of aromatic compounds, 334–337
 of carbohydrates, 459, 460
 definition, 148

Tartaric acid/ copper (II) sulfate, 462, 463
Tautomerism, 127, 128, 383
Tautomerization, and decarboxylation, 308
Temperature, 35
Tert-butylhydroperoxide, 244
Tertiary structure, peptides, 445, 446
Tethered base, 178, 180
Tetrafluoroboric acid, as a catalyst, 175
Tetrahedral intermediates, 294
Tetrahedral shape, 20, 24
Tetrahedron, 20, 24, 26, 62, 67, 77, 80, 84, 143
Tetrahydridoborate, 266
Tetrahydrofuran, *see* THF
Tetrahyridoaluminate, 265
Tetramethylsilane, 205, 213
Theobromine, 426
Thermodynamic control, alkenes, with bromine, 392, 393
 dienes, with aqueous acid, 392
 dienes, with HCl, 391
 enolate reactions, 373, 382
Thermodynamic enolates, 360–362, 367
Thermodynamic stability, 95
Thexylborane, 120
THF, 106, 125, 140, 146, 418
Thiazolones, 443
Thiohydantoins, 442, 443
Thiols, 27, 143, 227, 228
 with aldehyde or ketones, 227, 228
Thionyl bromide, 145
 with alcohols, 145
 with carboxylic acids, 290
Thionyl chloride, 145
 with alcohols, 145
 with alcohols and amines, 421
 with carboxylic acids, 290
 with triethylamine + alcohols, 145
Thiophene, 318, 348, 424
 S_EAr reactions, 350
Three-dimensional shape, 24
Three letter code, amino acids, 431
Through-bond effects, 42, 278
Through-space field effect, 279
Through-space inductive effects, 43
Thymidine, 466
Thymidine triphosphate, 467
Thymine, 425, 465
TMS, *see* Tetramethylsilane
Tollen's test, 464
Toluene, 331
Torsion strain, 68
Transannular steric interactions, 70, 73
Transesterification, 296, 297, 372, 379
 mechanism, 296, 297
Transfer RNA, 468, 469
Transition metals, 189; *see also* Metals
Transition state, 36, 100, 137, 138, 168–170
 decarboxylation, 307
 E2, 166
 epoxidation, 112
 hydroboration, 118–120
 pentacoordinate, 136, 137
 reaction curves, 138
 rearrangement, 103
 six-centered, 405
 S_N2 reaction, 136, 137
 stability, 100, 101
Transoid conformations, 390
Trans-stereoisomer, 96, 97
Triglyceride, 303
Trioxolanes, 247, 402
Triphenylphosphine, 233, 263
Triphenylphosphine oxide, 234
tRNA, *see* Transfer RNA
Twist boat conformation, 70, 71

Ultraviolet light, 191
Ultraviolet spectroscopy, 406–409; *see also* UV
Upfield signal, nmr, 206
Uracil, 425, 465
Urea solutions, 446
Uric acid, 426
Uridine triphosphate, 467
UV, and conjugated dienes, 408
UV, and functional groups, 407–409
UV light, and radical halogenation, 159
UV spectrum, 407

Valence, 8, 19, 21, 50, 183
Valence electrons, 8, 12, 19, 24
Valence number, 28
Valence shell, 8
Valence Shell Electron Pair Repulsion model, *see* VSEPR model
van der Waals attraction, 10
van der Waals forces, 29, 30
Vaska's catalyst, 263
Vibration, molecular, 61
Vic-dimethyl, 52
Vicinal dihalides, 176
Vicinal dimethyl, 52
Vicinal diols, 113
Vinyl carbocations, *see* Carbocations
Vinyl ethers, 405, 406
Vinyl halides, *see* Halides
Vinylogy, 369
VSEPR model, 23–26, 143

Walden inversion, 137
Water, 19, 24, 31, 45, 105, 108, 117, 127, 128, 140, 151, 155, 166, 171, 173, 196, 222, 224, 225, 251, 266–269, 385
Watson–Crick model, DNA, 470
Wavefunction, 3, 191
Wavelength, and infrared spectroscopy, 197
Wheland intermediate, 320
Wilkinson's catalyst, 263
Williamson ether synthesis, 147, 148
Wittig reaction, 233–235
  mechanism, 234
Wohl degradation, 460
Wolff–Kishner reduction, 333, 334
Wolff–Kishner reduction, mechanism, 334

Xylenes, 332

Ylids, 233–235
Yids, with aldehydes or ketones, 234

Z-stereoisomer, 97
Zaitsev elimination, 170
Zeolites, 225
Zero point, nmr, 205
Zig-zag conformation, 67
Zinc, and acetic acid, with ozonides, 249
Zinc amalgam, 334
Zinc enolate, ester, 381
Zusammen, 98
Zwitterions, 234, 430

Printed in the United States
by Baker & Taylor Publisher Services